5

9.95

1.99

Principles of Nutrition

SECOND EDITION

PRINCIPLES
OF NUTRITION

Eva D. Wilson Professor of Food and Nutrition
Ohio State University

Katherine H. Fisher Nutritionist, HRB - Singer Inc.
State College, Pennsylvania

Mary E. Fuqua Professor and Chairman,
Department Foods and Nutrition
Purdue University

John Wiley & Sons, Inc., New York • London • Sydney

Library of Congress Catalog Card Number: 65-24299
Printed in the United States of America
ISBN 0 471 94975 2

PREFACE

This edition is intended, as was the first, to provide basic information in nutrition at the elementary level. It is written primarily for the college student; however, the point of view of the professional nutritionist has also been kept in mind.

Most of the features previously used for a simplified approach to chemistry have been omitted in this edition. The change is made on the assumption that students enter college today better prepared in the sciences than they were six years ago when the first edition was published.

Three new sections are introduced in the current edition: one on dietary standards and allowances of this and other countries; dietary interrelationships are discussed in a separate chapter in order to emphasize to the student the magnitude and importance of this little-explored area of basic nutrition; and a chapter on new developments in food and nutrition, that is, space nutrition, new methods of food preservation, food additives, and strontium-90 as a problem in nutrition.

Appreciation is expressed to Mrs. Mary A. Howell and Miss Helen M. King for assistance in the collection of data for the preparation of the manuscript; Dr. Thomas Allen, Dr. Robert Cowan, Mr. Emery Keck, Dr. Paul A. Lachance, Dr. Raymond W. Swift, and Dr. John E. Vanderveen for their review and critical evaluation of portions of the manuscript; and Dr. Paul A. Lachance and Dr. Bernice K. Watt for the use of prepublication data for the manuscript. Also we are particularly grateful to those persons whose suggestions helped improve the quality and usefulness of the revised book.

Once again we wish to express our appreciation to those investigators whose research is reported here. The challenge of selecting only those investigations that are significant to a study of elementary nutrition in college is very real because the field of nutrition has become so vast.

We hope the introduction to nutrition as presented in this text will create an interest on the part of the reader for study of the subject in greater depth. Nutrition research, which is in progress in many parts of the world and intensively so in the United States, brings continuously new information.

Eva D. Wilson
Katherine H. Fisher
Mary E. Fuqua

July 1965

CONTENTS

Principles of Nutrition

CHAPTER 1

Introduction to nutrition

Nutrition is the science of nourishing the body. Nutrient substances for this purpose are provided by food. Many of the nutrients have been isolated and identified and are now available as pure chemical compounds. The provision of one of the nutrients, vitamin D, differs from all others since in addition to food as a source, the body can on exposure to sunlight or other source of ultraviolet rays, produce it.

An individual's nutritional status is dependent on the provision of sufficient nutrient substances and the good utilization of these nutrients. Poor status of nutrition may be caused by eating food that is inadequate in amount or kind or it may be caused by failures in digestion and the utilization of these nutrients.

The desire to eat is natural in normal, healthy individuals, and we are capable of some discernment as to how much we should eat. However, there is another aspect of eating for which man, even with his capabilities, has not a natural judgment, at least to our knowledge, and that is the selection of an adequate diet for himself. The attributes of an adequate diet must be learned; the information is provided through research studies.

An individual's selection of food is influenced by many factors, such as the habits of his family and associates, his religion, where he lives, and his attitude as to the appropriateness of the substance for use as food. A common denominator, however, is that people like the foods which they are accustomed to eating—whether it be rice, olive oil, or roast beef.

Some of the benefits of good nutrition are readily recognized. Good posture, firm muscles, and abundant vitality are the result of an adequate diet over a period of time.

Nutrition does make a difference. Children who are malnourished fail to grow at a normal rate. Poor food habits of adults are associated with fatigue and decreased work output. The performance of an athlete can be impaired significantly by a faulty or an inadequate diet, even before clinical signs of a deficiency appear (8). It was observed among women factory workers that those who showed a high incidence of absenteeism ate less adequate diets than those who were not absent in over a year's time. Although there were undoubtedly other factors, the dietary difference is believed to have played an important role (5). Industrial workers in the office and in the factory achieved a greater output of work if a good breakfast was eaten in contrast to eating none at all (7).

A good diet helps to assure more vitality in health. It is a bulwark against illness and essential in recovery from illness.

▶ THE BEGINNING OF THE STUDY OF NUTRITION

The first record of man's effort to probe the mysteries of nourishment of the body was in ancient times, and the search has continued ever since (1–4, 6). Many observations made by the early philosophers were indeed prophetic. In the first century B.C. Egyptians believed that excessive eating was the cause of many diseases. In the ancient world the Greek philosopher Hippocrates (460–359 B.C.) pondered the problems of medicine and of the body's reaction to food. Even without the advantage of experiment, this brilliant philosopher made observations which modern science has upheld. Among his aphorisms is the statement, "Growing bodies have the most innate heat; they require the most food, for otherwise their bodies are wasted. In old people the heat is feeble and they require little fuel, as it were, for it would be extinguished by much." His pronouncement that "Persons who are naturally very fat are apt to die earlier than those who are slender" is not unfamiliar in current literature (2). Another contributor from the ancient Greek world was Aristotle (384–322 B.C.), who carried out investigations in physiology as well as other areas.

The Italian Renaissance produced a genius of many talents, Leonardo da Vinci (1452–1519). At the same time artist, anatomist, biologist, and aeronautical engineer, he made statements about nutrition that have a modern connotation.

Concerning the need for nourishment—

... if you do not supply nourishment equal to the nourishment departed, life will fail in vigor; and if you take away this nourishment, life is utterly destroyed (2).

the need for oxygen—

Where flame cannot live no animal can sustain its existence (2).

Born shortly after the death of da Vinci, Sanctorius (1561–1636), a professor at Padua, Italy, went to great trouble to investigate a question that troubled many of that era and which, to be sure, is still under study. Sanctorius experimented: he spent much of his life weighing himself. He found that he lost weight during periods "when no additional food or drink was taken and no sensible evacuations from the body occurred." He termed this loss "insensible perspiration."

When Sanctorius was performing his experiments, there was no science of chemistry. In the years that followed, chemical discoveries were made that also paved the way for nutrition discoveries. In the seventeenth century the mysteries of "air" and of processes of respiration were under investigation. Most significant were the experiments of John Mayow (1643–1679). He placed a small animal and a burning candle in a closed jar. He observed that the candle burned a longer time without the animal in the jar, and that the animal lived a longer time in the jar without the burning candle. Mayow at the age of 25 wrote a treatise on respiration. With perceiving vision he stated that "the particles of the air absorbed during respiration are designed to convert the black or venous blood into the red or arterial." This young scientist died when he was only 36, cutting short his brilliant career.

About a century elapsed before others took up the studies of respiration. In a period of about 15 years four men were born who made discoveries that laid the groundwork for the science of nutrition.

Joseph Black (1728–1799), a physician and professor at the University of Edinburgh, discovered what he termed "fixed air," later identified as carbon dioxide. He found that by breathing through a tube into lime water, it became cloudy; also when poured into a jar in which a candle had been burned, the lime water became cloudy. Black proposed that all kinds of animals expire "fixed air."

Joseph Priestley (1733–1804) and Karl Scheele (1742–1786) independently discovered oxygen at about the same time. Priestley was a Unitarian clergyman in England, Scheele a Swedish apothecary and chemist.

Priestley thought that both animals and flames exhausted the air. He wondered how the air once "exhausted" could be revitalized. He found the answer by burning a candle in a jar until it went out, and then placing a living plant (a sprig of mint) in the jar. Ten days later he placed another candle in the enclosed space and found that it burned perfectly well; the living plant had revitalized the air. Priestley produced oxygen by heating red oxide of mercury in a closed vessel with the heat of the sun focused by means of a burning glass.

Scheele performed an experiment in which he placed two large bees with a little honey in a small box fitted in the top of a glass cylinder. He immersed the cylinder in limewater after filling it with "fire-air" (his term for oxygen), that he had obtained by heating mercuric oxide. After eight days the bees were both dead and the limewater had risen in the container. The "fire-air" had been used up by the bees and the carbon dioxide given off was absorbed in the limewater.

It was the Frenchman Antoine Laurent Lavoisier (1743–1794) who brought together the findings of his predecessors to explain the phenomenon of respiration. He studied the respiration of animals, and also of his associate, Armand Seguin. Lavoisier supported the theory that ordinary air is a mixture of oxygen and nitrogen gases, that during respiration the nitrogen returns unchanged, but the oxygen is diminished. He found that when Seguin had eaten food, he absorbed more oxygen than without it, and that exercise increased the absorption of oxygen.

The achievements that lead to the modern era of nutrition often did not bring honor to the men with the brilliant minds. Priestley unhappy with the reception of his work on the continent, came to America in 1794, making his home in Northumberland, Pennsylvania, where he spent the remainder of his life. Lavoisier was executed at the age of fifty-one for alleged criminal acts during the French Revolution. One of Lavoisier's friends said of him, "It took but a second to cut off his head; a hundred years will not suffice to produce one like it."

During the nineteenth century great strides were made in identifying the nutrient materials needed in the diet for life and well-being. Only a very few of the noted scientists of the time are mentioned here. François Magendie (1783–1855), a French scientist who observed that when he fed dogs only sugar, or butter, or olive oil, or gum arabic, plus distilled water, the animals died. He concluded that the protein element was necessary. Not only was Magendie distinguished for his own research, but for being the teacher of Claude Bernard, (1813–1878), who discovered glycogen and also proclaimed that pancreatic juice performs some function that is necessary for the absorption of fats. In Germany Baron Justus von Liebig (1803–1873) taught that fats and carbohydrates were fuel foods and termed the nutrient that formed body tissues during growth "plastic food"; and Karl von Voit (1831–1908) believed that "the requirement of protein is dependent on the organized mass of the tissues; the requirement for fat and carbohydrate is dependent on the amount of mechanical work accomplished" (2).

That brings us to the twentieth century and our own times. Never in the whole history of nutrition have the strides of this century been paralleled. Studies of this era have encompassed the discovery and the identification of certain nutrients (the vitamins, amino acids, and certain minerals), the nutrient needs of the body in health and in disease, the

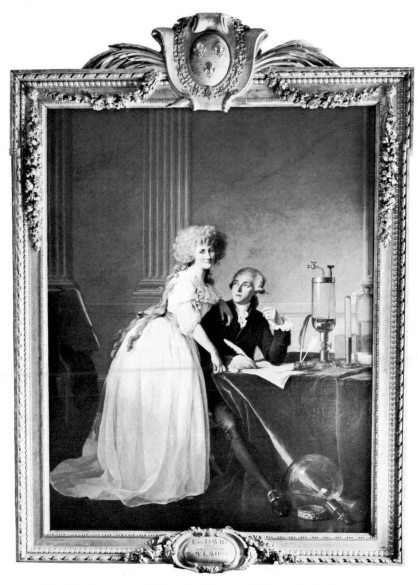

Fig. 1.1.   Lavoisier and his wife. (Courtesy of The Rockefeller Institute.)

specific and interrelated functions that these nutrients play, sources of these nutrients, and their use to enrich food to a higher nutritive value— all for the benefit of mankind. The twentieth century ushered in the "one world" concept also and with it, concern not only for an adequate diet for our nation, but for enough food to feed the world. Some of the scientists and certain of their contributions will be cited in the chapters to follow.

▶ THE CHAPTERS TO FOLLOW

The remaining chapters are devoted to the essentials of an adequate diet, the energy, the protein, mineral, and vitamin needs, with methods for planning a food intake to supply these nutrients. The benefits of good nutrition, the disadvantages of poor nutrition, the nutritional needs of children, women during pregnancy and lactation, and older persons are all discussed in succeeding chapters. The appendix includes a glossary of terms that may be new to the reader and tables to supplement the reading.

REFERENCES

1. Hawley, E. E., G. Carden, and E. D. Munves (1955). *The Art and Science of Nutrition.* 4th ed. The C. V. Mosby Co., St. Louis.
2. Lusk, G. (1933). *Nutrition.* Paul B. Hoeber, New York.
3. McCollum, E. V. (1957). *A History of Nutrition.* Houghton Mifflin Co., Boston.
4. McCollum, E. V., E. Orent-Keiles, and H. G. Day (1939). *The Newer Knowledge of Nutrition.* The Macmillan Co., New York.
5. Peel, R. M., and M. L. Dodds (1957). Nutritive intake of women factory employees. Comparison of non- and high-absence groups. *J. Am. Dietet. Assoc.* **33:** 1150.
6. Taylor, C. M., G. Macleod, and M. S. Rose (1956). *Foundations of Nutrition,* 5th ed. The Macmillan Co., New York.
7. Tuttle, W. W., and E. Herbert (1960). Work capacity with no breakfast and a mid-morning break. *J. Am. Dietet. Assoc.* **37:** 137.
8. Van Itallie, T. B., and L. Sinisterra (1956). Nutrition and athletic performance. *J. Am. Med. Assoc.* **162:** 1120.

CHAPTER 2

The functions of food

Eating is an essential part of the daily lives of everyone. Colleges and universities, recognizing the importance of food for the students, provide food service facilities on the campus. Even though the chief function of the food is to supply materials to meet physiological needs, it serves other functions also. Food plays an integral role in social life, whether on the college or university campus, in the homes of the land, or in the affairs of the convening diplomats of the world. Still another function of food is that of the psychological or emotional influence. Familiar foods are favorite foods, imparting a sense of well-being and satisfaction unrelated to food value but reminiscent of past experiences.

▶ THE PHYSIOLOGICAL FUNCTION OF FOOD

The physiological function of food may be divided into three general categories: the need for food materials to supply energy, the need for food materials to build and maintain the cells and tissues, and the need for food materials to regulate body processes. These needs are satisfied by substances called *nutrients* which are found in the food man eats. The nutrients themselves have been subdivided into six general classes: carbohydrates, lipids, proteins, minerals, vitamins, and water. The discussion of the part that these food factors play in the maintenance of good health will follow in subsequent chapters.

The Need for Food Nutrients to Supply Energy

Inasmuch as the primary function of food is to supply the body with energy-producing materials, the energy demand must be satisfied before the body uses food for building and maintenance, or regulation. The nutrients in foods which supply energy are called the *energy nutrients;* they include the carbohydrates, fats, and proteins. Carbohydrate in the diet is the chief source of energy. This is true of diets around the world. Fat follows carbohydrate as a source of energy, with protein providing the least amount. There will be further discussion in Chapter 4 about this topic.

The Need for Food Nutrients to Build and Maintain Body Tissue

Nutrients used in the building and maintenance of the body are proteins, minerals, and water. The most abundant body-building nutrient is water, followed by protein, with minerals occurring in the least amount. Each cell and tissue contain some of each of the body-building nutrients. The specific location and structural function will be discussed in the chapters concerning the respective nutrients.

The Need for Food Nutrients to Regulate Body Processes

All of the nutrients, with the exception of carbohydrate, play a role in the regulation of the body processes. The essential fatty acids present in certain fats, the proteins, the minerals, the vitamins, and water each perform certain regulatory functions essential to normal body operation, such as the movement of fluids, the control of the balance between acid and base, the coagulation of blood, the activation of enzymes, and the maintenance of normal body temperature. The role of the respective food nutrients in these physiological functions and others will be discussed in later chapters.

▶ THE SOCIAL FUNCTION OF FOOD

Food has always served an important function in the social exchanges of people. In the ancient world guests could be invited only when there was enough food for current needs and future wants (1). The social occasions centering around food in our country are many—the sugaring off parties of Vermont and New Hampshire at maple sugar time, the "at homes" at Christmas and New Year's in the South, the food festivals of the Middle West, and the outdoor hospitality of the Far West (2).

Inasmuch as food is an integral part of the social phase of college or university living, this function is important to college men and women. (See Fig. 2.1.) Food is served at many social events: teas, breakfasts, banquets, athletic award dinners, dances, and meetings of all sorts. At all of these affairs, food indirectly serves as an instrument to develop social rapport. The indirect purpose of refreshments after a club meeting may be to attract more students to the meeting, but the main function is to create an atmosphere where social relationships may be fostered. When a college man or coed is asked to plan a menu for a social function, the criterion for selection will probably *not* be whether the food will provide important nutrients needed for good nutrition but rather whether it will be popular with the guests.

▶ THE PSYCHOLOGICAL FUNCTION OF FOOD

In addition to nourishing the body and filling a need in social life, food satisfies certain emotional needs. Even though a meal may be adequate nutritionally, it may not give a sense of genuine satisfaction. People who travel or live in a new land often find adjusting to the unfamiliar food customs a problem. With time the strange becomes familiar and new likes are formed. Traditional habits are characterized by certain foods pleasing persons of one culture and being distasteful to those of another.

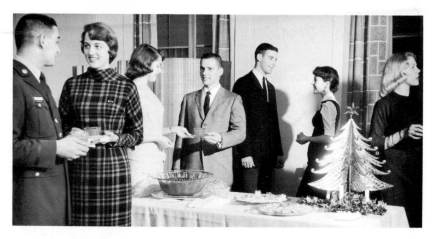

Fig. 2.1.   Food as part of college social functions. (Courtesy of Laverne Henderson, The Pennsylvania State University.)

Food is also used to express feelings. The giving of food is a token of friendship; the serving of favorite foods an expression of special attention and recognition; and the withholding of wanted foods a means of punishment.

REFERENCES

1. Nichols, N. B. (1952). *Good Home Cooking across the U.S.A.* Iowa State College Press, Ames.
2. Prentice, E. P. (1939). *Hunger and History.* Harper and Brothers, New York, p. 83.

CHAPTER 3

Dietary allowances and standards

The general term used to describe the "yardstick" of man's nutritional needs is the dietary standard. It has been defined as a compilation or a summary of nutrient requirements, stated quantitatively (8).

The first expression of a dietary standard for man is sometimes credited to E. Smith, who in 1862 recommended food needs in terms of carbon and nitrogen to prevent starvation diseases among unemployed cotton workers (6). Using data from extensive studies with German laborers, Karl von Voit in 1880 proposed that man's daily requirement would be provided by a diet which contributed about 3055 Cal. and contained 500 gm of carbohydrate, 56 gm of fat, and 118 gm of protein (7). Since that time other scientists (e.g., Rubner, Atwater, Lusk) and scientific groups (e.g., League of Nations, British Medical Association, National Academy of Sciences-National Research Council, Food and Agriculture Organization of the United Nations) have formulated and proposed dietary allowances and standards.

The accumulation of pertinent data on nutritive function and requirement, as well as experience gained in the formulation and use of statements on dietary needs through the past several decades, have resulted in the expression of modern-day formulas of dietary recommendations that are in effect in some countries of the world. Australia, Canada, Central America and Panama, India, Japan, the Netherlands, Norway, the Philippines, South Africa, the U.S.S.R., the United Kingdom, and the United States all have dietary allowances for their population groups.

11

Energy and protein recommendations for use on an international basis have been proposed by scientific groups of the Food and Agriculture Organization (FAO). International calcium requirements have also been suggested by a combined group from the FAO and the World Health Organization (WHO).

Dietary standards in various parts of the world vary from country to country. Dr. L. A. Maynard (10) has prepared an interesting table which compares the dietary recommendations for adults in twelve countries and the FAO. (See Table 3.1.) Most of the countries listed show dietary allowances for nine nutrients, the exception being the FAO requirements, India, and the U.S.S.R.

Only the Recommended Dietary Allowances of the United States, the Dietary Standards for Canada, the British Medical Association Standards, and the International Recommendations of the FAO and the FAO-WHO will be presented here.

▶ RECOMMENDED DIETARY ALLOWANCES OF THE UNITED STATES

Over 20 years ago the term "Recommended Allowances" was coined by the Food and Nutrition Board of the National Academy of Sciences—National Research Council (NRC) to describe the suggested nutritional needs in the United States. This term was chosen "to avoid any implication of finality of standard or of minimal or optimal requirement." The first edition of the Recommended Dietary Allowances was issued in 1943 followed by revisions in 1945, 1948, 1953, 1958, and 1963. The allowances are "intended to serve as goals toward which to aim in planning food supplies and as guides for the interpretation of food consumption records of groups of people." Furthermore, the allowances are believed to be values that "will maintain good nutrition in essentially all healthy persons in the United States under current conditions of living."

Table A-1, in the appendix of this book, is taken from the *Recommended Dietary Allowances, Sixth Revised Edition* (10). The nutrients for which recommendations have been made in this table are energy (Cal.), protein (gm), calcium (gm), iron (mg), vitamin A activity (IU), thiamine (mg), riboflavin (mg), niacin equivalents (mg), and ascorbic acid (mg). A vitamin D allowance (IU) has been recommended for periods of growth, pregnancy, and lactation. Allowances for American men and women are expressed in terms of age: 18–35 yr, 35–55 yr, and 55–75 yr, while separate allowances are given for infants, boys, girls, and adolescents.

A detailed presentation of the Recommended Allowances is found in the sections devoted to the study of the nutrients (Chapters 4–6, 8,

10–17) and to the study of the needs for growth, pregnancy, lactation, and old age (Chapters 24 and 25).

▶ DIETARY STANDARD FOR CANADA

The Dietary Standard for Canada was revised in 1963 by a committee of the Canadian Council on Nutrition (5) to replace the recommendations issued by the Council in 1950. This modern statement of dietary needs is designed to be used in planning diets and food supplies for groups of healthy people or healthy individuals, as well as in establishing the need for or the evaluation of a public health nutrition program. These recommended daily nutrient intakes are considered to be adequate for the maintenance of good health among the majority of Canadians.

The nutrient intakes recommended for adult Canadians, 25 to 29 years, of different body size and activity are shown in Table A-2 (appendix). The three weight categories, males (144, 158, and 176 lb) and females (111, 124, and 136 lb), are further subdivided into five activity levels: maintenance, A, B, C, and D. A description of types of work in each of the five activity levels is presented in terms of general occupations: home or household, office, industry, and recreation. For example, in industrial occupations supervising or monitoring work corresponds to maintenance activity whereas heavy work, like the felling of trees by hand or the shoveling of gravel or coal is classified as category D activity.

The need for energy in the Canadian Standard for adults is related to body size, activity, age, environmental temperature, and physiological state (pregnancy and lactation). Regardless of age, the body size of the individuals is based on the desirable weight at age 25 to 29. The relationship of activity to the energy need has been described above. With advancing age, a decrease in the need for energy (based upon the energy need at age 25) has been recommended: 3 per cent (25–35 yr), 5 per cent (35–45 yr), 9 per cent (45–55 yr), 13 per cent (55–65 yr), and 17 per cent (over 65 yr). For the most part, environmental temperature is not considered to be a varying factor in the energy need of the Canadian because it is customary to adjust shelter and clothing to match the climate.

Because the dietary needs for thiamine, riboflavin, and niacin are related to the energy expenditure, values for these nutrients have been derived from factors expressed as units per 1000 Cal. Factors of 0.3 mg per 1000 Cal. and 0.5 mg per 1000 Cal. are used to calculate the need for thiamine and riboflavin, respectively. The recommended intakes for niacin, which represent only the intake of the "preformed vitamin" (see Chapter 16), are calculated from the factor of 3 mg per 1000 Cal.

The standard for protein is based on the FAO statement of human pro-

Table 3.1. Comparative Dietary Standards for Adults in Selected Countries and FAO with Explanations

Country	Sex	Age, Years	Weight, kg	Activity	Calories
U.S.A.[1]	M	18–35	70	Footnote[2]	2900
	F	18–35	58	Footnote[2]	2100
FAO[1]	M	25	65	Footnote[2]	3200
	F	25	55	Footnote[2]	2300
Australia[1]	M	25	65	Footnote[2]	2700
	F	25	55	Footnote[2]	2300
Canada[1]	M	25	72	Footnote[2]	2850
	F	25	57	Footnote[2]	2400
Central America and Panama[1]	M	25	55	Moderate work	2700
	F	25	50	Moderate work	2000
India[1]	M	25.4	55	Moderate work[2]	2800
	F	21.5	45	Moderate work[2]	2300
Japan[1]	M	Footnote[2]	56	Moderate work[3]	3000
	F	Footnote[2]	48.5	Moderate work[3]	2400
Netherlands[1]	M	20–29	70	Light work	3000
	F	20–29	60	Light work	2400
Norway[1]	M	25	70	None	3400
	F	25	60	Given	2500
The Philippines[1]	M	None	53	Moderate work	2600
	F	Specified	45	Moderate work	2300
South Africa[1]	M	None	73	Moderate work	3000
	F	Specified	60	Moderate work	2300
United Kingdom[1]	M	20 up	65	Medium work[2]	3000
	F	20 up	56	Medium work[2]	2500
U.S.S.R.	M and F			Moderate work	

The purpose for establishing a national dietary standard is not the same in all countries. Therefore, some variation in nutrient allowances from country to country is to be expected. At the same time, it must be recognized that the "reference" individual will vary from country to country. Furthermore, even in instances when there are presumed similar objectives among countries as to the purpose and usefulness of proposed standards, it can be seen that there is by no means uniform agreement as to the nutrient allowances considered desirable as national

Table 3.1. (continued)

Protein, gm	Calcium, gm	Iron, mg	Vitamin A Activity, IU	Thiamine, mg	Riboflavin, mg	Niacin Equiv.[3], mg	Ascorbic Acid, mg
70	0.8	10	5000	1.2	1.7	19	70
58	0.8	15	5000	0.8	1.3	14	70
43[3]	0.4–0.5[4]						
36[3]	0.4–0.5[4]						
65	0.7	10	2500[3]	1.1	1.6	18[4]	30
55	0.6	12	2000[3]	0.9	1.4	15[4]	30
50[3]	0.5	6	3700[4]	0.9	1.4	9	30
39[3]	0.5	10	3700[4]	0.7	1.2	7	30
55	0.7	10	4333[2]	1.4	1.4	14	50
50	0.7	10	4333[2]	1.0	1.2	10	45
55[3]							
45[3]							
70[4]	0.6	10	2000[5]	1.5	1.5	15	65
60[4]	0.6	10	2000[5]	1.2	1.2	12	60
70[2]	1.0	10	5500[3]	1.2	1.8	12	50
60[2]	1.0	12	5500[3]	1.0	1.5	10	50
70	0.8	12	2500[2]	1.7	1.8	17	30
60	0.8	12	2500[2]	1.3	1.5	13	30
55	0.7	6	4000[2]	1.6	1.4[3]	16	75
45	0.7	10	4000[2]	1.4	1.1[3]	14	70
65	0.7	9	4000[2]	1.0	1.6	15	40
55	0.6	12	4000[2]	0.8	1.4	12	40
87[3]	0.8	12	5000[4]	1.2	1.8	12	20
73[3]	0.8	12	5000[4]	1.0	1.5	10	20
			5000[2]	2.0[3]	2.5	15	70[3]

guides. Standards are also subject to revision as newer knowledge becomes available. Particular attention should be paid to the footnotes, which explain, in brief form, the basis for nutrient allowances in the various countries and those of FAO. The original publications should be consulted for detailed explanations. The Board is indebted to Dr. L. A. Maynard for the preparation of this table.

(Footnotes continued on page 16.)

Table 3.1. (continued)

U.S.A.:

[1] Source: Recommended Dietary Allowances, Revised 1963. NAS-NRC Publ. 1146. Washington (1964).

[2] Allowances are intended for persons normally active in a temperate climate.

[3] Niacin equivalents include dietary sources of the preformed vitamin and the precursor, tryptophan. 60 mg tryptophan represents 1 mg niacin.

FAO:

[1] Source: Calorie Requirements, FAO. Nutritional Studies, No. 15, Rome (1957).

Protein Requirements, FAO. Nutritional Studies, No. 16, Rome (1957).

Calcium Requirements, FAO. Nutrition Meetings Report Series No. 30, Rome (1962).

Mean annual temperature, 10°C.

[2] The activity for the reference man is described as "on each working day he is employed 8 hours in an occupation which is not sedentary, but does not involve more than occasional periods of *hard* physical labor. When not at work, he is sedentary for about 4 hours daily and may walk for up to 1½ hours. He spends about 1½ hours on active recreations and household work." The activity of the reference woman is described as "she may be engaged either in general household duties or in light industry. Her daily activities include walking for about 1 hour and 1 hour of active recreation, such as gardening, playing with children, or non-strenuous sport."

[3] The protein value is defined as a safe practical allowance and is based on an average minimum requirement for a reference protein: increased by 50% to allow for individual variability, and by a further percentage in accordance with the estimated protein score of the protein of the diet. The values given in the table are for a diet similar to that of the USA, using a coefficient of 1.25 to allow for differences in protein quality, thus arriving at an allowance of 0.66 gm per kilogram body weight.

[4] The value is considered a safe practical allowance. A range is given to emphasize that present knowledge does not permit any greater accuracy as to a safe allowance.

Australia:

[1] Dietary allowances for Australia, 1961 revision, *Med. J. Australia*, Dec. 30, 1961. The allowances are designed to be used as a basis for planning food supplies for persons or groups.

[2] The activities specified are similar to those of the reference man and woman (Calorie Requirements, FAO Nutritional Studies No. 15, Rome). Mean annual external temperature, 18°C.

[3] Three I.U. of carotene equivalent to one I.U. of vitamin A activity.

[4] Preformed niacin plus (grams of protein $\times$ 0.16).

Canada:

[1] "Recommended daily intakes of nutrients adequate for the maintenance of health among the majority of Canadians." Issued 1963.

[2] Five categories of activity are listed and described. The values for calories and nutrients here given apply to "most household chores," "office work," "laboratory work," "shop and mill work," "mechanical trades or crafts," various sports.

[3] Based on normal mixed Canadian diets.

[4] Based on mixed Canadian diet supplying both vitamin A and carotene. As preformed vitamin A the suggested intake would be two-thirds of amounts indicated.

Central America and Panama:

[1] Institute of Nutrition of Central America and Panama (INCAP), Boletin de la Oficina Sanitaria Panamericana, Supplemento No. 2, Noviembre, 1955, page 225. The figures for nutrients are designed to meet the needs of all individuals. Average annual temperature, 20°C, activity not defined.

[2] This figure is given in the INCAP table as 1.3 mg of vitamin A and assumes that two-thirds of the activity is supplied from vegetable sources. International units shown were derived by converting as follows: one I.U. = 0.0003 mg vitamin A alcohol.

India:

[1] Patwardhan, V. N., Dietary allowances for India. Calories and Protein. Indian Council of Medical Research, Special Report Series No. 35, New Delhi, 1960. The data are 1958 revisions of earlier figures.

[2] The activities corresponding to the calorie recommendations are detailed in the above publication. "Moderate" refers to activity in a "light industrial occupation."

[3] "An allowance of one gm of protein per kilogram body weight of vegetable proteins in properly balanced diets."

Japan:

[1] Nutrition in Japan, 1962, Ministry of Health and Welfare, Tokyo, 1962. Data adopted by the Council on Nutrition in 1960. The allowances are believed to be sufficient to establish and maintain a good nutritional state in typical individuals.

[2] Age not specified.

[3] Five categories of activity are specified for men and four for women, with corresponding intakes for calories and B vitamins.

[4] Higher intakes are specified for heavy and very hard work.

[5] Requirement for both sexes specified as 2000 I.U. of preformed vitamin A or 6000 I.U. of carotene.

Netherlands:

[1] Recommended quantities of nutrients, Committee on Nutritional Standards of the Nutrition Council Voeding 22, 210–214, 1961. The figures for nutrients are set to cover individuals having high requirements. The figures for calories are average requirements.

[2] Assumes one-third is from animal sources. Figures are increased for heavy and very heavy work.

[3] Assumes 1500 I.U. as preformed vitamin A and 4000 I.U. of activity as carotene.

Norway:

[1] Evaluation of nutrition requirements, State Nutrition Council, 1958. Figures are "somewhat higher than average requirements."

[2] Vitamin A as present in animal foods.

The Philippines:

[1] Recommended daily allowances for specific nutrients, Food and Nutrition Research Center, 1960, "Objectives toward which to aim in planning practical diets."

[2] Assumes two-thirds contributed by carotene.

[3] Grams protein × 0.025.

South Africa:

[1] Recommended minimum daily dietary standards, National Research Council, S. A. Med. J., 30: 108, 1956.

[2] Assumes two-thirds contributed by carotene.

United Kingdom:

[1] Report of the Committee on Nutrition, British Medical Association, 1950. The levels of nutrients recommended are believed to be sufficient to establish and maintain a good nutritional state in representative individuals or groups concerned.

[2] Values are given for 6 levels of activity for males and 5 for females. Medium work is described as 8 hours at 100 Calories per hour and traveling (130 Calories per hour).

[3] The protein allowance is increased with calories on the basis that the protein in the diet should provide not less than 11% of the energy for adults not engaged in hard work.

[4] A mixed diet containing one-third vitamin A and two-thirds carotene.

U.S.S.R.:

[1] New daily vitamin supply standards in man, 1961, Yarusova, N. S., Vop. Pitan., 20: 3, 1961.

[2] I.U. is equivalent to 0.3 μg of natural vitamin.

[3] To be increased up to 50% in far north.

From *Recommended Dietary Allowances Sixth Revised Edition.* Natl. Acad. Sci.—Natl. Res. Council, Publ. 1146, 58–59, 1964.

tein requirement with the necessary adjustment for protein quality in the typical national diet of Canada.

The recommended nutrient intakes of calcium, vitamin A, and ascorbic acid are the same for men and women; however, the iron need suggested for Canadian men is about 60 per cent of the value suggested for Canadian women.

Pregnancy and lactation demand extra nutrients. Additional amounts of the nine nutrients plus a supplementary intake of vitamin D have been recommended for these periods of stress.

The recommended daily nutrient intakes for boys and girls are shown in Table A-3 (appendix). Up to the age of 15 years the activity of boys and girls is considered to be "usual," but from age 16 through 19 the weight and activity categories listed for adults are used to determine the need for Calories by the older adolescent. For the adolescent male and female (16–19 yr), the energy need is 113 per cent and 104 per cent, respectively, of their adult counterpart of the same weight and activity. The committee has recommended a daily intake of vitamin D for all children through the age of 19 years.

▶ BRITISH MEDICAL ASSOCIATION STANDARDS

As early as 1934 the British Medical Association issued a *Report on Nutrition* (1) that was followed by *Family Meals and Catering* (1934) and the *Doctor's Cookery Book* (1938). In 1948 a special committee was set up to examine the nutrition in the United Kingdom, particularly the adequacy of wartime and postwar diets. The work of this committee was divided into four subsections: nutritional requirements, food consumption, clinical assessment, and psychological and practical aspects of nutrition. This report was issued in 1950 (11). The level of nutrients recommended in the 1950 British Standard is believed to be sufficient to establish and maintain a good nutritional state in representative individuals or groups concerned. Only the daily dietary allowances recommended for five specific groups are shown in Table A-4 (appendix).

The basic energy needs for men and women "for 24 hours of ordinary living" are estimated to be 2200 and 1800 Cal., respectively. Extra Calories are either added or subtracted to account for variations in grade of work, for the physiological demands of pregnancy and lactation, and for old age. Thus five different categories of energy needs are proposed for men (sedentary, moderately active, active, very active, and over 65 yr), and six different ones for women (sedentary, moderately active, active, pregnancy, lactation, and over age 60).

The British Dietary Standard for infancy and childhood is given in the following age groups: up to 1 yr, 1–3 yr, 4–6 yr, 7–9 yr, 10–12 yr, 13–15 yr (males), 13–15 yr (females), 16–20 yr (males), and 16–20 yr (females). The recommendation for protein in the British Standard is based on the energy content of the diet. For the stress periods of growth, pregnancy, and lactation, 14 per cent of the Calories in the form of protein is suggested. Not less than 11 per cent of the energy allowance has been recommended as the protein requirement for adults.

A daily allowance for dietary fat ("visible" and "invisible") has been proposed by the committee. At least 25 per cent of the total Calories and up to 35 per cent, with increasing physical activity, has been recommended.

As in the NRC Recommended Allowances and the Canadian Standards, the dietary allowances for thiamine, riboflavin, and niacin are related to the energy need; however, the allowances stated for calcium, iron, and vitamin A are neither weight nor energy related.

The committee believes that 20 mg of ascorbic acid per day is an adequate amount of this nutrient for adults and 30 mg undoubtedly provides a good margin of safety. An extra amount of ascorbic acid has been recommended for pregnancy and lactation.

A dietary allowance for vitamin D is recommended for pregnancy, lactation, and growth. Also, a value for the mineral iodine has been proposed.

▶ INTERNATIONAL REQUIREMENTS OF THE FAO AND FAO-WHO

Committees within the FAO and the FAO-WHO have formulated and published assessments of requirements to meet the energy, protein, and calcium needs of persons of different countries and population groups throughout the world.

The need for a system of international energy standards was realized during the period of the Second World War. Since that time two reports have been prepared by the Committee on Calorie Requirements of the FAO (3, 4) for assessing caloric requirements, which, with appropriate adjustments, can be applied to different people in different parts of the world. The FAO system derives caloric requirements for adult populations from the measurements of two reference persons—the "Reference Man" and the "Reference Woman." Tables of numerical values are then used to assess energy needs of populations based on variations in body size, age, and environmental temperature (see Table 8.5, Chapter 8). The FAO energy requirements for childhood and early adolescence are assessed independently of the reference requirements, except as they pertain to environmental temperature. In late adolescence, ages 16 to 20, the caloric requirements are based on body size, taking into account also the influence of climate.

In 1957 the Committee on Protein Requirement of the FAO (9) presented a method to estimate the protein need of people throughout the world. The committee adopted a provisional pattern of essential amino acids for man, and expressed these requirements in terms of a "reference protein" value as part of the procedure in the assessment of protein needs. The FAO provisional pattern of essential amino acids, expressed in terms of amino acids per 100 gm of protein, is shown in Table 6.5 (Chapter 6). The steps involved in the estimation of a "safe practical allowance" for protein are the adjustment for individual variation in protein requirements, and the adjustment to allow for differences in protein quality.

After the assessment of requirements for energy and protein, the next logical step in the development of world dietary allowances was the study of needs for calcium. This task was undertaken by a FAO-WHO Expert Group who presented a report on calcium requirements in 1962 (2). To express values for calcium, the group adopted the term "suggested practical allowance," which has been defined as "the intake at which the needs of the great majority of persons in any defined population group are likely to be adequately met." The "suggested practical allowance" for different age groups, expressed as milligrams per day, is presented in Table 10.2 (Chapter 10). In the opinion of this group, there was neither evidence for recommending different allowances for males and females, except during the third trimester of pregnancy and lactation, nor sufficient evidence to warrant a special allowance for older persons at the time of this report.

These modern statements of assessing energy, protein, and calcium needs on an international basis are highly tentative and are open to testing and further research.

REFERENCES

1. Adequacy of the national diet, B. M. A. Nutrition Committee's Report (1950). *Brit. Med. J.* **4652:** 541.
2. *Calcium Requirements* (1962). World Health Organ., WHO Tech. Rept. Series 230, Geneva.
3. *Calorie Requirements* (1950). Food Agr. Organ. U.N., FAO Nutr. Studies 5, Rome.
4. *Calorie Requirements* (1957). Food Agr. Organ. U.N., FAO Nutr. Studies 15, Rome.
5. Dietary Standard for Canada (1964). *Can. Bull. Nutr.* **4:** no. 1.
6. Leitch, I. (1942). The evolution of dietary standards. Historical outline. *Nutr. Abstr. Rev.* **11:** 509.

7. McCollum, E. V. (1957). *A History of Nutrition.* Houghton Mifflin Co., Boston, p. 192.

8. McHenry, E. W. (1957). *Basic Nutrition.* J. B. Lippincott Co., Philadelphia, p. 217.

9. *Protein Requirements* (1957). Food Agr. Organ. U.N., FAO Nutr. Studies 16, Rome.

10. *Recommended Dietary Allowances Sixth Revised Edition* (1964). Natl. Acad. Sci.—Natl. Res. Council, Publ. 1146, Washington, D.C.

11. *Report of the Committee on Nutrition* (1950). British Medical Association, London.

CHAPTER 4

The carbohydrates

Carbohydrates serve a unique function in nature because they are the chief source of nutriment for the animal kingdom. Through the process of photosynthesis, which involves a series of complex chemical reactions, the chlorophyll of the plant is able to use the sun's energy to synthesize carbohydrates from the carbon dioxide of the air and the water from the soil. Thus it is through the medium of the plant that animals are able to have food. This nutrient also is the main source of food energy for the peoples of the world. The rice, cassava, sugars, potatoes, corn, wheat, and other cereal grains found in the international food supplies are all rich in carbohydrate.

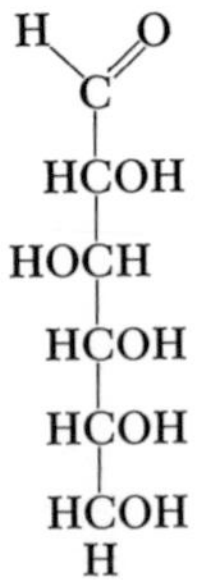

```
     H    O
      \  /
       C
       |
     HCOH
       |
    HOCH
       |
     HCOH
       |
     HCOH
       |
     HCOH
       H
```

Fig. 4.1. The chemical formula of glucose.

All carbohydrates contain carbon, hydrogen, and oxygen. In a simple carbohydrate unit, there are six carbon atoms arranged in a chain with atoms of hydrogen and oxygen attached to the carbons in the same ratio as found in water, two to one. The chemical formula of glucose is presented in Fig. 4.1. The energy value of carbohydrates is 4 Cal. of energy per gram of the nutrient.

A simple classification of some carbohydrates important in nutrition, based on the number of single carbohydrate units found in each chemical structure, is presented in Fig. 4.2. Compounds with one carbohydrate unit are called *monosaccharides*, those with two units are designated as *disaccharides*, and *polysaccharide*

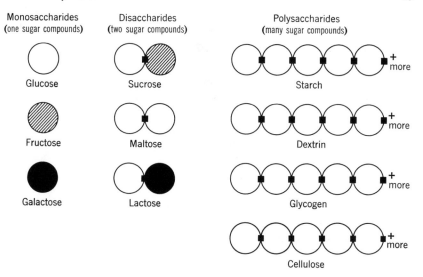

Fig. 4.2.   A simple classification of the carbohydrates.

is the term used to describe a compound with more than two carbohydrate units in its chemical structure. The three illustrated monosaccharides are the carbohydrate units contained in the structures of the di- and polysaccharides. The mono- and disaccharides are soluble in water, crystalline in structure, and have a sweet taste; they are called sugars and all have the characteristic name ending, -*ose*. In contrast, most polysaccharides are insoluble in water; they do not form crystals, do not taste sweet, and have neither a group name nor a characteristic ending. The approximate composition of various sweetening agents is presented in Table 4.1.

The Monosaccharides

The three monosaccharides that are important to the study of nutrition are glucose, fructose, and galactose.

Glucose. This monosaccharide, sometimes called dextrose or grape sugar, is widely distributed in nature. In the plant kingdom glucose is found in fruits, vegetables, and sap. It is the most abundant carbohydrate found in corn sugar and is present in corn sirup, honey, and molasses (Table 4.1). In the animal body it is an end product of digestion of starch, sucrose, maltose, and lactose.

Glucose is the carbohydrate found in the blood stream of animals and man, where it serves as a source of immediate fuel or energy for the body

Table 4.1. Approximate Composition of Various Sweetening Agents, in Percentages

Sugar Product	Water	Total Sugar	Sucrose	Dextrose	Levulose	Invert Sugar[1]	Maltose	Dextrins	Ash
Corn sirup	17.7	47.6	—	21.2	—	—	26.4	34.7	—
Corn sugar (cerelose)	9.0	91.0	—	87.5	—	—	3.5	0.5	0.04
Golden sirup	22.5	68.5	31.0	—	—	37.5	—	—	3.9
Honey	17.7	76.9	1.9	34.5	40.5	—	—	1.5	0.2
Invert sugar[1]	20.0	80.0	6.0	—	—	74.0	—	—	—
Maple sugar	35.0	64.1	62.6	—	—	1.5	—	—	0.6
Molasses	20.0	70.4	53.6	8.8	8.0	—	—	—	4.0
Sorghum sirup	23.0	63.0	36.0	—	—	27.0	—	—	2.5
Sucrose	—	100.0	100.0	—	—	—	—	—	—

[1] A mixture of sugars (glucose and fructose) formed by the process of inversion.

From Triebold's *Food Composition and Analysis*. Copyright 1963, D. Van Nostrand Co., Inc., Princeton, N.J.

cells and tissues. Man's normal level of blood glucose is about 80 mg of glucose per 100 ml of blood and is maintained within a narrow range by the balance of glucose entering and leaving the blood stream. Blood glucose originates from dietary carbohydrate, from stores of glycogen, or from carbohydrate synthesis. In diabetes, a disorder caused by the body's inability to use glucose, the blood glucose level is elevated. A more detailed discussion of diabetes and of the role of glucose in metabolism is presented in Chapter 7.

Fructose and Galactose. These two monosaccharides have the same chemical formula as glucose ($C_6H_{12}O_6$) but differ in the arrangement of chemical groups along the chemical chain.

Fructose, which has the sweetest taste of all the sugars, is also known as levulose or fruit sugar. It is found in the nectar of flowers, in fruits, and in vegetables and is produced during the hydrolysis of sucrose in digestion. This monosaccharide is found both in honey (40 per cent) and in molasses (8 per cent).

Galactose, however, does not occur free in nature like glucose and fructose but is produced in the body during the digestion of the disaccharide, lactose. The lack of an enzyme to convert galactose to glucose results in a disorder in infants known as galactosemia (see Chapter 7).

The Disaccharides

Sucrose, maltose, and lactose are the three disaccharides that are contained in the foods of the diet.

Sucrose. This disaccharide, the white and brown sugar that we use every day, is produced from sugar cane and sugar beets. Although cane and beet sugar differ slightly in texture and color, they have the same caloric value and can be used interchangeably. This almost pure carbohydrate is consumed in large quantities by the American people. The consumption of cane sugar in the United States increased markedly after the First World War and has remained at a high intake level throughout the years except when it was rationed during the Second World War. A 1963 report from the U.S. Department of Agriculture on food consumption shows the average per capita consumption of sucrose to have been 97.2 lb for the year 1962, approximately 1.9 lb per week (2). This amount of sucrose represents about 3447 Cal. per week, or the number of Calories recommended to met the energy needs of college men (2900 Cal. per day) and women (2100 Cal. per day) over 18 years for approximately 1.2 and 1.6 days, respectively.

Sucrose occurs in some fruits and vegetables but is found more frequently in sweetening agents. Maple sirup and molasses contain more than 50 per cent sucrose whereas lesser amounts are found in sorghum sirup, golden sirup, and honey (Table 4.1). Glucose and fructose are formed when sucrose is hydrolyzed during digestion.

Maltose and Lactose. Maltose and lactose, unlike sucrose, do not occur in large amounts in the average diet.

Maltose or malt sugar occurs in sprouting grains, malted cereals, and malted milk. Of the commonly used sweetening agents this disaccharide is found only in corn sirup (26 per cent) and corn sugar (4 per cent). The most important source of maltose for the body, however, is as an intermediate product of starch digestion. When hydrolyzed, maltose yields two molecules of glucose.

Lactose or milk sugar is found only in the milk of mammals. The amount of lactose in human and cow's milk has been reported to be about 6.8 and 4.9 per cent, respectively (7). Glucose and galactose are the two monosaccharides formed when lactose is hydrolyzed.

The Polysaccharides

The polysaccharides are complex carbohydrates that may contain as many as 2000 simple carbohydrate units arranged in long chains in either a straight or a branched structure. Starch, dextrin, glycogen, and cellulose are four polysaccharides that are important in the study of nutrition.

Starch. The plant products—roots, seeds, and tubers—that are easily produced, and produced in abundance, contain starch. Throughout the world starch is the most important carbohydrate in man's diet.

The seeds of plants are nature's richest storehouses of starch. Corn, millet, rice, rye, and wheat, the important cereal grains, contain as much as 70 per cent of this carbohydrate, whereas the percentage of starch found in the dried seeds of leguminous plants (*e.g.*, beans, peas) averages about 40 per cent.

Starch is found in the cells of plants in the form of granules. These granules, different in size and shape and markings, are typical of the plants in which they occur. Wheat starch granules are oval-shaped; the granules of cornstarch are small, rounded, and angular.

The starches are not soluble in cold water but when boiled with water they form pastes. In starch cookery, as the temperature of the liquid increases, the granules begin to swell and the mixture becomes viscous; this change is called gelatinization. Cooking makes starch-containing foods more palatable and more easily digested. Glucose is the end product of all starch hydrolyzed in the body.

Dextrins. The second group of polysaccharides, known as the dextrins, occur as metabolic products in animals and plants, and are particularly abundant in germinating seeds. Actually the dextrins are not too important as a source of carbohydrate because they are produced as in-between products in the hydrolysis of starch to maltose and finally glucose, both in the preparation of foods and digestion of starch. An appreciable amount of dextrin is found in corn sirup, but corn sugar and honey contain less (Table 4.1).

Glycogen. This polysaccharide is found in the liver of all animals and in small aquatic animals called mussels. Like starch, glycogen yields molecules of glucose on hydrolysis.

The term *animal starch* is another name given to glycogen, the storage polysaccharide of animals. Because the body does not have the capacity to store glycogen as it does fat, only about 350 gm or ¾ lb of it are found in the body as reserve. Muscle glycogen, which represents about two-thirds of the total reserve, is designated solely for the use of muscle tissue whereas liver glycogen is available as a source of energy to any of the body cells.

The formation and breakdown of glycogen in the body, which involve a series of complex chemical reactions, are directly related to several physiological factors. The formation of glycogen takes place when the blood glucose is increased beyond its normal level and extra amounts of glucose are present in the blood stream. In contrast the breakdown of glycogen takes place when carbohydrate is not being absorbed from the intestinal tract, and to meet this deficit the emergency supply of body energy, liver glycogen, must be utilized until the cells can begin to synthesize glucose from noncarbohydrate sources (glyconeogenesis). On the average about 100 gm of glycogen, or 400 Cal. of energy, are stored as liver glycogen. If the process of formation of glucose from non-carbohydrate sources were to cease (a hypothetical example), this amount of glycogen would supply the energy needs of college men and women over 18 years old for only about 3.3 and 4.5 hours, respectively.

Cellulose. Another carbohydrate, known as cellulose, occurs only in plants where it is the structural constituent of the cell wall that makes up the skeletal parts of all plants. Cellulose, commonly referred to as fiber in the human diet, is not important to most mammals as a direct source of food because they lack enzymes necessary to hydrolyze it to glucose. However, the *Herbivora* or ruminant animals (*e.g.*, cows, sheep) have bacteria in their rumens or stomachs that activate the breakdown of cellulose to useable carbohydrate products. Thus when man ingests products from these animals, he is indirectly using cellulose as a source of food.

Cellulose or fiber is important in the diet of man to aid in the maintenance of the normal peristaltic action of the intestines and in the removal of waste products from the intestinal tract. This polysaccharide provides a source of roughage to the intestinal tract which absorbs moisture and provides bulk to stimulate the normal evacuation of the large intestine.

The best food sources of cellulose or fiber are dried fruits, whole-grain cereals, nuts, fresh fruits, and vegetables. (See Fig. 4.3) Milk, meat, eggs, cheese, and highly refined foods (*e.g.*, white flour and sugar) are poor in fiber. Because the fiber in meat is protein, it is digestible and provides little if any bulk to the intestinal tract. Using the average values in Fig. 4.3, one can estimate the fiber content of a diet. The daily need for fiber, estimated to be 4 to 7 mg, may be easily obtained if the diet includes a serving of whole-grain cereal or bread, two servings of vegetables, and two servings of fruit.

Function of Carbohydrate

Carbohydrate has a variety of functions in the animal organism: it supplies energy for the body functions, it aids in the utilization of body fats, it exerts a sparing effect on protein, it plays an important role in the function of the intestinal tract, and it adds flavor to the diet.

The main function of carbohydrate is to supply energy for the body processes. Even though fats yield more than twice as much energy per unit weight as do carbohydrates (9 Cal. per gm as compared to 4 Cal.

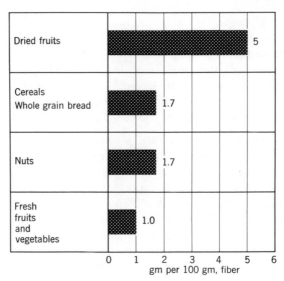

Fig. 4.3.   Average values for fiber content. (Courtesy of Rosenthal, Baker, and McVoy, *Stern Applied Dietetics*, 3rd ed., Williams and Wilkins Co., Baltimore, p. 79, 1949.)

per gm), the intake of carbohydrate is ordinarily greater than fat in the average diet. About 47 per cent of the energy value of the average American diet is provided by carbohydrate.

To describe the role of carbohydrate in the utilization of body fats, the expression "fat burns in a flame of carbohydrate" is often used. The complete oxidation of fats to the metabolic end products of carbon dioxide and water depends on an organic acid, pyruvic acid, formed during the oxidation of carbohydrates. When insufficient amounts of carbohydrates are available, greater than normal amounts of ketone bodies are produced. The accumulation of ketone bodies increases the acidity and reduces the alkalinity of the blood. This condition, called *ketosis,* may result in a coma if the alkalinity of the blood is reduced appreciably. Ketosis may occur in diabetes where the cells cannot utilize carbohydrate and in starvation where the cells must use the fat stores of the body for energy.

At the expense of tissue building and maintenance, relatively more protein is used for energy when the carbohydrate and fat content of the diet is below the desirable caloric level than when it is sufficient. This has been shown to occur during periods of weight reduction (8) and periods of semistarvation (3). The explanation of this metabolic effect is that the first physiological demand of the body, the energy need, must be satisfied before nutrients are used for other functions. Thus another important function of carbohydrate is to spare protein for its primary purpose, that is, the building and repairing of body tissue.

The relationship between the energy intake and its sparing action on protein in man has been studied in the laboratory. Leverton and her group (4) were among the first to report a definite sparing action on protein in college women when the caloric intake was increased from 1800 to 2400 Cal. per day. Other workers (1) have shown that a deficit of 7.5, 10, 15, and 20 per cent of the established Calories in man causes a distinct decrease in the sparing action of carbohydrate on the protein metabolism.

The carbohydrates also play important roles in the function of the mammalian intestinal system. They serve as a source of energy for the microorganisms that synthesize some of the B-complex vitamins in the intestinal tract, and the celluloses provide fiber and bulk that promote healthy intestinal hygiene.

Carbohydrate foods add flavor to the diet, and the cereals and breads furnish the body with protein.

Recommended Allowances for Carbohydrate

At this time there appears to be no basis for the formulation of a dietary allowance for carbohydrate in the human diet (5). It has been suggested, however, that normal adults need about 500 carbohydrate Calories per day either provided by the diet or derived from body stores of protein or glycogen.

Food Sources of Carbohydrate

The sugars, cereal grains, legumes, and dried fruits are the richest sources of carbohydrate found in the foods of the diet (Table 4.2). White sugar is almost pure carbohydrate, but cereal grains, legumes, and dried fruits vary in their carbohydrate content. Some of the processed foods that contain appreciable quantities of carbohydrate are noodles, dried nonfat milk solids, pretzels, jams, jellies, pastries, breads, cakes, and candies. Although most fresh fruits and vegetables are considered low in carbohydrate, bananas, dates, white potatoes, and sweet potatoes are rich in this nutrient. Eggs, fish, poultry, cheese, fresh milk, and meats (with the exception of liver) contain little carbohydrate, and the animal and vegetable fats none.

Carbohydrates in the World's Food Supply

At the beginning of the chapter it was stated that carbohydrate is the main source of food energy for the peoples of the world. To substantiate the importance of this nutrient in the world's food supply, data on the energy derived from cereals, starchy roots, and sugar as a percentage of

Table 4.2. The Percentage of Carbohydrate in Some Typical Foods

Carbohydrate	The Foods			
Per cent between 100–91	brown sugar white sugar			
90–81	corn flakes honey maple sugar	marshmallows peanut butter rice cereals		
80–71	bran flakes cookies crackers	dates fudge oat cereals	popcorn shredded wheat sirups	wheat flakes
70–61	chocolate sirup dried apricots jellies and jams	molasses		
60–51	cakes chocolate bars dried nonfat milk solids	white bread		
50–41	potato chips rolls whole-wheat bread			
40–31	apple pie French fried potatoes sweet potatoes			
30–21	baked potato banana cooked macaroni	noodles	rice	spaghetti
20–11	apple corn grapes	ice cream Lima beans pears	peas	
10–0	beef liver broccoli butter	carrot Cheddar cheese egg	green beans melons milk	orange peaches tomatoes
none	beef chicken fats oils	lamb pork salmon	veal	

Adapted from values in *Composition of Foods—Raw, Processed, Prepared.* U.S. Dept. Agr., Agr. Handbook 8, revised 1963.

the total Calories available for various geographical regions are presented in Table 4.3. These values are expressed in three ways: values before the Second World War (prewar), values after the Second World War (postwar), and values of recent years (recent).

The African countries derive about 74 per cent of their total Calories from carbohydrate-type foods. Prewar and postwar values for Africa are not available.

The percentage of Calories derived from carbohydrate sources ranges from 72 to 83 per cent for the peoples of Asia. The countries of the Near East (72 per cent) obtain about 10 per cent less of their food energy from carbohydrates than do those of the Far East (81 per cent).

Table 4.3. Calories Derived from Cereals, Starchy Roots, and Sugar as a Percentage of Total Food Calories Available throughout the World

	Prewar Value, %	Postwar Value, %	Recent Value, %
Africa:			
East and southern Africa	—	—	73
North Africa	—	—	75
West and central Africa	—	—	74
Asia:			
China, mainland	77	78	83
Eastern Asia	85	90	80
Near East	78	78	72
South Asia	76	76	78
Southeastern Asia, mainland	—	—	78
Southeastern Asia, major islands	83	81	81
Europe:			
Eastern Europe and U.S.S.R.	76	76	71
Western Europe	60	61	55
Oceania:			
Australia and New Zealand	50	50	48
North America:			
Canada and United States	48	43	40
Caribbean	66	64	60
Central America	62	75	71
Mexico	70	73	85
South America:			
Brazil	59	65	64
North and western countries	69	70	66
River Plate countries[1]	53	56	54

[1] Argentina, Paraguay, and Uraguay.

From *Third World Food Survey*. Food Agr. Organ. U.N., Basic Study No. 11, pp. 88–93, 1963.

Western Europe consumes about 20 per cent less carbohydrate Calories (55 per cent) than does the area of Eastern Europe and the U.S.S.R. (71 per cent). It has been reported that about two-thirds of the food energy in Europe, as a whole, comes from cereals, starchy roots, and sugars (63 per cent).

Like Canada and the United States, the countries of Oceania, Australia and New Zealand, produce large amounts of food, and their consumption of carbohydrate Calories is similar to ours (about 48 per cent).

In North America the percentage of Calories derived from cereals, starchy roots, and sugars ranges from 40 to 85 per cent within the regions of the continent. Less than one-half of the total food energy comes from carbohydrate sources in Canada and the United States (40 per cent), whereas the people of Mexico obtain about 85 per cent of their Calories from carbohydrate foods.

The countries of South America obtain between one-half and two-thirds of their food energy from carbohydrates. In Argentina, Paraguay, and Uraguay (River Plate Countries), the national diets contain about 54 per cent carbohydrate Calories; in Brazil and the north and western countries they contain somewhat more, about 65 per cent.

Comparisons have been made on the basis of "high-Calorie countries" and "low-Calorie countries" (6). In "high-Calorie countries" (Canada, Europe, Oceania, River Plate Countries, United States) about 57 per cent of the total energy comes from cereals, starchy roots, and sugars; in "low-Calorie countries" (Africa, Far East, Latin America, and Near East) over three-fourths of the Calories come from these same food sources (78 per cent).

When all these data are accumulated to represent the world as a whole, about 70 per cent of the total Calories come from carbohydrate foods (6).

REFERENCES

1. Clark, H. E., E. T. Mertz, and S. P. Yang (1958). Influence of caloric intake on urinary nitrogen excretion in man. *Federation Proc.* **17:** 473.
2. *Consumption of Food in the United States 1909–52. Supplement for 1962* (1963). U.S. Dept. Agr., Agr. Handbook 62, Washington, D.C.
3. Fisher, K. H., E. D. Huang, V. A. Campbell, and R. W. Swift (1962). *Dietary Conditioning for Nutrient Restriction in Humans.* Artic Aeromedical Lab., Tech. Doc. Rept. AAL–TDR–62–1, Fort Wainwright, Alaska.
4. Leverton, R. M., M. R. Gram, and M. Chaloupka (1951). Effect of the time factor and caloric level on nitrogen utilization of young women. *Federation Proc.* **10:** 386.
5. *Recommended Dietary Allowances Sixth Revised Edition* (1964). Natl. Acad. Sci.—Natl. Res. Council, Publ. 1146, Washington, D.C.

6. *Third World Food Survey* (1963). Food Agr. Organ. U.N., Basic Study 11, Rome.
7. Triebold, H. O., and L. W. Aurand (1963). *Food Composition and Analysis*. D. Van Nostrand Co., Princeton, N.J.
8. Young, C. M., A. M. Brown, B. A. Gehring, and B. M. Morris (1960). Stepwise weight reduction in obese, young women; clinical and metabolic responses. *J. Nutr.* **70:** 391.

SUPPLEMENTARY REFERENCES

Harper, A. E. (1959). Carbohydrates. In *Food. The Yearbook of Agriculture 1959*. (A. Stefferud, ed.), U.S. Dept. Agr., Washington, D.C.
Sinclair, H. M. (1964). Carbohydrates and fats. In *Nutrition, a Comprehensive Treatise*, Vol. I. (G. H. Beaton and E. W. McHenry, eds.), Academic Press, New York.

CHAPTER 5

The lipids

The lipids are an important group of chemical compounds that are widespread in nature and are characterized by their insolubility in water and their solubility in ether, chloroform, benzene, and other fat solvents. Like the carbohydrates, the lipids contain carbon, hydrogen, and oxygen, and some also have phosphorus and nitrogen in their chemical structure. The lipids are classified into three groups according to their chemical structure: the simple lipids, the compound lipids, and the derived lipids. The *fatty acids, fats* and *oils, phospholipids,* and *sterols,* are several of the groups of compounds found among the lipids which are important in the study of nutrition.

► **THE FATTY ACIDS**

Fatty acids are composed entirely of carbon, hydrogen, and oxygen and are found in all the simple and compound lipids. The simplest fatty acid is acetic acid, familiar as the substance that gives vinegar its sour taste. The fatty acids have interesting names; a few of the common ones found in fats are butyric, caproic, myristic, palmitic, stearic, oleic, and linoleic (Table 5.1).

There are short-chain (under 12 carbon atoms), long-chain (16 to 18 carbon atoms), and extra long-chain fatty acids (more than 20 carbon atoms), but in the average diet most of them are of the long-chain

34

Table 5.1. Some of the Fatty Acids Found in Fats

Name	Number of Carbon Atoms	Length of Carbon Chain	Type	Occurrence in Food
Acetic	2	short	saturated	vinegar
Butyric	4	short	saturated	butter
Caproic	6	short	saturated	butter
Caprylic	8	short	saturated	coconut
Myristic	14	long	saturated	nutmeg and mace
Palmitic	16	long	saturated	lard and palm oil
Stearic	18	long	saturated	beef tallow
Oleic	18	long	monounsaturated	olive oil
Linoleic	18	long	polyunsaturated	corn oil
Clupanadonic	22	extra long	polyunsaturated	fish oils

variety. Short-chain fatty acids are found in coconut oil, milk fat, and butterfat; the extra long-chain ones occur in fish oils and peanut oil (Table 5.1).

The three general types of fatty acids found in foods are classified according to their degree of saturation or unsaturation (Table 5.1 and Fig. 5.1). Certain fatty acids, such as stearic acid, contain as many hydrogen atoms as the carbon chain can hold, and these are called *saturated fatty acids*. There are others that have only one "double-bond" linkage (two hydrogen atoms missing) in the carbon chain; these are referred to as *monounsaturated fatty acids*. A third group, the *polyunsaturated fatty acids*, may have 2, 3, 4, or more "double-bond" linkages in the carbon chain with 4, 6, 8, or more hydrogen atoms missing. This group of fatty acids is sometimes further classified as *dienoic, trienoic, tetraenoic,* and so forth, to identify the number of "double-bond" linkages. Linoleic acid is classified as a dienoic acid, linolenic and arachidonic acids as trienoic and tetraenoic, respectively.

The saturated fatty acids comprise about 40 per cent of the fatty acids contained in the average American diet. For the most part these acids are concentrated in foods from animal sources. However, the plant products, chocolate and coconut, both contain appreciable amounts of the saturated fatty acids. The most common ones found in foods are stearic acid and the long-chain fatty acid, palmitic (Table 5.2). Butter and cow's milk contain about 12 per cent stearic acid; other animal products contain larger amounts. The palmitic acid content of most animal fats ranges from 20 to 30 per cent.

The quantity of the monounsaturated fatty acids in the average American diet matches that of the saturated ones, about 40 per cent. The best example of this type is the long-chain fatty acid, oleic, which

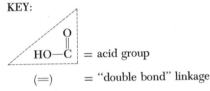

Stearic acid (saturated) $C_{18}H_{36}O_2$

Oleic acid (monounsaturated) $C_{18}H_{34}O_2$

Linoleic acid (polyunsaturated) $C_{18}H_{32}O_2$

KEY:

HO—C ‖ O = acid group

(=)   = "double bond" linkage

Fig. 5.1.   The chemical structure of a saturated, monounsaturated, and polyunsaturated fatty acid.

is found in appreciable amounts in most foods (Table 5.2). Oleic acid comprises nearly one-half of the fatty acid content of bacon and more than 75 per cent of the fatty acid content of olive oil.

The polyunsaturated fatty acids comprise a family of compounds that include the essential fatty acids and the extra long-chain fatty acids. The quantity of these acids in the average American diet is much less than either the saturated or monounsaturated ones (Table 5.2). Although corn oil and safflower oil are among the richest food sources of this fatty acid group, fats from nuts, peanuts, poultry, legumes, and leafy-green vegetables are also important sources.

▶ THE FATS AND OILS

Fats are composed of fatty acids and glycerol, a compound which like the fatty acids is composed of carbon, hydrogen, and oxygen. The ratio of carbon and hydrogen to oxygen in the fat molecule, however, is much

Table 5.2. Fatty Acid Content of Food Fats

(gram per 100 gm ether extract or crude fat)[1]

Food Fat or Oil	Saturated Fatty Acids			Unsaturated Fatty Acids		
	Total[2]	Palmitic	Stearic	Total[3]	Oleic	Linoleic
Animal Products						
Meats:						
Beef	48	28	19	47	44	2
Buffalo	66	34	28	30	24	1
Deer	63	24	34	32	24	3
Goat	57	26	24	37	33	2
Horse	30	24	5	60	30	6
Lamb	56	29	25	40	36	3
Luncheon meats	36	24	11	59	45	7
Pork:						
Back, outer layer	38	26	12	58	46	6
Bacon	32	21	9	63	48	9
Liver	34	13	18	61	27	5
Other cuts	36	21	13	59	42	9
Rabbit, domesticated	38	28	4	58	35	11
Milk Fat:						
Buffalo, Indian	62	29	15	33	26	1
Cow	55	25	12	39	33	3
Goat	62	27	8	33	25	5
Human	46	22	7	48	34	7
Poultry and Eggs:						
Chicken	32	24	7	64	38	20
Turkey	29	22	6	67	43	21
Chicken eggs	32	25	7	61	44	7
Fish and Shellfish:						
Eel, body	23	17	2	73		36(−2.6H)
Herring, body	19	11	1	77		19(−3.5H)
Menhaden, body	24	15	3	71	15	3
Salmon, body	15	12	2	79		26(−2.8H)
Tuna, body	25	18	3	70		25(−3.2H)
Turtle	44	16	7	51		31(−2.6H)
Separated Fats and Oils:						
Butter	55	25	12	39	33	3
Lard	38	31	7	57	46	10
Codfish liver	15	12	1	81		25(−3.3H)
Halibut liver	17	13	Trace	72	31	—
Whale blubber	15	9	1	41		21(−2.4H)
Plant Products						
Cereals and Grains:						
Cornmeal, white	11	8	1	82	34	44
Millet (Foxtail)	31	10	14	61	20	35

Table 5.2. (continued)

(gram per 100 gm ether extract or crude fat)[1]

Food Fat or Oil	Saturated Fatty Acids			Unsaturated Fatty Acids		
	Total[2]	Palmitic	Stearic	Total[3]	Oleic	Linoleic
Cereals and Grains:						
Oats, rolled	22	13	4	74	32	41
Rice	17	12	2	74	39	35
Sorghum	12	7	5	81	37	44
Wheat flour, white	14	10	4	76	31	42
Wheat germ	15	11	4	77	23	48
Fruits and Vegetables Including Seeds:						
Avocado pulp	20	18	2	69	45	13
Cantaloupe seed	15	10	4	79	26	53
Chickpea	9	4	2	87	50	36
Chocolate	56	23	33	39	37	2
Olives	11	9	2	84	76	7
Pigeon pea	33	—	—	57	6	46
Pumpkinseed	17	9	8	78	37	41
Rapeseed	6	2	2	89	16	14
Sesame seed	14	8	4	80	38	42
Soybeans	20	11	7	75	16	52
Squash seed	18	12	6	77	35	42
Watermelon seed	17	10	6	78	18	59
Nuts and Peanuts:						
Almond	8	7	1	87	67	20
Beechnut	8	5	3	87	54	31
Brazil nut	20	14	6	76	48	26
Cashew	17	6	11	78	70	7
Coconut	86	10	2	8	7	Trace
Filbert (Hazelnut)	5	2	2	91	54	16
Hickory	8	6	1	87	68	18
Peanut	22	11	4	72	43	29
Peanut butter	26	11	6	70	45	25
Pecan	7	6	1	84	63	20
Pistachio	10	8	2	85	65	19
Walnut, black	6	3	2	90	35	48
Walnut, English	7	5	2	89	15	62
Separated Fats and Oils:						
Cacao butter	56	23	33	39	37	2
Corn oil	10	8	2	84	28	53
Cottonseed oil	25	22	2	71	21	50
Margarine[4]	26	21	3	70	57	9
Olive oil	11	9	2	84	76	7
Palm oil	45	39	4	49	40	8
Peanut oil	18	8	6	76	47	29

Table 5.2. (continued)

(gram per 100 gm ether extract or crude fat)[1]

Food Fat or Oil	Saturated Fatty Acids			Unsaturated Fatty Acids		
	Total[2]	Palmitic	Stearic	Total[3]	Oleic	Linoleic
Separated Fats and Oils:						
Safflower oil	8	3	4	87	15	72
Sesame oil	14	8	4	80	38	42
Shortening (animal and vegetable)	43	27	12	53	41	11
Shortening (vegetable)	23	14	6	72	65	7
Soybean oil	15	9	6	80	20	52
Sunflower oil	12	6	5	83	20	63

[1] To calculate fatty acids in foods, multiply amount (gm) of fat in food portion by value of each fatty acid. Trace is used to indicate values of 0.5 or less.
[2] Includes other saturated fatty acids in addition to palmitic and stearic.
[3] Includes other unsaturated fatty acids in addition to oleic and linoleic.
[4] Varies widely depending on the fats used.

From *Fatty Acids in Food Fats*. U.S. Dept. Agr., Home Econ. Res. Rept. 7, 1959.

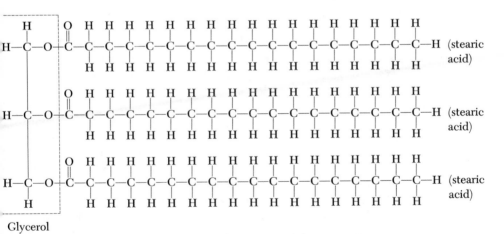

Glycerol

Fig. 5.2. The chemical formula of tristearin (a fat found in beef): $C_{57}H_{110}O_6$.

greater than that in a carbohydrate. For example, a fat found in beef which is called tristearin (Fig. 5.2) has 110 atoms of hydrogen to 6 atoms of oxygen, as compared to the two-to-one ratio of the same elements in the carbohydrate glucose (Fig. 4.1). The chemical term for a fat is *triglyceride.*

When a fat is burned in the body additional oxygen must be supplied by the cells to combine with all the carbon and hydrogen atoms, thus producing more heat. For this reason a gram of pure fat gives the body 9 Cal. of energy, whereas a gram of pure carbohydrate yields only 4 Cal.

There are essentially four parts to every fat molecule. (See Fig. 5.2.) The core of the molecule is *glycerol,* a three-carbon compound which is related to the family of alcohols. Then a fatty acid is attached to each of the three carbon units of the glycerol molecule.

The nature of a fat depends on the kinds of fatty acids linked to the glycerol core, the length of the carbon chain of the fatty acids, and the degree of saturation or unsaturation of the fatty acids. The fatty acid pattern of a fat may be three identical acids, three different ones, or a combination of two alike and one different. The three fatty acids found in the fat tristearin (Fig. 5.2) are identical, that is, the long-chain, saturated stearic acid. When all of the fatty acids in a fat molecule are the same, the fat is called a simple glyceride. A mixed glyceride is the term used to identify a fat with different fatty acids in its chemical structure. Tristearin is designated as a simple glyceride.

The form of a glyceride, whether it is liquid or solid, depends on the kind of fatty acids in its structure. A glyceride that is liquid at room temperature is called an oil and contains more of the unsaturated fatty acids, whereas a glyceride that is solid at room temperature contains more of the saturated fatty acids in its structure and is called a fat. Oils are the predominant glycerides in plants; fats are the predominant glycerides in animals.

The fats of animals differ from species to species and even vary in composition in the different parts of the body of the same species (4). Lard, the fat of swine, melts at 28°C (82°F), beef fat at 46°C (115°F), and sheep fat at 51°C (124°F). These values show that swine produce a fat that is softer and richer in unsaturated fatty acids than do either beef or sheep. A comparison of the melting point of the typical body fat of swine (lard) with the fat of swine kidney, 43°C (109°F), shows the latter to be of a firmer consistency and higher saturated fatty acid composition. This difference is to be expected because the fat around the kidneys cushions these vital organs to protect them from injury. As a general rule the fats in the more active parts of the animal organism have a lower melting point and are more unsaturated, which means they are more easily oxidized than those stored as fatty tissues.

Chemical substances, known as *antioxidants*, delay the oxidation of "double-bond" linkages in a glyceride, thus prolonging the shelf life of a fat or oil. There are both natural and synthetic antioxidants. Vitamins C and E are examples of natural antioxidants; gallates and BHT (butylated hydroxytoluene) are examples of synthetic ones. Antioxidants apparently function in that they themselves are more easily oxidized than the glycerides they protect. "As a rule, it can be said that these substances have little effect on vegetable oils but a pronounced action on being added to animal oils and fats" (33).

Hydrogenation of Fats and Oils

The oils from plants may be hardened to form solid glycerides, or "soft" fats may be hardened to increase their melting point by a process known as *hydrogenation*. In this chemical process hydrogen enters the "double-bond" linkages of the unsaturated fatty acids to make the glycerides more saturated. At one time (12) a fraction of the oil was completely hydrogenated, and this saturated mass was then mixed with other glycerides to obtain a product of desired consistency (nonselective hydrogenation). Today, because of the market demand for unsaturated fat products, a processing method is used in which all the oil or fat undergoes partial hydrogenation to increase the firmness of the glyceride without producing saturated fatty acids (selective hydrogenation). In selective hydrogenation the polyunsaturated fatty acids are changed to monounsaturated rather than saturated fatty acids.

Hydrogenation has helped to alleviate the shortage of solid fat in the world food market. By means of this process a hardened fat product can be manufactured that will meet the needs which the climate imposes. For example, a hydrogenated oil to be marketed in northern Alaska would be designed to have a lower melting point than one to be sold in Panama. Also the decrease in the degree of unsaturation (from polyunsaturate to monounsaturate) increases the keeping quality of a glyceride.

The influence of hydrogenated versus unhydrogenated fats on the growth rate of the rat and on the serum cholesterol level in man has been reported. Aaes-Jorgensen and his group (1) have observed a slight decrease in the growth of rats which are fed a ration containing a high percentage of hydrogenated fat; however, the presence of 3 to 4 per cent linoleic acid in a ration rich in hydrogenated fats appears to support satisfactory growth in this animal (33). In man the blood cholesterol response to a dietary intake of partially hydrogenated vegetable fats and oils has been observed to be equivalent to the response from unhydrogenated vegetable oils (24).

Function of Fats and Oils

Fats and oils play an important role in human nutrition because they are sources of energy and of the essential fatty acids in the diet. In addition fat deposits in the body serve as insulation and provide protective cushions for the organs.

Source of Energy. Fats are the most concentrated form of energy in foods, yielding more than twice as much energy as equal portions of either carbohydrates or proteins. Moreover, the greatest supply of reserve energy in animals and man is found in the fat stores of the body which may be mobilized to meet the body's need for energy.

Sources of Essential Fatty Acids. Although it is known that fatty acids can be synthesized from extra amounts of carbohydrates in the body, there are certain fatty acids which man needs for good health that the body cannot produce. These are called the *essential fatty acids,* and include the following three acids: linoleic, linolenic, and arachidonic. The importance of these factors in nutrition was first demonstrated when rats who were fed a ration devoid of fat developed a scaly condition of the skin and tail, failed to grow, and eventually died (Fig. 5.3). All the known fatty acids were added to the fat-free diet of the animals, but only linoleic, linolenic, and arachidonic acids were

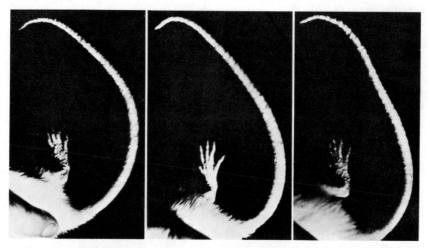

Fig. 5.3.   The scaly condition of the skin and tail of a rat fed a low-fat diet and the effects of humidity on the skin lesions. (Left) Low-fat rat from colony. (Center) Same animal after 48 hours at 97 per cent relative humidity. (Right) Same animal after 3 weeks at 50 per cent relative humidity. (Courtesy of Burr, Hawaii Agriculture Experimental Station.)

effective in preventing this disorder (7). It now appears that a dietary source of the essential fatty acids is required by the mouse, the dog, and probably man.

It has been found from studies with normal children that there is no dietary requirement for arachidonic acid when linoleic acid is supplied in optimal amounts (34). Thus it has been established that arachidonic acid is not a true dietary essential because it can be formed in the body from linoleic acid. It has also been confirmed that linolenic acid has a different and less important function than linoleic. Because of these findings, the view is now held that the term "essential fatty acids" should be reserved only for those members of the linoleic family (21).

In the animal organism linoleic acid has been shown to play an essential role in reproduction and lactation (13). Furthermore, it has been reported to serve as a protective agent against radiation effects and to prevent the excessive loss of water from the body by preventing the development of the permeability of the skin capillaries.

Attempts to produce a fatty acid deficiency in man have not been successful. However, a tendency toward skin disorders is a characteristic response to a low-fat diet in infants (22). This condition can be alleviated in a short time, however, by adding 2 per cent of the total Calories of the diet as linoleic acid (18). Hansen and his group (19) have observed unsatisfactory growth records for infants maintained on low linoleic acid intakes.

Little is known about the essential fatty acid requirement of man. It has been reported, however, that optimal levels of serum fatty acids are attained in children when the linoleic acid intake is about 4 per cent of the total Calories (35).

Protection of the Body. Fats are known to protect the body in two ways. The deposits of fat under the skin act as nonconductors of heat, helping to insulate the body and prevent the rapid loss of heat. Furthermore, the viscera and certain organs of the body, such as the kidneys, are supported and cushioned by fat.

Recommended Allowance for Fat

The 1963 revision of the NRC Recommended Dietary Allowances does not suggest an allowance for either the desirable amount of fat or patterns of fatty acids in the average diet. However, it is stated that "for many Americans, moderate reduction in total fat and some substitution of polyunsaturated for saturated fat may be indicated. This has to be judged on an individual basis and, in the adjustment of the diet, other changes in calorie and nutrient balance must be taken into account" (28).

The U.S. Department of Agriculture reported for 1962 that the amount of fat available for consumption per capita in the United States was about 147 gm or 5 oz per day (11). The percentage of fat contributed by the major food groups (2) was 15.3 (dairy products, excluding butter), 3.6 (eggs), 25.0 (meats, poultry, and fish), 49.4 (fats and oils, including pork fat cuts and butter), 4.0 (dry beans and peas, nuts, soya flour, and cocoa), 0.1 (potatoes and sweet potatoes), 0.2 (citrus fruit and tomatoes), 0.2 (leafy-green and yellow vegetables), 0.7 (other vegetables and fruits), 1.5 (flour and cereal grains), and 0 (sugar and sirups).

Food Sources of Fat

The richest sources of fat in the diet are the vegetable oils, such as corn oil, peanut oil, olive oil, and vegetable shortenings, and the animal fats, such as lard and butter (Table 5.3). Nuts rank high as contributors of fat to the diet, with pecans having the most fat, peanuts the least. Meat, poultry, and fish vary in their fat content; bacon contains about twice as much as beef and salmon (an example of fatty fish). All cheeses with the exception of cottage cheese contain appreciable amounts of the nutrient. The fat in an egg is found only in the yolk. Processed and prepared foods made with fats and oils such as potato chips, cakes, pastries, cookies, and candy bars may contain appreciable amounts of the nutrient. Most fruits and vegetables contain little fat; however, avocados and coconuts, which contain about 20 per cent fat, are exceptions.

The Effect of Food Preparation on Fats and Oils

The effect of food preparation on the fats and oils of food products has been studied in the laboratory. There apparently is little alteration in the essential fatty acids of meat and poultry when prepared by conventional cooking methods (8). However, when meat is fried in a very hot pan, the glycerol of the fat molecule may decompose to form a substance known as acrolein, which has a very pungent odor. Baking does not appear to affect the fatty acid composition of the fat used in baked products, but slight losses of linoleic acid occur when vegetable oil is used for several hours in deep-fat frying (9). A series of experiments conducted to study the decomposition of fats during home frying procedures (30) showed that changes in fat composition are related to the method of frying, kind of fat used, and kind of food fried. Several of the recommendations made to avoid these changes were to discard a frying fat when it begins to foam severely when food is added, to discard a frying fat when the color changes become pronounced, and to use the largest amount of fat the container will hold and add fresh fat to maintain this volume each time the fat is reused.

Fats and Oils in the World's Food Supply

The amounts of fat and oil in the per capita food supplies of the various regions of the world reflect the areas of food shortages and food abundance (Table 5.4). These values, expressed both in kilograms and

Table 5.3. The Percentage of Fat in Some Typical Foods

Fat	The Foods			
Per cent between 100–91	lard salad and cooking oils vegetable fats			
90–81	butter fat salt pork margarine			
80–71	mayonnaise pecans			
70–61	walnuts			
60–51	bacon baking chocolate			
50–41	peanuts peanut butter			
40–31	Cheddar cheese chocolate bar coconut	egg yolk heavy cream pork chop	potato chips salad dressing	
30–21	beef pattie frankfurter ham	sirloin steak		
20–11	apple pie avocado chocolate cake	doughnut egg	lamb roast luncheon meats French fried potatoes	veal cutlet
10–0	apple baked potato beef liver	bread carrot chicken	cottage cheese halibut ice cream	milk oatmeal salmon
none	sugars and sirups			

Adapted from values in *Composition of Foods—Raw, Processed, Prepared.* U.S. Dept. Agr., Agr. Handbook 8, revised 1963.

Table 5.4. Fats and Oils in the Food Supplies of the World

	Kilograms per Capita Per Year			Pounds per Capita per Year		
	Prewar Value	Postwar Value	Recent Value	Prewar Value	Postwar Value	Recent Value
Africa	—	—	7	—	—	15.4
Europe	13	11	16	28.6	24.2	35.2
Far East	4	5	3	8.8	11.0	6.6
Latin America	6	8	9	13.2	17.6	19.8
Near East	4	4	7	8.8	8.8	15.4
North America	21	20	21	46.2	44.0	46.2
Oceania	16	15	16	35.2	33.0	35.2

From *Third World Food Survey*. Food Agr. Organ. U.N., Basic Study No. 11, pp. 88–93, 1963.

pounds per year, are given for the prewar and postwar years of the Second World War, as well as for recent times (32).

The countries of Africa, the Far East, Latin America, and the Near East have less than 20 lb of fat and oil per person per year. In the Far East, where the supplies of fats and oils are the shortest (6.6 lb or 3000 gm per person per year), the daily intake of this nutrient would average only about 8 gm per day.

The people of Europe, Canada and the United States (North America), as well as Australia and New Zealand (Oceania), have available more than 35 lb of fats and oils per person per year. In Europe and Oceania the daily per capita intake of fat would average about 44 gm and about 58 gm in North America.

A comparison of the fat supplies between the "low-Calorie" countries (Africa, Far East, Latin America, and Near East) and the "high-Calorie" countries (Europe, North America, and Oceania) shows a wide difference in the availability of these energy-rich foods: 8.8 lb per person per year as compared to 39.6 lb per person per year. In terms of daily supplies an individual in a "high-Calorie" country (about 50 gm) would have access to about five times as much fat as an individual in a "low-Calorie" country (about 11 gm).

If the world's supply of fats and oils were divided equally among the world's population, each person would have about 17.6 lb or 8 kg per year, or about 22 gm per day.

▶ THE PHOSPHOLIPIDS AND STEROLS

Two important groups in the lipid family are the phospholipids and the sterols.

The phospholipids are found in every living cell. These complex lipids aid in the transport of fatty acids in the body. The three types of phospholipids (the lechithins, cephalins, and sphingomyelins) are formed from glycerol, fatty acids, phosphoric acid, and a nitrogenous base. Choline is one of the nitrogenous bases found in the phospholipids.

Ergosterol, 7-dehydrocholesterol, and cholesterol are three important compounds found in the group of derived lipids known as the sterols. Ergosterol, a plant sterol, and 7-dehydrocholesterol, an animal sterol, are two preforms of vitamin D. Cholesterol, the best known of the sterols, has attracted attention in scientific circles throughout the world because of the association of elevated blood cholesterol levels with atherosclerosis and coronary heart disease.

Cholesterol, a natural constituent of animal tissues, is found in the cells and body fluids. Some of it is combined with fatty acids to form bound cholesterol, but for the most part it is found in the body as free cholesterol. The sum of the free and bound forms is referred to as total cholesterol.

The body's supply of cholesterol is derived in two ways: from the foods in the diet (exogenous cholesterol) and by synthesis in the tissues, particularly in the liver (endogenous cholesterol). It has been stated that the average American adult ingests between 500 and 800 mg of cholesterol per day and that the body synthesis of cholesterol approaches 1500 mg per day (20). Almost three-fourths of this is excreted as bile acids, and a portion of the remainder is excreted also, both in the feces.

Blood cholesterol values vary from species to species (26) and vary with age in the same species (5). The average serum cholesterol value, expressed as milligrams per 100 ml, is about 80 for the rat, 120 for the monkey, 140 for the dog, and 220 for man. In man the total cholesterol value (milligram per 100 ml) increases with advancing age: 65 in fetal cord blood, 190 among young adult men and women (18 to 35 years), and 245 among middle-aged men and women (45 to 65 years).

The cholesterol values of some commonly used foods are presented in Table 5.5. Eggs, butter, lard, and meats are examples of foods rich in cholesterol whereas foods from plant sources are devoid of the sterol.

▶ CONCEPTS OF THE RELATIONSHIP OF DIETARY FAT
TO ATHEROSCLEROSIS

There is a great deal of interest in the causes of atherosclerosis, a disease in which the walls of the arteries thicken owing to deposits of fats and mineral salts. It is believed that this condition in man makes him more susceptible to heart attacks and strokes. In part the basis for the present concepts on the relationship of dietary fat to atherosclerosis, and thus

Table 5.5. Cholesterol Content of Foods

Food	Cholesterol per 100 gm Edible Portion, in mg	Food	Cholesterol per 100 gm Edible Portion, in mg
Beef, raw	70	Kidney, raw	375
Butter	250	Lamb, raw	70
Cheese:		Lard and other	
Cheddar	100	animal fat	95
cottage, creamed	15	Liver, raw	300
cream	120	Lobster	200
other (25 to 30% fat)	85	Margarine:	
Cheese spread	65	all vegetable fat	0
Chicken, raw	60	two-thirds animal	
Crabmeat	125	fat, one-third	
Egg, whole	550	vegetable fat	65
Egg, white	0	Milk:	
Egg yolk:		fluid, whole	11
fresh	1500	dried, whole	85
frozen	1280	fluid, skim	3
dried	2950	Mutton	65
Fish, steak or fillet	70	Pork	70
Heart, raw	150	Shrimp	125
Ice cream	45	Veal	90

From *Composition of Food—Raw, Processed, Prepared.* U.S. Dept. Agr., Agr. Handbook 8, revised 1963.

to heart disease, originated with the observations made in Norway during the years of the Second World War as well as with more recent interracial studies made in other parts of the world. In Norway, when the fat content of the diet was markedly reduced by wartime rationing, the incidence of atherosclerosis was also greatly reduced. Moreover, atherosclerosis is not prevalent in countries such as Japan, Spain, Italy, or parts of Africa where the total of fat Calories is much lower than in the average American diet. Because the incidence of atherosclerosis is associated with high cholesterol levels in the blood and with altered values of other blood lipids, notably the triglycerides (fat), intensive research has been directed to identifying influences of the blood level of these substances (37, 23, 3). Although these controversial issues must be clarified by further research, some of the important studies and explanatory theories are presented.

The influence of cholesterol in the diet on the blood level of this constituent is uncertain. Before it was discovered that the body could synthesize cholesterol, food of course was considered its only source. Using radioactive isotopes (29), Rittenberg and Schoenheimer learned that the body could synthesize cholesterol and does so at the rate of 2 to 3 gm per day. Because the amount in an average diet is only about 0.5 gm daily, dietary cholesterol has been considered fairly inconsequential. However, indications that the fat fed with the cholesterol may be a factor in its absorption have once again directed attention to food sources. Cholesterol fed with butterfat at the level of 30 per cent of the total Calories raised the blood level of the young adults serving as subjects above that of the butterfat alone. This was not observed when cholesterol was fed with coconut oil. The fats that tend to elevate the cholesterol level in the blood are the ones in which cholesterol is most soluble (36). Conclusive evidence of the cholesteremic effect of dietary cholesterol as related to the accompanying dietary fat needs further research.

The total fat content of the diet has not as marked an effect on the serum cholesterol level as do diets which are unchanged in amount of fat but increased in polyunsaturated fatty acid content. Fats high in polyunsaturated fatty acids produce and maintain lower cholesterol levels in the majority of human beings and experimental animals than do diets high in saturated fatty acid content (15).

The mechanisms by which polyunsaturated fatty acids lower plasma cholesterol are being explored. An increased excretion of bile acids and sterols in the feces occurs in individuals on diets high in polyunsaturated fatty acids (15). Because bile acids are the principal end products of cholesterol metabolism, this would seem to indicate one manner in which the fats high in polyunsaturated fatty acids might exert a lowering influence on the plasma cholesterol level.

Dietary nutrients other than fat are found to influence cholesterol blood levels. Low protein intakes have been found to be hypercholesteremic (6, 25); increased niacin intake is effective in reducing blood cholesterol (27, 14).

Factors other than nutrients of the diet influence the cholesterol level of the blood. Important among them is exercise. Some believe exercise to be more important than amount and kind of fat in the diet in the control of cholesterol. In Switzerland a study of active farm families on a higher intake of fat than less active city families revealed similar levels of plasma cholesterol in the two groups (16).

New research suggests that feeding patterns may influence the level of blood cholesterol in the animal organism. The response of blood cholesterol concentration in human subjects to the daily intake of the same diet in 3 feedings (3-meal pattern), 10 feedings (nibbling), and 1 feeding (gorging) has been studied (17). The dietary shift from 3 meals to nibbling produced a decrease in total blood cholesterol values whereas an increase was noted when the pattern of the diet was shifted from nibbling to gorging. In another study (10), made to compare the effect of 6 feedings versus 3 feedings per day of isocaloric diets, healthy young adults had significantly lower cholesterol values during the 6-meal-a-day pattern than during the pattern of 3 meals a day. Cohn (10) has written that "if the preliminary data are substantiated by additional experiments, a new factor in the pathogenesis of human atherosclerosis might be man's eating habits."

Although no direct relationship between diet or serum lipid concentration and the cause of atherosclerosis has been proven yet, the regulation of dietary fat is now a suggested medical procedure in the treatment of certain diseases. The Council of Foods and Nutrition of the American Medical Association (31) has recommended to the medical profession that the diet's total fat content in gall bladder disease, certain types of malabsorption, and hypertriglyceridemia be restricted, as well as an increase of dietary polyunsaturated fats in hypercholesteremia.

REFERENCES

1. Aaes-Jorgensen, E., J. P. Funch, P. F. Engel, and H. Dam (1956). The role of fats in the diet of rats. 9. Influence on growth and histological findings of diets with hydrogenated arachis oil or no fat, supplemented with linoleic acid or raw skim milk, and of crude casein compared with vitamin test casein. *Brit. J. Nutr.* **10:** 292.
2. *Agriculture Statistics 1962* (1963). U.S. Dept. Agr., Washington, D.C., p. 584.
3. Albrink, M. J. (1963). The significance of serum triglycerides. *J. Am. Dietet. Assoc.* **42:** 29.
4. Anderson, A. K. (1953). *Essentials of Physiological Chemistry*, 4th ed. John Wiley and Sons, New York, p. 112.
5. Barr, D. P. (1953). Some chemical factors in pathogenesis of atherosclerosis. *Circulation* **8:** 641.
6. Beveridge, J. M. R., W. F. Connell, and C. Robinson (1963). Effect of the level of dietary protein with and without added cholesterol on plasma cholesterol levels in man. *J. Nutr.* **79:** 289.
7. Burr, G. O., and M. M. Burr (1930). On the nature and role of the fatty acids essential in nutrition. *J. Biol. Chem.* **86:** 587.
8. Chang, I. C. L., and B. M. Watts (1952). The fatty acid content of meat and poultry before and after cooking. *J. Am. Oil Chemists' Soc.* **29:** 334.
9. Chang, I. C. L., and L. I. Y. Tchen, and B. M. Watts (1952). The fatty acid content of selected foods before and after cooking. *J. Am. Oil Chemists' Soc.* **29:** 378.
10. Cohn, C. (1964). Feeding patterns and some aspects of cholesterol metabolism. *Federation Proc.* **23:** 76.
11. *Consumption of Food in the United States. Supplement for 1962* (1963). U.S. Dept. Agr., Agr. Handbook 62, Washington, D.C.
12. Coons, C. M. (1959). Fats and fatty acids. In *Food. The Yearbook of Agriculture 1959.* (A. Stefferud, ed.) U.S. Dept. Agr., Washington, D.C., p. 78.

13. Deuel, Jr., H. J. (1955). Newer concepts of the role of fats and the essential fatty acids in the diet. *Food Res.* **20:** 81.
14. Goldsmith, G. A. (1962). Mechanisms by which certain pharmacologic agents lower serum cholesterol. *Federation Proc.* **21:** 81.
15. Goldsmith, G. A. (1962). Highlights on the cholesterol-fats, diets, and atherosclerosis problem. *J. Am. Med. Assoc.* **176:** 783.
16. Gsell, D., and J. Mayer (1962). Low blood cholesterol associated with high calorie, high saturated fat intakes in a Swiss Alpine village population. *Am. J. Clin. Nutr.* **10:** 471.
17. Gwinup, G., R. C. Byron, W. H. Roush, F. A. Kruger, and G. J. Hamwi (1963). Effect of nibbling versus gorging on serum lipids in man. *Am. J. Clin. Nutr.* **13:** 209.
18. Hansen, A. E. (1958). The problem of the essential fatty acids in relation to human nutrition. *Am. J. Clin. Nutr.* **6:** 625.
19. Hansen, A. E., H. F. Wiese, A. N. Boelsche, M. E. Haggard, D. J. D. Adams, and H. Davis (1963). Role of linoleic acid in infant nutrition. *Pediatrics* **31:** 171.
20. Hodges, R. E., and W. A. Krehl (1963). *Cholesterol as Related to Atherosclerosis— A Review of the Literature*, July 1961 to July 1962. Cereal Institute Inc., Chicago, p. 8.
21. Holman, R. T. (1961). How essential are fatty acids? *J. Am. Med. Assoc.* **178:** 930.
22. Holt, Jr., L. E. (1957). Dietary fat—its role in nutrition and human requirements. In *Fats in Nutrition*. American Medical Association, Chicago.
23. Kagan, A., T. R. Dawber, W. B. Kannel, and N. Revotakie (1962). The Framingham study: a prospective study of coronary heart disease. *Federation Proc.* **21:** 52.
24. McOsker, D. E., F. H. Mattson, B. Seringen, and A. M. Klegman (1962). The influence of partially hydrogenated dietary fats on serum cholesterol levels. *J. Am. Med. Assoc.* **180:** 380.
25. Nath, N., A. E. Harper, and C. A. Elvehjem (1959). Diet and cholesteremia. III. Effect of dietary proteins with particular reference to the lipids in wheat gluten. *Can. J. Biochem. Physiol.* **37:** 1375.
26. Olson, R. E. (1958). Atherosclerosis—a primary hepatic or vascular disorder. *Perspectives Biol. Med.* **2:** 84.
27. Parsons, Jr., W. B. (1960). The effect of nicotinic acid on serum lipids. *Am. J. Clin. Nutr.* **8:** 471.
28. *Recommended Dietary Allowances Sixth Revised Edition* (1964). Natl. Acad. Sci.—Natl. Res. Council, Publ. 1146, Washington, D.C.
29. Rittenberg, D., and R. Schoenheimer (1937). Further studies on the biological uptake of deuterium into organic substance, with special reference to fat and cholesterol formation. *J. Biol. Chem.* **121:** 235.
30. Stasch, A. R., and L. Kilgore (1963). *Influences of Repeated Use for Cooking on Some Changes in Composition of Frying Fats*. Mississippi State Coll. Agr. Expt. Sta., Bull. 662, State College.
31. The regulation of dietary fat (1962). *J. Am. Med. Assoc.* **181:** 411.
32. *Third World Food Survey* (1963). Food Agr. Organ. U.N., Basic Study No. 11, Rome.
33. van der Steur, J. P. K. (1961). Nutritional aspects of processing and chemical additives on fats and oils. *Federation Proc.* **20:** 217.
34. Wiese, H. F., R. H. Gibbs, and A. E. Hansen (1954). Essential fatty acids and human nutrition. I. Serum level for unsaturated fatty acids in healthy children. *J. Nutr.* **52:** 355.
35. Wiese, H. F., A. E. Hansen, and D. J. D. Adams (1958). Essential fatty acids in infant nutrition. I. Linoleic acid requirements in terms of serum di- , tri- , and tetraenoic acid levels. *J. Nutr.* **66:** 345.
36. Wilkens, J. A., H. de Wit, and B. Bronte-Stewart (1962). A proposed mechanism for the effect of different dietary fats on some aspects of cholesterol metabolism. *Can. J. Biochem. Physiol.* **40:** 1091.

37. Wilkinson, Jr., C. F., E. A. Hand, and M. T. Fliegelman (1948). Essential familial hypercholesterolemia. *Ann. Internal Med.* **29:** 671.

SUPPLEMENTARY REFERENCES

Coons, C. M. (1959). Fats and fatty acids. In *Food. The Yearbook of Agriculture 1959.* (A. Stefferud, ed.) U.S. Dept. Agr., Washington, D.C.

Panel III. Lipids in Health and Disease (1961). Proc. Fifth Intern, Congr. Nutr. (Washington, D.C.). *Federation Proc.* **20:** 115.

Proceedings of the International Conference on Diet, Serum Lipids, and Atherosclerosis (1962). (Rye, N.Y.). *Federation Proc.* **21:** Supplement 11.

Rathmann, D. M. (1957). *Vegetable Oils in Nutrition.* Corn Products Refining Co., New York.

Sebrell, Jr., W. H. (1962). An over-all look at atherosclerosis. *J. Am. Dietet. Assoc.* **40:** 403.

Sinclair, H. M. (1964). Carbohydrates and fats. In *Nutrition a Comprehensive Treatise.* Vol. I. (G. H. Beaton and E. W. McHenry, eds.) Academic Press, New York.

The Role of Dietary Fat in Human Health (1958). Natl. Acad. Sci.—Natl. Res. Council, Publ. 575, Washington, D.C.

Van Itallie, T. B., and S. A. Hashim (1961). Diet and heart disease—facts and unanswered questions. *J. Am. Dietet. Assoc.* **38:** 531.

CHAPTER 6

The proteins and amino acids

The word *protein,* derived from the Greek language, means "to come first." Gerardus Mulder, the famous Dutch chemist (1802–1880), proposed use of the term because he believed that proteins were "unquestionably the most important of all known substances in the organic kingdom."

The early chemists sought to learn something of the nature of vegetable and animal substances by submitting the samples to distillation. Thus the invention of a "steam digestor" by the French physicist Denis Papin (1647–1712) prepared the way for the study of protein; he invented the apparatus to soften bones in order to extract gelatin from them (22). The *jelly* from bones and meat also attracted the attention of scientists; they considered it "the true animal substance." The term *albuminous* was used to designate *animal matter.* Mulder was the first to propose a theory that all albuminous substances contained a common structural unit which he called protein. Later Justus von Liebig, too, supported this theory.

These and many other studies of early scientists led the way for the advances that followed in the nineteenth century and in the current era. Today man is trying to understand the formation of proteins in body tissues, and ultimately to synthesize them.

▶ PROTEINS AND THEIR CLASSIFICATION

Protein is one of the most abundant components in the body. It is exceeded in amount only by one other compound—water. The major portion of the protein is located in muscle tissue; the remainder is widely distributed in blood, other soft tissues, bones, and teeth.

The chemical elements found in each protein are carbon, hydrogen, oxygen, and nitrogen. Sulfur is present in many of the molecules, as is phosphorus, iron, iodine, and cobalt. Of the elements present in protein, nitrogen is the distinguishing one because it does not occur in fat and carbohydrate and is always present in protein.

The number of different proteins found in nature is infinite. They vary from tissue to tissue within the plant or animal and in the corresponding tissues among different species. However, within a species the same proteins are synthesized by all members. Protein specificity is the term applied to this property of proteins of being characteristic of the animal species in which they occur.

Proteins are classified chiefly on the basis of their solubilities and other physical properties. Because of the complexity of the protein molecule, a chemical classification is not used. Proteins may be grouped in three classes (20):

(1) *Simple proteins*—protein substances that yield amino acids after complete hydrolysis. Examples are albumen of egg, zein of corn, keratin of hair, and globin of hemoglobin.

(2) *Compound or conjugated proteins*—compounds of a protein with some other nonprotein molecule or molecules or with a metal. Examples are hemoglobin (protein + heme) of blood, casein (protein + phosphoric acid) of milk, mucin (protein + carbohydrate) of saliva, and lipoprotein (protein + lipid) in blood plasma.

(3) *Derived proteins*—products formed from the partial breakdown of proteins by the action of heat and other physical forces, or by hydrolytic agents. Examples are peptones, polypeptides, and peptides which are mixtures of amino acids with decreasing numbers of amino acids in the chain length.

▶ THE AMINO ACIDS

Proteins are made up of amino acids, often called "building stones" of protein. As the name suggests, an amino acid is a compound which contains an amino group (—NH_2) and carboxyl or acid group (—COOH). The chemical structure of the amino acid glycine is given in Fig. 6.1.

Most food proteins are comprised of 12 to 22 amino acids linked together in one large molecule; however, some proteins may have as many as 280 amino acids in a single molecule. Listed below are 22 of the amino acids that occur commonly in foods and in body proteins, and although there are many more amino acids, they are not of recognized importance in nutrition:

alanine	hydroxyproline	serine
arginine	isoleucine	threonine
aspartic acid	leucine	thyroxine
cystine	lysine	tryptophan
glutamic acid	methionine	tyrosine
glycine	norleucine	valine
histidine	phenylalanine	
hydroxyglutamic acid	proline	

Amino acids are white crystalline substances, each with an individual microscopic structure. They differ in taste; some are sweet (glycine, alanine, and serine), some are tasteless (tryptophan and leucine), others are bitter (arginine).

Proteins are formed from amino acids by the amino group of one acid linking to the carboxyl group of another with the elimination of a molecule of water. This grouping which joins the amino acids together is called the peptide linkage (Fig. 6.1). A dipeptide results when two amino acids are joined by the peptide bond; three amino acids joined by two peptide bonds result in a tripeptide; and a large number of amino acids joined together are polypeptides.

▶ FUNCTIONS OF PROTEIN

An important function of dietary protein is the provision of amino acids for the body to build new tissue and to maintain the tissue already formed. In addition, amino acids are used to form nitrogen-containing substances

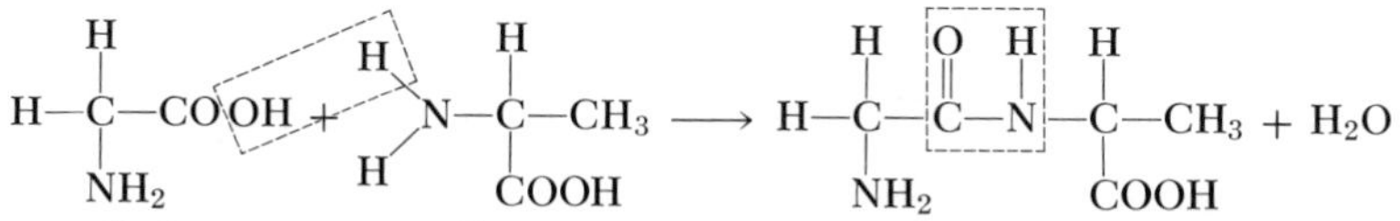

Glycine Alanine Glycyl-alanine (a dipeptide)

Fig. 6.1. Chemical formulas of two amino acids, glycine and alanine, showing the formation of a dipeptide by the peptide linkage.

essential to body function, such as the enzymes, antibodies, and some of the hormones. Protein serves also in certain body regulating capacities and provides energy.

Body-Building and Maintenance Substance

Protein is present in every cell in the body. The nature and behavior of protein in cells of various tissues differ, each contributing certain distinguishing characteristics. The protein in muscle allows for contractibility and the capacity of muscle for holding fluid which gives that tissue a certain firmness even though it is composed of at least 75 per cent water; the protein in epithelial tissue is hard and insoluble, providing a protective covering for the body; in the walls of the blood vessels, the protein contributes elasticity, essential for the maintenance of normal blood pressure; the mineral matter of bones and teeth is embedded in a framework composed of protein. The above functions, and others, demonstrate the significant and specific role of protein as a tissue-building substance.

The need for protein to build new tissue and to maintain and repair the old continues throughout life. The need for new tissue is greatest in the young, but there is also a continuing minimal need for the adult. The hair and the nails continue to grow; the outer layer of skin scales off and is replaced. In pregnancy there is need for the formation of new tissue in the developing fetus and certain tissues of the mother.

Proteins in the body tissues are not stable chemical combinations that remain static once formed. They are in a state of dynamic equilibrium, which means that body proteins are continually being broken down and replaced by new protein synthesized from amino acids from both dietary and tissue sources. Cantarow and Trumper (7) stated that more than one-half of the protein of the liver and intestinal mucosa may be broken down and resynthesized in ten days. This constant exchange of protein explains a daily need of protein for adults as well as children.

Protein Synthesis. Research scientists continue to study how the synthesis of protein in the tissues takes place, a process which has challenged investigators for a long time. So intense is the research pursuit, that information is changing rapidly in this field. The preparation of amino acids in which the carbon or nitrogen is radioactive made possible the initial breakthrough on the phenomena of protein synthesis. Research studies on the metabolism of the cell itself, conducted chiefly in the research laboratories of the United States and England, have extended the knowledge of this important biochemical process.

Amino acids "tagged" with radioactive elements can be followed throughout the body and distinguished from those already present in the body that normally have no radioactivity. From such ingenious studies it has been learned that the amino acids released from the degraded proteins are replaced by new ones from the blood in a continuous interchange between tissue and blood (1, 24). Also for a particular protein to be synthesized, all of the amino acids needed for its formation must be available simultaneously and in the required proportion (10, 13). If even one of the needed amino acids is missing in the diet or the amount provided is insufficient, growth failure occurs in the young. In the adult if the amino acid is not available when needed, body tissue is broken down in an effort to supply it.

The necessity of having available simultaneously all amino acids essential for the synthesis of tissue proteins has practical implications in the planning of diets. If the protein and caloric intake are limited, then better use of protein is realized by providing a source of protein that supplies all of the amino acids needed for tissue formation (complete protein) such as meat, milk, or eggs at each meal of the day. In a study with college women whose diets contained 43 gm of protein (58 gm equals Recommended Daily Dietary Allowance) and 1959 Cal. (2100 Cal. equals Recommended Daily Dietary Allowance) more nitrogen was retained in the body, indicating better use of the dietary protein when all three meals included a source of complete protein than if protein was included in only two meals (21). If the protein and the energy intake were adequate, omission of a source of complete protein at one of the day's meals made less difference.

What is it that determines the alignment of the amino acids so that the right protein is formed each time? A simplified explanation follows, derived from results of metabolism studies of the cell. It is now believed that information necessary for all functions of the living cell, including protein synthesis, resides in the deoxyribonucleic acids (DNA) found in the chromosomes of the cell, which in turn are located in the nucleus. DNA operates through an intermediate set of ribonucleic acids (RNA) known as messenger-RNA (M-RNA). Imprinted or coded on M-RNA are the directions for making one kind of protein. Apparently there are at least as many different kinds of M-RNA's as there are different proteins. Other RNA's, known as transfer RNA's, pick up and move specific amino acids to M-RNA. The M-RNA then lines up the amino acids for the synthesis of a specific protein in a manner as dictated by the code it carries from DNA (8, 9). The code is under intensive study; the pattern it dictates is basic to protein synthesis.

Building Substance for Enzymes, Hormones, and Antibodies

Some of the compounds essential in vital processes in the body are made from amino acids. In this group of nitrogen-containing compounds are the body enzymes, including the digestive enzymes and those that function in processes of oxidation in the tissue cells. Some of the hormones are nitrogen-containing compounds; among them are insulin, thyroxine, adrenalin, the hormone of the parathyroid gland, and certain of the secretions of the pituitary gland.

Man is trying to understand the living cell's secret of enzyme manufacture. In 1963 Hofmann (17) of the University of Pittsburgh achieved the first partial synthesis of a working enzyme. His model was ribonuclease, a much-studied natural enzyme that breaks down the ribonucleic acid found in all cells. Hofmann took natural ribonuclease and split it into two parts, one containing 20 amino acids, the other containing 104. He built a copy of the smaller fragment using 13 amino acids rather than 20. This synthetic segment was joined to the 104 unit natural fragment and the reconstituted enzyme proved to have 70 per cent of the activity of the natural substance.

The hormones are both simple and complex in chemical structure. Thyroxine is a rather simple structure made from two units of the amino acid tyrosine plus the mineral iodine. Sanger (30) won the Nobel prize in 1959 for his explanation of the sequence of amino acids in insulin. He showed that this hormone which is manufactured in the pancreas consists of two parts, one fraction containing 21 amino acid residues and the other 30.

Still another protein compound of particular significance is *gamma globulin*, a normal protein in the blood which has been identified as an antibody. Animals subjected to prolonged protein undernutrition exhibit a pronounced loss of the ability to manufacture antibodies and consequently are less able to resist infection. The antibody-producing capacity is quickly restored when adequate amounts of high-quality proteins are ingested. Cannon (6), who did extensive research on gamma globulin, suggested that the increased susceptibility to infection shown by starving persons is likely to be attributable to protein depletion and the consequent inability to produce new supplies of antibodies.

Body Regulating Substance

Movement of Fluid. Protein is one of the factors that contributes to the control of fluid movement in and out of cells and movement to and from the blood stream. The large size of the protein molecule prevents its passage through membranes, whereas water and materials in solution pass readily. Fluids move from a medium of lesser concentration to one of greater concentration. The process (osmosis) is one of the means the body has of maintaining normal composition of the blood and other body fluids.

Maintenance of Normal Reaction in the Tissues. There are several mechanisms for maintaining a normal balance between acidic and basic substances in the body. Blood proteins help to maintain the normal, slightly alkaline reaction of the blood by the buffering action of protein in the blood plasma and the action of hemoglobin in the red cells (1). Hemoglobin, a conjugated protein, carries CO_2 to the lungs to be eliminated as a gas. If CO_2 was not eliminated it would dissolve in water and form carbonic acid. Thus hemoglobin and the lungs work together in the regulation of the acid-base balance of the blood and extracellular fluid.

Source of Energy

One gram of protein supplies approximately 4 Cal. In the average American diet 10 to 15 per cent of the energy value of the diet comes from protein sources. The extent protein is used for energy depends on the amount of carbohydrate and fat in the diet as well as the total intake of protein. Even though protein is primarily considered a body-building and body-regulating substance, the function of providing energy takes precedence when the carbohydrate and fat in the diet furnish insufficient Calories. There are several pathways that this fraction may take; it may be oxidized directly; it may be converted to either carbohydrate or fat; or it may be changed back to certain amino acids (the nonessential amino acids) by adding an available amino group, a process by which amino acids can be synthesized in the body. As for the nitrogen removed from the protein, most of it is eliminated as waste by way of the kidney. (Protein metabolism is discussed further in Chapter 7.)

▶ THE NUTRITIONAL VALUE OF PROTEINS

Proteins differ in their nutritive value due to the difference in their amino acid content. This was demonstrated in the classic studies of T. B. Osborne and Lafayette B. Mendel at Yale University in which single proteins were fed to young albino rats as the only source of the nutrient. Certain of the proteins could not support growth of the young animals (gliadin of wheat and rye) and others not only did not support growth, but failed even to maintain weight (zein of corn). When the amino acid lysine was added to the ration containing gliadin growth in the animals resumed; addition of the amino acid tryptophan to the ration containing zein permitted maintenance of body weight; and when both tryptophan and lysine were added to the zein ration growth became satisfactory.

As a result of such studies as those of Osborne and Mendel and others, the following classification of proteins based on nutritive quality was proposed.

Incomplete proteins neither maintain life nor support growth. Most vegetable proteins are incomplete; the glycinin of soybeans is an exception. The zein of corn and the animal protein gelatin are incomplete.

Complete proteins maintain life and provide for normal growth of the young when used as the only protein in the diet of experimental animals. As a general rule, the proteins of animal source are complete including those of meat, fish, fowl, eggs, and milk; gelatin is an exception. Some proteins in legumes, grains, and nuts are complete such as glycinin of soybeans, glutenin of wheat, glutelin of corn, and excelsin in Brazil nuts.

Partially complete or incomplete proteins maintain life but fail to support normal growth. Examples include gliadin of wheat, hordein of barley, and prolamin of rye.

The above classification is not absolute. When limited quantities of complete protein are fed, the response is like the feeding of partially incomplete protein, with failure of the young to grow. Cereals as a source of complete protein illustrate this point. Wheat, for example, contains a complete protein and also one that is incomplete. Although each of the grains is a source of complete protein, the amount is relatively small and makes it impossible to consume enough of the grain alone to provide an adequate intake of protein of good quality.

Essential Amino Acids

By 1938 a new type of study became possible for assessing the nutritive value of proteins. Instead of feeding proteins as in the Osborne and Mendel studies (1911–1924), a mixture of chemically pure amino acids was used. This kind of study could not have been conducted, of course, until the amino acids found in proteins had been isolated. As many as nine new ones were identified during the intervening years between 1924 and 1938. William Rose of the University of Illinois pioneered in these early classic studies using young albino rats as the experimental animal. In order to assess the nutritional value of each amino acid, one by one they were omitted from the mixture and the effect on growth was observed. When certain amino acids were removed, growth was impaired; the omission of others had no effect. There were ten amino acids found to be needed in the food intake; the body was unable to synthesize them at a rate sufficiently rapid to provide for the needs of growth. They are called "essential" or "indispensable" amino acids. The ten amino acids essential for growth of young rats are listed in Table 6.1. Those amino

Table 6.1. Amino Acids Essential for Growth in the Young Rat, Growth in Children, and for Maintenance in Adult Men

Amino Acids	Essential for Growth in Young Rats	Essential for Growth in Children	Essential for Maintenance in Young Men
Arginine	x		
Histidine	x	x	
Isoleucine	x	x	x
Leucine	x	x	x
Lysine	x	x	x
Methionine	x	x	x
Phenylalanine	x	x	x
Threonine	x	x	x
Tryptophan	x	x	x
Valine	x	x	x

acids not needed in the diet are the ones the body is able to synthesize at the rate needed. They are designated as "nonessential" or "dispensable."

After identifying the amino acids essential for growth in young rats, the next questions naturally concerned the need for specific amino acids in the human being. Again Rose pioneered, this time using graduate students as his subjects. The experimental diet bore little resemblance to our customary meals but was still adequate in nutrient content. A mixture of pure amino acids supplied the protein content of the diet; the remainder of the food was free of all protein. The complete diet consisted of the amino acids, cornstarch, sucrose, corn oil, inorganic salts, and vitamin concentrates. One by one the amino acids were removed from the mixture as in the earlier studies, and the effect on the *nitrogen balance* was observed. If the removal of an amino acid from the mixture resulted in a greater excretion than intake of nitrogen, it was an indication that the amino acid was *essential* for the adult, and the body could not synthesize it at the rate needed. If the balance was unchanged by the removal of an amino acid, that particular amino acid was considered *nonessential*. Eight amino acids were found to be essential for maintenance in young men, as indicated in Table 6.1.

Nine amino acids were considered essential for the human during periods of growth. These are histidine, isoleucine, leucine, lysine, methionine, phenylalanine, threonine, tryptophan, and valine. There has been a question concerning the need of arginine. In a recent study with infants (18) Holt found arginine not to be essential for normal growth.

Nonessential Amino Acids

The term nonessential as applied to amino acids should not mislead us as to the importance of these amino acids in the body. It simply means that they do not have to be provided "ready-made" in the diet; the body can supply them as it needs them. To demonstrate that they are important, it may be pointed out that they comprise 40 per cent or more of the tissue protein. When they are supplied in the food intake, as they always are in an ordinary diet, less of the essential acids are needed. The nonessential amino acids can supply nitrogen for the synthesis of some body compounds for which essential amino acids would otherwise be used.

Experiments have shown that diets containing only the essential amino acids support a slow rate of growth. Currently there is interest in the ratio of essential to nonessential amino acids which promotes a normal rate of growth. Stucki and Harper (31) reported the growth of rats that were fed diets having essential-nonessential amino acid ratios between 4.0 and 1.0 was generally satisfactory.

Digestibility of Proteins

Fundamental to the nutritive value of a protein, in addition to the amino acid composition, is its digestibility. Proteins from the animal group of foods are the most available for absorption, those from dried legumes least available because of less complete digestion (Table 6.2).

The digestibility of a given protein is influenced not only by the fiber content of the food containing the protein but also by the amount of

Table 6.2. Average Digestibility of Proteins from Different Food Groups

Food Group	Coefficients of Availability, per cent[1]
Animal foods	97
Cereals	85
Fruits	85
Vegetables	83
Legumes, dried	78

[1] Approximations for an average mixed diet.

From W. O. Atwater, and A. P. Bryant, *Twelfth Ann. Rept. Storrs Agr. Expt. Sta.*, University of Conn., p. 73, 1899.

fiber in the remainder of the diet (15). There are several reasons for the interfering effect of fiber on digestion. Motility of the gastrointestinal tract is increased by the presence of fiber; the more rapid the movement of the intestinal content along the tract, the shorter the time allowed for digestive enzymes to act. Also it is presumed that cellulose may further detract from the completeness of digestion by preventing the protein from coming in contact with the digestive enzymes.

▶ THE REQUIREMENT OF PROTEIN AND AMINO ACIDS

Method of Study

The method commonly used in determining protein requirement is the nitrogen balance study. In determining the nitrogen balance, the nitrogen content of the food eaten and of the urinary and fecal excretion are determined quantitatively. One of the steps in the procedure for nitrogen analysis is shown in Fig. 6.2. The nitrogen values can be converted to protein by multiplying by the factor 6.25 because, on the average, food proteins are 16 per cent nitrogen. The findings are interpreted in this manner. If the intake of nitrogen exceeds the outgo, the retention of nitrogen in the body is designated as a *positive* balance. If the outgo is greater than the intake, the loss of nitrogen is termed a *negative* balance. When the intake and outgo are approximately the same, the individual is said to be in nitrogen *equilibrium.* The lowest nitrogen intake that will permit a state of nitrogen equilibrium is considered the *minimum* nitrogen (protein) need. Nitrogen equilibrium can be obtained at any level of protein intake above minimum. Therefore, the nitrogen balance method is useful in determining the minimum protein requirement but does not answer the question as to what is optimal.

Factors Influencing Minimum Protein Need

Among the factors influencing the nitrogen balance are (1) the physiological state of the individual, (2) adequacy of energy intake from carbohydrates and fats, and (3) the capacity to adjust to level of intake. The amount of protein required in the diet to maintain equilibrium varies with the state of the nitrogen stores or reserves. As the limited amounts that can be stored are progressively depleted, dietary nitrogen is utilized more efficiently. When consuming a diet comparable in nitrogen content, a malnourished person retains more than one who is well nourished (26). Certain physiological conditions increase the need for protein. During pregnancy and childhood there is need for nitrogen

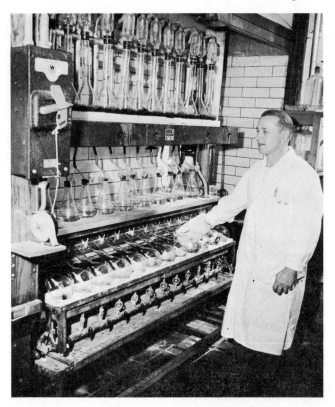

Fig. 6.2.   Analyzing food for nitrogen. (Courtesy of Swift, Department of Animal Nutrition, The Pennsylvania State University.)

for building new tissue; as a consequence, at those periods the balances are normally positive.

There are differences of opinion about the presence of protein stores (reserves) or a labile supply in the body (2, 19). It is agreed that there are no special cells to store protein as fat is stored or special substances like glycogen, the storage form of carbohydrates. However, there are blood and tissue proteins that increase or decrease in quantity as the dietary nitrogen is raised or lowered, respectively. Labile proteins are said to be present in internal organs and glands such as liver, pancreas, intestinal wall, and plasma albumin. Studies of hepatic enzymes have shown that the activity of a number of enzymes is reduced when protein privation occurs. Holt and associates (19) believe that the term protein reserve is incorrect because it indicates a reservoir of protein that can be filled up to be emptied again in case of need.

The adequacy of the energy intake makes a difference in the amount of protein required. Although the interdependence of energy intake and protein requirement is not clearly defined, it is recognized that insufficient energy in the diet can limit the utilization of protein. Sparing protein the necessity of being used exclusively for energy is called the *sparing effect* of carbohydrate and fat. There have been many investigations of the comparative effectiveness of carbohydrate and fat in their sparing action (25, 32). From experimental studies with animals on a restricted caloric intake, it now appears that on a caloric basis carbohydrate and fat are used equally well if some of each is present in the diet.

In an adult, the body with its profound capacity for adaptability tends to maintain nitrogen equilibrium even though the intake may vary widely. When the intake is lowered, the excretion also decreases, chiefly in the urine. The converse takes place when the intake is increased; the excretion likewise increases. Table 6.3 shows the adaptation made by an individual whose diet was changed from one providing an unrestricted intake amounting to approximately 75 gm of protein daily to one almost protein free. On an unrestricted protein intake the nitrogen excretion in the urine was approximately 12 gm; after four days on an almost protein-free diet the excretion was reduced to 1.41 gm of nitrogen.

Increased Need for Protein Under Conditions of Stress

After surgery or injury, during a wasting illness, or while recovering from extensive burns, excessive loss of nitrogen from the body occurs. It is generally felt that these losses should be replaced through a liberal intake of protein.

Table 6.3. The Effect of Extremely Low Protein Intake on Nitrogen Excretion

Days on Diet	Average Daily Nitrogen Intake, gm	Average Daily Excretion, gm	
		Urine	Feces
7	Unrestricted diet	12.03	1.03
6	0.27	4.85	0.85
7	0.77	3.55	0.73
8	0.94	2.21	0.83
4	0.32	1.41	0.89
2	Unrestricted diet	9.21	—

Adapted from Smith, *J. Biol. Chem.* **68:** 15, 1926.

Table 6.4. Influence of Work on Nitrogen Excretion

| Activity | Period, Days | Food/Day | | Nitrogen Excreted, Daily Average, gm |
		Nitrogen, gm	Energy, Cal.	
Bed rest	6	5.9	2300	4.77
Light exercise	5	6.0	3000	4.40
Heavy exercise	4	5.9	3200	3.94

Adapted from Shaffer, *Am. J. Physiol.* **22**: 445, 1908.

Influence of Exercise on Protein Need

It is unexpected perhaps that exercise does not increase the protein need. If the caloric intake is sufficient to cover the increased energy requirement during exercise, little, if any, additional protein is needed. The finding is logical because during exercise glycogen, not protein, is the ultimate constituent used up in muscle contraction. The data in Table 6.4 are taken from an early experiment in which a subject was maintained on the same nitrogen intake with adjustments in energy intake to take care of different degrees of exercise. No increase in the excretion of nitrogen resulted with exercise, reflecting no additional need for protein.

Recommended Allowance for Protein

For young men and women 18 to 35 years of age, the Recommended Daily Dietary Allowance is one gm per kg of body weight. Approximately 10 to 12 per cent of the total Calories are from protein in diets that are adequate in this nutrient. The needs for infancy, childhood, and during pregnancy and lactation are discussed in those respective chapters.

Findings from nitrogen balance studies are the basis for the recommended daily intake. However, when the quantitative findings on which the original recommendations were made are examined, it is found that an average intake of approximately 0.6 gm per kg of body weight was the minimal amount sufficient for maintenance of nitrogen equilibrium in normal adults. Henry Sherman, who summarized the earlier work, proposed that an allowance for safety be added and recommended that the daily intake be increased to one gm per kg for normal adults.

There is a growing feeling among nutritionists, who now have the advantage of more recent studies, that the protein need may be less than was previously supposed. In a study with college women at the University of Illinois (5), nitrogen equilibrium was maintained at an intake of 0.55 gm per kg even though the protein in the diet was predominantly from cereal sources. Also in a study done by Hegsted and his coworkers at the Harvard School of Public Health, nitrogen equilibrium in healthy adults was possible on intakes of 0.43 gm to 0.57 gm per kg with cereals, vegetables, and fruits providing the protein (16). Replacing one-third of the protein in the diet with protein of animal sources made it possible to maintain equilibrium at an intake of only 0.39 gm per kg.

The FAO Reference Protein

In 1957 an FAO committee reported its recommendation on protein requirements (27). Because of the large differences in the nutritive value of individual proteins or combinations of proteins, the committee thought that any expression of protein requirements must be related to proteins of a specific kind. Therefore, a hypothetical protein called a "reference protein" was used for the committee's standard. This reference protein is similar to the proteins contained in milk, eggs, and meat. The "provisional pattern" of amino acids set up for the reference protein is compared with those in three animal proteins in Table 6.5. The FAO committee suggests 0.35 gm per kg of body weight as the average minimum requirement of adults for the reference protein. It was suggested that the provisional pattern of amino acids be used in appraising the protein (amino acids) value of diets and for indicating appropriate methods of supplementing diets deficient in protein (amino acids).

Table 6.5. Essential Amino Acids in Provisional Pattern and Milk and Egg Proteins

Amino Acids	Amino Acids per 100 gm Protein			
	Provisional Pattern	Cow's Milk	Human Milk	Egg
Isoleucine	4.2	6.4	6.4	6.8
Leucine	4.8	9.9	8.9	9.0
Lysine	4.2	7.8	6.3	6.3
Phenylalanine	2.8	4.9	4.6	6.0
Tyrosine	2.8	5.1	5.5	4.4
Methionine	2.2	2.4	2.2	3.1
Threonine	2.8	4.6	4.6	5.0
Tryptophan	1.4	1.4	1.6	1.7
Valine	4.2	6.9	6.6	7.4

From *Protein Requirements.* Food Agr. Organ. U.N., FAO Nutr. Studies No. 16, p. 26, 1957.

The Quantitative Need for Amino Acids

After it was established that the adult man needs certain amino acids for the maintenance of nitrogen equilibrium, the next step was to study the amount of each acid needed daily. Sufficient research (28, 29) has been done with both women and men so that quantitative amounts needed daily can be proposed as summarized in Table 6.6.

In considering the practical use of this information, it must be borne in mind that for the most part pure amino acids were used in these studies. Indications are that an equivalent amount of nitrogen is better utilized when the amino acids are provided in food protein than in amino acid mixtures (33). The reasons for the difference are not clear at present. Rose (29), who proposed the *minimum* daily need for the essential amino acids from his research studies, has suggested that the *safe* amount should be twice the minimum values.

An Interpretation of Protein Need

To summarize certain aspects of the daily protein need, a generous allowance for protein is justified in that it provides for individual differences in need and differences in the quality of proteins in the diet. On the other hand, there is evidence that the body adjusts to the intake and that nitrogen equilibrium can be maintained on amounts much lower, as well as much higher, than the Recommended Daily Dietary Allowance. From the practical standpoint, the capacity of the body to maintain equilibrium at a lower intake is reassuring, for in parts of the world the more generous allowance is unattainable.

Table 6.6. Minimum Amounts of Essential Amino Acids Required Daily for Maintenance of Nitrogen Equilibrium in Adults

Essential Amino Acid	Women, gm	Men, gm
Isoleucine	0.45	0.70
Leucine	0.62	1.10
Lysine	0.50	0.80
Methionine	0.29	1.10
Phenylalanine	0.22	1.10
Threonine	0.31	0.50
Tryptophan	0.16	0.25
Valine	0.65	0.80

Adapted from M. S. Reynolds, *J. Am. Dietet. Assoc.* **33:** 1016, 1957.

► PROTEIN DEFICIENCY

Insufficient protein in the diet results in stunted growth in the young. The growth effect is readily demonstrated in experimental animals by feeding a diet deficient in either quantity or quality of protein. Farmers and stock feeders are well aware of the necessity of providing adequate protein for the best growth of their livestock. If the limitation is severe and prolonged, the protein content of the blood may be reduced below normal (hypoproteinemia) (3).

Protein deficiency is widespread in large sections of the world and especially in many developing countries. The Food and Nutrition Board of the National Research Council of the United States manifested its interest in this problem by organizing the Committee on Protein Malnutrition. In 1960 this committee sponsored an international conference to study the problem of meeting protein needs of infants and preschool children (23), and another in 1963 to determine where urgent research was needed (12).

Four syndromes associated with protein deficiency in the human (12) are described by the Food and Nutrition Board: hunger edema, pellagra, kwashiorkor, and nutritional liver disease. Only nutritional liver disease is of consequence today in the United States. This disease is often seen in the alcoholic whose diet is low in essential nutrients, including protein; less frequently it occurs in individuals who are losing or destroying proteins at an abnormal rate or who are failing to synthesize adequate protein. The simplest form of nutritional liver disease is characterized by an enlarged fatty liver, which may be cured by eating an adequate diet.

With the advent of the Second World War and the reappearance of mass semistarvation in civilian populations and in prison camps, hunger edema came into prominence. Protein deficiency is only one of the factors giving rise to the excessive retention of fluid in body cells, the most prominent manifestation of hunger edema.

A severe deficiency disease, *kwashiorkor*, found among the children of Africa and parts of Central and South America, is caused by a shortage in total amount of protein and also a shortage of protein of good quality (34). This disease is most prevalent in populations whose protein supply is chiefly of vegetable origin. If the diet is inadequate in protein, it is most certain to be so in other nutrients; for that reason the condition has been described as a "multiple-deficiency syndrome." Children between the ages of 1 and 4 are most commonly afflicted, although sporadic cases do occur among older children.

The children suffering with kwashiorkor manifest certain characteristic symptoms: they are stunted in growth; the skin shows hyperpigmentation and is frequently ulcerated; the children are apathetic showing marked lassitude, but at the same time are irritable and restless; the digestive system is impaired by continuous diarrhea; the children have poor appetites; anemia is always present; the incidence of dental caries is high; and the muscles are underdeveloped and lacking in tone. Children suffering with kwashiorkor are shown in Fig. 6.3.

Treatment of the disease is essentially dietary. Sources of good-quality protein such as skim milk and other animal proteins have been effective in alleviating the condition. In Central America a discussion of preventive measures for the disease resulted in the following suggestions: that varieties of maize higher in methionine and tryptophan content be developed; that the production of certain protein-producing plants now being consumed, such as beans, be increased; and that the use of soybean milk be promoted to substitute for milk unavailable in those areas.

▶ THE SUPPLEMENTARY VALUE OF PROTEIN

Foods differ in the nutritive value of the protein they contain. Each food, with the exception of gelatin, contains more than one kind of protein, each with a characteristic number and concentration of amino

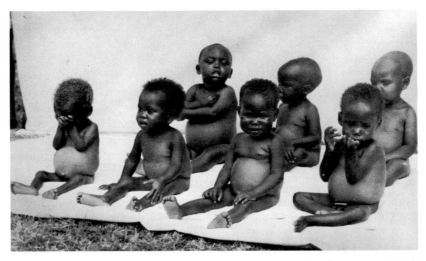

Fig. 6.3. African children with typical symptoms of kwashiorkor. (Courtesy of World Health Organization, Monograph Series 8, Geneva.)

acids. The proteins of some foods contain limited amounts of certain essential amino acids, generous amounts of others. Therefore, a combination of foods in which the amino acids contained in the proteins supplement each other is of higher nutritive quality than either alone. Early studies with experimental animals demonstrated that the proteins of milk are superior in quality to those of cereals. Nevertheless, cereal and milk fed together in the right proportions, with cereals replacing some of the milk, were as effective as milk alone. Cereals are limited in lysine; milk provides it generously.

An examination of the table of amino acid content of foods (Table A–9, appendix) shows possibilities of combining foods so that amino acids may supplement each other. For example, tryptophan is limited in corn and white flour, whereas foods of animal origin provide tryptophan generously. Two-thirds cup of cooked corn meal (25 gm dry) contains 0.056 gm of tryptophan, whereas a serving of pork, chicken, or beef provides approximately four times that amount. Legumes (beans and peas) are deficient in tryptophan and methionine and need to be supplemented by animal protein.

As more complete analyses are available, further possibilities of supplementation will be realized. Final conclusions on the supplementary value of certain proteins cannot be drawn, however, until it is known how well the human being is able to use the amino acids in different foods. The use of protein combinations to improve the nutritional quality of the diet holds greatest significance for persons living in parts of the world where foods of animal origin are scarce, and the diet is chiefly cereal.

▶ FOOD SOURCES AND SUPPLY OF PROTEINS AND
   AMINO ACIDS

Although protein is widely distributed in nature, few foods provide highly concentrated amounts (Table 6.7). Cheese, eggs, fish, meats, nuts, and poultry are the primary sources in the United States with a range of 12 to 29 per cent. Cereal grains rank second as protein contributors to the diet. Fruits and vegetables are low-protein foods. Those containing no protein are the sugars and sirups and the pure fats and oils.

Animal foods have protein high in nutritive quality and in amounts that make them first in order of importance, but this knowledge should not minimize our appreciation of the role of plants in providing protein. Soybeans and some nuts, such as Brazil and almonds, contain protein of good quality, and most cereals provide a limited amount. In addition,

Table 6.7. Protein Values of Some Typical Foods

Food	Measure	Protein, gm
Chicken, breast	2.7 oz	25.0
Tuna fish	3 oz	24.0
Beef, round	3 oz	24.0
Lamb, leg	3 oz	22.0
Pork loin	3 oz	20.0
Milk, whole	1 c	9.0
Beans, red kidney	½ c	7.5
Cheese, process	1 oz	7.0
Egg	1 med	6.0
Lima beans, immature	½ c	6.0
Bacon	2 sl	5.0
Peanut butter	1 tbsp	4.0
Ice cream	⅛ qt	3.0
Potato	1 med	3.0
Oatmeal	½ c	2.5
Broccoli	½ c	2.5
Bread, whole wheat	1 sl	2.0
Green beans	½ c	1.0
Lettuce, head	½ c	0.6
Orange juice	4 oz	0.5

From *Nutritive Value of Foods*. U.S. Dept. Agr., Home Garden Bull.
72, revised 1964.

plants are fundamental to the production of animal proteins for human
consumption. Nature has equipped plants with the capacity to take
nitrogen available in the soil for the synthesis of amino acids and
protein. Ruminant animals consume the proteins in plants and are able
to use them as a source of nitrogen for the synthesis of their tissue
proteins.

A Guide to the Selection of Foods to Meet the Protein
Needs of College Men and Women

A practical approach to assuring an adequate provision of protein is
to include certain types of foods in the diet each day. This does not
mean, however, that such a pattern is inflexible but rather that it is a
useful guide. Such a pattern includes a pint or more of milk, an egg, a
serving of meat, and a serving of another protein food (such as beans)
or a second serving of meat. The importance of animal protein foods in
meeting man's amino acid needs is shown in Table 6.8. The combined

contribution of 100 gm of beef round, 1 egg, and 1 pint of milk generously exceeds the minimum requirement for adults.

The menus in Table 6.9 are planned to provide an adequate intake of protein at three levels of cost. It is assumed that for the most part prices are relatively the same everywhere, except, of course, when the season and the supply alter the price. In the low-cost meal, nonfat milk solids, beans, peanut butter, and a cheaper selection of meat provide the protein. Irrespective of cost the protein of meat, fish, and poultry is of good quality. It is fortunate that the supplementary value of proteins makes it possible to combine cereals and legumes with dairy and meat products to provide a diet adequate in protein at comparatively low cost. The high-cost menu includes a more expensive source of meat than the moderate- and low-cost meals, that is, a rib roast as compared to a rump roast or meat loaf.

Proteins and Amino Acids in Diets in the United States

Available food supplies in the United States during the last 50 years have provided generous amounts of protein, averaging between 90 and 100 gm per person per day. There has been a gradual increase in the proportion of dietary protein from animal sources, from about one-half in 1909–1913 to two-thirds in 1961. This change reflects the increase in consumption of dairy products, eggs, and meat with a decrease in consumption of grain products (Table 6.10). The U.S. Department of Agriculture reported for 1962 that the amount of protein available for consumption per capita in the United States was 95 gm per day.

Although protein foods are plentiful in the United States, individuals do not share these supplies equally or in accordance with their nutritional need. This is due to differences in food choices, total food consumed, and income level. Usually more of the diets of younger

Table 6.8. Essential Amino Acid Composition of Certain Food Proteins in Grams

Food	Isoleucine	Leucine	Lysine	Methio-nine	Phenyl-alanine	Threo-nine	Trypto-phan	Valine
100 gm beef round	1.02	1.60	1.70	0.48	0.80	0.86	0.23	1.08
1 egg	0.42	0.56	0.41	0.20	0.37	0.32	0.10	0.48
1 pt milk	1.09	1.68	1.33	0.42	0.83	0.79	0.24	1.17
Total	2.53	3.84	3.44	1.10	2.00	1.97	0.57	2.73
Minimum requirements for men	0.70	1.10	0.80	1.10	1.10	0.50	0.25	0.80

From *Amino Acid Content of Foods*, U.S. Dept. Agr., Home Econ. Res. Rept. 4, 1957.

Table 6.9. Meeting the Daily Protein Need of an Adult at Three Cost Levels

Food	Protein, gm	Food	Protein, gm	Food	Protein, gm
		Low-Cost Menu			
Tomato juice, ½ c	1.0	Bean soup, ⅔ c	7.2	Meat loaf, 3 oz	21.0
Oatmeal, ⅔ c	3.3	Sandwich, peanut		Msh. potatoes, ¾ c	3.0
Bread, enriched or		butter, 2 T, enriched	8.0	Cabbage, ½ c	0.7
w. w., 2 sl	4.0	or w. w.	4.0	Bread, w. w. or	
Nonfat milk, solids,		bread, 2 sl		enriched, 2 sl	4.0
1 c	9.0	Carrot sticks, ½ c	0.6	Vanilla pdg., ½ c	4.3
		Raw apple, 1 med	tr		
		Nonfat milk, solids,			
		1 c	9.0		
Total	17.3		28.8		33.0
		Moderate-Cost Menu			
Orange juice, frozen,		Mushroom soup,		Rump pot rst., 3 oz	23.0
½ c	0.5	canned, ⅔ c	5.4	Msh. potatoes, ½ c	2.0
Egg, 1	6.0	Sandwich, cheese,	7.0	Gr. beans, ½ c	1.0
Bread, enriched or		1 oz, enriched or		Celery sticks, ½ c	0.7
w. w., 2 sl	4.0	w. w. bread, 2 sl	4.0	Pan rolls, 1	3.0
Milk, 1 c	9.0	Lettuce wedge, ⅛ hd	0.5	Apricots, 2	0.5
		Apple betty, ½ c	2.0		
		Milk, 1 c	9.0		
Total	19.5		27.9		30.2
		High-Cost Menu			
Orange juice, fresh,		French onion soup,		Roast rib beef, 3 oz	20.0
½ c	0.5	⅔ c	0.0	Baked potato, 1	3.0
Egg, 1	6.0	Sandwich, ham, 2 oz,	12.0	Asparagus, ⅔ c	2.6
Bacon, 2 sl	5.0	w. w. bread, 2 sl	4.0	Chef's salad, ⅔ c	1.0
Blueberry muffins,		Relish plate		Cloverleaf roll, 1	3.0
1 ea	4.0	olives, pickles,		Fresh pineapple, ⅔ c	0.6
Milk, 1 c	9.0	celery, carrots	0.2		
		Apple betty, ½ c	2.0		
		Milk, 1 c	9.0		
Total	24.5		27.2		30.2

From *Nutritive Value of Foods*. U.S. Dept. Agr., Home Garden Bull. 72, revised 1964.

children meet the recommended intake than do those of older children, and in general boys' diets are better than girls. The adolescent girl, the homemaker, and the elderly person tend to consume the least adequate amount of protein.

Some consideration is being given to adding the essential amino acids that are supplied in limited amounts in commonly used foods, such as cereals, in an effort to improve their nutritional quality as a source of protein; however, the idea is viewed with skepticism by some nutritionists (11). The average American diet appears at present to provide the essential amino acids adequately without fortification of foods. The estimated essential amino acid content of the average diet exceeds even the *safe* level, which is twice the minimum need for maintenance in the adult (Table 6.11). It should be noted that the average diet in the year 1959 was high in protein content, made possible by the general high level of purchasing power among the people and an abundance of food available.

Another reason, and one more fundamental for delaying the adoption of amino acid fortification of foods, is that the addition might bring about an imbalance in the relative proportion of amino acids a complex dietary problem not yet completely clarified (14). It is known from studies with experimental animals that the addition of one amino acid may alter the need for others, and instead of achieving the desired effect of improved well-being, the animal may be less well-off than without the addition. On the other hand, fortification of foods with amino acids may be found, with further study, to be a desirable way of providing more protein of good quality. If the process should prove to

Table 6.10. Sources of Protein in U.S. Food Supply (Selected Years)[1]

Foods	Percentage of Protein from Specified Sources					
	1909–13	1925–29	1935–39	1947–49	1957	1962[2]
Dairy products	17.7	20.0	22.2	24.8	25.4	23.6
Eggs	5.2	6.1	5.7	7.0	6.6	6.1
Meat, poultry, fish, fats, oils	29.0	28.4	28.2	31.5	35.0	37.0
Grain products	35.7	31.6	28.6	23.0	19.5	19.6
Legumes, nuts	4.5	5.1	6.1	5.3	5.5	5.8
Other vegetable sources	7.9	8.8	9.2	8.4	8.0	7.9
Total	100.0	100.0	100.0	100.0	100.0	100.0
Total animal sources	51.9	54.5	56.1	63.3	67.0	66.7
Total vegetable sources	48.1	45.5	43.9	36.7	33.0	33.3
Protein per person per day, gm	102	95	91	95	96	95

Sources:
[1] *Evaluation of Protein Nutrition.* Natl. Acad. Sci.—Natl. Res. Council Publ. 811, 35, 1959.
[2] *1963 Outlook Issue—Natl. Food Situation.* U.S. Dept. Agr., pp. 22–23, Oct., 1962.

Table 6.11. Essential Amino Acid Content of the "Average" American Diet Compared with "Safe" Levels for Men

Essential Amino Acid	"Average" American Diet, gm/day	"Safe" Levels for Men, gm/day
Isoleucine	4.2	1.40
Leucine	6.5	2.20
Lysine	4.0	1.60
Methionine	3.0	2.20
Phenylalanine	4.1	2.20
Threonine	2.8	1.00
Tryptophan	0.9	0.50
Valine	4.2	1.60

From M. S. Reynolds, *J. Am. Dietet. Assoc.* **33:** 1017, 1957.

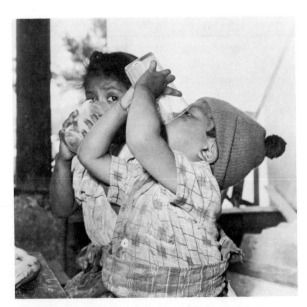

Fig. 6.4. Preschool children of a rural village in Guatemala drinking "Incaparina." (Courtesy of Instituto de Nutrición de Centro América y Panamá.)

be practical, the people of many parts of the world, where a lack of adequate protein is a serious dietary problem, would benefit.

Proteins and Amino Acids Worldwide

In large sections of the world and in many developing countries protein deficiency is widespread. Two-thirds of the world's population subsists almost entirely on vegetable diets such as rice, corn, wheat, and cassava. In these countries the lack of animal proteins makes it necessary to develop agricultural products that will provide a mixture of plant proteins with a high nutritive value for animals and man. Much interest has been displayed in the development of an all-vegetable mixture high in protein (4) by investigators at the Institute for Nutrition of Central America and Panama (INCAP). One of these, *Incaparina*, is being produced commercially at low cost and requires little or no readjustments in the eating habits of the native families. This formula contains 29 per cent whole ground corn, 29 per cent whole ground sorghum, 38 per cent cottonseed flour, 3 per cent Torula yeast, 1 per cent calcium carbonate, and 4500 IU of vitamin A per 100 gm. The product is sold for 3 cents for a 75 gm bag sufficient for 3 glasses (when reconstituted with water), with a protein content comparable to that of a similar amount of milk (Fig. 6.4).

REFERENCES

1. Allison, J. B. (1955). Biological evaluation of proteins. *Physiol. Rev.* 35: 664.
2. Allison, J. B., and W. H. Fitzpatrick (1960). *Dietary Proteins in Health and Disease.* Charles C. Thomas, Springfield, Ill., pp. 10–13.
3. Berg, C. P. (1948). Protein deficiency and its relationship to nutritional anemia, hypoproteinemia, nutritional edema, and resistance to infection. In *Proteins and Amino Acids in Nutrition* (M. Sahyun, ed.), Reinhold Publishing Corp., New York, p. 290.
4. Bressani, L. B. Elias, A. Aguire, and N. S. Scrimshaw (1961). All-vegetable protein mixture for human feeding III. The development of INCAP vegetable mixture nine. *J. Nutr.* 74: 201.
5. Bricker, M. L., R. F. Shively, J. M. Smith, H. H. Mitchell, and T. S. Hamilton (1949). The protein requirements of college women on high cereal diets with observations on the adequacy of short balance periods. *J. Nutr.* 37: 163.
6. Cannon, P. R. (1950). *Recent Advances in Nutrition with Particular Reference to Protein Metabolism.* University of Kansas Press, Lawrence, p. 27.
7. Cantarow, A., and M. Trumper (1962). *Clinical Biochemistry,* 6th ed. W. B. Saunders Co., Philadelphia, p. 123.
8. Conn, E. E., and P. K. Stumpf (1963). *Outlines of Biochemistry.* John Wiley and Sons, New York, p. 269.
9. Curtis, H. J. (1963). Biological mechanisms underlying the aging process. *Science* 141: 686.

10. Dalgliesh, C. E. (1957). Time factors in protein biosynthesis. *Science* 125: 271.
11. Deshpande, P. D., A. E. Harper, and C. A. Elvehjem (1957). Nutritional improvement of white flour with protein and amino acid supplements. *J. Nutr.* 62: 503.
12. *Evaluation of Protein Quality* (1963). Natl. Acad. Sci.—Natl. Res. Council Publ. 400, Washington, D.C.
13. Geiger, E. (1950). The role of the time factor in protein synthesis. *Science* 111: 594.
14. Harper, A. E. (1958). Balance and imbalance of amino acids. *Ann. N.Y. Acad. Sci.* 69: 1025.
15. Hegsted, D. M., M. F. Trulson, and F. J. Stare (1954). Role of wheat and wheat products in human nutrition. *Physiol. Rev.* 34: 221.
16. Hegsted, D. M., A. G. Tsongas, D. B. Abbott, and F. J. Stare (1946). Protein requirements of adults. *J. Lab. Clin. Med.* 31: 261.
17. Hofmann, Klaus, et al. (1963). Studies on polypeptides. XXVI. Partial synthesis of an enzyme possessing high Rnase activity. *J. Am. Chem. Soc.* 85: 833.
18. Holt, L. E., and S. E. Synderman (1961). The amino acid requirements of infants. *J. Am. Med. Assoc.* 175: 100.
19. Holt, L. E., E. Halac, and C. N. Kajdi (1962). The concept of protein stores and its implications in diet. *J. Am. Med. Assoc.* 181: 699.
20. Kleiner, I. S., and J. M. Orten (1962). *Biochemistry,* 6th ed. C. V. Mosby Co., St. Louis, pp. 108–110.
21. Leverton, R. M., and M. R. Gram (1949). Nitrogen excretion of women related to the distribution of animal proteins in daily meals. *J. Nutr.* 39: 57.
22. McCollum, E. V. (1957). *A History of Nutrition.* Houghton Mifflin Co., Boston.
23. *Meeting Protein Needs of Infants and Children* (1961). Natl. Acad. Sci.—Natl. Res. Council Publ. 843, Washington, D.C.
24. Mitchell, H. H. (1955). The validity of Folin's concept of dichotomy in protein metabolism. *J. Nutr.* 55: 193.
25. Munro, H. N. (1951). Carbohydrate and fat as factors in protein utilization and metabolism. *Physiol. Rev.* 31: 449.
26. Pollack, H., and S. L. Helpern (1952). *Therapeutic Nutrition.* Natl. Acad. Sci.—Natl. Res. Council, Washington, D.C., p. 22.
27. *Protein Requirements* (1957). Food Agr. Organ. U.N., FAO Nutr. Studies No. 16, Rome.
28. Reynolds, M. S. (1958). The amino acid requirements of adults. *Am. J. Clin. Nutr.* 6: 439.
29. Rose, W. C., C. H. Eades, Jr., and M. J. Coon (1955). The amino acid requirements of man. XII. The leucine isoleucine requirements. *J. Biol. Chem.* 216: 225.
30. Sanger, F. (1959). The chemistry of insulin. *Science* 129: 1343.
31. Stucki, W. P., and A. E. Harper (1962). Effect of altering the ratio of indispensable to dispensable amino acids in diets for rats. *J. Nutr.* 62: 278.
32. Swanson, P. P. (1951). Influence of non-protein calories on protein metabolism. *Federation Proc.* 10: 660.
33. Vivian, V. M. (1964). Relationship between tryptophan-niacin metabolism and changes in nitrogen balance. *J. Nutr.* 82: 395.
34. Williams, R. R. (1956). Kwashiorkor and the future. *Williams-Waterman Fund, A History of the Period 1935 through 1955.* Research Corp., New York, p. 78.

CHAPTER 7

Digestion, absorption, and metabolism

When a hamburger or milk shake is eaten, nutrients that will ultimately be used to nourish the cells of the body are being ingested. Yet, before the nutrients contained in these foods finally reach the cells, the foods themselves must be digested and the nutrients absorbed. The *digestion* of the food involves the subdivision of the complex molecules into simple, soluble materials (the nutrients) which can pass through the lining of the digestive tract into the blood and lymph streams. After absorption the nutrients enter into the chemical processes of the body known as metabolism.

▶ DIGESTION

The Beginning of the Study of Digestion

As indicated in earlier chapters, the mystery of what happens to food in the body led philosophers of the prescientific era and the scientists who followed them to the study of respiration. The study of digestion also began in quest of an answer to that mystery. The first notable contribution was made by René de Reaumur (1683–1757), a French scientist who studied changes of the food in the stomach (8). He performed his experiments on his pet buzzard, a bird that swallowed its food in large pieces and later regurgitated indigestible portions. Reaumur took advantage of this unique opportunity and trained his pet to swallow sponges. When the sponges were brought up, they were soaked with gastric juice. He found that the juice squeezed from the sponge would liquefy meat.

The next important investigations were made by Lazzaro Spallanzani (1729–1799), who studied the action of saliva on foodstuffs and verified Reaumur's observations on gastric digestion. He performed a number of daring experiments on himself. He was impelled to use himself as a subject because of his conviction that because certain observations on digestion in animals had been made he should try to do the same with man. He wrote of his plans:

> I intended to make these experiments on myself but I admit that those involving the use of tubes seemed to me to be rather dangerous, for I knew that bodies held up in the stomach without being digested had led to dire consequences and after a considerable time had been vomited up. . . . However, the various contradictory facts that are current encouraged me to try these experiments; I knew that very hard stones, like those of cherries, morellas, medlars, and plums were swallowed with impunity by children and country people and they passed through the anus very easily without causing the slightest discomfort: in the midst of this struggle the previous events which I recorded induced me to overcome my reluctance (8).

Spallanzani swallowed little linen bags containing food; he found to his satisfaction that digestion takes place in the human stomach.

Most important were the contributions of William Beaumont (1785–1853), a physician stationed at a military post in the forest of Northern Michigan. He took advantage of the unique opportunity of studying the processes of digestion in the victim of a gunshot wound which left a permanent opening (fistula) into the stomach. His subject, Alexis St. Martin, was a trapper. During the first two years after the accident Beaumont tried to close the wound. Failing to do so, he grasped the opportunity of making studies of gastric digestion. It took infinite patience and ingenuity to maintain the cooperation of Alexis St. Martin through the years of study. His epoch-making observations were of movements of the stomach during digestion and of the normal appearance of the gastric mucosa.

These studies were fundamental to the advances that followed in the study of digestion in the nineteenth and twentieth centuries and lead to present-day knowledge.

The Processes of Digestion

Even though most of the food eaten is composed of complex molecules, there are certain factors in food like the simple carbohydrates, the minerals, and water that can be absorbed directly because of their elementary chemical structures. The digestion of the more complex food molecules, however, takes place in the gastrointestinal tract between the mouth and the end of the small intestine (Fig. 7.1). Digestion is brought about by both mechanical processes and chemical action.

Food processing methods and cooking procedures actually begin the breakdown of factors in food before the food itself is ingested. Cellulose is softened and the hydrolysis of starch and collagen begin during food processing. Also cooking enhances the digestibility of some foods (egg white) and improves the flavor of others (onions). The aroma and taste of

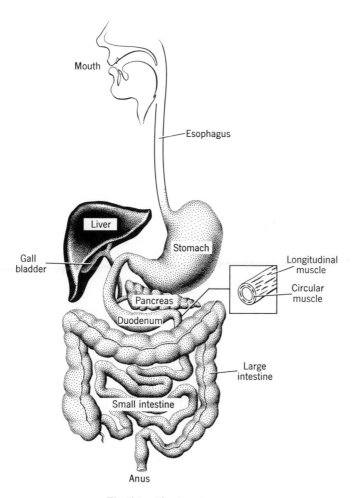

Fig. 7.1. The digestive tract.

flavorful, well-prepared foods may initiate the chemical phase of digestion by stimulating the secretions of the digestive tract.

The Mechanical Phase of Digestion

The mechanical phase of digestion, which is responsible for the mixing, subdividing, and moving of the food along the digestive tract, is brought about by chewing in the mouth and by the muscular activity of the walls of the tract itself. These walls contain two types of muscular tissue: muscle fibers that run in a circular direction and muscle fibers that run in a longitudinal direction (Fig. 7.1). When the circular fibers contract, the squeezing process results in the food being mixed and subdivided into smaller pieces. The contraction of the longitudinal fibers, on the other hand, causes the food mass to be pushed on through the tract. The coordinated movement of these two kinds of muscle fibers results in a wavelike motion all along the digestive canal called *peristalsis*.

The movements of the stomach are interfered with by nervousness and anxiety. Eating when fatigued, agitated, or worried may give rise to gastrointestinal disturbances. Hurried meals under tense conditions are not conducive to normal digestive movements.

The Chemical Phase of Digestion

The chemical phase of digestion, which is responsible for the chemical breakdown of the food, is brought about by the action of a group of complex chemical substances called *enzymes.* An enzyme is an interesting substance because it can become involved in a chemical reaction without undergoing any change in itself. The sketch (Fig. 7.2)

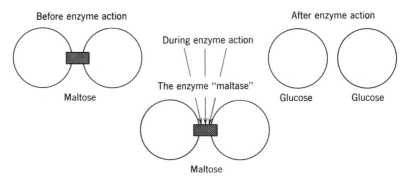

Fig. 7.2. A sketch showing the action of an enzyme.

illustrates how the enzyme, maltase, aids in breaking down the disaccharide, maltose, into two molecules of the monosaccharide, glucose, without changing its own chemical structure. Although in this chapter only the enzymes concerned with digestion are discussed, there are many others that are important in the body's overall function.

The Digestive Enzymes

The digestive enzymes are produced by the organs of the digestive tract. They aid in the breakdown of the complex carbohydrates to simple sugars, the fats or lipids to glycerol and fatty acids, and the proteins to amino acids. A distinctive feature of an enzyme is that it is specific; those that act on carbohydrates are not capable of acting on fats or proteins and vice versa. Even though a naming system for the enzymes has been adopted, certain names which were chosen before this system was established are still in use, such as pepsin and trypsin. In the new system of enzyme nomenclature, the root of the enzyme name is derived from the substance that it acts upon (the substrate) plus the suffix "ase," the characteristic designation of an enzyme. Enzymes that subdivide a carbohydrate, a fat or lipid, and a protein are called *carbohydrases, lipases,* and *proteases,* respectively. For a specific carbohydrate such as starch, the root of the enzyme name is derived from the word "amylum" meaning starch, thus *amylase* is the root of this enzyme name. However, the root names of the disaccharide-splitting enzymes are derived from the sugars themselves, that is, *sucrase, maltase,* and *lactase.* Because the steps in digestion for one nutrient may occur in different parts of the digestive tract, an adjective that describes the source of the enzymatic secretion is used before the root word to complete the enzyme name (Table 7.1). For example the fat-splitting enzyme which acts in the small intestine is secreted by the pancreas, and is called pancreatic lipase.

Digestion in the Mouth

Food enters the digestive tract through the mouth where it is chewed, broken into small pieces, and mixed with saliva. The fluid secreted by the salivary glands contains the first of the digestive enzymes, salivary amylase (ptyalin), which hydrolyzes starch or dextrin by splitting off molecules of maltose from the long carbohydrate chain (Fig. 7.3). Furthermore the lubricating action of the saliva aids in the swallowing of the food when it passes from the mouth to the stomach by way of the *esophagus.*

Table 7.1. The Digestive Enzymes

Source of the Enzyme Secretion	Site of Enzyme Reaction	Names of Enzymes and the Substances They Act Upon			
		Starches	Sugars	Fats	Proteins
Salivary glands	Mouth	Salivary amylase (ptyalin)			
Stomach	Stomach			Gastric lipase	Gastric protease (pepsin)
Pancreas	Small intestine	Pancreatic amylase		Pancreatic lipase	Pancreatic proteases
Wall of small intestine	Small intestine		Sucrase Maltase Lactase		Intestinal proteases

Digestion in the Stomach

When food enters the stomach it remains temporarily in the upper portion of the organ, though most of the digestive action occurs in the lower part of the stomach. Here, the action of the salivary amylase (ptyalin) continues until the pH of the mixture is too acid. Gastric juice, which contains hydrochloric acid, pepsinogen, and gastric lipase, is secreted in the lower part of the stomach and is mixed with the food by the churning action of the stomach walls.

Hydrochloric acid plays an important role in gastric digestion. It converts the inactive form of the protein-splitting enzyme, pepsinogen, to the active enzyme, pepsin; creates the optimum acidity in the stomach for the digestion of protein; and acts as a bactericide to prevent the entrance of bacteria into the lower digestive tract. In addition to these functions hydrochloric acid also may hydrolyze some of the disaccharides contained in the food mass as well as increase the solubility of calcium and iron, which results in the optimum absorption of these essential nutrients in the small intestine.

The protein-splitting enzyme, pepsin, is present in its inactive form, pepsinogen; otherwise when the stomach is empty of food the enzyme would begin to digest the stomach wall. In this first step of protein digestion the long chain of a protein is split into smaller units called *polypeptides* by the enzymatic action of pepsin (Fig. 7.4). The polypeptides, which vary in size, may contain as few as three amino acids linked together or as many as several hundred.

Because gastric lipase is inactive at the normal acidity of the gastric content, there is little fat digestion in the stomach. For this reason the enzyme may be of little physiological importance to man. Only the fats that are in a highly homogenized form as found in milk or egg yolk can be digested in the stomach.

For a long time the clotting of milk in the human stomach has been attributed to the action of the enzyme *rennin*. Some authorities now believe, however, that rennin is not present in the stomach of the adult, but that it may be present in the infant gastric secretion and only functions in the early period of life.

The length of time that food remains in the stomach differs with the composition of the diet and varies widely between individuals eating comparable food mixtures. An ordinary mixed meal leaves the stomach

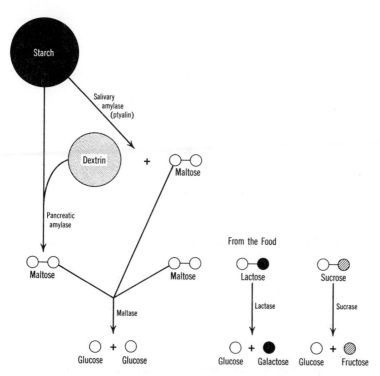

Fig. 7.3. A sketch showing starch and disaccharide digestion.

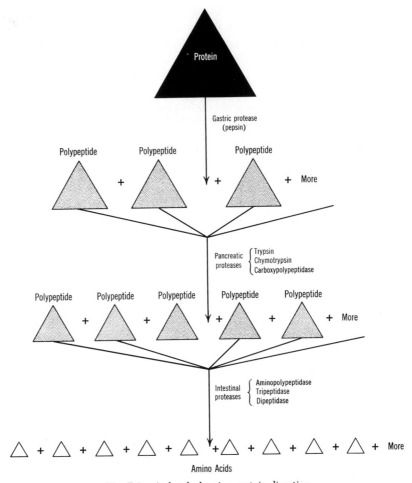

Fig. 7.4. A sketch showing protein digestion.

in three to four and one-half hours. Carbohydrate foods leave the stomach most rapidly, followed by protein, with fat foods remaining in the stomach for the longest length of time. The sensation of hunger occurs more quickly after a meal relatively high in carbohydrate than after a meal containing adequate protein and fat.

Digestion in the Small Intestine

After leaving the stomach the highly liquefied food mass which is referred to as *chyme* passes into the first section of the small intestine, the *duodenum*. Into this area flow the intestinal juices, the pancreatic juices, and the bile. The secretions of the pancreas and the small intestine contain enzymes necessary for the complete digestion of carbohydrates, fats, and proteins.

Carbohydrate digestion, which began in the mouth, is resumed in the duodenum. Here nature has provided a second amylase to convert any remaining starch or dextrin to maltose, thus completing the conversion of starch to the disaccharide maltose (Fig. 7.3). Pancreatic amylase appears to be more potent in this action than is salivary amylase. Even uncooked or raw starch, which was not acted upon by the amylase of the saliva, may be digested by the pancreatic form of the enzyme. It should be noted, however, that raw starches are less digestible than cooked starches because of the nature of the starch granules. Raw potato starch is rather poorly digested and if consumed in large quantities a significant amount of this particular starch may pass through the digestive tract without change. Other carbohydrates, the disaccharides, which are found in the food intake or as end products of amylase action must also be changed to simple sugars before they can be absorbed by the body. The three carbohydrases in the intestinal secretion (sucrase, maltase, and lactase) complete the hydrolysis of the carbohydrates to glucose, fructose, and galactose (Fig. 7.3).

Because there is little enzymatic action produced by gastric lipase, the digestion of fats from the practical standpoint actually begins in the small intestine. The two secretions which are involved in this fat-splitting process are the bile, a secretion of the liver, and the pancreatic lipase (Fig. 7.5). A fraction of the bile fluid, the bile salts, acts as emulsifying agent. The bile also functions to accelerate the action of the pancreatic lipase and to neutralize the acidity of the chyme. In the process of emulsification the fats are broken up into small globules which are more easily hydrolyzed by the pancreatic lipase. Not all of the fat is digested to the glycerol and fatty acid stage by lipase; some of it is hydrolyzed only to di- or monoglycerides, which are compounds composed of glycerol and two or one fatty acid(s), respectively.

Trypsin is one of the three protein-splitting enzymes contributed to the "digestive pool" by the pancreatic secretion. As in the case of the gastric protease (pepsin), trypsin is also secreted in its inactive form, trypsinogen, which prevents digestion of the intestinal tissue. Trypsin, chymotrypsin, and carboxypolypeptidase attack the links of the polypeptide chains and further subdivide them into polypeptides of smaller units (Fig. 7.4). Finally the complete breakdown of the polypeptides to amino acids is brought about by the action of three additional protein enzymes, aminopolypeptidase, tripeptidase, and dipeptidase, secreted in the intestinal juice (Fig. 7.4).

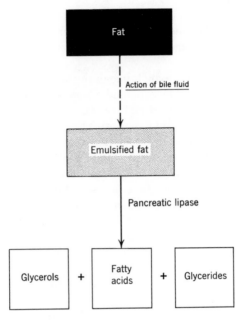

Fig. 7.5.   A sketch showing fat digestion.

The Large Intestine

The material entering the large intestine (colon) contains undigested residues, some of the end products of digestion that had escaped absorption, bile pigments and other waste materials, and water. No digestive enzymes are secreted in the colon. Little change occurs except for the absorption of water.

▶ ABSORPTION

Before the body can use the soluble products formed during digestive action, the nutrients must be absorbed through the lining of the digestive tract. Even though water and small amounts of simple sugars pass through the mucosa of the stomach into the blood stream, most of the absorption takes place in the small intestine. The absorptive area of this section of the digestive passage is increased an estimated 600 fold by the *villi* (20), which are fingerlike projections in the lining of the small intestine. Each villus contains a lymph vessel surrounded by a network of capillaries (Fig. 7.6). The nutrients absorbed into the lymph vessel pass into the lymphatic system, and those absorbed by the capillaries empty into the portal vein and are carried directly to the liver. The lymph vessels are the "connecting passageways" in the body, between the blood and tissues, by which food material and oxygen are brought to the individual cells.

Absorption of End Products of Carbohydrate Digestion

Most of the simple sugars, the end products of carbohydrate digestion, are absorbed directly into the capillaries and are carried by way of the portal vein to the liver where those not needed for energy may be converted to glycogen for storage. Small amounts of the monosaccharides may be absorbed by way of the lymphatic system. Carbohydrates other than monosaccharides are not absorbed through the intestinal wall.

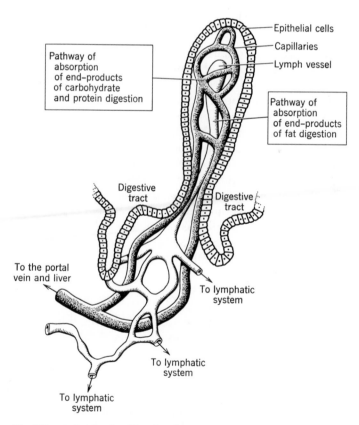

Fig. 7.6. A sketch of a villus, the absorptive organ of the small intestine.

Absorption of End Products of Fat Digestion

At the present time it is believed that the end products of fat digestion are absorbed in two forms: one-third to one-half is completely
hydrolyzed to glycerol and fatty acids, and the remainder are partially
hydrolyzed to monoglycerides (7). Moreover, after the glycerol and fatty
acid molecules pass into the intestinal wall, the two may recombine to
form a fat molecule. Then the glycerides and the reformed fat molecules,
as well as any glycerol and most of the fatty acids that may be present,
pass into the lymph vessels. It is believed that bile salts aid in fat
absorption because of the property of emulsification. They bypass the
liver and later enter the blood stream. Then the end products are trans-
ported directly to the tissues where they are either used for energy or
stored as body fat.

Absorption of End Products of Protein Digestion

The amino acids formed during protein digestion are readily absorbed
from the intestinal tract into the capillaries and pass to the liver by way
of the portal vein. From here they are carried by the blood to the tissues
where they are used in protein metabolism as needed.

It is now known, however, that protein derivatives larger than amino
acids may be absorbed into the blood stream. The etiology of food
allergies suggests that small amounts of intact or partially hydrolyzed
proteins from foods must be absorbed by the body. This appears to be
true because the allergy-produced reactions (asthma, skin eruptions,
etc.) are no longer present when the proteins causing the allergy are
completely hydrolyzed to amino acids. A conclusive explanation for the
abnormal absorption of protein has not been established. One proposal
is that "transient local defects exist in the intestinal epithelium" and
that they may be responsible (20).

Absorption of Other Nutrients

Minerals and vitamins are absorbed from the small intestine. Water
can be absorbed from the stomach, the small, and the large intestine.

▶ METABOLISM

Metabolism may be described as all the chemical changes that nutrients
undergo from the time they are absorbed until they become a part of

the body or are excreted from the body. The two general phases of metabolism are referred to as *anabolism* and *catabolism*. The anabolism phase involves all the chemical reactions that the nutrients undergo for the construction or building up of body materials such as blood, enzymes, various tissues, hormones, glycogen, and others. The catabolism phase involves the reactions in which various compounds of the tissues are broken down, such as carbohydrates into carbon dioxide and water, releasing energy. In the cell both processes go on simultaneously. *Energy metabolism* is the general term that has come to be used to describe all the changes, both chemical and physical, that the energy nutrients undergo in the release of energy for the body's use.

Carbohydrate Metabolism

After the end products of carbohydrate digestion (the monosaccharides) reach the liver, they are used for energy or stored, depending on the body's immediate need.[*] There is evidence that monosaccharides, except glucose, are changed to glucose in the liver cells (4). These glucose molecules are sent to all parts of the body via the blood stream and pass from it into the tissues and cells by way of the fluids that surround the cells. The carbohydrate is oxidized in the cell to supply energy needed for the body processes.

The Formation of Glycogen. The formation of glycogen from glucose in either the liver or muscle cells involves a series of enzymatic reactions. In one of these chemical steps, the catalytic agents involved are ions of magnesium. The glycogen formed, often referred to as animal starch, is stored both in the liver and in the muscle (Fig. 7.7). However, only limited amounts of this complex carbohydrate can be stored as compared to the body's storage capacity for fat. It has been estimated that the liver can store up to 10 per cent of its weight in glycogen or about 100 gm, and the storage capacity of the muscle is only about 2 per cent of its weight.

Insulin plays an essential role in carbohydrate metabolism. This hormone, which is secreted by the Islets of Langerhans of the pancreas, aids not only in the oxidation of glucose in the body, but also accelerates the conversion of blood glucose to glycogen.

---

[*] Sinclair (18) has written of the wrong usage of "glycogenic" and "glycogenesis" as terms in intermediary metabolism. He states that these terms refer to the production of glucose from any source and have nothing to do with glycogen by derivation. According to this author, glyconeogenesis, glycogenolysis, and glycogenesis are defined as follows. *Glyconeogenesis* (or *gluconeogenesis*) is the production of glucose from noncarbohydrate suorces, the proteins or fatty acids; *glycogenolysis* is the breakdown of glycogen; *glycogenesis* is the formation of glucose from other monosaccharides and other compounds along the glycolytic pathway.

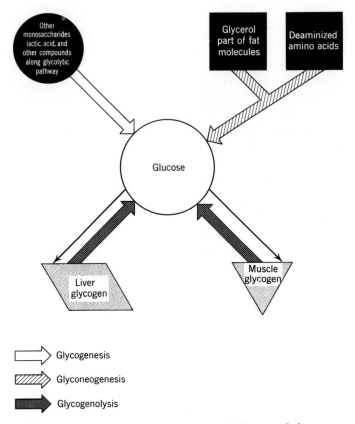

Fig. 7.7.   A sketch depicting the formation of glucose and glycogen.

The Breakdown of Liver and Muscle Glycogen. When extra energy is needed by the body, the liver glycogen is mobilized and changed to glucose by a process called glycogenolysis (Fig. 7.7). This reaction occurs only in the liver cells. *Epinephrine,* commonly referred to as *adrenalin,* is the hormone produced by the adrenal glands which stimulates the breakdown of liver glycogen. After the glucose has been formed, it leaves the liver and passes to the tissues for immediate use.

The breakdown of muscle glycogen also is accelerated by adrenalin. However, the end product of this conversion is not glucose but a closely related compound, glucose-1-phosphate.

Glucose Formation from Noncarbohydrate Sources. Although most of the glucose in the body comes from dietary carbohydrates, it may be formed in the liver from noncarbohydrate molecules by a process called glyconeogenesis (Fig. 7.7). The three sources of noncarbohydrate molecules, which may be precursors of liver glycogen and finally blood glucose, are the glycerol part of fat molecules, *deaminized amino acids,* and other compounds along the glycolytic pathway (e.g., lactic acid). A deaminized amino acid is one in which the amino group (NH_2) has been removed.

Oxidation of Carbohydrate for Energy. The steps in the oxidation of carbohydrate for energy are pictured in Fig. 7.8. The first stage in the oxidation process involves the breakdown of glycogen or glucose to pyruvate (pyruvic acid) and lactate (lactic acid). This conversion is not a simple chemical change but occurs in many complex enzymatic reactions. In addition to this a derivative of the glycerol part of the fat molecule enters the oxidation cycle along the glycolytic pathway.

The second stage in the oxidation process involves the breakdown of pyruvate to carbon dioxide and water with the release of energy. Energy is released when one molecule of pyruvate goes through the complete cycle of the chemical changes known as the Kreb's Cycle. Oxygen is required in these reactions.

Even though the exact mechanism found in the oxidation process is complicated and involved, the sketch gives an idea of the series of known reactions that take place in this complex process.

Conversion of Carbohydrates to Fats and Amino Acids. When carbohydrates are ingested in quantities greater than the energy needs of the body, the excess amount is converted to fat and stored in the tissues. This fact has been demonstrated by controlled experiments with both animals and man. From the sketch (Fig. 7.8) it can be seen how a fat may be formed from a carbohydrate. The glycolytic pathway from carbohydrate to glycerol and from the "acetyl CoA" (a coenzyme concerned with enzymatic processes involving two-carbon compounds) to fatty acid are both two-way reactions. Derivatives of either glycogen or glucose may be diverted from the main pathway and travel along these side reactions to glycerol and fatty acids. These two substances then combine to form a fat which is stored in the body tissue.

Besides being converted to fat, extra carbohydrate may also assist in the formation of amino acids. It can be seen how it is possible for this to occur from the sketch of the chemical system (Fig. 7.8). For example, pyruvate may be (1) oxidized to release energy, (2) reconverted to carbohydrate, (3) used for the synthesis of fat, or (4) synthesized into an amino acid. It is here that the synthesis of the amino acid alanine occurs. Two other amino acid derivatives, glutamate (glutamic acid) and aspartate (aspartic acid), are synthesized also from pyruvate. Then glutamate

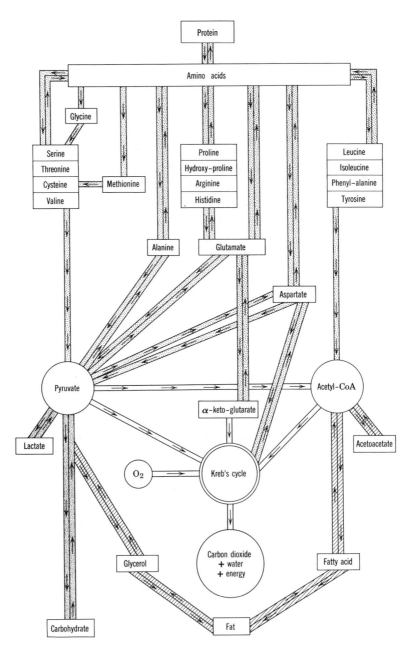

Fig. 7.8. A sketch depicting the chemical system which represents the pathway of oxidation for carbohydrates, fats, and proteins in the body. (Adapted from *Biology Data Book*, P. L. Altman and D. S. Dietmer [eds.] (1964). Fed. Am. Soc. Expt. Biol., Washington, D.C., p. 203.)

gives rise to proline, hydroxyproline, arginine, and histidine. It is of interest that the chemical reactions involving four nonessential amino acids (serine, cysteine, glycine, and tyrosine) and the six essential amino acids (threonine, valine, methionine, leucine, isoleucine, and phenylalanine) constitute only one-way reactions to either pyruvate or acetyl-CoA.

Fat Metabolism

After the end products of fat digestion are absorbed through the walls of the intestinal tract, they pass into the lymph vessels on their way to the cells and tissues. Later they enter the blood stream, but before doing so some of the recombined fat molecules unite with molecules of phosphoric acid to form phospholipids, which aid in the transport of fatty acids in the body. The recombined fats, the phospholipids, the glycerides, the glycerol molecules, and the fatty acids go to all the body tissues, where they are either oxidized for energy or stored as adipose or fatty tissue.

Oxidation of Fats. The components of a fat molecule, the glycerol fraction, and the fraction of fatty acids, are oxidized separately to provide energy for the body processes. Before oxidation can begin, therefore, any fat or glyceride must first be hydrolyzed to glycerol and fatty acids.

The glycerol part of the fat molecule is first changed to a new compound before it enters the glycolytic pathway midway between the point marked "carbohydrate" and that marked "pyruvate" in Fig. 7.8. From here on the oxidation of glycerol is the same as the oxidation of carbohydrate.

The fatty acids, however, undergo several changes before they reach the acetyl-CoA reaction. From this point they travel the same route along the Kreb's Cycle as do the carbohydrates and the glycerol fraction of the fat in order to release carbon dioxide, water, and energy.

Fat Formation from Carbohydrates and Amino Acids. Both carbohydrates and amino acids may be used as sources of fat in the body. The formation of body fat from carbohydrates has already been mentioned. The conversion of protein to body fat, however, involves the amino acids along the metabolic pathway. As seen in Fig. 7.8, the amino acids are first deaminized and then proceed to acetyl-CoA. From this point they proceed to fatty acids as well as to pyruvate and then to the point where the reaction leads off to glycerol. The glycerol and fatty acid molecules then combine to form a glyceride.

Protein Metabolism

The amino acids, the end products of protein digestion, are readily absorbed into the blood stream from the intestinal mucosa, pass to the liver, and from there are carried to all the cells of the body. There are three ways in which the amino acids are used by the body. First, some are synthesized to proteins and are used by the body to build new cells and to replace worn-out ones and to form body regulators, that is, hormones, enzymes, antibodies. Second, some of the amino acids may exchange amino groups with other amino acids or even contribute amino groups to nonprotein materials to form new amino acids. Finally, amino acids may undergo oxidation for energy production.

Formation of Body Protein. A discussion of factors related to protein formation in the body is presented in Chapter 6.

Oxidation of Amino Acids. Before amino acids enter the metabolic pathway to be oxidized the amino groups must be removed. This reaction of deaminization occurs in several steps and in many of the tissues of the body but primarily in the liver and kidney. The amino group that is removed forms ammonia before it is converted to *urea* in order to be excreted from the body. The urea, which is the major nitrogenous product in the decomposition of proteins in the body, is then carried to the kidneys where it is eliminated in the urine. The oxidation of the remainder of the amino acid, however, follows the pathway of carbohydrate metabolism (Fig. 7.8). After the amino acids have been oxidized for energy, the end products are excreted from the body as carbon dioxide, water, urea, and other nitrogenous constituents. The kidneys are the pathway of excretion of the nitrogenous end products of protein metabolism.

Conversion of Amino Acids to Carbohydrate and Fat. As has been noted in the discussion of carbohydrate and fat metabolism, amino acids may be converted to either carbohydrate or fat in the normal processes of metabolism (Fig. 7.8).

Some Disorders that may Interfere with Metabolism

Disorders may occur caused by faulty metabolism of the food nutrients. These disorders which are related to heredity are now referred to as *inborn errors of metabolism.* Diabetes mellitus is the most common one; others, phenylketonuria and galactosemia, occur less frequently.

Diabetes Mellitus. Diabetes mellitus, which is estimated to affect more than two million people in the United States alone, is caused by the inability of the pancreatic cells to produce sufficient insulin to oxidize and store body glucose (Fig. 7.7). The characteristic symptoms of diabetes are excessive hunger, thirst, and urine output; accumulation of organic acids and acetone in the blood; weakness; and loss of body weight. With adequate treatment even severe diabetics are able to carry on active, productive lives.

The treatment of diabetes consists essentially of adjusting the patient's diet to his limited supply of endogenous insulin. In general the type of diet recommended contains approximately 40 per cent of the total Calories as carbohydrate, 45 per cent as fat, and 15 per cent as protein. If, however, the supply of endogenous insulin is markedly insufficient for dietary control, insulin then must be administered hypodermically. Oral hypoglycemic agents have been developed that sometimes aid in the control of diabetes. "Orinase" and "Diabinese" are two of the oral hypoglycemic agents now used.

Other Inborn Errors of Metabolism. At the present time over fifty inborn errors of metabolism have been identified (12). They are all transmitted in a hereditary manner, caused by an abnormality in one or more of the genes, and all are rare. These disorders have been found to involve the metabolism of carbohydrates, lipids, amino acids, purines, pyrimidines, and minerals as well as defects in the renal tubular transport, and blood and blood-forming tissues. The expression of the metabolic error may vary from no symptoms whatsoever, as in the case of pentosuria, to the severe symptoms encountered in phenylketonuria or galactosemia. The therapy for the control of these metabolic anomalies may involve dietary measures or pharmaceutical agents, depending upon the nature of the disorders.

To illustrate the different kinds of inborn errors of metabolism, a brief description of a carbohydrate defect, a mineral defect, and two amino acid defects are presented here. For a more comprehensive review of inborn errors of metabolism, however, the paper by Sinclair (17) is suggested.

Galactosemia is a disorder resulting from the deficiency of a specific enzyme (galactose-1-phosphate-uridyl-transferase) involved in the conversion of galactose to glucose. This disorder, which usually manifests itself shortly after birth, results in failure to thrive, enlargement of the liver, galactose in the urine, jaundice, cataracts, and mental retardation. A restricted intake of foods containing lactose is the treatment now described for galactosemia (1, 15). It has been observed that although diet therapy did not appear to improve the cataracts of galactosemia, children whose diets were vigorously restricted in lactose were more intelligent than those whose diets were restricted little or not at all (13).

Wilson's disease is a metabolic error associated with a disturbance in copper metabolism characterized by an enzymatic deficiency in the production of the copper protein ceruloplasmin (2, 6). In this disorder, copper deposition occurs in the brain, liver, and other organs with the result that the normal function of the cells is inhibited. An oral therapeutical agent, penicillamine, is now used to accelerate the removal of the excess copper from the body.

Phenylketonuria is an inborn error of metabolism that develops soon after birth and involves a deficiency of an enzyme in the liver necessary for the conversion of the amino acid, phenylalanine, to another amino acid, tyrosine (5). Motor disorders, eczema, sometimes fair skin and hair, musty-smelling urine, and mental retardation are some of the typical symptoms of this disorder. A restricted intake of foods containing phenylalanine is used to control this disorder (14, 19). Because phenylalanine is widespread in all protein foods, synthetic amino acid products low in the amino acid ("Ketonil" and "Lofenalac") have been developed to treat the PKU patient. The improvement of the mental retardation in PKU children is apparently related to the early use of the restricted diet (3, 10, 11). There is some evidence that dietary treatment of phenylketonuria can be relaxed in the early school years of the patient.

Histidinemia, an inborn error of metabolism that involves a deficiency of the enzyme, histidase, which catalyzes the transfer of the amino acid, histidine, to urocanic acid was first described in 1962 (9, 16). In the five known cases of histidinemia, the only serious clinical manifestation of the disorder appears to be a speech defect; none are mentally retarded.

REFERENCES

1. Acosta, P. B. (1963). Dietary treatment of galactosemia. In *Report of Institute on Nutrition Services in Mental Retardation Programs.* U.S. Dept. Health, Education, and Welfare, Washington, D.C., p. 47.
2. Bearn, A. G. (1961). Wilson's disease. *Am. J. Clin. Nutr.* 9: 695.
3. Berman, P. W., F. K. Graham, P. L. Eichman, and H. A. Waisman (1961). Psychologic and neurologic status of diet-treated phenylketonuric children and their siblings. *Pediatrics* 28: 924.
4. Best, C. H., and N. B, Taylor (1961). *The Physiological Basis of Medical Practice,* 7th ed. Williams and Wilkins, Co., Baltimore.
5. Centerwall, W.R. (1960). Phenylketonuria. A general review. *J. Am. Dietet. Assoc.* 36:201.
6. Cumings, J. N. (1962). The metabolism of copper and Wilson's disease. *Proc. Nutr. Soc. (London)* 21: 29.

7. Danielson, H. (1963). Influence of bile acids on digestion and absorption of lipids. *Am. J. Clin. Nutr.* **12:** 214.

8. Fulton, J. F. (1930). *Selected Readings in the History of Physiology.* Charles C. Thomas, Baltimore.

9. Histidinemia—A new inborn error of metabolism (1963). *J. Am. Dietet. Assoc.* **42:** 51.

10. Horner, F. A., C. W. Streamer, D. E. Clader, L. L. Hassell, E. L. Binkley, Jr., and K. W. Dumars, Jr. (1957). Effect of phenylalanine-restricted diet in phenylketonuria. *J. Dis. Child.* **93:** 615.

11. Horner, F. A., and C. W. Streamer (1959). Phenylketonuria treated from earliest infancy. Report of three cases. *AMA J. Diseases Children* **97:** 345.

12. Hsia, D. Y. Y. (1960). Recent developments in inborn errors of metabolism. *Am. J. Public Health* **50:** 1653.

13. Hsia, D. Y. Y. (1961). Variability in the clinical manifestations of galactosemia. *J. Pediat.* **50:** 872.

14. Koch, R., P. Acosta, N. Ragsdale, and G. N. Donnell (1963). Nutrition in the treatment of phenylketonuria. *J. Am. Dietet. Assoc.* **43:** 212.

15. Koch, R., P. Acosta, N. Ragsdale, and G. N. Donnell (1963). Nutrition in the treatment of galactosemia. *J. Am. Dietet. Assoc.* **43:** 216.

16. La Duc, B. N., R. R. Howell, G. A. Jacoby, J. E. Seegmiller, and V. G. Zannoni (1962). An enzymatic defect in histidinemia. *Biochem. Biophys. Res. Commun.* **7:** 398.

17. Sinclair, H. M. (1962). Historical aspects of inborn errors of metabolism. *Proc. Nutr. Soc. (London)* **21:** 1.

18. Sinclair, H. M. (1964). Carbohydrates and fats. In *Nutrition a Comprehensive Treatise,* Vol. I. (G. H. Beaton and E. W. McHenry, eds.) Academic Press, New York, pp. 46–48.

19. Umbarger, B. (1963). Phenylketonuria—low phenylalanine diet. In *Report of Institute on Nutrition Services in Mental Retardation Programs.* U.S. Dept. Health, Education, and Welfare, Washington, D.C., p. 38.

20. Wilson, T. H. (1962). *Intestinal Absorption.* W. B. Saunders Co., Philadelphia.

SUPPLEMENTARY REFERENCES

Best, C. H., and N. B. Taylor (1961). *The Physiological Basis of Medical Practice.* 7th ed. Williams and Wilkins Co., Baltimore.

Conn, E. E., and P. K. Stumpf (1963). *Outlines of Biochemistry.* John Wiley and Sons, New York.

Holum, J. K. (1962). *Introduction to General and Biological Chemistry.* John Wiley and Sons, New York.

Wilson, T. H. (1962). *Intestinal Absorption.* W. B. Saunders Co., Philadelphia.

CHAPTER 8

The need for energy

The energy nutrients, their digestion, absorption, and metabolism have been discussed. The next step in the energy story is to present the factors which comprise the total energy need as well as the caloric requirement of man.

▶ **HISTORY OF ENERGY METABOLISM**

Lavoisier, who is called the "Father of Nutrition," laid the foundations for the basic principles of energy metabolism in the eighteenth century through his discoveries of the importance of oxygen gas in the process of combustion. The period of the development of the concepts of energy metabolism, however, extended throughout the nineteenth century with the work of many German scientists including Justus von Liebig and Max Rubner. Yet the instruments used to measure the energy expenditures of men and animals, as well as the potential energy value of food products were only perfected in this century by men like Wilbur Atwater, Henry Armsby, and others. Since their efforts Lafayette Mendel, Elmer McCollum, Francis Benedict, Henry Sherman, Raymond DuBois, H. H. Mitchell, Leonard Maynard, Raymond Swift, and other scientists have advanced the knowledge of potential energy in foods and energy metabolism by obtaining quantitative data on both.

Attention was diverted from work in the field of energy metabolism when the first vitamins were discovered, shortly before the First World War. During the period of the Second World War, however, when this country began to help feed the war-distressed nations of the world as well as its own armies, it became apparent that the available information on the energy composition of food substances and the energy needs of man was inadequate. In contrast to this, an increasing awareness of the problems of overweight and obesity (caloric overnutrition) further stimulated the interest and focused attention on the need for new energy research. As a consequence there has been a broader study in this area of nutrition. There has been a reawakening of interest in energy metabolism during the past two decades.

▶ FACTORS WHICH DETERMINE THE TOTAL ENERGY NEED

The three factors that determine the total energy need of an individual are the basal metabolism, the physical activity, and the specific dynamic effect of food. The basal metabolism, which usually represents the largest fraction of the total energy expenditure, is the minimum amount of energy needed to carry on the vital life processes of the body when awake. The regulation of body temperature is an important entity in the basal metabolism. Energy for the performance of all types of physical activity ranks next to basal metabolism in amount of energy expended. The extra energy required to metabolize food (with a resulting increase in heat production, small as it may be, which is known as the specific dynamic effect) is the third factor that is part of the total energy requirement.

Definition of Terms

Some of the specific terms used in the study of energy metabolism are calorie, calorimetry, and calorimeter.

A *calorie* has been defined as the standard unit used to measure energy. The calorie used in nutrition is called the kilocalorie or large calorie and is written with a capital letter (Calorie or Cal.). This unit is one thousand times greater than the small calorie (calorie or cal.) used in chemistry or physics. To distinguish between the size of the large and small calorie, the example of the energy value of a pat of butter is cited. A pat of butter contains 50 Cal. or 50,000 cal. Although the word "Calorie" is often used to describe the potential energy in food, it is not a nutrient but rather a unit of measure of heat.

Calorimetry is the measurement of the amount of heat given off or absorbed. The energy value of a particular food and the daily energy needs of a person are both determined by calorimetry, and expressed in terms of Calories. If the measurement is made from the actual heat produced, this is referred to as *direct calorimetry*. On the other hand, if the amount of oxygen consumed and/or the carbon dioxide produced is used as a basis to indirectly measure heat production, this is called *indirect calorimetry*.

A *calorimeter* is the instrument or apparatus used to measure the calories of heat produced. The energy value of foods is measured by either the oxy- or bomb calorimeter (Chapter 9). Examples of instruments used to measure the heat production of man, directly or indirectly, are the Armsby Calorimeter and the Benedict-Roth apparatus.

▶ THE ENERGY NEED FOR BASAL METABOLISM

The *basal metabolism*, which may be defined as the amount of heat given off by an individual during physical, digestive, and emotional rest, represents the amount of energy needed to carry on the vital life processes of the body (the activity of the heart, kidney, and other organs as well as the metabolic processes within the cells). It excludes the energy needed for physical activity and the specific dynamic effect of food.

The basal metabolism determination, which has a definite value in medicine, is used in many hospitals and clinics as a tool in diagnosing certain disorders and diseases. From the measurement of the basal metabolism, the conditions of *hypothyroidism* (an undersecretion of the thyroid gland) and *hyperthyroidism* (an oversecretion of the gland) are recognized. The basal metabolic rate may be depressed 30 to 40 per cent below normal in hypothyroidism and elevated as much as 80 per cent in hyperthyroidism. The most valuable test in the evaluation of thyroid disease, however, is the serum protein-bound iodine determination (2), which reflects the activity of the thyroid by the quantitative measure of iodine bound to serum proteins.

Methods of Determining Basal Metabolism

The measurement of the basal metabolism of an individual may be either by indirect or direct calorimetry. Indirect calorimetry, the procedure universally used, involves the determination of either the amount of oxygen consumed and/or the amount of carbon dioxide produced, which indirectly measures the amount of heat produced by oxidation in the cells of the body. A unit measure of oxygen is equivalent to a given number of Calories when certain food and food nutrients are oxidized.

It is assumed that under the conditions of the basal metabolism determination that the individual is oxidizing a mixed diet.

The machine used most widely to measure the basal metabolism is the Benedict-Roth apparatus which involves the measurement of the amount of oxygen used by an individual. The short time required for a measurement and its operating simplicity have made it a most satisfactory instrument for medical diagnosis. The Tissot apparatus, which involves the collection and analysis of expired air of an individual, has been found to be a desirable instrument for determining the basal metabolism in experimental studies. This method is expensive both in operating time and cost of equipment, but because a greater accuracy in the basal measurement is possible, it is a valuable tool in energy research. Direct calorimetry, which is used most frequently in the study of energy need during exercise, is discussed later in this chapter.

Conditions Under Which the Basal Metabolism Should Be Measured

There are certain conditions under which the basal metabolism of an individual should be measured. First, the test should be made 12 to 18 hours after the last intake of food. To eliminate any effect of food on the heat production, the morning hours are generally used for the measurement. Second, the subject should be awake and lying quietly in a room of comfortable temperature. The metabolism of an individual is lowered approximately 10 per cent during sleep. Any activity on the part of the subject or need to produce heat to maintain the body temperature will increase the metabolic processes and result in an extra energy expenditure beyond the basal metabolism. Third, the subject should be relaxed because nervousness or tension may cause an increase in the heat production.

A Way to Compute the Basal Metabolism

A simple procedure for approximating the basal metabolism under normal conditions is the "rule of thumb," 1 Cal. per kilogram per hour.

Basal metabolism = 1 Cal. $\times$ body weight in kilograms $\times$ 24 hr (in Cal./24 hr).

The kilograms of body weight are found by dividing the weight in pounds by the factor 2.2. The calculation for the energy needed for the basal metabolism of a college man weighing 176 lb would then be:

$$\text{Basal metabolism} = 1 \times \frac{176}{2.2} \times 24$$

$$= 1920 \text{ Cal./24 hr}$$

For a more accurate estimate of the basal metabolism, laboratory methods previously described are used.

Factors Which May Affect the Basal Metabolism

The factors which may affect the basal metabolism are body size, type of body composition, age, climate, status of health (fever and malnutrition, or semistarvation), secretion of the ductless glands, pregnancy, and growth. In the past studies involving the Eskimo, the New Orleans and West Indian Negro, and the Egyptian have shown the

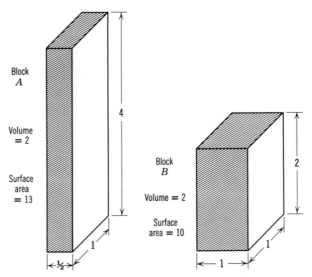

Fig. 8.1.   Blocks *A* and *B* represent two men of the same age and body weight (volume = 2). Yet the surface area of Block *A* (the tall, thin man) is 30 per cent greater than that of Block *B* (the short, stout man).

basal metabolism of these racial groups to be within the normal expected limits. Recent evidence from the Arctic Aeromedical Laboratory (12) indicates that the Eskimo (46 Cal./hr/m²) and the Arctic Athapascan Indian (42.5 Cal./hr/m²) have higher basal metabolic rates than Caucasians (about 37 Cal./hr/m²).

Body Size.   The basal metabolism of individuals of the same height and age or people of the same weight and age may differ or be influenced by the variation in the body form of the individuals. These differences can be explained by borrowing an idea from Best and Taylor (1) who illustrated the principles by using pieces of wood to represent the area of body surface. In the first example (Fig. 8.1) Block A and B represent two men of the same age and body weight but who are different in shape, one being tall and the other short. Even though Block A and B are identical in volume and weight, the surface area of Block A is about one-third greater than that of Block B. Thus the tall man will have a higher basal metabolism per unit of body weight than the shorter man of the same weight. In the second example (Fig. 8.2), where Block C represents the thin man and Block D represents the stout man, the two men are of the same height and age but the thin man weighs

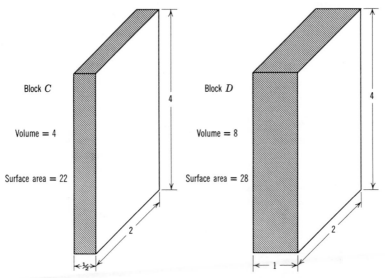

Fig. 8.2.   Blocks C and D represent two men of the same age and height. Block D (volume $= 8$) weighs twice as much as Block C (volume $= 4$), yet the surface area of Block D is only one and one-quarter times greater than Block C, not twice as great.

one-half as much as the stout man. Here the surface area of the stout block is only about one and one-fourth times greater than the thin block, not twice as great. These examples serve to show the important relationship of body size and shape to the actual basal heat production of an individual.

The reader is referred to Best and Taylor (1) or to Swift and Fisher (24) for a more comprehensive treatise of ways to determine the surface area of man as well as tables and formulas for predicting the basal metabolism.

The concept that basal metabolism is proportional to surface area has been accepted by most students of nutrition. However, within recent years the relationship between body composition and the basal metabolism has been studied, with the result that some scientists are doubting the validity of the surface-area basal metabolism concept and propose instead the "active tissue mass" basal metabolism concept. For more details on this relationship the reader is referred to the monograph of the Conference on Techniques for Measuring Body Composition (21).

Types of Body Composition. The kinds of tissue that make up the body have a direct influence on the basal metabolism. In muscle tissue, for example, where oxidative processes are constantly taking place, more energy is expended than in fatty tissue. It has been estimated that an athletic-type man with well-developed muscular tissue will have a basal metabolism about 6 per cent higher than a nonathlete of comparable body surface. Men have a 5 per cent higher heat production than do women of comparable body size and age, the higher value, however, is not a sex difference, per se, but is attributed at least in part to the smaller amount of fatty tissue found in men as compared to women.

Age. Age is still another factor which affects the basal heat production of an individual. The caloric requirement, which is based on area of body surface, reaches its highest point at about 18 months of age. Then there is a slight decrease in the caloric need from this time until the period of adolescence when another peak occurs. After the completion of growth there is a gradual decline in the basal heat production which extends from about age 20 throughout life. It has been estimated that the basal metabolism of a man at 75 years is about 20 per cent lower than that of a man at 20 years.

Climate. Living in a cold climate does not appear to affect the basal metabolism of an individual to any extent because of the protection provided by clothing and shelter. Lewis and his group (8) found that during a period of more than two years in the Arctic the basal metabolism of 29 young adults remained quite stable. The effect of a hot climate on the basal metabolism has not yet been satisfactorily investigated. In some of the earlier studies where lower basal metabolism values were found among people living in the tropics, it is difficult to conclude whether the differences reported were real or due to the use of trained subjects. Recent reports, however, confirm the earlier indications that people living in the tropics have "lower" metabolic rates (based on body weight) than do those living in the areas of the temperate zones (6).

At this time there is considerable interest in the effect of altitude on metabolic processes in man. Altitude, however, does not appear to alter the basal metabolism. Subjects living at altitudes above 5000 and 15,000 feet have been found to have basal metabolic patterns well within the limits found in man at sea level (9, 14).

Status of Health. The measurement of the basal metabolism as defined, involves a normal, healthy subject. Such a measurement will be lower when the subject has been malnourished (the extent depending on the degree of undernutrition) and will be higher when the subject has a body fever.

Illnesses involving an elevation of body temperature may markedly increase the basal heat production. For each degree rise in temperature above 98.6°F the basal rate is increased about 7 per cent. For example, with a body temperature of 103.6°F, which is 5 degrees above normal, the basal metabolism will be increased 35 per cent.

Malnutrition will lower the basal metabolism, depending upon the degree of undernutrition. It has been observed that undernourished children whose diets were inadequate in Calories had lower basal metabolic rates per unit of body weight than did adequately fed children of the same age (11).

The classic studies by Keys and co-workers at the University of Minnesota (7) have shown the effect of semistarvation on the basal metabolic rate. Thirty-six healthy young men were the subjects for this fourteen-month experiment. The plan of the study included a 3-month control period followed by a 6-month semistarvation period and ended with 3 months of restricted rehabilitation and 2 months of unrestricted rehabilitation. The number of Calories ingested daily during these periods were approximately 3492, 1570, between 1931 and 2944, and then an unrestricted amount, respectively. Although the restricted caloric pattern of the diet for the semistarvation period resulted in a loss of about one-fourth the total body weight of the subjects, the basal consumption of oxygen was decreased only as much as 10 per cent below the prestarvation values. However, the transfer to an energy intake of 3200 Cal. or above per day during the unrestricted rehabilitation period resulted in a gradual restoration of the basal metabolism to the normal level.

Secretion of the Ductless Glands. The secretion of the thyroid gland has more influence on the regulation of the metabolic rate than do the secretions of any of the other ductless glands. Increases in the basal metabolism, as much as 80 per cent, have been found in cases of *exophthalmic goiter* (hyperthyroidism), whereas in cases of *myxedema* (hypothyroidism) the metabolic rate may be lowered as much as 30 to 40 per cent. Adrenalin, secretion of the adrenal glands, causes a temporary rise in heat production. Certain fractions of the pituitary secretion, the thyrotropic and also the adrenotropic, exert an influence by stimulating the thyroid and adrenal glands to function. The secretions of other endocrine glands, however, have a less marked effect, if any, on the basal heat production.

Pregnancy and Growth. The increase in total active tissue during pregnancy and growth results in an increase in the basal metabolic rate. Comparisons of the metabolic rates of pregnant women just before delivery showed increases of 15 to 23 per cent above their pre-pregnant rates (10). The additional active tissue is accounted for by the developing fetus and enlargement of certain maternal tissues. Indications are that lactation, however, does not cause an increase in the basal heat production.

Periods of rapid growth are associated with an increase in the basal metabolism. The period of most rapid growth in childhood is in infancy; a baby during the first 6 months of life will double his birth weight, and triple it by the end of 12 months. At the end of the second year of life or the early part of the third, the basal rate per square meter of body surface is the highest in the lifetime of an individual. At adolescence, when the growth rate again speeds up markedly, the basal metabolic rate increases also. A comprehensive evaluation of basal metabolic data for infants as well as for children and youth has been published by the U.S. Department of Agriculture (17, 18).

▶ THE REGULATION OF BODY TEMPERATURE

The body maintains its normal temperature at about 98.6°F (37°C) by both chemical and physical means. The chemical regulation involves the production of heat within the cells from the metabolism of the energy nutrients, whereas the physical regulation involves the loss or conservation of this heat in order to maintain a normal thermal balance.

Manner of Heat Loss from the Body

Heat is lost from the body in a variety of ways: by *radiation, convection,* and *conduction;* by *evaporation* of water from the skin and lungs; via the urine and feces; through the warming of the inspired air; and the warming of liquids and food consumed. In the processes of radiation and convection, the heat actually radiates from the body to the outside air when the environmental temperature is below that of the body. In man conduction (contact with a cold object or immersion in water) plays only a minor role in heat loss. About 5 per cent of the heat loss is attributed to loss in the urine and feces and to the warming of air, liquids, and food.

The environmental temperature affects the rate of heat loss, and the manner of heat disposal is affected by the humidity of the air. When the environmental temperature is lower than that of the body, most of the heat will be lost by radiation and conduction. When the temperature of the environment is equal to or above body temperature, all the heat must be eliminated by perspiration and evaporation of water from the lungs, because heat will neither radiate nor be conducted from a body of equal or lower temperature than its environment. Furthermore, dry air will favor a more rapid rate of evaporation of water from the body than will moist or humid air. It is for this reason that during the summer months a 100°F temperature reported from a low-humidity area like Arizona will not cause as much discomfort to an individual as an 85°F temperature reported from a humid area along the seacoast.

Regulation of Body Temperature

There is a range of environmental temperature for man and animals in which the metabolism is not affected. This range, referred to as the zone of thermal neutrality, is between 27°C (81°F) and 30° to 31°C (86° to 88°F) for men and 27°C (81°F) and 32° to 33°C (90° to 91°F) for women. As the environmental temperature is lowered, the point at which the body must deliberately produce extra heat to maintain a normal body temperature is referred to as the *critical temperature* (25° to 27°C or 77° to 81°F for man). It has been reported, however, that shivering begins when the skin temperature reaches 19°C or 66°F (22). Between the critical temperature and the point of shivering there is a gradual increase in the heat production which may be as high as 36 per cent and associated with a progressive tensing of the entire musculature. Shivering is an involuntary contraction of the skeletal muscles to produce heat for the maintenance of body temperature.

There are groups of native people in the world who have lived in cold climates for generations. Studies have been made with the Lapps, the Eskimos, and the Aborigines of Australia to observe how they adapt to the cold. Scholander (19) has reported that the nomadic Lapps living in northern Norway have a cultural adaptation to the cold through their clothing inasmuch as they are not normally subjected to cold stress. In the Eskimo the regulation of body temperature has been found to be adapted more to heat loss than to heat conservation because of their lower skin insulation (16). In contrast to the Lapp and the Eskimo, the naked or poorly clad Aborigine from central Australia is able to withstand his cold environment because of three factors: a low tissue thermal conductance, a tolerance for low-body temperatures, and a greater psychological tolerance for cold discomfort (20).

▶ THE ENERGY NEED FOR PHYSICAL ACTIVITY

Any kind of physical activity increases the energy expenditure above the basal caloric need. The amount of energy needed for physical work by the moderately-active man or woman usually comprises the second largest caloric expenditure after the expenditure for basal metabolism. This, however, would not be true for a very active individual, such as a football player or a lumberjack; his caloric expenditure for physical activity would rank ahead of that for basal metabolism.

The Energy Cost of Physical Activities

The energy cost of a physical activity is related to three factors: the amount of work done, the intensity of the work performed, and the body size of the individual.

Different kinds of activities require different amounts of energy. For example, it takes almost three times as much energy to walk upstairs (2.540 Cal./kg/10 min) as it does to walk downstairs (0.976 Cal./kg/10 min), about twice as much to play tennis (1.014 Cal./kg/10 min) as to play ping-pong (0.566 Cal./kg/10 min), and sitting writing a theme (0.268 Cal./kg/10 min) requires about 1.5 times as much energy as sitting reading a book (0.176 Cal./kg/10 min).

The caloric cost of the same activity will vary with the intensity of the task. For example, a college man walking on the level on a treadmill requires over three times as much energy walking at a speed of 5.80 mph (1.667 Cal./kg/10 min) as he does at a speed of 2.27 mph (0.513 Cal./kg/10 min).

The body size of the individual performing a task is related to the total cost of the activity. For example, the cost of the activity involved in sitting and participating in a one-hour college lecture class would be 43 per cent greater for a 176-lb (80 kg) college football player (118 Cal.) than for a 123-lb (56 kg) college coed (82 Cal.).

The energy expenditures in different kinds of physical activities have been compiled and listed by several groups of workers. The list presented in Table 8.1 (in terms of Calories per kilogram of body weight per 10 min.) was compiled by Consolazio, Johnson, and Pecora. To convert these figures to Cal./kg/min, one simply divides the value by 10 (e.g., showering = 0.466 Cal./kg/10 min or 0.0466 Cal./kg/min). Another

Table 8.1. Metabolic Costs of Various Activities Including Basal Metabolism and Specific Dynamic Effect

Activity	Cal./kg/ 10 min	Activity	Cal./kg/ 10 min
Archery	0.754	Running	5.514
Bicycling on level roads	0.734	Running long distance	2.203
Bowling	0.975	Running on grade (treadmill)	
Calisthenics	0.734	8.70 mph on 2.5% grade	2.652
Canoeing, 2.5 mph	0.441	8.70 mph on 3.8% grade	2.803
Canoeing, 4.0 mph	1.029	Running on level (treadmill)	
Carpentry	0.564	7.00 mph	2.045
Chopping wood	1.101	8.70 mph	2.273
Classwork, lecture	0.245	11.60 mph	2.879
Cleaning windows	0.607	Shining shoes	0.437
Conversing	0.269	Shooting pool	0.299
Cross-country running	1.630	Showering	0.466
Dancing, fox trot	0.650	Sitting, eating	0.204
Petronella	0.681	normally	0.176
Waltz	0.750	playing cards	0.210
Rumba	1.014	reading	0.176
Eightsome reel	1.000	writing	0.268
Moderately	0.612	Sled pulling (87 lb) 2.27 mph	1.242
Vigorously	0.831	Snowshoeing 2.27 mph	0.835
Dressing	0.466	Sprinting	3.423
Driving car	0.438	Stacking lumber	0.856
Driving motorcycle	0.531	Standing, light activity	0.356
Driving truck	0.342	normally	0.206
Farming, haying, plowing		Stone masonry	0.930
with horse	0.979	Sweeping floors	0.535
Farming, planting, hoeing,		Swimming (pleasure)	1.454
raking	0.686	Back stroke 25 yd per min	0.566
Farming chores	0.564	Back stroke 30 yd per min	0.778
Gardening, digging	1.365	Back stroke 35 yd per min	1.000
Gardening, weeding	0.862	Back stroke 40 yd per min	1.222
Golfing	0.794	Breast stroke 20 yd per min	0.704
House painting	0.514	Breast stroke 30 yd per min	1.056
Ironing clothes	0.627	Breast stroke 40 yd per min	1.408
Lying, quietly	0.195	Crawl 45 yd per min	1.278
Making bed	0.572	Crawl 55 yd per min	1.556
Metal working	0.514	Side stroke	1.222
Mopping floors	0.665	Truck and automobile repair	0.612
Mountain climbing	1.470	Volleyball	0.505
Personal toilet	0.278	Walking on level (treadmill)	
Pick-and-shovel work	0.979	2.27 mph	0.513
Pitching horseshoes	0.518	3.20 mph	0.690
Playing baseball		3.50 mph	0.733
(except pitcher)	0.686	4.47 mph	0.969

Table 8.1. (continued)

Activity	Cal./kg/ 10 min	Activity	Cal./kg/ 10 min
Playing football (American)	1.178	4.60 mph	1.212
Playing football (association)	1.308	5.18 mph	1.382
Playing Ping-Pong	0.566	5.80 mph	1.667
Playing pushball	1.122	Walking downstairs	0.976
Playing squash	1.522	upstairs	2.540
Playing tennis	1.014	Washing and dressing	0.382
Repaving roads	0.734	Washing and shaving	0.419
Resting in bed	0.174		
Rowing for pleasure	0.734		

From *Physiological Measurements of Metabolic Functions in Man* by Consolazio, Johnson, and Pecora. Copyright 1963. McGraw-Hill Book Co., New York. Used by permission.

compilation of energy expenditure data has been published by Passmore and Durnin (13). This compilation is based on new data from German and British surveys and other expenditure data over the past 50 years, including thirty-eight tables of energy expenditures for many kinds of activities and work.

That the cost of a physical activity may vary with the environmental temperature has been the subject of a human study (5). Consolazio and his group measured the energy expenditures of young men performing three levels of physical activity at three environmental temperatures (70°, 85°, and 100°F) and found that the metabolic cost of a fixed physical activity increased significantly in the heat.

Methods of Determining the Energy Needs for Physical Activity

One of the early ways devised to measure the energy used for a particular activity was the Douglas method, an indirect method. The expired air of the individual performing the activity is collected in a large bag and analyzed for carbon dioxide and oxygen content. Although an accurate method, its usefulness is limited because of the cumbersomeness of the collecting bag.

A new type of apparatus called the *respiration gas meter* was designed and constructed at the Max-Planck Institute in Germany. It consists of a lightweight box, containing a meter for recording the volume of the expired air, which straps on the back. The machine samples the expired air, portions of which are collected in a small bag attached to the meter. This eliminates the cumbersomeness of the Douglas method and increases the span of time for activity measurements. After the expired air collected during the activity performance test has been analyzed for carbon dioxide and oxygen, the caloric expenditure can be calculated. The respiration gas meter can be used to measure the energy expenditure of an individual either at rest or at work.

Today indirect calorimetry methods are used to study the energy cost of man's physical expenditures. Yet many of the early values on the cost of physical activities were obtained by the use of direct calorimetry methods which involved the use of respiration chambers. These chambers, which were used by laboratories in Germany and in this country, ranged in size from small ones that would accommodate only a man in either a standing or a reclining position to those that would house large farm animals. The Armsby Calorimeter (Fig. 8.3), which is the largest respiration calorimeter ever constructed, is still in existence on the campus of The Pennsylvania State University. In the past decade this calorimeter was used to study human energy problems.

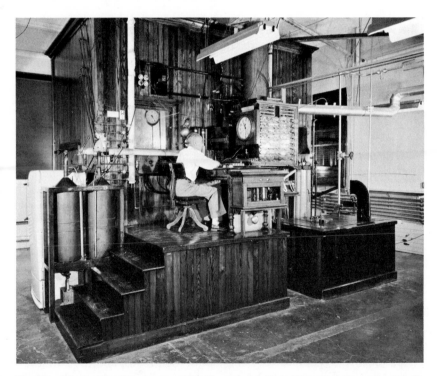

Fig. 8.3. The Armsby Calorimeter at The Pennsylvania State University. (Courtesy of Swift, Department of Animal Nutrition, The Pennsylvania State University.)

The respiration calorimeter, as the name indicates, combines the direct and indirect methods of energy determination. The complex apparatus includes an airtight, well-insulated chamber where the experimental subject stays during a test period. The heat evolved from the occupant is absorbed by water that circulates in metal coils located near the ceiling of the chamber. The amount of heat given off is computed from the rise in temperature of the water during its passage through the chamber and the amount of water that flows through the coils during the period of observation. Direct calorimetry also requires a knowledge of the amount of water that evaporates from the skin and lungs. This is determined by a comparison of the water contents of the air entering and leaving the chamber.

The indirect method of determining energy expenditure involves an analysis of the air entering and leaving the chamber for content of oxygen and carbon dioxide.

► THE ENERGY NEED FOR THE SPECIFIC DYNAMIC EFFECT

The increased heat production brought about by the ingestion of food itself is referred to as the *specific dynamic effect*. It is possible to explain the relationship of the specific dynamic effect to food eaten by comparing it to the system of tax withholding in this country. For example, if a man earns $400.00 per month, his "take-home" pay is not $400.00 but only $360.00 after taxes. The $400.00 salary represents the caloric value of a meal, and the $40.00 tax represents the heat increment of the specific dynamic effect.

In the past, the specific dynamic effect of food on the total metabolism has been greatly overrated. Early workers observed a dramatic increase in heat production by feeding test meals of individual portions of each of the three energy nutrients (carbohydrate, fat, or protein) as the sole nutrient in the diet. They assumed, moreover, that the dynamic effect of a mixed diet would be the sum of the increases brought about by each of its individual components and failed to study the actual heat production of diets which contained portions of all three of the energy nutrients.

The energy expenditure for the specific dynamic effect has been found in human experiments to be a small part of the total expenditure. Experiments have been conducted on college men to study the dynamic effects of long-time intakes of both high (about 122 gm daily) and low (about 34 gm daily) protein diets of equal Calorie value (23). These mixed diets were composed of commonly used foods, and the two levels of protein used represent the two extremes of protein intake which might be encountered within a population group. The Armsby Calorimeter was used to measure the total heat production of the subjects at selected 48-hour periods throughout the study. It was found that the specific dynamic effect on the high-protein diet, which furnished about 122 gm of protein per day, was about 8 per cent higher than that of the low-diet, where the protein content was only about 34 gm. An average estimate of the specific dynamic effect is 6 to 8 per cent of the sum of the energy expenditure of the basal metabolism and physical activities.

▶ THE TOTAL CALORIC REQUIREMENT

The total Calorie needs of an individual are directly related to the energy expenditures for the basal heat production, for physical activity, and for the specific dynamic effect of food eaten. It is possible to estimate these needs either by the use of the factorial method of calculation, or by the use of tables of recommended energy allowances. Both procedures have certain limitations. However, if these shortcomings are realized and the results interpreted in the light of their limitations, an approximate energy requirement obtained by either method can be used satisfactorily.

The Factorial Method of Determining Total Energy Needs

In this method of estimating energy requirement, the caloric need is calculated from the individual's basal metabolism, his physical activity, and the specific dynamic effect of his food. To illustrate the use of the factorial method, the energy need of a young male college student (19 years old, weighing 154 lb, and 66 in. tall) who participates in long-distance running is used.

Calculation of the Energy Expenditure for the Basal Metabolism. Basal metabolism may be calculated by the use of the simple formula (basal metabolism = kilograms of body weight × 1 Cal. per hour × 24 hr per day) which was presented early in this chapter. Using this formula, the first step in the calculation is to convert pounds to kilograms of body weight. The 154-pound college student used in this example therefore weighs 70 kilograms. By the substitution of this value in the formula, the energy expenditure for the basal metabolism of this college man is as follows:

$$= 70 \text{ kg} \times 1 \text{ Cal./hr} \times 24 \text{ hr/day}$$
$$= 1680 \text{ Cal./24 hr}$$

Table 8.2. The Daily Total Energy Expenditure of a Young Male College Student as Estimated by the Factorial Method

The total energy expenditure is 2800 Cal. for a 16-hr day	
The basal metabolism, uncorrected for sleep, is 1680 Cal. per 24 hr or 70 Cal. per hr and is included in the 16-hr activity day	
The remaining 8 hr, the uncorrected basal metabolism is 1680 − (16 × 70) = 1680 − 1120 = 560 Cal. Corrected for sleep, 560 − 56 = 504 Cal.	
Total energy expenditure during 16 hours of activity including basal metabolism and specific dynamic effect	2800 Cal.
8-hr basal metabolism corrected for sleep	504
Total energy expenditure per 24-hr day	3304 Cal.°

° Specific dynamic effect about 6% of total or 198 Cal.

Because the metabolic rate is lower than the basal during sleep, a correction must be made for the hours of sleep. The formula for the correction for sleep is 0.1 Cal. × kilograms of body weight × number of hours of sleep. After the substitution of numerical values in this formula (0.1 Cal. × 70 kg × 8 hr = 56 Cal.), the 56 Cal. difference must be deducted from the calculated basal metabolism for a 24-hour period (Table 8.2).

Calculation of the Energy Expenditure for Physical Activities. In order to estimate the energy expenditures for the physical activities of an individual, it is necessary to keep an accurate record of the kind and duration of all activities. There are two limitations, however, in the calculation of this part of the total energy need. First, it is difficult to determine correctly the amount of time spent in any activity, and second, data on the caloric expenditure for different kinds and intensities of activities are limited. It has been suggested that if energy expenditures of activities are expressed in Calories per minute rather than Calories per hour, there might be less error involved because few activities are carried on steadily for long periods of time (13). The development and the use of the respiratory gasmeter for determining the caloric expenditures for activity, rather than the Douglas method, has increased the variety and intensities of activities which can now be measured satisfactorily (13).

Using the energy costs of various activities given in Table 8.1, the Calories used for physical activity by the college student can be estimated. The number of Calories used for an activity per unit of body weight per minute, multiplied by the kilograms of body weight and the number of minutes of performance, give the energy expended for a particular physical activity. A list of the student's activities for a 7-day period follows:

	Time per Week		
Sleep	56 hr	0 min	
Washing and dressing	7	30	450 min
Washing and shaving	1	48	108
Showering	2	20	140
Eating meals and snacks	14	50	890
Sitting in classes	20	0	1200
Standing in chemistry lab	6	0	360
Running with the track team	6	25	385
Swimming (pleasure)	0	50	50
Studying, sitting reading	19	20	1160
Studying, sitting writing	10	20	620
Walking (about 2.27 mph)	10	15	615
Walking rapidly (5.80 mph)	0	10	10
Driving an automobile	10	0	600
Attending a movie	2	12	132
	168	0	

The caloric expenditure for the physical activities of this 70-kg college student is estimated then as follows:

	Energy Cost of Activity	Time Spent	Energy Expended
	Cal./kg/min	min	Cal./kg
Washing and dressing	0.0382	450	17.19
Washing and shaving	0.0419	108	4.53
Showering	0.0466	140	6.52
Eating meals and snacks	0.0204	890	18.16
Sitting in classes	0.0245	1200	29.40
Standing in chemistry lab	0.0356	360	12.82
Running with track team	0.2203	385	84.82
Swimming (pleasure)	0.1454	50	7.27
Studying, sitting reading	0.0176	1160	20.42
Studying, sitting writing	0.0268	620	16.62
Walking (about 2.7 mph)	0.0513	615	31.55
Walking rapidly (5.80 mph)	0.1667	10	1.67
Driving an automobile	0.0438	600	26.28
Attending a movie	0.0206	132	2.72
			279.97

Total energy expanded in physical activity per week =
    279.97 Cal./kg × 70 kg (body weight) = 19597.9 Cal. or 2800 Cal./day.

Estimation of the Specific Dynamic Effect of Food Eaten. The estimation of the specific dynamic effect of the food eaten is one of the
limiting factors in the determination of the total energy need. At this
time, however, it seems appropriate to allot between 6 and 8 per cent
of the sum of the energy expenditure of the basal metabolism and physical activities for this factor (Table 8.2).

*The Daily Total Energy Expenditure as Estimated by the Factorial
Method.* The daily total energy expenditure of this college student as
estimated by the factorial method is 3304 Cal. per day (Table 8.2).

► THE USE OF TABLES OF RECOMMENDED ENERGY
   ALLOWANCES OR SYSTEMS FOR DETERMINING TOTAL
   ENERGY NEED

Another approach to assessing the caloric need of an individual is
to use accepted tables of recommended energy allowances or systems
which have been developed by nutritionists on the basis of research and
their experienced judgment. The table of recommended daily dietary
allowances, which includes the need for Calories, was prepared for use
in this country by the Food and Nutrition Board of the National Research
Council (NRC), whereas the Calorie requirements proposed by the
Food and Agriculture Organization of the United Nations (FAO) are
designed for use on an international scale (4). Here as with the factorial
method, there are certain limitations in the use of either the NRC tables
or the FAO system for assessing energy need.

The Recommended Allowances for Energy

The allowances for Calories adopted by the Food and Nutrition
Board in the 1963 revision of the NRC Recommended Dietary Allowances (15) are based on the formula of the "Reference Man" and "Reference Woman" proposed by the first FAO Committee on Calorie
Requirements (3). The Reference Man weighs 70 kg, and the Reference
Woman, 58 kg. Both individuals are 25 years old, live in an environment
with a mean temperature of 20°C, and are considered to be moderately-
active. In the new NRC allowances, however, the caloric values for
adult persons are lower than those proposed in previous revisions (Table
8.3). The basis for lowering the energy values stems from the fact that
the caloric expenditure of the average American adult was found to be
lower than the energy as derived from the mathematical expression used
to calculate the value. For example, the daily allowance for a 20-year-

Table 8.3. The Daily Recommended Calorie Allowances of the NRC

Age, years	Males Cal.	Both Sexes Cal.	Females Cal.
Infants, up to 1 yr		kg × 115 ± 15	
1–3		1300	
3–6		1600	
6–9		2100	
9–12	2400		2200
12–15	3000		2500
15–18	3400		2300
18–35[1]	2900		2100
35–55[1]	2600		1900
55–75[1]	2200		1600
			add 200 Cal. for 2nd and 3rd trimesters of pregnancy
			add 1000 Cal. for lactation

[1] 70-kg (154 lb) man and 58-kg (128 lb) woman.

From *Recommended Dietary Allowances Sixth Revised Edition.* Natl. Acad. Sci.—Natl. Res. Council, Publ. 1146, p. vii, 1964.

old college man (70 kg) and woman (58 kg) has been lowered from 3200 to 2900 Cal. and 2300 to 2100 Cal., respectively.

The energy allowances for adults of different ages as well as for the stress periods of pregnancy, lactation, and growth are presented (Table 8.3).

The Adjustments for Age, Body Size, and Climate. The energy allowances proposed at this time incorporate adjustments for age, body size, and climate. The allowances as they are derived represent the average needs of persons for the age 25 years or to cover the years from 18 to 35. Because the energy requirements decline steadily throughout life (a decrease in the basal metabolism and physical activity), the allowance for Calories also must be reduced. The energy allowances are reduced by 5 per cent per decade between ages 35 and 55, by 8 per cent per decade between ages 55 and 75, and by 10 per cent beyond the age of 75.

Individuals whose body size is greater or less than the reference formula will have caloric requirements above or below the standard allowance. In order to adjust for differences in body size, a table of Calorie allowances based on body weights and age has been compiled

(Table 8.4). For example, a 20-year-old college woman whose desirable weight is 110 lb (50 kg) has a daily allowance of 1900 Cal., whereas another girl of the same age weighing 154 lb (70 kg) will need about 2400 Cal. per day.

Most individuals in the United States live in an area where the mean environmental temperature averages 68°F (20°C); however, when there is exposure to cold or heat, adjustment in the energy allowance may be necessary (15).

Table 8.4. Adjustment of Calorie Allowances for Adult Individuals of Various Body Weights and Ages[1]

Desirable Weight			Calorie Allowance[2]		
kg	lb		25 years	45 years	65 years
		Men	(1)	(2)	(3)
50	110		2,300	2,050	1,750
55	121		2,450	2,200	1,850
60	132		2,600	2,350	1,950
65	143		2,750	2,500	2,100
70	154		2,900	2,600	2,200
75	165		3,050	2,750	2,300
80	176		3,200	2,900	2,450
85	187		3,350	3,050	2,550
		Women	(4)	(5)	(6)
40	88		1,600	1,450	1,200
45	99		1,750	1,600	1,300
50	110		1,900	1,700	1,450
55	121		2,000	1,800	1,550
58	128		2,100	1,900	1,600
60	132		2,150	1,950	1,650
65	143		2,300	2,050	1,750
70	154		2,400	2,200	1,850

Formulas

(1) 725 + 31W	(2) 650 + 28W	(3) 550 + 23.5W
(4) 525 + 27W	(5) 475 + 24.5W	(6) 400 + 20.5W
W = weight in kg		

[1] At a mean environmental temperature of 20°C. (68°F.) assuming average physical activity.
[2] Values have been rounded to nearest 50 calories. To convert formulas for weight in pounds, divide factor by 2.2.

From *Recommended Dietary Allowances Sixth Revised Edition*. Natl. Acad. Sci.—Natl. Res. Council, Publ. 1146, p. 5, 1964.

Table 8.5. The Calorie Requirements of the FAO[1]

Age Group	Males Cal.	Both Sexes Cal.	Females Cal.
0–1		1120	
1–3		1300	
4–6		1700	
7–9		2100	
10–12	2500		2400
13–15	3100		2600
16–19	3600		2400
20–29	3200		2300
30–39	3104		2231
40–49	3008		2162
50–59	2768		1990
60–69	2528		1817
70+	2208		1587

[1] Based on FAO reference standards of body size and environmental temperature (Adult weights: male, 65 kg; female, 55 kg. Temperature: 10°C.)

From *Calorie Requirements*. Food Agr. Organ. U.N., FAO Nutr. Studies No. 15, p. 46, 1957.

The FAO System

The need for a system of international energy standards was recognized during the Second World War. Since that time two reports (3, 4) have been prepared by the Committee on Calorie Requirements of the FAO for assessing the caloric requirement, which with appropriate adjustments can be applied to different people in different parts of the world.

The FAO system derives caloric requirements for adult populations from the measurements of two "reference" persons as does the NRC system. Tables of numerical values are then used to assess energy needs of populations based on variations in body size, age, and environmental temperature. For example, according to the FAO system, the energy allowance for 21-year-old women weighing 55 kg and living in a climate where the annual temperature averages 10°C is 2300 Cal. (Table 8.5). If these same women lived in a part of the world where the average temperature was 20°C rather than 10°C, their energy requirement would be 5 per cent less or 2185 Cal. At age 64, these same women would have a caloric allowance 21 per cent less (1817 Cal.) than their needs at age 21.

The FAO energy requirements for childhood and early adolescence are assessed independently of the reference requirements, except as they pertain to environmental temperature. In late adolescence, ages 16 to 20, the caloric requirements are based on body size as well as climate. The additional energy allowance for reproduction and lactation has been assessed as 40,000 extra Cal. per pregnancy and 180,000 extra Cal. per lactation. This modern statement of assessing energy needs is highly tentative and open to testing and further research. However, it has been used satisfactorily in providing for the periodic evaluation of the world food situation as well as in planning for the food production programs in many countries.

The Limitations of the NRC Table and the FAO System

The caloric allowances as proposed by the NRC table and the FAO system are tentative guides to estimate the energy needs of populations and population groups. They are not directed to individuals. The most variable factor in estimating energy needs is the difference in physical activity among people. The activity definition of the "Reference Man and Woman" in both the NRC and FAO systems corresponds generally to the average activity of the population. In cases of greater activity, the caloric allowances must be increased. The NRC system suggests that a maximum of 25 per cent increase above the standard level should account for the extra Calories needed for the usual type of heavy work. For example, 19-year-old football players in the United States may need 725 more Cal. each day during football season than will moderately active men of the same age. In contrast to this, caloric levels should be reduced when the activity is less than that defined for "the Reference Man or Woman." It has been suggested that the allowance is best judged for adequacy by weight change and status of health.

▶ A GUIDE TO THE SELECTION OF FOODS TO MEET THE ENERGY NEEDS OF COLLEGE MEN AND WOMEN

In view of the present downward trend in Calorie allowances, greater care must be taken by college men and women to select foods that contribute other nutrients as well as energy to the diet. Some foods contribute only Calories to the food intake (e.g., 1 tsp sugar = 15 Cal. and an 8-oz carbonated beverage = 95 Cal.). These types of foods are said to contain "empty Calories" and should be used in limited amounts by college-age individuals.

Of all the nutrients, the need for energy is most easily obtained by man because all foods carry Calories; and in this country because of our overabundance of food, it is sometimes difficult for a person not to exceed his energy need.

REFERENCES

1. Best, C. H., and N. B. Taylor (1961). *The Physiological Basis of Medical Practice*, 7th ed. Williams and Wilkins Co., Baltimore.
2. Blackburn, C. M., and M. H. Powell (1955). Diagnostic accuracy of serum protein-bound iodine determination in thyroid disease. *J. Clin. Endocrinol. Metab.* 15: 1379.
3. *Calorie Requirements* (1950). Food Agr. Organ. U.N., FAO Nutr. Studies No. 5, Rome.
4. *Calorie Requirements* (1957). Food Agr. Organ. U.N., FAO Nutr. Studies No. 15, Rome.
5. Consolazio, C. F., L. O. Matoush, R. A. Nelson, J. B. Torres, and G. J. Isaac (1963). Environmental temperature and energy expenditure. *J. Appl. Physiol.* 18: 65.
6. Galvao, P. E. (1950). Human heat production in relation to body weight and body surface. III. Inapplicability of surface law on fat men of tropical zones. IV. General interpretation of climatic influences on metabolism. *J. Appl. Physiol.* 3: 21.
7. Keys, A., J. Brozek, A. Henschel, O. Mickelsen, and H. L. Taylor (1950). *The Biology of Human Starvation*. Vol. I. University of Minnesota Press, Minneapolis.
8. Lewis, H. E., J. P. Masterton, and S. Rosenbaum (1961). Stability of basal metabolic rate on a polar expedition. *J. Appl. Physiol.* 16: 397.
9. Lewis, R. C., A. Iliff, and A. M. Duval (1943). Further consideration of the effect of altitude on basal metabolism. *J. Nutr.* 26: 175.
10. MacLeod, G., C. Taylor, E. Robb, D. Baker, M. O'Donahoe, and P. McCrery (1939). The basal metabolism of pregnancy. *J. Nutr.* 17: suppl. 20.
11. Mann, A., W. S. Dreizen, and T. D. Spies (1947). The determination of status and progress in children with nutritive failure. *J. Pediat.* 31: 161.
12. Milan, F. A., J. P. Hannon, and E. Evonuk (1963). Temperature regulation of Eskimos, Indians, and Caucasians in a bath calorimeter. *J. Appl. Physiol.* 18: 378.
13. Passmore, R., and J. V. G. A. Durnin (1955). Human energy expenditure. *Physiol. Rev.* 35: 801.
14. Picon-Reategui, E. (1961). Basal metabolic rate and body composition at high altitudes. *J. Appl. Physiol.* 16: 431.
15. *Recommended Dietary Allowances Sixth Revised Edition* (1964). Natl. Acad. Sci.—Natl. Res. Council, Publ. 1146, Washington, D.C.
16. Rennie, D. W., B. G. Covino, M. R. Blair, and K. Rodahl (1962). Physical regulation of temperature in Eskimos. *J. Appl. Physiol.* 17: 326.
17. Sargent, D. W. (1961). *An Evaluation of Basal Metabolic Data for Children and Youth in the United States*. U.S. Dept. Agr., Home Econ. Res. Rept. No. 14, Washington, D.C.
18. Sargent, D. W. (1962). *An Evaluation of Basal Metabolic Data for Infants in the United States*. U.S. Dept. Agr., Home Econ. Res. Rept. No. 18, Washington, D.C.
19. Scholander, P. F., K. L. Anderson, J. Krog, F. V. Lorentzen, and J. Steen (1957). Critical temperature in Lapps. *J. Appl. Physiol.* 10: 234.
20. Scholander, P. F., H. T. Hammel, J. S. Hart, D. H. LeMessurier, and J. Steen (1958). Cold adaptation in Australian aborigines. *J. Appl. Physiol.* 13: 211.
21. *Techniques for Measuring Body Composition* (1961). Natl. Acad. Sci.—Natl. Res. Council, Washington, D.C.

22. Swift, R. W. (1932). The effects of low environmental temperature upon metabolism. I. Technique and respiratory quotient. *J. Nutr.* **5**: 213.
23. Swift, R. W., G. P. Barron, Jr., K. H. Fisher, N. D. Magruder, A. Black, J. W. Bratzler, C. E. French, E. W. Hartsook, T. J. Hershberger, E. Keck, and F. P. Stiles (1957). *Relative Dynamic Effects of High Versus Low Protein Diets of Equicaloric Content.* Penn. State Univ. Agr. Expt. Sta., Bull. 618, University Park.
24. Swift, R. W., and K. H. Fisher (1964). Energy metabolism. In *Nutrition a Comprehensive Treatise.* Vol. I. (G. H. Beaton and E. W. McHenry, eds.) Academic Press, New York.

SUPPLEMENTARY REFERENCES

DuBois, E. F. (1936). *Basal Metabolism in Health and Disease.* Lea and Febiger, Philadelphia.
Swift, R. W., and C. E. French (1954). *Energy Metabolism and Nutrition.* The Scarecrow Press, Washington, D.C.
Swift, R. W. (1959). Food energy. In *Food. The Yearbook of Agriculture 1959.* (A Stefferud, ed.) U.S. Dept. Agr., Washington, D.C.
Taylor, C. M., G. MacLeod, and M. S. Rose (1956). *Foundations of Nutrition,* 5th ed. The Macmillan Co., New York.

CHAPTER 9

The energy value of foods

The amount of carbohydrate, fat, and protein in a food determines its energy value. The source of energy in these compounds is energy from sunlight. The plant has a unique capacity to convert solar energy into the chemical energy of a variety of organic compounds. Water and carbon dioxide through the process of photosynthesis combine to form carbohydrate. Photosynthesis takes place through the catalytic influence of the green pigment chlorophyll located in chloroplasts, small granules in the cell, visible in an electron microscope.

By means of radioactive carbon (isotopic carbon) and refined analytical methods, it has been possible to follow the pathway of carbon in the photosynthetic process. In addition to carbohydrate, the radioactive carbon has been found in lipids and amino acids. All of this takes place in the minute chloroplast of the cell through many reactions and the formation of many intermediary compounds.

Animals are dependent on food as the source of energy to do work and maintain body temperature. It thus becomes obvious that the process of photosynthesis is basic to life itself (1, 2, 3).

The potential energy stored in the chief organic compounds of food (carbohydrate, fat, and protein) is released on combustion. When these compounds are burned in the laboratory or oxidized in the body, energy is released through a series of reactions. One of the prime designations between organic compounds (those containing carbon) and inorganic compounds (minerals) is that organic compounds are combustible, inorganic ones are not. For instance, water (H_2O), an inorganic compound, has no fuel value.

Foods with relatively large proportions of carbohydrate, fat, and protein per unit of weight are high in energy content (caloric value) whereas those with small proportions are low in caloric value (Fig. 9.1). An ordinary pat of butter has an energy value of 50 Cal. because of its high fat content. In contrast, the portion of tomato juice equivalent to the energy value (in Calories) of the pat of butter is 35 times greater by weight, or one cup.

The caloric values of some favorite foods of college students are shown in Table 9.1; those of other commonly used foods are listed in Table A-8 (appendix).

Determination of Food Energy

In the laboratory, the *bomb calorimeter* and the *oxycalorimeter* are the two instruments used to determine the energy value of a food. The former measures the heat produced when a food is actually burned, whereas the latter measures the oxygen used and the carbon dioxide produced during the burning of a food. Because the bomb calorimeter is more widely used in energy determinations of foodstuffs, it will be the only method described here.

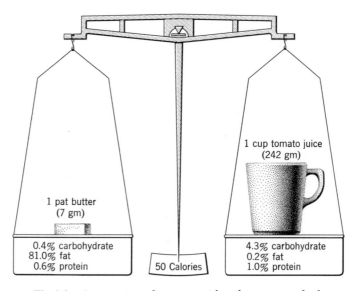

Fig. 9.1. A comparison of an energy-rich and energy-poor food.

Table 9.1. Caloric Value of Some Favorite Foods of College Students

Food	Portion	Cal./Serving
Apple	1 med	70
Beef, steak, sirloin	8-oz steak	460
Cake, chocolate with fudge icing	2-in. sector	445
Candy, chocolate almond bar	1-oz bar	176[1]
Carbonated beverage, cola type	8 oz	95
Catsup	1 tbsp	15
Chicken, broiler, fried	¼ bird, no bone	232[1]
Crackers, saltines, 2-in. square	4 crackers	70
Doughnuts, cake type	1 doughnut	125
Frankfurter in a roll	1 frank, 1 roll	270
Hamburger in a roll	3 oz beef, 1 roll	360
Ice cream	⅛ qt	145
Lobster, broiled or boiled	1 (¾ lb) lobster, 2 tbsp butter	308[1]
Milk, chocolate	8 oz	190
Milk, nonfat (skim)	8 oz	90
Milk, whole	8 oz	160
Milkshake, chocolate	8 oz whole milk, 2 tbsp chocolate sirup, ⅛ qt ice cream	405
Peanut butter	1 tbsp	95
Pickle relish	1 tbsp	14[1]
Pie, apple	4-in. sector	345
Pizza, cheese	5½-in. sector	185
Potato chips	10 chips	115
Potatoes, French fried	10 pieces	155
Salad, fresh fruit	3 hp tbsp, 2 lv lettuce	174[1]
Salad, potato	½ c with French dressing	184[1]
Spaghetti, Italian-style	1 serving with grated cheese	436[1]

[1] From Church, C. F., and H. N. Church. *Food Values of Portions Commonly Used—Bowes and Church*, 9th ed. J. B. Lippincott Co., Philadelphia, 1962.

Adapted from *Nutritive Value of Foods*. U.S. Dept. Agr., Home and Garden Bull. 72, revised 1964.

The bomb calorimeter apparatus consists of two parts: the bomb, in which the food is burned, and the water-bath arrangement, which measures the heat produced from the combustion (Fig. 9.2). After the sample of food to be analyzed is weighed, compacted, and placed in the bomb, the two halves of the bomb are screwed together and oxygen is introduced into it. Then the bomb is placed in the insulated water bath which contains a known amount of water. The water is agitated by a

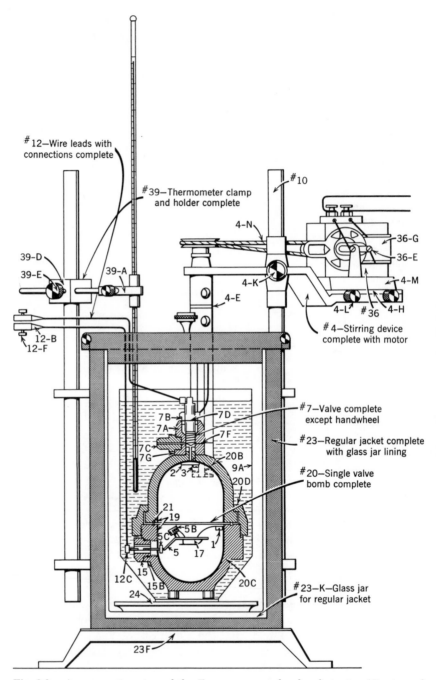

#12—Wire leads with connections complete

#39—Thermometer clamp and holder complete

#10

4-N

39-D
39-E
39-A

4-K
4-E

36-G
36-E
4-M

12-B
12-F

4-L #36 4-H

#4—Stirring device complete with motor

7B 7D
7A
7C 7F
7G
2 3   20B
9A
20D

#7—Valve complete except handwheel

#23—Regular jacket complete with glass jar lining

#20—Single valve bomb complete

21
19
5C 5B
5C 1
5 17

12C
15
15B
24
20C

#23-K—Glass jar for regular jacket

23F

Fig. 9.2. A cross-section view of the Emerson oxygen bomb calorimeter. (Courtesy of Arthur H. Thomas Company, Philadelphia.)

128

mechanical stirrer. A thermometer, which can be read to a thousandth of a degree, is used to measure the temperature of the water before and after combustion. The bomb is "fired" when an electric current is passed through the fine iron-wire fuse that is attached to the food sample within the bomb chamber. Here when the excess amount of oxygen present causes complete combustion of the food, the heat is conducted from the bomb to the water, and the increase in temperature is measured. From the temperature readings, the energy value or *fuel value* of the food can be calculated. The energy value of foods in food composition tables is based on bomb calorimeter measurements.

The fuel values of the three energy nutrients are different. A gram of fat yields 9.45 Cal. whereas only 4.10 Cal. of energy are obtained when a gram of carbohydrate is burned in the bomb calorimeter. The fuel value of a gram of protein, 5.65 Cal., is higher than the fuel value of a gram of carbohydrate.

The Physiological Fuel Values of Foods

The animal body does not derive as much energy from the food it ingests as is released in the bomb calorimeter. During the combustion of a food in the bomb calorimeter, all the available energy can be measured because the carbon, hydrogen, and nitrogen of the energy nutrients contained in the foodstuffs are completely changed to the simplest components: carbon dioxide, water, and nitrous oxide. The body, however, is not as efficient in its use of food because the energy foods are not completely digested and absorbed from the digestive system, and the nitrogen from protein is not completely changed to nitrous oxide. For these reasons, the amount of energy that one obtains from the carbohydrate, fat, and protein of the diet is somewhat less than the bomb calorimeter fuel values that have been presented. These values, based upon the body's use of energy, are referred to as the *physiological fuel values*

When one knows the correction factors for the energy losses due to the incomplete digestion and absorption of energy foods as well as the incomplete combustion of nitrogen in proteins, it is easy to calculate the physiological fuel values of the energy nutrients (Table 9.2). The first step is to subtract 1.25 Cal. per gm from the fuel value of protein, which accounts for the energy lost from the incomplete combustion of the nitrogen. Because it has been found that about 98 per cent of the carbohydrate, 95 per cent of the fat, and only 92 per cent of the protein ingested is absorbed by the human digestive mechanism, the second step in the calculation is to multiply each of the remaining fuel values by its percentage of digestibility. The final values of 4 Cal. per gm for

Table 9.2. The Calculation of the Physiological Fuel Values of Carbohydrate, Fat, and Protein

	Carbohydrate, Cal./gm	Fat, Cal./gm	Protein, Cal./gm
Fuel values	4.10	9.45	5.65
Loss due to incomplete combustion of nitrogen			−1.25
	4.10	9.45	4.40
Percentage of digestibility	×0.98	×0.95	×0.92
Physiological fuel values	4	9	4

carbohydrate, 9 Cal. per gm for fat, and 4 Cal. per gm for protein are the physiological fuel values that can be used with reasonable accuracy to calculate the energy content of any food.

The Limitations in the Use of the Physiological Fuel Values. During and after the Second World War, the first step in the food rehabilitation of the hungry nations of the world was to meet their energy needs. It was found, however, that the energy evaluation procedures used in the United States did not always apply to the national diets of other countries. It was pointed out that the physiological fuel values 4-9-4 were based on data applicable only to the foods of the average mixed American diet, and not to single foods or foods of different mixed diets eaten by other nations. To illustrate the significance of this international problem in planning for the food needs of the world population, an example is cited concerning the energy value of rice. According to the values 4-9-4, 100 gm of polished rice used in this country averages 351 Cal. whereas the values for the same amount of the undermilled and brown rice used in the Orient averages 340 and 320 Cal. respectively. On an international scale where millions of tons of rice are involved, the 4-9-4 figures would overvalue the caloric content of this food. In order to overcome this problem it was recognized that a universal method for the determination and expression of food energy values, as well as for other food nutrients, was needed. Since that time several publications have become available which have used specific factors as the basis for the calculations of the available energy in foods (4).

Calculations of the Energy Value of Foods

Although the physiological fuel values may not be valid to use in calculating the caloric value of international food supplies, they are useful in this country. If the percentage of carbohydrate, fat, and protein is known, it is easy to calculate its energy value by using the 4-9-4 figures.

The amount of carbohydrate, fat, and protein in a food is determined by chemical analysis. Most foods contain fractions of all three of the energy nutrients (Table A-8, appendix). For example, whole milk contains 4.9 per cent carbohydrate, 3.9 per cent fat, and 3.5 per cent protein. Yet there are some foods in the diet, such as white sugar and salad oil, that are rich in just one of the nutrients. Salad oil contains 100 per cent fat; 99.5 per cent of sugar is in the form of carbohydrate.

To find the approximate caloric value of 50 gm of salad oil, the percentage of fat in the oil (100 per cent) would be multiplied by the amount of oil (50 gm). The amount of fat is thus found to be 50 gm. Fifty times the physiological fuel value of 1 gm of fat (9 Cal.) equals 450 Cal., the caloric value of the oil. If the energy value of 100 gm of whole milk was calculated by using the 4-9-4 values, the procedure would be as follows:

	Per gm	Physiological Fuel Value, Cal./gm	Cal./gm
Carbohydrate	0.049	4	0.196
Fat	0.039	9	0.351
Protein	0.035	4	0.140
			0.687

1 gm whole milk = 0.687 Cal.

100 gm whole milk = 0.687 × 100 = 68.7 or 69 Cal.

Methods for Measuring or Estimating the Caloric Value of a Diet

The two ways in which the Calories of the food intake can be measured are by bomb calorimeter assays of the food eaten or by calculations of diet records from food tables. Distinction should be made here that the laborious bomb calorimeter assay is the actual true measure of food energy and is used in research studies where the exact caloric value of the food eaten is important. If, however, a college student wanted to know the number of Calories that he ate in one day, he could calculate this by using either a long or a short method of dietary analysis. In the long method an accepted table of food values would be used to count the Calories contributed by the amounts of the individual foods eaten. The use of a condensed table of caloric values in the short method proves to be a time saver in calculating dietary energy.

It is interesting to compare the energy values of a typical breakfast meal using these three methods of evaluation: the bomb calorimeter

Table 9.3. A Comparison of the Energy Value of a Typical Breakfast Meal
as Assessed by Bomb Calorimeter Assays, Long, and Short Methods of Dietary
Calculation

		Method of Dietary Assessment		
Food	Measure	Bomb Assay,[1] Cal.	Long Method,[2] Cal.	Short Method,[3] Cal.
Orange juice	1 serving (100 gm)	42	45	50
Scrambled eggs	1 serving (100 gm)	200	163	160
White enriched bread	2 sl (46 gm)	129	124	130
Butter	1 tbsp (14 gm)	107	100	100
Grape jelly	2 tbsp (40 gm)	102	109	120
Whole milk	8 oz (244 gm)	181	161	160
		761	702	720

[1] Relative Dynamic Effects of High versus Low Protein Diets of Equicaloric Content. Penn.
State Univ. Agr. Expt. Sta. Bull. 618, 1957.
[2] Composition of Foods—Raw, Processed, Prepared. U.S. Dept. Agr., Agr. Handbook 8,
revised 1963.
[3] Food Composition Table for Short Method of Dietary Analysis (3rd revision). J. Am. Dietet.
Assoc. Nov., 1965.

assay, the long method, and the short method of calculation (Table 9.3).
The foods analyzed and calculated were orange juice, scrambled eggs,
white bread, butter, grape jelly, and whole milk. The meal actually
contained 761 Cal. as assayed by the bomb calorimeter. When calculated
by the long method, a value of 702 Cal. was obtained, and the short
method of calculation gave a value of 720 Cal. According to these data,
there is good agreement between the values for the bomb assay and the
long and short method of calculation. The energy values calculated by
the long and short method, however, were approximately 8 and 5 per cent
lower respectively.

REFERENCES

1. Calvin, M. (1962). The path of carbon in photosynthesis. Science 50: 436.
2. Downes, H. R. (1962). The Chemistry of Living Cells. Harper and Row, New York, p. 609.
3. Galston, A. W. (1961). The Life of the Green Plant. Prentice-Hall, Englewood Cliffs, N.J.
4. Watt, B. K., and A. L. Merrill (1963). Composition of Foods—Raw, Processed, Prepared.
   U.S. Dept. Agr., Agr. Handbook 8, revised, Washington, D.C.

SUPPLEMENTARY REFERENCES

Chatfield, C. (1953). Food Composition Tables for International Use. Food Agr. Organ. U.N.,
   FAO Nutr. Studies No. 3, Rome.

Church, C. F., and H. N. Church (1962). *Food Values of Portions Commonly Used—Bowes and Church*. 9th ed. J. B. Lippincott Co., Philadelphia.

Leung, W. W., R. K. Pecot, and B. K. Watt (1952). *Composition of Foods Used in Far Eastern Countries*. U.S. Dept. Agr., Agr. Handbook 34, Washington, D.C.

Leung, W. W., and M. Flores (1961). *Food Composition Table for Use in Latin America*. Interdepartmental Committee on Nutrition for National Defense, National Institutes of Health, Bethesda, Md.

Lowenberg, M. E., and E. D. Wilson (1959). *Nutrients in Frozen Foods*. Natl. Assoc. Frozen Food Packers, Washington, D.C.

McCance, R. A., and E. M. Widdowson (1960). *The Composition of Foods*. Her Majesty's Stationery Office, London.

Miller, C. D., and B. Branthoover (1957). *Nutritive Values of Some Hawaii Foods*. Hawaii Agr. Expt. Sta., Cir. 52, Honolulu.

Watt, B. K., A. L. Merrill, and M. L. Orr (1959). A table of food values. In *Food. The Yearbook of Agriculture 1959*. (A. Stefferud, ed.) U.S. Dept. Agr., Washington, D.C.

CHAPTER 10

Introduction to minerals: calcium and phosphorus

► INTRODUCTION TO MINERALS

Thus far the organic compounds, carbohydrates, lipids, and proteins have been discussed. The chief chemical elements in these compounds are carbon, oxygen, hydrogen, and nitrogen. With water, these compounds comprise about 96 per cent of the body weight (Table 10.1), and the remainder, approximately 4 per cent, is made up of the mineral elements.

The mineral elements are also referred to as inorganic or ash constituents. On combustion of a substance such as coal or wood, for example, the organic matter burns, the inorganic remains; hence the terminology, ash constituents. In the body the minerals provided in food remain after the organic compounds of which they are a part have been oxidized. All of the nutrients listed in Table 10.1 have an established purpose in animal nutrition. More is known about the nutritional significance of some minerals than others. There has been less extensive research with the human, and as a consequence, the significance of some elements for man is less well established.

At this time, it is known that animals and man require fourteen different mineral elements for good health and growth. Certain ones, calcium, phosphorus, sodium, chlorine, potassium, magnesium, and sulfur, are needed in appreciable amounts; others, iron, manganese, cop-

Table 10.1. Elementary Composition of the Adult Human Body

Chemical Elements	Percentages
Oxygen	65
Carbon	18
Hydrogen	10
Nitrogen	3.0
Calcium	1.5–2.2[1]
Phosphorus	0.8–1.2[2]
Potassium	0.35
Sulfur	0.25
Sodium	0.15
Chlorine	0.15
Magnesium	0.05
Iron	0.004
Manganese	0.0003
Copper	0.00015
Iodine	0.00004
Cobalt	trace
Zinc	trace
Others found in minute traces	

[1] Estimates of normal calcium content vary widely.
[2] Phosphorus varies with calcium. (Adapted from Sherman, *Chemistry of Food and Nutrition*, 8th ed., The Macmillan Co., New York, p. 227, 1952.)

per, iodine, zinc, cobalt, and molybdenum, are needed only in very small amounts or traces. This latter group, therefore, has come to be referred to as the "trace elements." Furthermore, traces of mineral elements such as aluminum, boron, vanadium, and others have been found in animal tissues, but as yet there is not conclusive evidence that any of these has a specific biological function.

Mineral elements are present in the body in combination with organic compounds, in combination with other inorganic ions, and as free ions. For example, some of the calcium present in blood is bound to protein, some is present as free ions. In bone, phosphorus exists in combination with the mineral calcium. In body cells phosphorus is in organic combination with lipids to form phospholipids, with proteins to form phosphoproteins, and with other compounds to form substances important in the metabolic processes of the body.

▶ FUNCTIONS OF THE MINERALS

The mineral elements function in two general roles, as building substances and as regulatory substances. As structural constituents they serve in three general ways:

(1) As building constituents in the hard tissues of the body, the bones and teeth, giving rigidity to these structures.

(2) As components in soft tissue: muscle protein contains sulfur; other substances in muscle tissue contain phosphorus; nervous tissue contains phosphorus.

(3) As components in compounds essential to the functioning of the body: iodine is present in thyroxine, zinc in insulin, cobalt in vitamin B_{12}, sulfur in thiamine, iron in hemoglobin, and other compounds in tissue cells.

As components in body fluids the minerals have important regulatory functions. Some of the ways in which the minerals aid in the regulation of body processes are discussed more fully with the appropriate mineral but are enumerated here:

(1) They contribute to the osmotic pressure of body fluids.

(2) They contribute to the maintenance of approximate neutrality in the blood and body tissues by helping to protect against the accumulation of either too much acid or too much base (alkali).

(3) They make possible normal rhythm in the heart beat.

(4) They help to maintain a normal response of nerves to stimuli.

(5) They are essential for blood clot formation.

Three chapters have been devoted to the study of the minerals: calcium and phosphorus (Chapter 10), iron and iodine (Chapter 11), and the other minerals (Chapter 12). The role of fluorine in nutrition is discussed in Chapters 12 and 23, and Strontium-90 in the diet is presented in Chapter 26.

▶ CALCIUM

The body contains more calcium than any other mineral. It accounts for approximately 2 per cent (2 to 3 lb) of the body weight of the adult. In the newborn the skeleton is only partly mineralized and the total amount of calcium is 25 to 30 gm. About 99 per cent of the total amount in the body is concentrated in the bones and teeth; the remainder is in the fluids and soft tissues.

Functions of Calcium

Calcium serves two important functions in the body—the building of bones and teeth and the regulation of certain body processes. The need for calcium for building the skeletal structure is, of course, greater during the years of growth, but the need does not cease when full growth is attained. Once bone is formed, it continues to change, with processes of building new bone and destroying old going on simultaneously. With such changes going on in the bone, it does not seem surprising that the calcium of bone interchanges readily with the calcium of blood and other tissues. Regulatory functions are carried on by calcium in tissue and blood. Normal behavior of heart muscles, nerves, and the blood clotting process all depend on the presence of calcium.

Building Bones and Teeth. Calcium, together with other mineral elements, gives rigidity and permanence to bones and teeth. These characteristics make it possible for bone to be the support of the body, providing the rigid structure to which muscle tissue is attached. Bone forms protective cavities for vital organs—heart and lungs in the chest cavity, the brain in the cranial cavity. Although bone will withstand almost as much weight as cast iron before breaking, it is itself light in weight.

The chief minerals in bone are calcium and phosphorus. Others include sodium, magnesium, chlorine, molybdenum, and zinc, all of which have known physiological functions in the body. In addition, a large number of minerals identified in bone which have no recognized physiological function are strontium, lead, fluorine, radium, barium, yttrium, uranium, plutonium, americium, cerium, zirconium, actinium, beryllium, and gallium (21).

The exact structure of the chief components in bone (calcium, phosphate, and carbonate) has not been determined. There is evidence that it may be a hydroxyapatite, a complex compound, containing calcium phosphate and calcium hydroxide (1). How the other elements take part in the unique mineral structure of bone is not known precisely.

The minerals in bone are deposited in an organic framework of protein called the organic matrix. Minerals comprise 60 to 70 per cent of the weight of dry bone, and organic matter 30 to 40 per cent of the dry bone; fresh bone is 15 to 25 per cent water. The protein is mainly collagen, which is quite insoluble. The combination of minerals and organic matter can be readily demonstrated by placing bone in a weak acid solution (ordinary household vinegar can be used), which dissolves the salts, leaving the flexible organic matter in the shape of the original bone.

Teeth, like bone, contain both inorganic and organic matter, with the inorganic portion comprising the major part. *Enamel*, the outermost covering, is approximately 99.5 per cent inorganic matter; *dentin*, the portion beneath the enamel and surrounding the tooth pulp, about 77 per cent; and *cementum*, the calcified portion covering the root of the tooth, is approximately 70 per cent inorganic matter. (See diagram of tooth, Chapter 23.)

Enamel, the hardest tissue in the body, contains 36 per cent calcium and 17 per cent phosphorus, which are more of the minerals than is contained in any other tissue. Dentin is 27 per cent calcium and 13 per cent phosphorus (Fig. 10.1). Although exchange of minerals between enamel and saliva occurs, unlike bone, the enamel of the tooth has no capacity to repair itself after a portion has been injured mechanically or through decay (26).

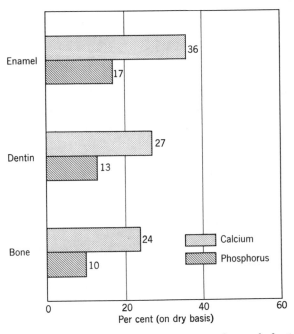

Fig. 10.1. The average calcium and phosphorous content of enamel, dentin, and bone. (Adapted from Harrow and Mazur, *Textbooks of Biochemistry*, 6th ed., W. B. Saunders Co., Philadelphia, p. 413, 1954.)

The organic matter of teeth is chiefly protein. In enamel the protein is a *keratin*, the most insoluble of proteins. In dentin, like bone, the protein is collagen.

Regulating Certain Body Functions. For the heart muscles to contract in a normal fashion, the tissue fluid that bathes them must contain an adequate amount of calcium. The role of individual minerals in heart muscle action was demonstrated in a classic experiment using a frog's heart removed from the body. The heart muscle could be made to continue to contract and relax if artificial circulation of a solution containing calcium, potassium, and sodium was maintained. If calcium salts were removed from the solution, the muscle failed to contract. On the other hand, if the concentration of calcium salts was too great, a state of continuous contraction or *calcium rigor* resulted. An excessive concentration of potassium caused continuous and extreme relaxation—potassium inhibition. A third element, sodium, was essential in the solution for the muscle to continue to contract and relax. However, when sodium salts alone were present in the solution, the muscle relaxed. The presence of these minerals in proper proportions makes possible the rhythmic characteristic of heart beats (25).

Calcium is indispensable for blood clot formation, which can be clearly demonstrated by adding oxalic acid to a blood sample. Oxalic acid forms an insoluble salt with calcium making it unavailable to function in the coagulation process. A simplified version of the clotting process is presented here to show the role of calcium. The clot is formed when fibrinogen, a soluble protein normally present in blood, is changed to fibrin, an insoluble protein. For this process to occur the enzyme thrombin, which normally is not present in blood, must be present. It is believed the process of its formation is as follows:

Prothrombin, an inactive form of thrombin (normally present in blood) + calcium + thromboplastin (a phospholipid released when cells are damaged) $\longrightarrow$ thrombin.

Fibrinogen (normally present in blood) $\xrightarrow{\text{thrombin}}$ fibrin.

▶ **ABSORPTION, STORAGE, AND EXCRETION OF CALCIUM**

Calcium absorption from the intestine is characterized by being incomplete. The extent of absorption varies widely among individuals, with greater absorption occurring when there is the greater need. Young growing animals, having a proportionately greater need for calcium than do older animals, absorb it much more completely (11). Infants fed human milk were found to absorb 50 to 70 per cent of the calcium ingested; adults absorb only 30 to 50 per cent of the calcium in a mixed diet (19).

Further evidence that the state of mineralization of bone in some way regulates calcium absorption comes from studies of adults with osteomalacia, a condition in which the mineral content of the bone is markedly diminished from what is normal. With vitamin D therapy absorption of calcium may increase, approaching that found in young infants, namely around 70 per cent. Also in an experiment with mature rats, greater intestinal absorption was observed in those animals previously depleted of calcium than in animals of the same age with normal mineral content.

Factors of the Diet Favoring Absorption of Calcium

Certain nutrients in the diet are found to improve the absorption of calcium; important among them are vitamin D, protein, and ascorbic acid.

Vitamin D. Vitamin D improves the efficiency of calcium absorption, particularly when the concentration of available calcium is low in the intestine. How vitamin D functions to improve the movement of calcium through the intestinal barrier is not known. However, an experiment of interest is the *in vitro* study, in which sacs made of segments of the intestine were used to observe transport of calcium. When the intestinal sac came from vitamin D deficient rats, the transport of calcium was markedly reduced from the rate when the sac was from the normal rat (13).

Vitamin D improves absorption of calcium when the need of the body for this mineral is comparatively greater, as in infancy, pregnancy, lactation, in children with rickets, and adults with osteomalacia. With normal adults absorption and retention of calcium are virtually unaffected by the addition of vitamin D to their diets (20).

Protein. The absorption of calcium is influenced by protein. Poor absorption occurs when diets are deficient in protein; increasing the protein content of a low-protein diet improves absorption (12). The amino acid lysine is found to improve absorption of calcium in the rat under certain conditions, that is, when the amino acid and calcium are present in the intestine at the same time and when the rats are fasted. Further research is needed to establish if this finding has significance for the human being (24).

Ascorbic Acid. Numerous studies have been done to explore the influence of ascorbic acid on absorption of calcium; the findings vary. In an experiment with college women absorption of calcium was improved by the addition of ascorbic acid under the conditions of the study, which were a low intake of both calcium (336 mg daily) and ascorbic acid (22 mg daily). Supplementation of the diet with an additional 25 mg of ascorbic acid significantly increased the absorption of calcium (16).

Factors of the Diet Interfering with Calcium Absorption

There is evidence that for calcium to be absorbed it must be in the ionic form. As a consequence, conditions that lessen the concentration of calcium ions in the intestine lessen absorption. The formation of insoluble salts lessens the ion concentration. Two normal constituents of the diet that form insoluble salts are oxalic acid and phytic acid.

Oxalic Acid. Oxalic acid combines with calcium to form insoluble calcium oxalate. Among the foods containing oxalic acid are beet greens, chard, rhubarb, spinach, and cocoa of lower than average grade. Although these foods contain calcium (particularly the leafy-green ones), it is present as the insoluble oxalate and cannot be absorbed (14). Even though the calcium in these foods cannot be used, it does not mean that they should be abandoned. The leafy-green vegetables are high in carotene and iron content, important nutrients in the diet.

There has been a question as to whether or not the free oxalic acid in these foods would combine with calcium from other foods consumed at the same time, making that calcium insoluble. In a study of children five to eight years of age with an adequate intake of calcium, no lessening of absorption of calcium was observed by the addition of a daily serving of spinach (2). So it would appear that with an adequate intake of calcium, the free oxalic acid makes no discernible difference in the absorption of calcium.

The effect of cocoa on calcium absorption has been of particular interest because of its use with milk in beverages. The adverse effect of cocoa on calcium absorption was observed in studies using experimental animals. Oxalic acid was identified as an interfering substance, as was cocoa butter. The amount of cocoa (16 per cent by weight) fed to the animals, however, was far above the relative amount customarily consumed in the human diet (22). Thus it was with much interest that the effect of cocoa on calcium absorption in the human being was sought. The question was investigated at the University of Illinois (4). College women were fed cocoa (moderate cost, American process) in amounts varying from approximately three-fourths tablespoon (5.6 gm) to a little more than one-half cup (58.2 gm) daily. The calcium content of the diets varied from 21 mg (milk-free diet) to 755 mg (a diet containing milk and ice cream). The cocoa had no discernible deleterious effect on calcium absorption in these studies.

Phytic Acid. Phytic acid occurs in the outer bran layers of whole wheat. Many studies have been conducted to discern the effect of phytic acid on calcium absorption. The findings indicate that if the diet is adequate in calcium, phytic acid will not have a detrimental effect (10). The influence of phytates is not a problem in this country, although in areas of calcium deprivation it may be of considerable importance.

Storage of Calcium

Bone serves as the storage place for calcium. When the supply of calcium in the body is sufficient, calcium may be stored in needle-like deposits called trabeculae in the ends of the bones. When calcium is needed in the tissues or the blood, these labile stores in the bones are drawn upon.

As the intake of calcium is lowered, the efficiency of the body to absorb and retain it increases whereas raising the intake may result in reduced absorption. In the adult the rejection of calcium by the intestine constitutes the chief means of adaptation; the same is true for the young. However, another adaptive mechanism available to the young, but not to adults, is deposition of calcium in the growing bone (5).

Excretion of Calcium

Calcium is excreted by way of the intestine, the kidney, and the skin. The relative amounts eliminated by the three pathways may be illustrated by findings from long-term studies (2 months to 1½ years) on men. On a calcium intake of approximately 1 gm, the mean daily fecal excretion was 622 mg, and the mean daily urinary excretion 235 mg (19). Under comfortable conditions, with sweating at a minimum, the average daily dermal excretion of the adult was 149 mg (23); when sweating was profuse the amount increased.

The fecal excretion of calcium is related to intake. As the amount of calcium consumed increases, the amount in the fecal excretion increases (19). Urinary calcium is on the average not greatly influenced by the daily intake. It is related to the process of reabsorption in the kidney tubules (renal tubular transport). Examples of conditions that influence renal reabsorption are hyperparathyroidism and hypervitaminosis D, both of which decrease re-absorption and increase the excretion.

The amount of calcium excreted differs widely among individuals but shows a characteristic constancy within each person (3, 15). Strangely enough, urinary calcium excretion appears to be independent of blood concentration.

Blood Calcium

The normal concentration of calcium in the blood is 9 to 11.5 mg per 100 ml. Fifty to 60 per cent of the blood calcium is present in the ionized form; the remainder is bound to protein (9).

The homeostatic mechanism for maintaining the blood at a normal level is more effective for calcium than for other minerals. Of major importance in the process is the hormone of the parathyroid glands, and also vitamin D. Parathormone functions by moving calcium from bone to blood. Vitamin D also mediates the movement of labile calcium from bone, under conditions of need for the mineral, to maintain the content of the blood at a normal level.

▶ INFLUENCE OF AMOUNT OF CALCIUM ON NUTRITIONAL WELL-BEING

An Improved Intake

It is of practical significance to know whether benefits are realized by increasing the calcium intake when the amount in the diet already allows for performance accepted as normal. Sherman did research on this question using rats as experimental animals. When calcium was added to the rations it produced beneficial effects. The unsupplemented ration had been adequate for what was considered normal growth, reproduction, and length of life. However, by increasing the amount of calcium in the diet by 75 per cent, growth was more rapid, the capacity to reproduce was longer, and the animals lived a longer life (Fig. 10.2). With these, as with other studies with animals, there are implications for the human being, but of course direct application cannot be made.

An Inadequate Intake

Insufficient calcium in the diet limits growth in the young. The stunting effect has been demonstrated in animal studies. In one such investigation twin rats were fed identical diets of meat and wheat except that

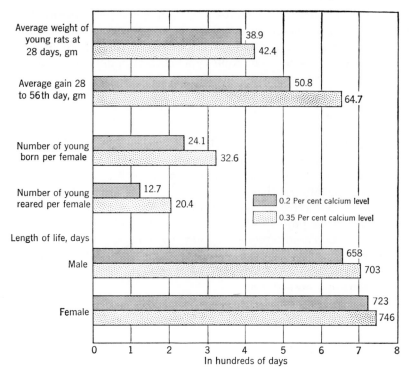

Fig. 10.2.   Influence of increased intake of calcium on behavior of experimental rats.
(Adapted from Sherman, *Chemistry of Food and Nutrition*, 8th ed., The Macmillan Co., New
York, p. 266, 1952.)

a supplement of milk was added to the ration of one. When milk was
added to the diet, the animal received many nutrients in addition to
calcium. However, of them calcium was the nutrient lacking in the
original diet that was most needed for bone development. The skeletal
growth of the rat with the added milk exceeded notably that of the rat
without the supplement (Fig. 10.3).

There is a need for the development of procedures for evaluating the
state of calcium nutrition in the human being and detecting the deficiency
at an early stage. In a deficiency state the concentration of calcium in
serum decreases to low levels (9). Tetany, the diagnostic clinical symptom
of calcium deficiency, is associated with rickets and osteomalacia and
occurs at an advanced stage of deficiency.

The incidence of osteoporosis is greater among individuals accustomed
to low calcium intakes than those who have had higher dietary intakes
of the mineral. Osteoporosis is one of the most common disorders of bone
and one associated with aging. The bone tissue is normal in composition

but reduced in amount. Resorption, a normal process in bone, proceeds at a greater rate than does bone formation in osteoporosis.

In addition to a low calcium intake, the lack of certain hormones (estrogens and androgens) and vitamin D are recognized as factors related to osteoporosis. In the treatment, therefore, it is recommended that not only dietary supplements of calcium be used but also the hormones and vitamin D be explored as curative agents (17).

Recommended Allowances for Calcium

The calcium balance study (Fig. 10.4) is the customary method used for estimating the amount of calcium needed to satisfy the daily recommendation. The approach to determining calcium needs for children differs from that for adults. For children intakes at which retention occurs are recommended in order to make allowances for growth; for adults the least intake that will assure a positive balance is considered sufficient.

The Recommended Allowance for calcium in late adolescence is 1.4 gm daily for older boys and 1.3 gm daily for older girls. The continued high intake recommended for the 15 to 18 years of age period satisfies the demands for growth, which for some young people is still great. For others, whose growth has tapered off, the generous intake affords an opportunity for them to make up whatever deficits in calcium intake they may have suffered in the preceding years. For adults of all ages the Recommended Allowance is 0.8 gm daily. The amount must be increased of course for women during pregnancy and lactation.

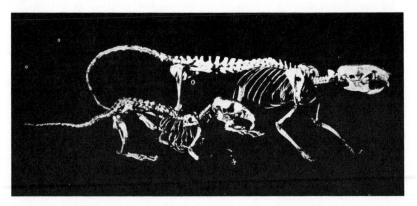

Fig. 10.3. Twin rats showing the effect on skeletal size of the addition of milk to the diet. (*J. Biol. Chem.,* **60:** 5, 1924.)

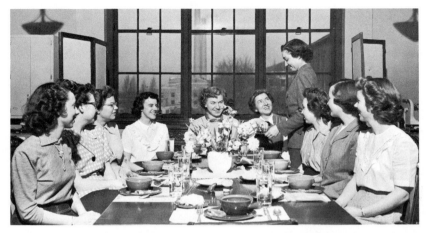

Fig. 10.4.   A group of students who are subjects in a calcium balance study. (Courtesy of Patton, Ohio Agricultural Experiment Station, Columbus. Photo by The Ohio State University.)

An expert group selected by the Food and Agriculture Organization (FAO) and the World Health Organization (WHO) reviewed calcium requirements. The group proposed and adopted the term "suggested practical allowances" which they define as "the intake at which the needs of the great majority of persons in any defined group or population are likely to be adequately met" (5). The Recommended Dietary Allowances are "designed for the maintenance of good nutrition of practically all healthy persons in the United States." Table 10.2 compares the Recommended Dietary Allowances of the NRC with the suggested practical allowances of the FAO/WHO Expert Group.

In summary, there are two fundamental factors that give reason for maintaining an intake of calcium that meets the Recommended Allowance. In the first place, wide differences exist in the capacity of individuals to utilize calcium; some people use it efficiently, others do not; the difference is not outwardly recognizable. Furthermore, factors adverse to calcium utilization that may characterize the diet are least detrimental when the intake of calcium is adequate.

Food Sources of Calcium

Few foods available to use are excellent sources of calcium. Milk and milk products are the most dependable ones. Fluid skim milk and non-fat milk solids have the added recommendation of being economical in cost. Without milk or milk products in the diet it is difficult to provide the Recommended Allowance for calcium, but including them in reasonable amounts practically assures meeting the allowance. In late adolescence or early adulthood 1½ pt of milk or its equivalent in the diet is usually sufficient, along with other foods, to meet the allowances. For adults a pint of milk is sufficient. Figure 10.5 illustrates the relative superiority of milk as a source of calcium as compared to other foods.

Leafy-green vegetables (excluding members of the goosefoot family, such as spinach and chard that contain oxalic acid) rank next to the dairy products in calcium content. Broccoli is a good source; citrus fruits and legumes are fair sources; meats, grains, and nuts provide the least calcium. The incorporation of milk in the bread formula improves this product as a source of calcium.

The calcium content of an average serving of some common foods is given in Table 10.3.

At times when there are certain dietary restrictions or a need for

Table 10.2. Comparison of Calcium Intakes Suggested by NRC and by FAO/WHO

		Recommended Dietary Allowances, NRC (mg/day)	Suggested Practical Allowances, FAO/WHO (mg/day)
Children, both sexes:	0–12 mo[1]	0–700[2]	500–600
	1–9 yr	800	400–500
	10–15 yr	—	600–700
	9–12 yr	1100	—
Males:	16–19 yr	—	500–600
	12–18 yr	1400	—
	Adults	800	400–500
Females:	16–19 yr	—	500–600
	12–18 yr	1300	—
	Adults	800	400–500
	Pregnancy	1300[3]	1000–1200[4]
	Lactation	1300	1000–1200

[1] Not breast fed.
[2] Increase proportionately with calories to the value shown.
[3] 2nd and 3rd trimeter.
[4] 3rd trimeter.

Recommended Dietary Allowances, Sixth Revised Edition. Natl. Acad. Sci.—Natl. Res. Council, Publ. 1146, 1964.

From Calcium Requirements. Food Agr. Organ. U.N. FAO Nutr. Meetings, Report Series No. 30, Rome, 1962.

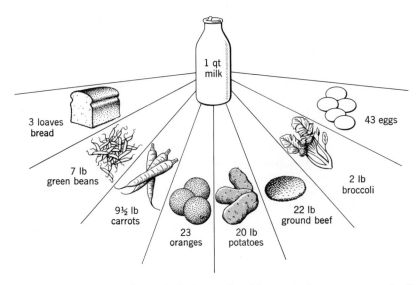

Fig. 10.5. Quantities of different foods that supply calcium equivalent to one quart of milk.

Table 10.3. Calcium Values of Some Typical Foods

Food	Measure	Calcium, mg
Milk	1 c, 8 oz	288
Cheese, American Cheddar	1 oz	212
Mustard greens	½ c	97
Ice cream	⅛ qt	87
Kale	½ c	74
Oranges	1 med	67
Broccoli	½ c	66
Cottage cheese, creamed	¼ c	53
Lima beans	½ c	38
Green beans	½ c	31
Egg	1 med	27
Bread, whole wheat	1 sl	23
Peas	½ c	19
Peanut butter	2 tbsp	18
Bread, white enriched	1 sl	16
Cream, light	1 tbsp	16
Oatmeal	½ c	11
Potato	1 med	9

From *Nutritive Value of Foods.* U.S. Dept. Agr., Home Garden Bull. 72, revised 1964.

calcium beyond that supplied by food, physicians may recommend the use of calcium salts. Numerous studies have been done using such salts as calcium gluconate, lactate, carbonate, and sulfate, with the general finding that calcium from the salts tested is utilized to approximately the same extent as that in milk.

Calcium in the Food Supply

The U.S. Department of Agriculture survey figures of food supplies show that approximately 980 mg of calcium are available per person per day in the United States (7). The males of the family, especially the father and adolescent boys, are most likely to eat foods that provide the Recommended Allowances for calcium. The mother and adolescent girls consume the lowest calcium intake of the family. After the age of twelve years, the calcium intake of the female starts to decrease and usually continues to do so with age.

In the United States milk products provide three-fourths of the calcium supply. Table 10.4 gives the sources of calcium in the American diet. Since few foods are excellent sources of calcium, diets tend to supply less than the recommended amount of calcium unless care is exercised in the selection of foods. This is especially true of diets that do not include milk products.

The total calcium supply available for human consumption varies widely from country to country; variations also exist in the relative

Table 10.4. Percentage of Total Calcium Contributed by Major Food Groups in the United States, 1962

Food Group	Calcium, per cent
Dairy products	76.3
Leafy-green and yellow vegetables	3.9
Other fruits and vegetables	3.7
Soya flour and cocoa	3.3
Flour and cereal products	3.1
Meat, poultry, and fish	2.6
Eggs	2.5
Citrus fruit and tomatoes	1.8
Potatoes and sweet potatoes	1.4
Sugar and sirups	0.8
Fats and oils	0.6

Consumption of Food in the United States 1909–52, Supplement for 1962. U.S. Dept. Agr., Agr. Handbook 62, p. 21, 1963.

contributions of different food groups to the calcium supply. It can be noted from Table 10.5 that milk may be the chief source of calcium in the United States, but in Japan the daily supply is derived fairly evenly from cereals, pulses, nuts, and vegetables.

▶ PHOSPHORUS

Phosphorus is an important constituent in every body tissue. The total amount constitutes about one per cent of the body weight. The amount of phosphorus in the body is exceeded only by calcium. It occurs in bones and teeth in combination with calcium and in fluids and soft tissues as a constituent of many compounds essential in active metabolism. Phosphorus is widely distributed in foods. A sufficient amount to satisfy the estimated needs of the body is easily supplied. For this reason phosphorus may not always be given its rightful share of consideration in nutrition discussions.

Functions of Phosphorus

Phosphorus combines with calcium to form a relatively insoluble compound which gives strength and rigidity to bones and teeth. The amount of phosphorus in bone is about one-half that of calcium. Although the extent of mineralization of bone may vary, the calcium-to-phosphorus ratio is rarely altered.

Phosphorus, like calcium, is needed not only for growth and development of the skeleton but also for its maintenance. Studies with radioactive phosphorus confirm the belief that the minerals of bone are in constant turnover. In comparable studies it was found that some mineral exchange also takes place in the teeth. Phosphorus in enamel interchanges with phosphorus in the saliva; dentin exchanges phosphorus with the blood supply in the tooth.

The full importance of the role of phosphorus in the functioning of the body has been more fully realized only within the past 20 years or so. The significance of phosphorus cannot be overemphasized, for the metabolic processes of all cells and the utilization of many nutrients that enter the body involve the formation and degradation of phosphorus-containing compounds. It is a component of enzyme systems essential to tissue respiration. A series of phosphorus compounds are formed in the utilization of carbohydrate. Fatty acids combine with phosphorus as a step in their use by the body. Phosphorus-containing nitrogenous compounds are broken down and rebuilt in the complex process of muscle contrac-

Table 10.5. Calcium in the Food Supplies of Selected Countries Based on FAO Food Balance Sheets

Country and Year	Cereals	Starchy Roots	Pulses and Nuts	Vegetables	Fruit	Meat and Poultry	Eggs	Fish	Milk and Milk Products	Total Calcium
United States (1958)										
Mg Ca/cap/day	29	10	18	135	21	18	5	5	856	1,116
Per cent of total Ca suppl.	3	1	2	12	2	2	2	—	75	100
Italy										
Mg Ca/cap/day	59	9	24	190	26	6	10	5	381	710
Per cent of total Ca suppl.	8	1	3	27	4	1	1	1	54	100
India										
Mg Ca/cap/day	98	6	67	23	5	—	—	1	147	347
Per cent of total Ca suppl.	28	2	19	7	1	—	—	—	43	100
Japan										
Mg Ca/cap/day	66	22	91	101	5	1	5	19	58	368
Per cent of total Ca suppl.	18	6	25	28	1	—	1	5	16	100

From *Calcium Requirements*. Food Agr. Organ. U.N., FAO Nutr. Meetings Report Series No. 30, pp. 39–41, 1962.

tion. Phosphorus is vital to the fundamental processes of metabolism in the body.

A complete discussion of the functions of phosphorus is beyond the scope of this book; however, two phosphorus-containing compounds might be mentioned—adenosine triphosphate (ATP) and nucleoproteins. ATP functions throughout nature as a link between processes releasing and those requiring energy. It is one of a group of compounds containing "energy-rich" or "high-energy" phosphate bonds. In the living cell the breakdown of organic compounds with the release of energy and the synthesis of others with the need for energy ensue at about the same time. The energy-rich compounds play an essential part in "coupling the production of energy from foodstuffs to the utilization of that energy by the cell for its multifold activities" (6).

Nucleoproteins constitute most of the nuclear material of all cells and also occur in the cytoplasm (8). The nucleoproteins are key compounds in the processes of cell division, reproduction, and the transmission of hereditary characteristics.

Absorption and Excretion of Phosphorus

Phosphorus is absorbed in the small intestine, chiefly as free phosphorus, to the extent of approximately 70 per cent of the amount ingested. As with calcium the less alkaline upper portion of the duodenum favors absorption of phosphorus. The kidney is the major pathway of excretion, influenced to some extent by the amount absorbed from the intestinal tract.

The normal inorganic phosphate concentration in blood is 2 to 4.5 mg per 100 ml in adults and 3 to 5 mg per 100 ml in children.

Deficiencies of Phosphorus

We are not concerned with phosphorus deficiencies in the human being because diets are seldom, if ever, inadequate in this nutrient; however, it has been a common deficiency in cattle and forage animals. In more recent years with increased knowledge of animal feeding, supplements are given to livestock to provide a more complete mineral ration. Animals suffering with phosphorus deficiency develop stiff joints, and the bones become fragile and break easily. Experimental phosphorus deficiency in rats, produced by limiting the intake, slows the rate of growth and causes subnormal deposition of calcium and phosphorus in the bones.

Recommended Allowances for Phosphorus

Diets that supply the Recommended Allowances of calcium and protein are quite certain to be adequate in phosphorus. The Food and Nutrition Board recommends that the phosphorus intake should be at least equal to that of calcium for children and for women during the latter part of pregnancy and the lactation period.

Food Sources of Phosphorus

Phosphorus is widely distributed in both plant and animal foods. Protein-rich foods such as meat, poultry, fish, and eggs are excellent sources of phosphorus, are abundant in supply, and are well-liked foods in the United States. Cereal grains provide phosphorus in good amount, whole grain more than the highly-milled product. The higher phosphorus

Table 10.6. Phosphorus Values of Some Typical Foods

Food	Measure	Phosphorus, mg
Liver, beef, fried	2 sl, 3″ × 2¼″ × ⅜″	311
Milk	1 c, 8 oz	234
Haddock, fried	3 oz	211
Pork chop, loin, fried	3 oz	200
Beef, round, cooked	3 oz	195
Lamb, chop, fried	3 oz	185
Cheese, American Cheddar	1 oz, 1″ cube	139
Baked beans, no pork	½ c	110
Cottage cheese	¼ c	106
Oatmeal	⅔ c	105
Egg	1 med	101
Shredded wheat	1 c	93
Ice cream	⅛ qt	78
Broccoli	⅔ c	76
Lima beans	½ c	62
Bread, whole wheat	1 sl	60
Corn	½ c	43
Orange	1 med	35
Grapefruit	½ med	32
Bread, white	1 sl	21

From C. F. Church and H. N. Church *Food Values of Portions Commonly Used*—Bowes and Church. 9th ed. J. B. Lippincott Co., Philadelphia, 1962.

content of the whole-grain products, however, may be misleading because of the greater content of phytin phosphorus which is not readily utilized by the body. Dried beans and eggs contain appreciable amounts of phosphorus, milk and dairy products are excellent sources. Vegetables and fruits, as a whole, are rather low in phosphorus content (Table 10.6).

REFERENCES

1. Bauer, C. H., A. Carlsson, and B. Lindquist (1961). Metabolism and homeostatic function of bone. In *Mineral Metabolism*, Vol. 1, Pt. B. (C. L. Comar and F. Bronner, eds.) Academic Press, New York, pp. 609–12.
2. Bonner, P., F. C. Hummel, M. F. Bates, J. Horton, H. A. Hunscher, and I. G. Macy (1938). The influence of a daily serving of spinach or its equivalent in oxalic acid upon the mineral utilization of children. *J. Pediat.* 12: 188.
3. Boyce, H., and J. King, Jr. (1959). Effects of high calcium intake on urine in human beings. *Federation Proc.* 18: 1102.
4. Bricker, M. L., J. M. Smith, T. S. Hamilton, and H. H. Mitchell (1949). The effect of cocoa upon calcium utilization and requirements, nitrogen retention and fecal composition of women. *J. Nutr.* 39: 445.
5. *Calcium Requirements* (1962). Food Agr. Organ. U.N., FAO Nutr. Meeting Rept. Series No. 30, Rome.
6. Conn, E. E., and P. F. Stumpf (1963). *Outlines of Biochemistry.* John Wiley and Sons, New York.
7. *Consumption of Food in the United States 1909–52*, Supplement for 1962 (1963). U.S. Dept. Agr., Agr. Handbook No. 62, Washington, D.C., p. 21.
8. Downes, H. R. (1962). *The Chemistry of Living Cells*, 2nd ed. Harper and Row, Evanston, Ill.
9. Goldsmith, G. A. (1959). *Nutritional Diagnosis.* Charles C Thomas, Springfield, Ill., p. 81.
10. Harris, R. S. (1955). Phytic acid and its importance in human nutrition. *Nutrition Rev.* 13: 257.
11. Harrison, H. E. (1959). Factors influencing calcium absorption. *Federation Proc.* 18: 1085.
12. Hegsted, D. M., I. Moscoso, and C. Collazos Ch. (1952). A study of the minimum calcium requirements of adult men. *J. Nutr.* 46: 181.
13. Intestinal absorption of calcium (1962). *Nutr. Rev.* 20: 46.
14. Johnston, F. A., T. J. McMillan, and G. D. Falconer (1952). Calcium retained by young women before and after adding spinach to the diet. *J. Am. Dietet. Assoc.* 29: 933.
15. Knapp, E. L. (1947). Factors influencing the urinary excretion of calcium. I. In normal persons. *J. Clin. Invest.* 26: 182.
16. Leichsenring, J. M., L. M. Norris, and M. L. Halbert (1957). Effect of ascorbic acid and of orange juice on calcium and phosphorus metabolism of women. *J. Nutr.* 63: 425.
17. Lutwak, K., and G. Whedon (1962). Osteoporosis—a disorder of mineral nutrition. *Borden's Rev. Nutr. Res.* 23: 45.
18. Macy, I. G. (1942). *Nutrition and Chemical Growth in Childhood*, Vol. I, Evaluation. Charles C Thomas, Springfield, Ill.

19. Malm, O. J. (1958). *Calcium Requirement and Adaptation in Adult Men.* Oslo University Press, Oslo, Norway, pp. 108–125.
20. McKay, H., M. B. Patton, M. S. Pittman, G. Stearns, and N. Edelbeute (1943). The effect of vitamin D on calcium retentions. *J. Nutr.* **26:** 153.
21. Mitchell, H. H. (1962). *Comparative Nutrition of Man and Domestic Animals.* Volume I. Academic Press, New York, p. 461.
22. Mitchell, H. H. (1964). *Comparative Nutrition of Man and Domestic Animals,* Volume II. Academic Press, New York, p. 681.
23. Mitchell, H. H., T. S. Hamilton, and W. T. Haines (1949). The dermal excretion under controlled environmental conditions of nitrogen and minerals in human subjects, with particular reference to calcium and iron. *J. Biol. Chem.* **178:** 345.
24. Raven, A. M., F. W. Lengernaun, and R. W. Wasserman (1960). Studies of the effect of lysine on the absorption of radiocalcium and radiostrontium by the rat. *J. Nutr.* **72:** 29.
25. Ringer, S. (1883–4). A further contribution regarding the influence of the different constituents of the blood on the contraction of the heart. *J. Physiol.* **4:** 29.
26. Sognnaes, R. F., and J. H. Shaw (1952). Salivary and pulpal contributions to the radiophosphorus uptake in enamel and dentin. *J. Am. Dental Assoc.* **44:** 489.

CHAPTER 11

Iron and iodine

Iron is of particular importance because it is essential to the processes of oxidation in the body. It is a constituent in compounds necessary for the transport of oxygen to the cells and for oxidation in the cells (1).

The total iron content of the body is relatively small. In an adult it is approximately 3 to 5 gm, whereas the total weight of the body is probably 65,000 gm or more. If we wish to visualize that amount of iron as a lump sum, we may think of it as being around one tenth of a teaspoon.

Functions of Iron in the Body

Iron is widely distributed throughout the body. The major portion is in the blood, approximately 55 to 60 per cent; muscle tissue contains about 3 per cent; and a variable amount is stored in the liver, spleen, kidney, and bone marrow.

In the Red Cells of the Blood. Most of the iron in the blood is located in the red cells (erythrocytes). It is present in the hemoglobin, a compound formed from the union of an iron-containing pigment, heme, and a protein, globin. If there is a deficiency of iron, the amount of hemoglobin that can be formed is limited. Even though iron constitutes less than 1 per cent of the total weight of the hemoglobin molecule, it is the keystone for its formation.

156

Soon after its absorption iron is incorporated into hemoglobin. This process takes place in the bone marrow where new red cells are formed. The time required for iron ingested in the food to be incorporated into the red cells has been studied with radioactive iron. Because radioactive iron is not normally found in the body, it is possible to identify it with certainty and differentiate it from the iron from other sources. After radioactive iron was administered intravenously to nine normal men, some of it appeared within 24 hours in the red cells in the blood. By the end of the fifteenth day, an average of 74 per cent of the injected radioactive iron was found in the circulating red cells (4).

In anemic dogs radioactive iron was identified in the red cells as early as 4 hours after its ingestion. It means that within those few hours the iron had (a) traveled to the bone marrow, (b) incorporated into the hemoglobin portion of new red cells, and (c) returned to the circulation.

The life span of erythrocytes is estimated to be approximately 120 days. Since the body contains 20,000 billion erythrocytes, this life span suggests that they are destroyed (and produced) at the rate of 115 million per minute (19).

Iron is not the only mineral necessary for the formation of hemoglobin, even though it is the only mineral in the molecule itself. Copper, too, is essential. This significant discovery was made at the University of Wisconsin. For several years the development of anemia in young animals (albino rats) restricted to a diet of milk had been under study. Copper was found to prevent this anemia; it was essential to the formation of hemoglobin but was not a constituent in the final product. In the average mixed diet that most people eat, sufficient copper is available to provide for normal hemoglobin formation.

Hemoglobin performs the important operation of carrying oxygen from the lungs to the tissues. In the lungs hemoglobin combines loosely with oxygen to form *oxyhemoglobin,* which carries the oxygen to the tissues and releases it there. In the lungs there is an abundance of oxygen, which facilitates the combination of atmospheric oxygen and hemoglobin. In the tissues there is little oxygen and as a need for it exists, it is readily released. Hemoglobin from which oxygen has been released is called *reduced hemoglobin.* The reduced hemoglobin then returns to the lungs by way of the venous circulation to again pick up oxygen in the formation of oxyhemoglobin, and the cycle is repeated (Fig. 11.1).

The release of oxygen to the tissues is accomplished by a transfer of carbon dioxide from the tissues to the blood stream. About 10 per cent of the carbon dioxide is carried by hemoglobin; the major portion, however, is carried as bicarbonate ion (3).

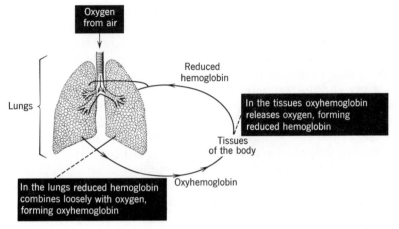

Fig. 11.1.   Diagrammatic presentation of the oxygen-carrying function of hemoglobin.

In the Blood Plasma. There is a small amount of iron in the plasma. It accounts for only about two-tenths per cent (0.2 per cent) of the total iron in the blood. Iron in the plasma is in transport. It may be newly absorbed iron, or iron moving from storage on its way for use by the body, for excretion, or for deposit for later use. Iron travels in the plasma bound to a protein, a specific globulin called transferrin.

Plasma iron comes from three sources: (*a*) that absorbed from the gastrointestinal tract of dietary origin, (*b*) that salvaged from the breakdown of hemoglobin, and (*c*) that released from stores in the body. In the normal individual the destruction (hemolysis) of red cells contributes by far the largest amount of iron of the three sources. It has been estimated that about 27 to 28 mg of iron per day comes from that source in the average man whereas only about 1 milligram comes directly from food (8). The amount used from storage is widely variable and depends on the need of the individual.

The level of iron in the plasma is considered a sensitive index of the state of iron metabolism in the body. Plasma iron determinations, however, are not often used in the usual clinical laboratory in diagnosing iron deficiency. Instead, the common practice is to determine the hemoglobin level and red cell count, which also give information on the status of the iron metabolism. Under normal conditions the plasma iron level may vary from 50 to 180 mcg per 100 ml of plasma. In iron-deficiency anemia, the level is reduced. On the other hand, there are certain abnormal conditions, such as excessive destruction of red cells, in which there is a pouring out of iron salvaged from the cells.

In Muscle Tissue. Iron is present in the muscle cells in two combinations as (*a*) myoglobin and (*b*) as a constituent of certain enzymes.

Myoglobin is a compound similar to hemoglobin in structure and in function. Like hemoglobin it is formed from the combination of an iron-containing pigment and a protein and is a carrier of oxygen. Myoglobin has the capacity of storing oxygen in the muscles for use in muscle contraction.

The iron-containing enzymes in muscle make possible the oxidation of carbohydrate, fat, and protein within the intact cell. These enzymes are the cytochromes, catalases, and peroxidases. Each has the same general function, but operates in a specific way in bringing about the oxidative changes within the tissue. Iron serves in a double capacity in cellular oxidation; it carries oxygen to the cells and makes possible oxidation in the cells through the iron-containing enzymes.

Absorption, Storage, and Excretion of Iron

Absorption of Iron. Iron is absorbed directly into the blood stream. The process may take place in all parts of the intestinal tract with the exception of the colon; absorption from that area is not definitely established. The duodenum is the location of greatest absorption, with the amount progressively decreasing from jejunum to ileum (2, 16).

In man iron is much more efficiently absorbed in the ferrous (reduced) state than in the ferric (oxidized) form. The iron in food, however, is predominantly in the ferric form. Reducing substances present in foods are believed to change some of the ferric iron present to the ferrous form. Bearing out this assumption is the finding that ascorbic acid, a reducing substance, when fed with ferric iron enhances absorption but has no effect on the absorption of ferrous iron (16).

Iron movement through the intestinal cell is unidirectional; that is, absorption from the intestine into the blood takes place, but re-excretion does not occur from the blood back into intestine (2).

The striking finding that some mechanism exists for the control of iron absorption was conclusively established through one of the most illuminating techniques in nutrition studies today, the use of radioactive elements. An ingenious study was done by Moore and his associates at Washington University (17). Persons in normal health and those with iron-deficiency anemia were fed a diet in which most of the iron was radioactive. Eggs containing radioactive iron were obtained by injecting radioactive iron into the laying hen. Vegetables were grown in nutrient solutions containing radioactive iron. The normal men and women on diets containing radioactive iron from these sources absorbed from 1 to

12 per cent of the iron intake; persons with iron-deficiency anemia absorbed as much as 45 to 64 per cent at the same level of intake. These values are from the one experiment; values in general for iron absorption suggested by Moore and Dubach are, for normal persons, 5 to 10 per cent (Fig. 11.2) and for iron-deficient persons 10 to 20 per cent of the iron in the food consumed. Individuals with a greater need for iron absorb a greater amount.

A relationship between iron absorption and the rate of erythrocyte formation has been observed. In a study performed in Peru, South America, the absorption of radioactive iron and its appearance in red blood cells was measured in individuals both at sea level and at an elevation of 15,000 ft (18). At the higher altitude absorption and red cell formation increased markedly over the values observed at sea level. By the end of a month at the higher altitude, however, the rates of absorption and cell formation had returned to the sea-level values; adaptation had occurred.

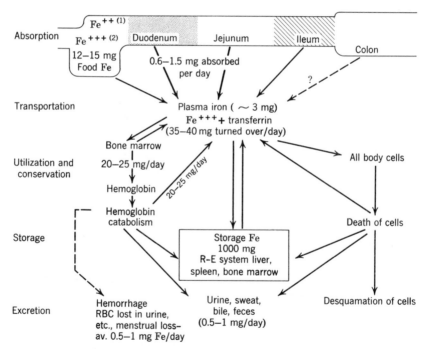

Fig. 11.2. Diagrammatic outline of iron metabolism in adults. (1) Fe + + − ferrous ion. (2) Fe + + + − ferric ion. (From C. V. Moore, "Iron and the Essential Trace Elements," *Modern Nutrition in Health and Disease*, [M. G. Wohl and R. S. Goodhart, eds.] Lea and Febiger, Philadelphia, p. 280, 1964.)

At present the mode of regulation of iron absorption is not understood. Absorption is of particular importance for iron because the capacity for elimination by the normal pathways, the kidney and re-excretion into the intestine, is negligible. Thus any control of the amount in the body must be at the time of absorption.

For the past quarter century the theory has been held that the ferritin content of the intestinal mucosa controlled the absorption of iron. More recent studies have not supported this theory.

Storage of Iron. Iron is stored chiefly in the liver, spleen, and bone marrow. The amount is variable, ranging from 1 to 2 gm. Storage iron is held in two compounds, ferritin and hemosiderin, both iron-containing proteins. Iron is first stored as ferritin, and it is ferritin that is first withdrawn when iron is needed by the bone marrow. The more stable stores are in the form of hemosiderin.

Excessive accumulation of iron in the body occurs among the Bantu people of South Africa. They consume diets containing as much as 200 mg of iron per day. Much of the dietary iron is derived from maize, the main food in the diet, which has been cooked in an iron pot. The condition, known as *siderosis,* is characterized by increased storage of iron in the liver and spleen (11).

Excretion of Iron. As indicated earlier in the discussion, very little iron is excreted. Once it has entered the blood stream the body holds tenaciously to it. Iron is excreted in the feces but it arises from the unabsorbed iron from food. The amount of iron that is re-excreted from the blood stream into the intestine is minute; for normal persons approximately 0.02 to 0.05 mg of iron per day (9, 17).

A very small amount of iron is excreted in the urine, usually less than 0.2 mg per day. It is evident from the amount excreted that iron liberated from the breakdown of hemoglobin is carefully saved and reused.

Loss of blood is really the only way in which significant amounts of iron can leave the body after absorption into the blood stream. Such loss may be through blood donations, abnormal hemorrhage resulting from casualties or illness, and in women through menstruation. A schematic outline of iron metabolism in adults is given in Fig. 11.2.

Menstruation results in an iron loss that is of such magnitude that care must be taken to provide a sufficient amount of the mineral in the diet for replacement. The extent of loss varies widely from person to person. In a study of all of the data in the literature in 1949, Frenchman and Johnston (6) found that almost one-half the women lost one-half milligram or less per day; 15 per cent lost more than 1.2 mg per day—an average spread over all days, not just for the menstrual period.

Effect of Inadequate Iron in the Diet

Insufficient iron in the body may result from (a) an inadequate intake, (b) poor absorption due to some disease complication, or (c) abnormal loss of blood from the body (7). Two forms of iron deficiency are commonly recognized; one is termed *latent*, the other *manifest* iron deficiency. The latent deficiency is not recognized by outward appearances but by the condition within the body; available iron stores are depleted, plasma iron level is reduced, and the "iron-binding" capacity of the blood is increased. In other words, more of the particular protein that takes on iron, transferrin, is free and uncombined. There is less iron to combine with it. In manifest deficiency outward symptoms are manifested as well as changes in the blood picture. A person with manifest iron deficiency is weak, pallid in appearance, and has frequent headaches. The hemoglobin level is lower than normal, and the red blood cells are smaller than normal (hypochromic microcytic anemia). The condition results in lowered oxygen-carrying capacity. The limited oxygen supply to the tissues results in the feeling of fatigue that characterizes anemia.

The iron and hemoglobin content of the blood in iron-deficiency anemia is markedly reduced. As shown in Table 11.1, the plasma iron level may be reduced to one-fourth that of normal. With hemoglobin although the level is found to vary widely among apparently healthy individuals, values 25 per cent or more below normal are generally considered to indicate a condition of anemia. For men the normal range is from 14.0 to 18.0 gm per 100 ml; for women it is lower, varying from 11.5 to 16.0 gm per 100 ml (Table 11.2). It is wise for persons to know the level of hemoglobin that is normal for them when in good health. Deviations can then be more readily recognized.

Clinically, iron-deficiency anemia is found chiefly in infants, young children, and women but rarely in men. The incidence of anemia has remained relatively high in young children of this country whereas other

Table 11.1. Plasma Iron Level

	Number of Cases	Microgram/100 ml
Normal	169	110 ± 31
Iron deficiency	40	26 ± 7

From Cartwright, Gubler and Wintrobe, *Methods for Evaluation of Nutritional Adequacy and Status.* Natl. Acad. Sci—Natl. Res. Council, p. 113, 1954.

Table 11.2. **Blood Erythrocyte and Hemoglobin Values**

Age	Erythrocyte Count, millions/cu mm		Hemoglobin, gm/100 ml	
	Mean	Range	Mean	Range[1]
End 6th month	4.6	3.9–5.3	12.3	10.0–15.0
End 12th month	4.6	4.0–5.5	11.6	9.0–14.6
End 4th year	4.7	3.8–5.4	12.6	9.6–15.5
End 8th year	4.7	3.8–5.4	12.9	10.3–15.5
End 12th year	4.8	3.8–5.4	13.4	11.0–16.5
14 years and over				
Males	5.4	4.6–6.2	15.8	14.0–18.0
Females	4.8	4.2–5.4	13.9	11.5–16.0

[1] Ninety-five per cent range.

From Albritton, *Standard Values in Blood*, W. B. Saunders Co., p. 38, 1952.

nutritional deficiencies have declined (13). In infants the prevalence of anemia may be due to two factors: the low iron stores in the newborn caused by low intakes of iron during pregnancy and the use of cow's milk formulas without sufficient supplementation of iron-containing foods. In women the condition may occur as a result of large menstrual losses or the increased requirement of pregnancy. In men, unless there is some abnormal blood loss, microcytic hypochromic anemia seldom, if ever, develops. On a global level a major cause of iron-deficiency anemia is hookworm infestation with the attendant blood loss. The parasites attach themselves to the mucosa of the small intestine and draw blood from the submucosal blood vessels (1, 10).

Blood donors experience a lowering of the hemoglobin level with each donation. The decrease may average 2.3 gm per 100 ml of blood with the removal of approximately 1 pint (555 ml), as found in a study of 200 persons at the University of Iowa (5). The mean hemoglobin level prior to the donation for this group was 12.8 gm. The length of time required for hemoglobin to return to the predonation level varies with individuals. It may be as short as 2 to 3 weeks for some or as long as 3 to 4 months for others. The average time required by the 200 Iowa persons was 50 days. For women the period of recovery is longer than for men. The differences among individuals is explained on the basis of variability in iron stores.

The administration of medicinal iron and the adherence to certain dietary precautions hasten the restoration of the hemoglobin level after giving blood. Medicinal iron administered as 1 gm of iron and ammonium citrate per day shortened the period from an average of 50 to 35 days after the first donation, with progressively less effect after subsequent donations.

Increasing the protein content of the diet was found to hasten the restoration of hemoglobin in a study of University of Nebraska college women. Diets containing 50, 75, and 90 gm of protein daily were fed to 129 young women who were contributors to the local blood bank. Only those who received 90 gm of protein daily had hemoglobin values of the predonation level in six week's time (14).

Other essential dietary nutrients play a role in maintaining the normal blood picture, including copper, ascorbic acid, and vitamin B_{12}. The function of each is discussed in Chapters 12, 15, and 17 respectively.

Recommended Allowances for Iron

The National Research Council has recommended a daily intake of iron of 15 mg daily for young people 15 to 18 years of age. For adult men, regardless of age, and women over 55 the amount recommended is 10 mg per day whereas 15 mg is the recommended amount for women between the ages of 18 and 55. The greater allowance for the 15 to 18 year group is needed to take care of growth and deficits in iron storage that may have developed in the preceding years of rapid growth. For women, menstruation imposes an extra demand for iron (12).

An approach to determining the iron need is measuring the loss from the body and the amount in the diet sufficient to replace this loss. An average value for the total excretion of iron in urine, sweat, and feces has been estimated to be 0.5 to 1.0 mg per day (17). An additional 0.5 mg was assumed to be needed daily by women to take care of menstrual losses. As less than 10 per cent of the iron in food is found to be absorbed on an intake of 15 mg, only 1.5 mg, using average values for the calculation, would be utilized.

The adequacy of the diet as a whole makes a difference in the amount of iron that is needed. In studies with college women at the University of Nebraska, Leverton and Marsh (15) found that with diets that supplied an abundance of essential nutrients, as little as 7 mg of iron daily was sufficient on the average to allow for some storage of the mineral; with suboptimal diets a loss of iron resulted at that level of intake. However, dietary studies reveal that few persons have a food intake that supplies the recommended amounts of all nutrients, making it desirable that the iron intake be above the minimum.

Food Sources of Iron

Liver is an excellent source of iron; other meat products are good sources. There is a generous amount of iron in the yolk of egg. Dried fruits, such as apricots and prunes, are good sources, as are leafy-green vegetables such as spinach. Fresh and canned fruits and other vegetables supply some of the mineral, but cannot be considered good sources. Enriched and whole-grain cereals furnish iron in amounts that are significant in the total day's dietary (Table 11.3).

Molasses is rich in iron content. It may be surprising that a concentrated sweet should be high in iron content. Molasses is the liquor remaining after the crystallization of raw sugar from the concentrated sap of sugar cane. On the market, molasses designated as "light" is that which comes from the first extraction of sugar. It is less concentrated, and consequently lower in iron content than subsequent extractions. The second extraction is designated as "dark." "Blackstrap" is the result of further extraction and although highest in iron content, it is not useful in human diets because of the strong flavor.

A Guide to Meeting the Daily Need for Iron

If a mixed diet of cereals, milk, meat, vegetables, and fruits is eaten each day, will the iron intake automatically approach 15 mg daily? Table 11.4 gives a list of foods that supply 10 and 15 mg of iron, respectively. In order to assure meeting the Recommended Allowance, foods that are *good* sources of iron must be eaten daily. In addition, *excellent* sources such as liver and leafy-green vegetables should be frequently included.

▶ IODINE

Iodine is recognized as an important dietary nutrient, chiefly because normal functioning of the thyroid gland depends on an adequate supply of it in the body. In this country we have seriously concerned ourselves with making certain that the intake of iodine is sufficient to prevent the damaging effect of long-continued iodine deficiency. Retardation, not only in physical development but in mental as well, results when generations are subjected to an insufficient intake of iodine (1).

Location in the Body

The amount of iodine in the body is infinitesimally small, with most of it concentrated in the thyroid gland. It occurs in the body bound to organic compounds to the extent of 99 per cent (1). Quantitative estimates of the total amount of iodine in the body vary widely. The

Table 11.3. Iron Values of Some Typical Foods

Food	Measure	Iron, mg
Cereal products		
Rice, white, cooked, enriched	½ c	0.7
Bread, white, enriched	1 sl	0.5
Bread, whole wheat	1 sl	0.6
Dairy products		
Cheese, Cheddar	1 cu in.	0.2
Milk, whole	1 c	0.1
Egg	1 med	1.1
Fish		
Salmon, cooked	3 oz	0.7
Fruit, fresh		
Orange	1 med	0.5
Apricot	3	0.5
Apple, pear	1 med	0.4
Fruit, dried		
Raisins	½ c	2.8
Apricot	½ c	2.5
Prunes, cooked	8–9 sm	2.2
Legumes		
Red kidney beans, canned	½ c	2.3
Meat		
Beef liver, cooked	2 oz	5.0
Beef, pork, cooked	3 oz	2.6
Chicken, cooked	3 oz	1.4
Nuts		
Peanut butter	1 tbsp	0.3
Molasses		
Blackstrap	1 tbsp	3.2
Light	1 tbsp	0.9
Vegetables		
Spinach, cooked	½ c	2.0
Peas, cooked	½ c	1.5
Potato, cooked	1 med	0.7
Tomato, raw and cooked	1 sm, ½ c	0.7
Broccoli, cooked	½ c	0.6
Carrots, cooked	½ c	0.5
Head lettuce, cabbage, raw	1 c	0.5

From *Nutritive Value of Foods*. U.S. Dept. Agr., Home Garden Bull. 72, revised 1964.

value accepted at present is 20 to 30 mg (11, 14). The amount in the thyroid gland is found by some investigators to be 70 to 80 per cent of the total and by others to be as high as 99 per cent. The remainder is widely distributed throughout the body. In fact, all tissues and secretions analyzed thus far for iodine are found to contain it.

The thyroid gland is located at the base of the neck. It consists of two lobes, one on either side of the trachea, connected by an isthmus across the front of the trachea. Normally the gland weighs 20 to 25 gm. An insufficient intake of iodine may result in an enlargement of the gland.

The thyroid is one of several endocrine glands. They are sometimes designated as *glands of internal secretion*, or *ductless glands*. Each produces one or more secretions which it pours directly into the blood stream. The secretions of the endocrine glands are known as hormones, a term derived from the Greek meaning to *excite* or *arouse*. They are chemical substances, each with a particular function within the body. The hormones influence growth, nutritional processes, and other specific physiological activities. Thyroxine is the main hormone secreted by the thyroid gland.

Table 11.4. Two Groups of Foods Supplying Approximately 10 and 15 mg of Iron, Respectively

Food	Measure		Iron, mg
Pork, loin	3 oz		2.6
Beef, hamburger	3 oz		2.7
Bread, white, enriched	2 sl		1.2
Egg	1 med		1.1
Potato	1 med		0.7
Carrots	½ c		0.5
Orange	1 med		0.5
Beans, green	½ c		0.4
Milk	1 pt		0.2
		Total	9.9
Beef, liver	3 oz		7.5
Beef, round	3 oz		2.6
Apricots, dried	½ c		2.5
Spinach	⅔ c		2.7
		Total	15.3

From *Nutritive Value of Foods.* U.S. Dept. Agr., Home Garden Bull. 72, revised 1964.

Metabolism of Iodine

Absorption. Iodine is readily absorbed both in organic and inorganic forms. Within 3 to 6 minutes after the administration of radioactive iodine to fasting individuals, it has been detected in the hand using the Geiger-Muller counter (9). Students in chemistry do a simple test to measure the speed of absorption. A capsule of (0.2 gm) potassium iodide is swallowed and in a few minutes the saliva gives a blue color with starch paste, indicating the presence of iodine.

Most of the iodine is absorbed from the small intestine. Some, however, enters the blood stream directly from the stomach. It can even be absorbed from the skin but not to any degree of practical importance.

Utilization. After absorption into the blood, the iodine is taken up by the thyroid gland and other tissues. The thyroid gland concentrates the element and serves as a storehouse for it. In man the ratio of iodine in the thyroid to that in the blood is about 25 to 1.

After the iodine is concentrated in the thyroid gland it is formed into these iodine-containing compounds: monoiodotyrosine, diiodotyrosine, thyroxine, diiodothyronine, and triiodothyronine. These compounds are present in the gland in a complex known as thyroglobulin. Of these compounds, thyroxine is the main one that leaves the gland to enter the blood stream and carries on the functions of the hormone throughout the body.

The body is conservative of its iodine supply. When thyroxine breaks down, as it does in the normal process of body function, it is believed that some of the iodine is saved for reuse. The salvaged iodine joins that absorbed from the gastrointestinal tract in a common pool for use.

Excretion. The chief pathway of excretion of iodine is by way of the kidney, with lesser amounts through the intestine, and in perspiration. During lactation some is secreted into the milk. During the laying season some of the iodine fed to hens is recovered in the eggs.

Functions of Iodine

So far as is known, the only function of iodine in the body is that of serving as an essential component of thyroxine and the other iodine-containing compounds of the thyroid gland. Consequently the physiological functions of thyroxine are those of iodine also.

Thyroxine was first isolated from the thyroid gland by Kendall at the Mayo Foundation, Rochester, Minnesota, in 1915. Not until eleven years later was it produced synthetically. Harington and Barger of England accomplished the feat.

There are four atoms of iodine in the thyroxine molecule. The basic structure of thyroxine is closely related to the amino acid tyrosine as shown in Fig. 11.3.

In Energy Metabolism. The primary function of the thyroid hormone is to influence the rate of oxidation in the cells of the body. An increased secretion of thyroxine speeds up the rate of energy metabolism, a lack of it retards the rate. Consequently the basal metabolic rate, which is an index of the rate of oxidation in the cells, is also an indicator of the normality of thyroid function. An elevated basal rate is associated with hypersecretion of the hormone, a low rate with hyposecretion.

In addition to basal metabolic rate as a method for assessing the state of thyroid function, two other laboratory procedures used are: a) determination of protein-bound iodine (PBI) in blood serum, and b) observations on the utilization of radioactive iodine. The protein-bound iodine is chiefly thyroxine. It is found to be low in hypothyroidism and elevated in hyperthyroidism.

Using radioactive iodine makes it possible to trace the utilization of an iodine dosage in the body; iodine normally present is not radioactive. An observation commonly made is the uptake of iodine by the thyroid gland. In general the hyperfunctioning gland takes up more iodine than the normal; the hypofunctioning gland takes up less.

In Growth and Development. Thyroxine is essential for the normal growth and development of the young of all species. With an under-secretion growth may be retarded, and if the reduction is severe and prolonged, will result in failure to mature both physically and mentally.

Children suffering from a severe deficiency of the thyroid secretion are known as cretins. Their growth is retarded and their development arrested; their facial features appear coarse and swollen; the skin is thick, dry, and pasty in appearance, and often deeply wrinkled. The tongue is enlarged, the lips are thickened and usually stay ajar (Fig. 11.4).

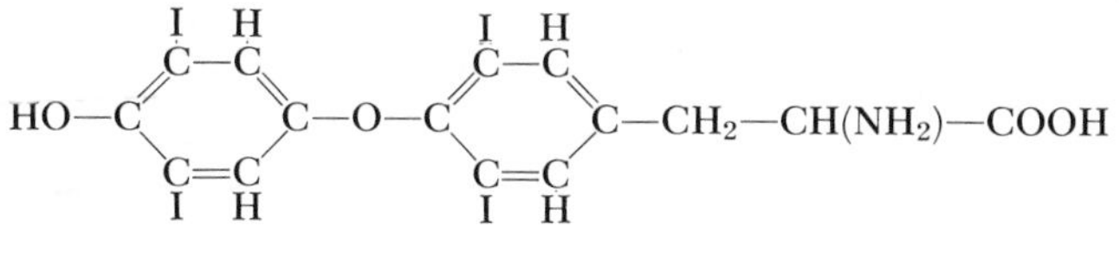

Fig. 11.3.   Thyroxine.

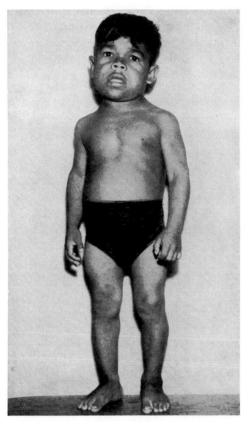

Fig. 11.4. A child suffering from cretinism. (Courtesy of Scrimshaw, Institute of Nutrition of Central America and Panama, Guatemala, C.A.)

Cretinism occurs today in those parts of the world where iodine shortage still exists.

One of the symptoms of thyroid deficiency in the adult is myxedema. The skin and subcutaneous tissues, particularly of the face and extremities, are thickened and puffy. The face is characteristically expressionless, the person lethargic and inactive.

In Pregnancy and Lactation. Iodine is essential for normal reproduction in both man and animal. Throughout time it has been observed that women frequently develop a goiter during pregnancy, indicating a greater need for the thyroid hormone.

Observations made of animals in low-iodine areas give evidence of the need for it for reproduction. A prolonged and severe lack may result in sterility, or if young are born they may be deformed. Farm animals in low-iodine regions showed abnormalities in reproduction that are now prevented by providing a sufficient amount of the mineral. Pigs were born without hair; sheep, swine, horses, and cattle developed enlarged thyroid glands during pregnancy, and the mortality rates were high among the young.

Endemic Goiter—the Result of an Inadequate Intake of Iodine

Goiter is a term applied to an enlargement of the thyroid gland. If the enlargement is due to a deficiency of iodine, it is "endemic" goiter, so named because the condition is common to certain geographic regions. These areas are characterized by low-iodine content in the soil. It is also known as "simple" goiter. In iodine deficiency the thyroxine level in the blood is lower than normal, which stimulates the thyroid gland to greater action, tending to cause it to enlarge. A young woman with endemic goiter is shown in Fig. 11.5.

Historical Incidence. As early as the first century A.D. endemic goiter was described among people living in the Alps. Burnt sponge was used as a treatment for the disorder in 1280, but it was more than five centuries later, in 1811, that the effective substance in the sponge was discovered to be iodine. This revelation was made by Bernard Courtois while extracting saltpeter from seaweed for gunpowder.

Geographic Incidence. The highest incidence has been observed in the Alps, the Pyrenees, the Himalayas, the Thames Valley in England, certain regions of New Zealand, a number of South American countries, and the Great Lakes and Pacific Northwest regions of the United States. Figure 11.6 shows the goitrous sections of the world.

Surveys show endemic goiter to be present in some 100 countries and territories (2, 6). Scrimshaw (13) believes, furthermore, that all of the goitrous areas in the world have not been identified as yet, and will not be until specific surveys are done.

Age and Sex Incidence. Women and girls are afflicted with endemic goiter more commonly than men and boys. Adolescence is the period of greatest susceptibility to limited iodine intake. Boys develop thyroid enlargement at this age but to a lesser extent than girls. The incidence of endemic goiter among Costa Rican school children illustrates the higher occurrence among adolescent girls, 23.8 per cent of whom were afflicted, in contrast to 19.4 per cent of the boys.

The Use of Iodine as a Preventive Measure. Although the use of iodine prophylactically was attempted in man as early as 1820, the

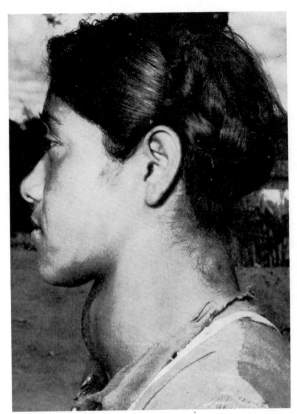

Fig. 11.5. A young woman showing endemic goiter. (Courtesy of Scrimshaw, Institute of Nutrition of Central America and Panama, Guatemala, C.A.)

effectiveness was not convincingly demonstrated until the experiments in the public schools of Akron, Ohio in 1917. Adolescent girls were selected for study because of the high incidence of thyroid enlargement in that age and sex group. Two grams of sodium iodide was administered twice yearly to 2190 girls during the 2½ years of observation. A group of 2305 with no additions of iodide was followed as controls. Among those taking iodine only 5 developed thyroid enlargement as contrasted to 495 in the control group.

In 1922 the state of Michigan, through the Medical Society and State Department of Health, surveyed the state for incidence of goiter among school children. An average incidence of 47.2 per cent indicated an urgent need for prophylaxis. Through the cooperation of the Wholesale Grocers' Association and the Salt Manufacturers' Association, table salt containing potassium iodide was put on the market. This pioneering

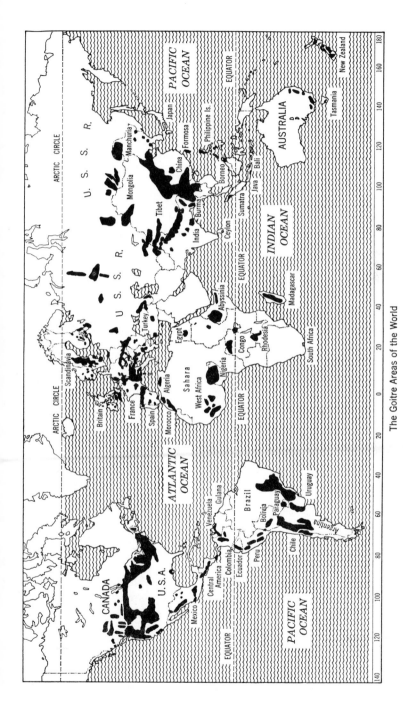

The Goitre Areas of the World

Fig. 11.6. Goiter areas of the world. (Courtesy of Iodine Educational Bureau, Chilean Nitrate Company, London.)

attempt to provide iodine for the people of Michigan was accompanied by an educational program emphasizing the need for this element in the diet.

The most recent resurvey of school children in Michigan to assess the effectiveness of iodized salt as a prophylactic measure was in 1952, 30 years after its introduction. In four counties 53,785 children were examined. The incidence of endemic goiter had fallen from 47.2 per cent to 1.4 per cent in that period (3). In 1954 the Department of Health in Ohio resurveyed the school children in the four counties that were first examined in 1925. The incidence among the boys in an earlier study was 24.2 per cent; in 1954, 2.2 per cent. Among the girls the incidence was 40.5 per cent in 1925 and was reduced to 5.8 per cent in 1954 (10).

The use of iodized salt is believed to be the major influence in the decline of endemic goiter in the United States. Another factor contributing to the decrease in the incidence of iodine deficiency is a marketing system that brings to any locality a food supply that originates from diverse areas of the country.

The 1960 report of the World Health Organization on Legislation on Iodine Prophylaxis indicated that only about ten countries at that time had legal measures making iodine prophylaxis compulsory (6). In Austria, the United Kingdom, and the United States, scientific committees recommended the use of iodized salt, but legislation has not been enacted making it compulsory. Canada, Guatemala, and Columbia are among the countries having mandatory salt-iodization programs.

The WHO Study-Group on Endemic Goiter recommended that ". . . all food salts should be iodized compulsorily in any country or area in which goiter is endemic, local variations in incidence of disease being disregarded" (16).

On occasion, rumors circulate that the use of iodized salt is harmful to health because of the iodine content. The World Health Organization Study Group on Endemic Goiter states this: "In no country in which iodine prophylaxis has been used on a community scale, has this measure had any adverse effects on the health of the population." From the report of The Third Conference on Nutrition Problems in Latin America, this statement concerning the prophylactic use of iodine explains further that " . . . all reports of unfavorable effects which have been investigated have proved to be false or explainable on the basis of coincidence" (13).

Recommended Allowances for Iodine

The National Research Council has recommended an intake of iodine of 100 to 150 μg daily for the adult. The need may be greater for the adolescent and pregnant or lactating woman.

Antithyroid Compounds

The term antithyroid compounds is applied to a number of substances which inhibit the formation of the thyroid hormone.

Drugs. One group of drugs functions by inhibiting the uptake of iodine by the thyroid gland. Thiocyanate is such a drug. However, if the level of iodine in the blood is sufficiently high, iodine may enter the thyroid, presumably by diffusion. A second group of drugs exerts its effect on the functioning of the thyroid gland a step beyond the process of iodine concentration. These compounds appear to block thyroxine synthesis even though the supply of the iodide ion is adequate. Such drugs include thiourea, thiouracil, phenol derivatives, and cobaltous chloride.

Antithyroid Compound in Foods. There seems to be little doubt but that there are factors in some foods that increase the need for dietary iodine (7). They are called "goitrogenic" because they increase susceptibility to goiter resulting from iodine deficiency. It is believed that these substances may be responsible, at least in part, for the simple goiters that appear in both man and animal at times, in spite of an intake of iodine that would normally be considered adequate.

The discovery that goitrogenic factors exist came from experimental studies with animals. It was in 1928 at Johns Hopkins University that rabbits fed almost exclusively on fresh cabbage were observed to develop enlarged thyroid glands (4). It was a fortuitous finding, for the investigators were actually seeking information on a certain disease condition unrelated to goiter.

Since the early study with cabbage, an antithyroid compound has been identified in the seeds of most of the mustard family and the edible portion of some plants (cabbage, kale, and rape) (8). The substance is known as goitrin and has been established as (−)-5-vinyl-2-oxazolidinethione. A precursor of goitrin, progoitrin, is present also in the seeds of some plants and has thus far been identified only in the edible portion of rutabagas and white turnips (12).

Progoitrin is active only when converted to goitrin. It was first believed that the enzyme which converts progoitrin to goitrin was present in the food but could be destroyed by heat. It is now known that progoitrin can be converted to goitrin by enzymes in the intestine. Thus cooked food as well as raw containing the compounds are potentially goitrogenic.

It may be that continuous ingestion of small amounts of goitrin or other unidentified goitrogens that may exist, may alter normal thyroid hormone synthesis. The effect would be expected to be more severe if only the minimal amount of iodine needed by the body were supplied in the diet.

Food Sources

The amount of iodine in most foods is exceedingly small, requiring sensitive chemical methods to determine it quantitatively. The content varies widely among foods, and even for the same food under different soil and fertilizer conditions. Vought and London (15) determined the iodine content of whole meals and individual foods served on metabolic diets and on regular house diets at the Clinical Center, National Institutes of Health. The metabolic diets contained from 15 to 219 μg and the regular house diets from 65 to 529 μg per day. The iodine content of food composites in each of seven food categories as determined by Vought and London is presented in Table 11.5. The authors stated that because of the skewed distribution, the median is a better centering constant than the mean.

Marine or deep-sea fish and shell fish are high in iodine content. The anadromous group of fish (those fish that spend a part of the time in sea water and a part in fresh), to which salmon and sea trout belong, contain more iodine than the fish that remain all the time in fresh water but less than most of the fish that remain at sea. The leaves and flowers of plants (spinach, turnip greens, and broccoli) appear to have higher iodine concentration than the roots.

A supplement to the iodine intake in goitrous regions becomes essential. Iodized salt is an effective means of providing the supplement. The amount of iodine added to salt in the United States is 0.01 per cent and

Table 11.5. Iodine Content of Composites of Food Categories

Food Category	No. of Samples	Iodine (mg/wet kg) Mean ± S.E.	Median
Sea foods	7	660 ± 180	540
Vegetables	13	320 ± 100	280
Meat products	12	260 ± 70	175
Eggs	11	260 ± 80	145
Dairy products	18	130 ± 10	139
Bread and cereal	18	100 ± 20	105
Fruits	18	40 ± 20	18

From Vought and London, *Am. J. Clin. Nutr.* **14**: 190, 1964.

is in the form of potassium iodide. It is not compulsory by law that iodine be added to salt, but it is voluntarily added by the manufacturers. A nationwide survey revealed that 20 per cent of the families never use iodized salt, 4 per cent use it a part of the time, and 76 per cent use it exclusively (5). Vought and London (15) reported that the median amount of salt added at the table by their subjects was 1.59 gm per day. If this were iodized salt, an estimated 122 μg of iodine per day would be added to the diet.

REFERENCES

IRON

1. Bothwell, T. H., and A. F. Clement (1962). *Iron Metabolism.* Little, Brown, an Co., Boston.
2. Brown, E. B. (1963). The absorption of iron. *Am. J. Clin. Nutr.* 12: 205.
3. Downes, H. R. (1962). *The Chemistry of Living Cells.* Harper and Row, New York.
4. Finch, C. A., J. G. Gibson, W. W. Peacock, and R. G. Fluharty (1949). Iron metabolism. Utilization of intravenous radioactive iron. *Blood* 4, 905.
5. Fowler, W. M., and A. P. Barer (1942). Rate of hemoglobin regeneration in blood doners. *J. Am. Med. Assoc.* 118: 421.
6. Frenchman, R., and F. A. Johnston (1949). Relation of menstrual losses to iron requirement. *J. Am. Dietet. Assoc.* 25: 217.
7. Goldsmith, G. A. (1959). *Nutritional Diagnosis.* Charles C Thomas, Springfield, Ill., p. 87.
8. Gubler, C. J. (1956). Absorption and metabolism of iron. *Science.* 123: 87.
9. Ingalls, R. L., and F. A. Johnston (1954). Iron from gastrointestinal sources excreted in the feces of human subjects. *J. Nutr.* 53: 351.
10. *Iron Deficiency Anemia* (1959). World Health Organ., WHO Tech. Rept. Series No. 182, Geneva.
11. Isaacson, C., H. Seftel, K. J. Keeley, and T. H. Bothwell (1961). Siderosis in the Bantu. The relationship between iron overload and cirrhosis. *J. Lab. Clin. Med.* 58: 845.
12. Johnston, F. A., and T. J. McMillan (1952). Iron requirement of six young women. *J. Am. Dietet. Assoc.* 28: 633.
13. Lahey, M. (1957). Iron and copper in infant nutrition. *Am. J. Clin. Nutr.* 5: 516–526.
14. Leverton, R. M., D. Schlaphoff, and M. Huffstetter (1948). Blood regeneration in women blood donors. II. Effect of protein, vitamin, and mineral supplements. *J. Am. Dietet. Assoc.* 24: 480.
15. Leverton, R. M., and A. G. Marsh (1942). The iron metabolism and requirement of young women. *J. Nutr.* 23: 229.
16. Moore, C. V., and R. Dubach (1962). *Iron in Mineral Metabolism,* Vol. 2, Pt. B. (C. L. Comar and F. Bronner, eds.) Academic Press, New York.
17. Moore, E. V., and R. Dubach (1956). Metabolism and requirements of iron in the human. *J. Am. Med. Assoc.* 162: 197.
18. Reynatarje, C., and J. Ramos (1961). Influence of altitude changes on intestinal iron absorption. *J. Lab. Clin. Med.* 57: 848.
19. Rogers, T. A. (1961). *Elementary Physiology.* John Wiley and Sons, New York.
20. Underwood, E. J. (1962). *Trace Elements.* 2nd ed. Academic Press, New York.

IODINE

1. Astwood, E. B. (1955). Iodine in nutrition. *Bordon's Rev. Nutr. Res.* **16:** 53.
2. Brock, J. F. (1961). *Recent Advances in Human Nutrition.* Little, Brown, and Co., Boston.
3. Brush, B. E., and J. K. Altland (1952). Goiter prevention with iodized salt; results of a thirty-year study. *J. Clin. Endocrinol.* **12:** 1380.
4. Chesney, A. M., T. A. Clawson, and B. Webster (1928). Endemic goiter in rabbits. *Bull. Johns Hopkins Hosp.* **43:** 261, 278, 291.
5. *Dietary Levels of Households in the United States Report No. 6* (1957). U.S. Dept. Agr., Washington, D.C., p. 63.
6. Endemic Goiter (1960). In *Legislation on Iodine Prophylaxis.* World Health Organ., Geneva, p. 14.
7. Greer, M. A. (1950). Nutrition and goiter. *Physiol. Rev.* **30:** 513.
8. Greer, M. A. (1960). The significance of naturally occurring antithyroid compounds in the production of goiter in man. *Borden's Rev. Nutr. Res.* **21:** 61.
9. Hamilton, J. G. (1948). The rates of absorption of the radioactive isotopes of sodium, potassium, chlorine, bromine, and iodine in normal human subjects. *Am. J. Physiol.* **124:** 667.
10. Hamwi, G. J., A. W. Van Fossen, R. E. Whetstone, and I. Williams (1955). Endemic goiter in Ohio school children. *Am. J. Public Health* **45:** 1344.
11. Riggs, D. S. (1952). Quantitative aspects of iodine metabolism in man. *Pharmacol. Rev.* **4:** 284.
12. Ruch, T. C., and J. F. Fulton (1960). *Medical Physiology and Biophysics,* 18th ed. W. B. Saunders Co., Philadelphia.
13. Scrimshaw, N. S. (1957). Endemic goiter. *Nutr. Rev.* **15:** 161.
14. Underwood, E. J. (1962). *Trace Elements.* 2nd ed. Academic Press, New York.
15. Vought, R. L., and W. T. London (1964). Dietary sources of iodine. *Am. J. Clin. Nutr.* **14:** 186.
16. World Health Organization, Study-group on endemic goiter (1953). *Bull. World Health Organ.* **9:** 293.

CHAPTER 12

The other mineral elements

Sodium, chlorine, potassium, magnesium, sulfur, manganese, copper, zinc, cobalt, molybdenum, selenium, chromium, and fluorine are all discussed in this chapter. Because of selenium's possible role as an essential trace element, information on it is presented. Chromium is included because of its apparent relationship to the glucose tolerance factor. Although fluorine is not classified as an essential mineral, it is discussed here and in Chapter 23 because of its role in the reduction of dental caries in man.

▶ SODIUM AND CHLORINE

It seems appropriate to discuss sodium and chlorine (as chloride) together inasmuch as they are closely related in both function and dietary intake.

It has been estimated that persons in the United States ingest 3 to 7 gm of sodium per day; the daily intake of chloride from food appears to be somewhat higher, about 6 to 7 gm per day. Although most of the sodium is found in the blood plasma and in the fluids outside the cells (extracellular), findings indicate that some of the body's sodium is found in the bones. As yet the nature of bone sodium is not well understood, but it appears to be important as a store of the element for emergency use. Chloride, like sodium, is found largely in the blood plasma and the fluids outside the cells of the body. In the foods we eat and in the body, some of the sodium and chloride are combined to form sodium chloride, ordinary table salt.

Functions of Sodium and Chloride

Sodium and chloride as major constituents in the extracellular fluid contribute to the osmotic pressure. They also help in the regulation of acid-base balance; sodium together with calcium, magnesium, and potassium in the extracellular fluid are basic in reaction; chloride with phosphate and sulfate groups, and protein are acidic in reaction. In addition, chloride is found in gastric juice as a component of the hydrochloric acid molecule; and in salivary amylase the chloride ion activates the starch-splitting enzyme of saliva.

The Effects of a Sodium and Chloride Deficiency and of a Sodium Chloride Excess

There are numerous studies that have shown the effects of sodium deficiencies in the animal organism, yet there are few available which deal solely with a chloride deficiency. Many of the data reported, however, demonstrate the combined effect of a sodium chloride deficiency.

A deficiency of sodium in the ration of rats produces retarded growth, perhaps related to the depressed appetite observed to accompany the deficiency (15). The effects of sodium inadequacies in the human have also been reported. A premature infant, ingesting a low-sodium feeding for a period of 49 days, lost weight throughout the seven weeks even though the energy intake was adequate (2).

A deficiency of chloride in the ration of the rat also produces retarded growth but to a lesser degree than has been shown with either a sodium or a combined sodium chloride deficiency. Slow growth in rats fed a chloride-free ration for a period of three months has been reported by workers at Johns Hopkins University.

There are evidences of the effects of low as well as high intakes of sodium chloride in both animals and man. Rats fed rations deficient in sodium chloride grew more slowly, lost hair about the back and shoulders, and showed signs of internal hemorrhages in the thymus gland and the liver. Moreover, slower growth rates have been observed in rats fed either a low or a high intake of sodium chloride. Studies with healthy men (9, 10) indicate that sodium chloride has an important influence on the capillary activity and on the consumption of oxygen of the body. After 14 days on a rich sodium chloride diet, one subject showed an increased blood pressure, an increased basal metabolic rate, and coarsened and thickened capillary walls of the fingernails, arm, and skin of the chest. The diet ingested by this man contained 15 gm of salt, 600 gm of meat, 100 gm of bread, 30 gm of cheese, and vitamins supplied by tablets. When this subject was shifted to a poor sodium chloride diet, which contained only 2 gm of salt per day, it was noted that all the symptoms described above regressed.

Recommended Allowances for Sodium and Chloride

Very little is known about the exact requirement for sodium and chloride. The National Research Council suggests that the normal requirement is more than met for these two minerals from the food and the salt added to the food in an average diet (28). However, the requirement is increased when environmental and climatic conditions cause increased sweating. In many industrial companies, employees who are exposed to excessive heat have salt tablets at their disposal in order to compensate for the sodium chloride lost in perspiration. The need for sodium chloride during the summer in the tropics was found to be 5.4 to 6.2 gm per day for the subjects studied by Malhorta and co-workers (22).

Food Sources of Sodium and Chloride

Sodium is widely distributed in the food inasmuch as the sodium-rich foods come from animal sources such as fresh meats, fish, poultry, eggs, and milk. In contrast, foods from plant sources are usually low in sodium. Such foods as ham, bacon, salted fish, bread, and crackers have a high sodium content because salt is added during processing. The theoretical sodium content of salt is 39,342 mg per 100 gm or about 2.8 gm per teaspoon. The sodium contents of 100-gm portions of some typical foods are listed in Table A-10 (appendix). For a more comprehensive list, the reader is referred to the revised edition of *Composition of Foods—Raw, Processed, Prepared* (46).

Besides food and salt, drinking water may be an important contributor of dietary sodium. For example, the public drinking water in Galveston, Texas, contains as much as 34 mg of sodium per 100 ml; that in Washington, D.C. contains about 0.3 mg per 100 ml. Suppose that a man in Washington, where the water sodium is low, ingests 2½ liters of water each day; he will have an intake of about 7.5 mg of sodium from water alone.

Owing to the abundance of chloride in the normal diet, it is most unlikely that a human deficiency from this mineral will occur. Pork, beef, eggs, certain cheeses, and clams are very rich sources of chloride, whereas fruits and vegetables contain only small amounts of this nutrient. Olives, crackers, ham, bacon, butter, and other similar foods contribute chloride because of the salt added during processing. The theoretical chloride content of salt is 60,300 mg per 100 gm or about 4.2 gm per teaspoon.

The Sodium-Restricted Diet

Studies in the last two decades have shown the therapeutic importance of dietary sodium restriction in certain pathological conditions such as congestive heart disease, hypertension, kidney disease, cirrhosis of the liver with ascites, and toxemia of pregnancy. Owing to the efforts of many dietitians and nutritionists, sodium-restricted diets have been developed and refined for use in these disorders (6, 7, 29, 30, 32).

The general pattern of a sodium-restricted regimen involves a menu plan comprised of food items low in the nutrient. Spices, herbs, and other flavorings, also low in sodium, are used to add variety to the food. The success of the diet is determined by the patient's acceptance of the meals.

Many of the early sodium-restricted diets used for therapeutic purposes proved to be unsatisfactory nutritionally. These diets were low in sodium but they were inadequate in other essential nutrients (protein, calcium, riboflavin). Robinson (30) has recommended the use of sodium-deficient milk to assure nutritional adequacy when sodium levels of 250 mg or less are prescribed.

▶ POTASSIUM

The adult human body contains more than two times as much potassium (about 9 oz) as it does sodium (about 4 oz), yet the normal daily intake of potassium is even a little less than sodium. Typical diets in the United States contain about 0.8 to 1.5 gm of potassium per 1000 Cal. (28). It is obvious that the body is more conservative of its potassium than of sodium. Potassium is concentrated primarily within the cells rather than in the extracellular or interstitial fluids as is sodium. Concentration of potassium within the cells contributes to the capacity of the body to conserve the mineral.

Function of Potassium

Like sodium and chloride, potassium functions in the maintenance of osmotic pressure and acid-base balance of the body—sodium and chloride functioning almost wholly in the extracellular fluid, potassium within the cell in the intracellular fluid. Recent findings suggest that potassium serves as an activator of enzymes and may be important in the use of amino acids following protein depletion as well as in optimal bone calcification.

The Effects of a Potassium Deficiency

The effects of inadequate potassium differ from species to species. Rats deprived of adequate potassium in their rations show slow but steady growth after 8½ months on low potassium intakes. Sexual maturity of these animals is delayed, and the fur is thin and rough. The symptoms of a potassium deficiency in chicks are retarded growth, followed by loss of the use of the legs, and finally death (Fig. 12.1). Like the chick, the dog fails to grow and develops paralysis when fed inadequate amounts of dietary potassium.

It is quite unlikely that a potassium deficiency occurs in man under normal conditions of health, but cases of hypopotassemia (potassium deficiency) have been reported in conditions of disease, body burns, and malnutrition.

At a large city hospital, during a period of one year, 309 of the surgical patients treated were found to have suboptimal serum potassium levels and

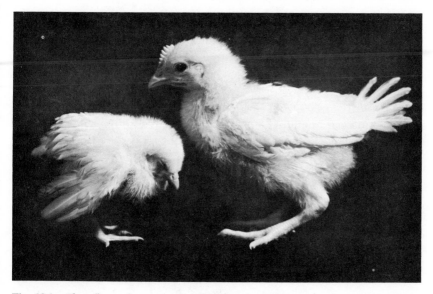

Fig. 12.1.   The effects of a potassium deficiency in chicks. (Courtesy of Gillis, *J. Nutr.*, **36**: 351, 1948.)

showed symptoms of hypopotassemia, muscular weakness, and lethargy (16). These symptoms were relieved by intravenous feedings of a solution containing potassium. A man who has been burned may show a negative potassium balance due to loss of large amounts of the mineral from the body cells. It has been demonstrated that a potassium and nitrogen intake in a ratio of 6 to 1, rather than the normal 4 to 1, was necessary to maintain equilibrium in the burned patients studied (27). In three cases of human starvation (48) the symptoms involved central nervous system damage which disappeared when potassium salts and vitamins were administered. The body's restoration of potassium within the cells, however, was very slow in spite of the fact that they were given large amounts of potassium chloride and had a potassium-rich diet. Also potassium deficiencies of major significance have been demonstrated in kwashiorkor, a childhood dietary deficiency disease related primarily to inadequate protein. It has been suggested that in the initial treatment of this disorder with skim milk, the high potassium content of the milk may be as important as its protein content in the relief of the symptoms of this disease (11).

Recommended Allowances and Food Sources of Potassium

At this time a human requirement for potassium has not been established (28). However, man's minimal potassium need, based on limited data, has been estimated to range from 0.8 to 1.3 gm per day. An adequate intake of the element is assumed inasmuch as a typical American diet contains 0.8 to 1.5 gm of potassium per 1000 Cal.

Potassium is found in almost all foods, both plant and animal, and occurs in very small amounts in drinking water (13, 46). Foods which contain more than 1 gm of potassium per 100 gm include bran, dried brewer's yeast, cocoa, coffee, dried legumes (peas, soybeans, and white beans), molasses, potato chips, spices, and tea (46). The potassium content of some typical foods is presented in Table A-10 (appendix).

▶ MAGNESIUM

The adult human body contains about 20 to 28 gm of magnesium concentrated primarily in the skeleton, with smaller amounts found in the soft tissues and extracellular fluids. Magnesium is closely allied to calcium and phosphorus, not only in body distribution but also in body function.

Function of Magnesium

The chief function of magnesium appears to be as an activator of certain enzymes in the body. In particular, it activates enzyme systems related to carbohydrate metabolism.

Magnesium apparently serves an important function in calcium and phosphorus metabolism. Although the teeth and bones contain about 70 per cent of the body's magnesium, little is known about the calcium-phosphorus-magnesium complex within these tissues.

A relationship between magnesium and endocrine function has been observed. It has been reported that with increased thyroid activity, the need for magnesium is also increased (45).

The Effects of a Magnesium Deficiency in Animals

Experimental magnesium deficiencies have been developed in several species of animals, including rats, rabbits, calves, ducks, guinea pigs, and dogs. Symptoms of the deficiency are similar, characterized by retarded growth, convulsive attacks, and finally death, if the deficiency is maintained. Rats in which a magnesium deficiency has been developed are hyperexcitable; the sound of paper rustling will precipitate a convulsive attack.

The Effects of a Magnesium Deficiency in Man

The magnesium deficiency syndrome in man has been observed in acute alcoholism and in cases of electrolytic imbalance. Magnesium deficiencies in adult patients resulting from chronic alcoholism, complicated by delirium tremens, have been observed (12, 40). The low blood serum magnesium values as well as the gross muscular tremors and delirium in these patients were relieved by magnesium therapy. An interesting observation in this work was the improvement of the muscular tremor after the administration of magnesium sulfate, as shown by samples of a patient's handwriting (Fig. 12.2). The intake of magnesium-free intravenous fluids over a long period of time has also resulted in a magnesium-deficient state in man.

In 1960 a group at Harvard Medical School described a new clinical disorder in man as "magnesium-deficiency tetany" (44). The clinical symptoms of this syndrome are similar to those observed in human "calcium-deficiency tetany," but the blood picture shows a normal

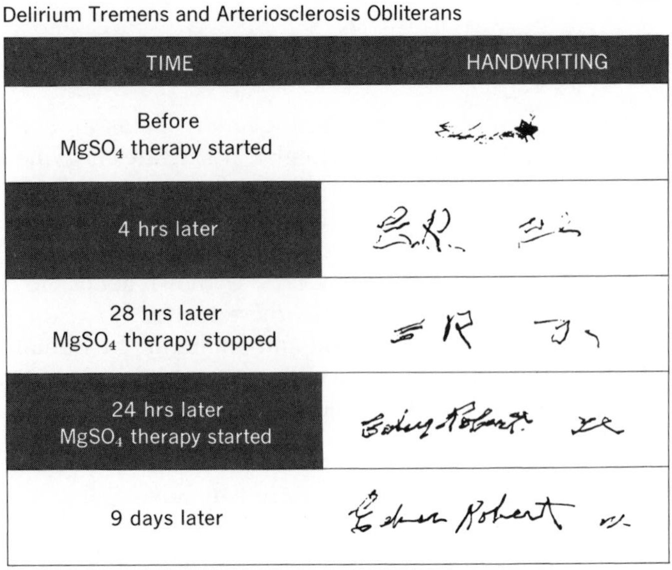

Delirium Tremens and Arteriosclerosis Obliterans

TIME	HANDWRITING
Before MgSO$_4$ therapy started	
4 hrs later	
28 hrs later MgSO$_4$ therapy stopped	
24 hrs later MgSO$_4$ therapy started	
9 days later	

Fig. 12.2. Signatures of handwriting obtained from a patient with low serum magnesium levels at various times as indicated. Part of the name has been obliterated. (Courtesy of Flink, *J. Lab. Clin. Med.*, **43:** 169, 1954.)

serum calcium and a very low level of serum magnesium. Intramuscular injections of magnesium sulfate proved to be beneficial to all the patients studied. As a matter of interest, it was reported that as the serum magnesium returned to normal levels, there was a prompt and dramatic relief from the symptoms of the tetany.

Recommended Allowances and Food Sources of Magnesium

At this time the National Research Council has made no recommendation for man's need of magnesium (28). Balance studies indicate, however, that the magnesium needs of young men range from 300 to 400 mg per day (20) whereas those for young women average about 300 mg per day (18). It is assumed that sufficient amounts of the mineral will be available to the body from the ingestion of an ordinary diet.

Because magnesium is found in so many foods that are common to any diet (13, 25, 46), a deficiency of the mineral is quite unlikely. The magnesium content of some typical foods is presented in Table A-10 (appendix).

▶ SULFUR

Sulfur is found in every cell of the body, located principally in the sulfur-containing amino acids; it is also present in body secretions, saliva and bile, and in the hormone, insulin.

Function of Sulfur

This element is related to protein nutrition because of its occurrence in the sulfur-containing amino acids and certain enzymes. The exact function of sulfur in the body, however, has not been fully established.

The Effects of a Sulfur Deficiency

Although little is known about the effects of inadequate sulfur in man and animals, studies have been made on the effect of sulfur-containing amino acids on wool production in sheep and hair growth in human beings. Because wool contains about 13 per cent cystine, one of the sulfur-containing amino acids, research has been done to study the influence of this amino acid on the wool production of sheep. Generally, the effects of feeding supplementary cystine to improve wool production have been negative. Also there is no evidence to warrant a relationship between a dietary deficiency of these amino acids, thus sulfur, and the lack of hair growth in the human being.

Recommended Allowances and Food Sources of Sulfur

Man's need for sulfur is not known. Because the mineral is so closely tied to protein nutrition, its requirement by man is undoubtedly related to the protein requirement. Organic sulfides are found in both plant and animal foods. Wheat germ, lentils, cheese, lean beef, kidney beans, peanuts, and clams are exceptionally rich food sources of this mineral.

▶ MANGANESE

Manganese is found in the liver, skin, bones, and muscles of animals. In fact all animal tissues thus far examined contain some manganese, but in very low concentrations. The relative amount of it found in the human body is about 12 to 20 mg in a 70 kg man.

Function of Manganese

Manganese functions in the animal organism as an activator of enzymes involved in the metabolism of carbohydrates, fats, and proteins.

The Effects of a Manganese Deficiency

Metabolism studies with the rat, chick, and rabbit have revealed the effects of a manganese deficiency in these species. The normal processes of reproduction and lactation in the rat are interfered with when they are fed rations low in manganese. Female rats fail to suckle their young, and in the male rat there is a degeneration of the reproductive organs. The long bones and bodies of the offspring of manganese-deficient rats have been found to be shorter than those of normal animals. A manganese deficiency in chicks is characterized by an abnormality of the leg bones known as *perosis* or slipped tendon (Fig. 12.3). Not only do the bones of the legs shorten and undergo other physical and chemical changes, but the crippling effect that results prevents the chick from securing food, and death soon follows. It is now known that choline is interrelated with manganese in the prevention of perosis in birds. An

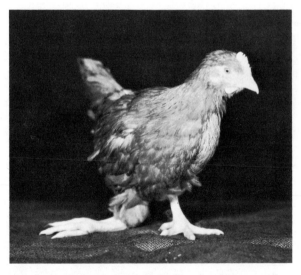

Fig. 12.3. A picture of a Rhode Island red chick afflicted with the type of perosis caused by manganese deficiency. (Courtesy of Poultry Husbandry Department, Cornell University, Ithaca, New York.)

impaired leg bone formation has also been observed in manganese deficient rabbits. In the front leg bones, the humeri are shorter and break more easily because of the low ash content of the tissue. In addition to the leg bone symptoms, the deficient rabbits showed less weight gain than did the ones that received an adequate amount of manganese.

Manganese Toxicity

Manganese toxicity has been reported in both animals and man. The animal studies of Chornock, Guerrant, and Dutcher (4) showed that high intakes of manganese retarded growth in rats in proportion to the amount of the mineral present in the ration. In dogs oral administration of large doses of manganese resulted in gastric disturbances but did not affect growth. Although cases of manganese poisoning are not common in man, toxicity was recognized as early as 1837 among men who worked loading ores rich in this mineral. Some of the symptoms of manganese poisoning found in these men were a peculiar mask-like expression of the face, involuntary laughing, a low voice with blurred speech, walking with a spastic gait, and tremors of the hands. A study (31) concerning 150 cases of manganese poisoning in Moroccan miners described the same symptoms (Fig. 12.4).

Recommended Allowances and Food Sources of Manganese

Man's requirement for manganese is not yet known (28). It has been reported, however, that young adult women retained about 1.54 mg or 41 per cent of the manganese ingested in a balance experiment (26). In view of this finding, it would seem that the average diet which contains about 4 mg of the mineral per day is more than adequate.

The manganese content of commonly used foods has been measured. Studies of the manganese content of one-hundred-twenty different foods has shown that wheat bran, blueberries, whole wheat, split peas, beets, and navy beans are the richest sources of the mineral in foods.

▶ COPPER

The importance of copper in nutrition was first demonstrated by Hart and others at the University of Wisconsin in a series of studies that began in 1925. When rats and rabbits were fed a milk diet, an anemia developed that iron supplementation did not correct and was relieved only when the copper-containing ash of certain foods was fed to the animals. This

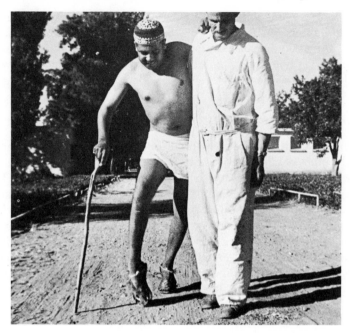

Fig. 12.4. The effects of manganese poisoning in Moroccan miners. The patient cannot walk without help. (From collection of Rodier, courtesy of the author and *Brit. J. Ind. Med.* 12, January 1955.)

work established the necessity of copper, along with iron, in the formation of hemoglobin in the body.

Function and Effects of a Deficiency of Copper

To this date the exact function of copper in animals and man is not understood; however, symptoms that develop in copper-deficient animals suggest certain functions. It is involved in the formation of red blood cells as a catalyst to the formation of hemoglobin. Copper is not a part of the hemoglobin molecule, even though essential for its formation. A diet deficient in copper is accompanied by a reduction of the oxidative enzymes, cytochrome oxidase and catalase in some species. On diets deficient in copper, lambs were found to manifest a failure in muscular coordination. Autopsy revealed demyelination (removal of outer tissue, myelin sheath) of nerve fibers. Dogs showed a crippling disorder of the bones (Fig. 12.5). Another manifestation of copper deficiency is the graying of hair in several species, the rat, rabbit, cat, dog, goat, and sheep.

A copper deficiency in human beings has only recently been observed. Although in the past a combined deficiency of copper and iron in children had been recognized, it was not until 1956 that a group of scientists at the University of Southern California demonstrated the use of copper sulfate in relieving an anemic condition in five young children (41). The need for copper in man apparently is most significant in the early months of life because low-copper blood levels are a characteristic pattern at birth. However, adult man does not develop a copper deficiency even during long periods of malnutrition. This fact has been substantiated by the observations made on thirty-eight American prisoners of the Second World War who had received a very inadequate food intake for an average period of 3⅓ years (3). An inborn error of metabolism in man that involves copper has been recognized. This hereditary disorder known as Wilson's disease is discussed in Chapter 8.

Recommended Allowances and Food Sources of Copper

As yet a copper requirement for man has not been stated (28). A comparison of the data from dietary analyses and from human balance studies indicate that the ordinary diet more than satisfies man's need for this nutrient. A typical diet provides about 2.5 mg of copper daily, and adults and children have been observed to maintain "copper balance" on 2 mg or less of the mineral per day.

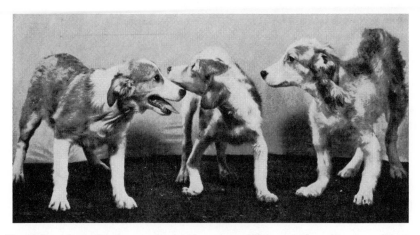

Fig. 12.5. A bone disorder associated with a copper deficiency in dogs. (Courtesy of Baxter and Van Wyk, *Bull. of the Johns Hopkins Hospital,* **93:** 1, 1953.)

The copper content of foods varies, but from a list of commonly used foods liver, oysters, mushrooms, currants, nuts, dried legumes, and chocolate are found to be the richest sources of copper.

▶ ZINC

Small amounts of zinc are found in both animals and plants. In animals most of the mineral is found in the liver, bones, and blood.

Function of Zinc

Even though the exact function of zinc in the animal body is unknown, it has been shown to be a component of several enzymes and hormones. The enzyme carbonic anhydrase contains zinc and is found in the red blood cells, where it speeds the breakdown of carbonic acid in the lungs during the exchange of carbon dioxide for oxygen. The mineral is also an essential part of one of the protein-splitting enzymes secreted by the pancreas and several dehydrogenases found in the liver. The presence of zinc in the crystalline structure of insulin, however, has been known since 1934. Although several types of insulin have been developed throughout the years, the one which has been most widely used is protamine-zinc insulin. This form, which is more slowly absorbed from the tissues than is plain insulin, requires less frequent injections to maintain the diabetic patient. It appears that the addition of zinc to the insulin solution has a retarding effect and therefore prolongs the activity of the hormone in the body.

The Effects of a Zinc Deficiency

The effects of a zinc deficiency have been reported in the rat, mouse, pig, chick, and calf. When suboptimal amounts of zinc are fed in the rations of rats and mice, the animals grow at a slower rate and lose hair around the neck and shoulders. A zinc deficiency in pigs is manifested by subnormal growth and a lesion of the horny layer of the skin known as parakeratosis. In addition to retarded growth and skin lesions, the chick shows symptoms of poor feathering and calcification on a zinc-free diet. Alopecia, extensive parakeratotic skin lesions, and low weight gains are a few of the symptoms observed in calves fed a low-zinc ration.

Zinc Toxicity

That high dietary levels of zinc interfere with the metabolism of copper in the young rat has been an accepted hypothesis for some time. Growth depression, anemia, and a decrease in liver copper are several of the characteristic symptoms of zinc toxicity in these animals. Newer experimental data (21) indicate that excess amounts of zinc in the diet also interfere with the metabolism of iron. It appears that zinc does not interfere with iron absorption but rather with its utilization.

Recommended Allowances and Food Sources of Zinc

The zinc requirement of man is unknown (28), but the results of balance studies have shown that there is a retention of the mineral in the body. From the difficulties experienced by research workers in preparing a zinc-deficient diet, it might be concluded that the possibility of this deficiency occurring in animals and man is very unlikely because most natural diets appear to contain an amount of the mineral sufficient to maintain good health.

Zinc is found in most foods of a normal diet. The richest food sources are oysters, wheat germ, and bran; fruits and vegetables contain only very small amounts of the mineral.

▶ COBALT

Cobalt is one of the mineral elements to be recognized recently as essential for the animal organism. It is needed in very small amounts and has been shown to be part of the vitamin B_{12} molecule.

Function of Cobalt

Cobalt functions in the animal organism as a constituent of proteins that carry oxygen in respiration reactions. Indirectly cobalt functions in the formation of red blood cells because of its important part in the vitamin B_{12} molecule. Observations with cattle and sheep have established the way that cobalt apparently functions in the animal organism. Those animals who eat only plant foods that contain little or no vitamin B_{12} need cobalt for the manufacture of the vitamin in their stomachs or rumen. If the intake of cobalt is low, then only a suboptimal amount of the vitamin will be available, and a deficiency will result.

The Effects of a Cobalt Deficiency

In New Zealand and Australia cattle and sheep have long suffered from a wasting disease that is now known to be caused by a deficiency of cobalt in the soils and as a consequence in the pastures where they graze. Animals ingesting these low-cobalt grains and grasses showed symptoms of listlessness, loss of appetite and weight, anemia, and finally death (Fig. 12.6).

Attempts to produce cobalt deficiencies in rats, guinea pigs, and rabbits have been unsuccessful; however, the addition of cobalt to the rations of rats and chicks has produced a growth-stimulating effect in both species.

Cobalt Toxicity

If cobalt is fed to animals and man in amounts greater than their requirement, an increase in the number of red blood cells results. The disorder is referred to as *polycythemia*. This condition has been produced in rats, mice, guinea pigs, rabbits, dogs, pigs, chickens, frogs, and man. Experimental polycythemia has been observed in normal men when fed daily intakes of 150 mg of cobalt salts (8). After ingesting the cobalt salts for a period of 7 to 22 days, the subjects showed increases in the number of red blood cells ranging from 16 to 21 per cent. Polycythemia is a natural condition in individuals throughout the world who live at very high altitudes. The extra production of red blood cells compensates for the lower percentage of oxygen in the air at high altitudes.

Recommended Allowances and Food Sources of Cobalt

The daily need for cobalt has not been established (28) but is probably quite small. Although there are few data on the cobalt content of foods, it appears that the average diet supplies more than adequate amounts for man.

▶ MOLYBDENUM

Even though the toxic effects of molybdenum in animals have been known for some time, the importance of the mineral in the nutrition of animals was established only in 1953.

Function of Molybdenum

Molybdenum has been demonstrated to be an essential factor for the rat, dog, lamb, turkey poult, and chick in the formation and maintenance of the intestinal enzyme called *xanthine oxidase*. This enzyme catalyzes

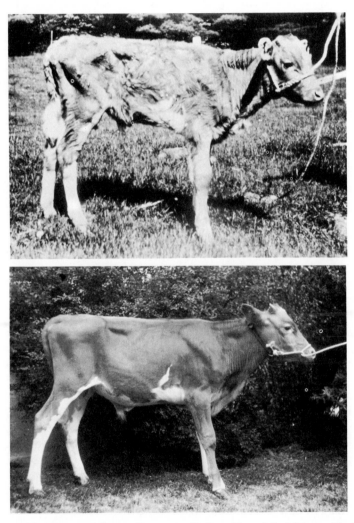

Fig. 12.6. The top picture shows a Guernsey calf affected by cobalt deficiency. The bottom picture shows the same calf after it was fed cobalt for a few weeks. (Courtesy of Keener, *Univ. N.H. Agr. Expt. Sta.*, Bull. 411, Durham.)

the oxidation of aldehydes and purines. No information is available yet on the function, if any, of molybdenum in man.

Molybdenum Toxicity

Even though the effects of inadequate molybdenum have not been observed in either animals or man, the effect of excess amounts of molybdenum have been reported in the rat, rabbit, and calf. Rats fed overabundant amounts of molybdenum show reduced growth rates and will die if the molybdenum content of the diet is too high. Symptoms of retarded growth, loss of weight, low hemoglobin and red blood cell counts, alopecia, and malformed leg bones have been reported in rabbits fed toxic levels of molybdenum. Chronic molybdenum poisoning in calves results in weight loss and changes in the hair coat. At first the hair is rough and thin, but as the toxicity continues the hair loses its pigment and greys.

Recommended Allowances and Food Sources of Molybdenum

As yet nothing is established about man's requirement for molybdenum (28). Like the other minerals discussed in this chapter molybdenum, too, is widely distributed in commonly used foods. However, legumes, cereal grains, some dark green vegetables, liver, and kidney are good sources of the mineral.

▶ SELENIUM

Schwarz and his coworkers found that certain foods (milk, brewer's yeast, meat, and certain cereals) contained an unidentified factor that prevented liver damage in rats. They called this unknown substance "Factor 3." In 1957 these workers isolated selenium from "Factor 3" as the third substance, in addition to cystine and vitamin E, that is effective in the prevention of liver necrosis in young rats (36). They further demonstrated that a minute amount of inorganic sodium selenite was equally as effective as "Factor 3" in relieving this disorder. Prior to this time the nutritional interest in selenium was directed solely to its toxic effect in animals.

Selenium-Vitamin E Relationships

The ability of selenium as an inorganic salt to prevent vitamin E deficiency conditions in the rat and chick has prompted investigations to compare the effects of selenium and vitamin E in animals.

A summary of the known effects of selenium and alpha-tocopherol (vitamin E) in the prevention of specific lesions in animals and birds is presented in Table 12.1. Selenium salts are effective in preventing liver necrosis (rat, mouse, and pig) and exudative diathesis (chick) but are ineffective in preventing infertility (rat) and encephalomalacia (chick). The ability of the mineral to prevent muscular dystrophy varies from species to species. Selenium salts are effective in preventing muscular dystrophy in lambs, for example, but ineffective in rats. Neither alpha-tocopherol nor selenium have been shown to be effective in the relief of human muscular dystrophy. As a matter of fact, nothing has been established concerning the role of this trace element in human nutrition (28).

Function of Selenium

At this time the function of selenium has not been defined, but evidence indicates that the mineral may act as a biological catalyst as part of an enzyme system in the animal organism (24). The range of selenium activity, as judged by the number of lesions prevented, appears

Table 12.1. The Prevention of Specific Lesions in Animals and Birds by Alpha-tocopherol and Selenium (1, 24, 35, 38)

Lesion	Species	Action of	
		Alpha-tocopherol	Selenium Salts
Infertility:			
Degeneration of testes	rat	effective	ineffective
Resorption of fetuses	rat	effective	ineffective
Liver necrosis	rat	effective	effective
	mouse	effective	effective
	pig	effective	effective
Exudative diathesis	chick	effective	effective
Depigmentation of teeth	rat	effective	ineffective
Encephalomalacia	chick	effective	ineffective
Muscular dystrophy	rabbit	effective	ineffective
	pig	effective	ineffective
	lamb	effective	effective
	calf	effective	partially effective
	chick	effective	effective
	mouse	effective	effective

to be quite narrow, yet it is effective in very small amounts. It has been reported that selenium is 500 times more active than alpha-tocopherol and 250,000 times more active than L-cystine in preventing liver necrosis (36).

Toxic Effects of Selenium

The toxic effects of selenium in farm animals fed rations grown on selenium-rich soils have been recognized for several decades. In this disorder, commonly referred to as "alkali disease," animals show symptoms of emaciation, loss of hair and hoofs, cirrhosis of the liver, and skeletal erosions.

Linseed oil meal as well as arsanilic acid and other organic arsenicals have been reported to be effective in counteracting chronic selenium poisoning in animals (43).

That selenium may be a factor contributing to an increased susceptibility to dental caries has been suggested from studies with Oregon school children (14, 42). The dental caries rate of the permanent teeth of children were significantly higher in seleniferous than in nonseleniferous areas. Also gingivitis was found to be more frequent among children living in the seleniferous areas. More research is needed, however, before this relationship can be confirmed.

▶ CHROMIUM

That chromium might be a dietary essential was suggested by Schwarz and Mertz (37) in 1959. They reported that chromium is concerned with the maintenance of the glucose tolerance level in the rat. This level refers to the amount of glucose that may appear in the blood without "spillage" into the urine.

It has been reported that chromium increased the growth rate of male and female mice and lessened the mortality of the male animals up to seventeen months of age (33). Data from a parallel study, using rats, have indicated that the growth pattern of the male rat also is stimulated by the element chromium (34).

At this time nothing is known about the relationship, if any, of chromium to human nutrition (28).

▶ FLUORINE

Inasmuch as fluorine has been shown to be valuable in combating tooth decay in children when ingested in very small amounts, it has gained prominence in nutrition even though at this time it cannot be considered an essential nutrient (23). The role of fluorine in dental health is presented in Chapter 23.

Effects of Minimal Levels of Fluorides in Man

Minimal amounts of fluoride have been shown to benefit man by providing an increased resistance to dental caries.

The effect of minimal amounts of fluorides on the skeletal tissues of man has been studied, both radiologically and histologically, in individuals who have been drinking water containing fluorides throughout their life (47). It has been reported that skeletal fluorosis has never been observed radiologically in persons drinking water containing less than 4 parts per million (ppm) of fluoride. Furthermore, no lesions characteristic of fluorosis have been found in the histological sections of rib bones from deceased persons who lived continuously in an area where the drinking water contained 1.9 ppm fluoride.

The effects of minimal levels of fluoride intake on the plasma fluoride have been studied in man. Singer and Armstrong (39) have found the fluoride content of the plasma to be constant for individuals who use fluoridated water within the range of 0.15 and 2.5 ppm.

Effects of High Levels of Fluorides in Animals and Man

Ingested fluorides accumulate in the hard tissues of the body, the teeth, and the bones. Changes in the teeth as well as pathological lesions of the bony tissues have been observed in animals when fed either toxic amounts of fluoride or lesser amounts that proved to be toxic after continuous ingestions for a period of time. In the rat the tooth enamel becomes chalky and brittle, and the incisor teeth continue to grow, forming an elongated tusk-like incisor that is no longer useful in securing food. The skull of the rat becomes thickened when excessive amounts of the mineral are fed to the rat. In cattle and swine the enamel of the teeth wears away, exposing the pulp cavity, and it becomes difficult for the animals to ingest food and water because of the sensitiveness of the teeth.

Balance studies involving the intake of large amounts of fluoride have been conducted with human beings. At intakes of 4 to 5 mg of a fluoride per day it has been shown that almost all of the fluoride ingested was eliminated (19), inasmuch as equilibrium in the body is maintained by the loss of the mineral through the kidney and skin. When as much as 12 to 25 mg per day was ingested, almost one-half of the absorbed amount was stored in the body tissues (17). After the individuals on these high levels of intake were returned to a normal intake pattern of the mineral, their body stores of fluoride were slowly depleted.

Food Sources of Fluoride

Fluoride analyses of some typical foods used in the American dietary have been made in nine field stations in the eastern, central, and western sections of the United States (5). Of all the foods tested, only fish and fish products, dry beans, and tea infusion contained more than 1 ppm of fluoride. Milk was very low in the mineral (0.09 ppm); most of the fruits, meats, and vegetables contained less than 0.30 ppm of fluoride.

Extra fluoride may be introduced to the diet from fluoride-containing insecticides and sprays that are used in fruit and vegetable pest control. In addition to this, vegetables absorb the mineral when they are cooked in fluoride-containing water.

REFERENCES

1. Blaxter, K. L. (1962). Muscular dystrophy in farm animals: its cause and prevention. *Proc. Nutr. Soc. (London)* **21:** 211.
2. Burke, E. C. (1954). Failure of premature infant to gain weight due to a low-sodium feeding: report of a case. *Proc. Staff Meetings, Mayo Clinic* **29:** 90.
3. Cartwright, G. E., and M. M. Wintrobe (1946). Hematologic survey of repatriated American military personnel. *J. Lab. Clin. Med.* **31:** 886.
4. Chornock, C., N. B. Guerrant, and R. A. Dutcher (1942). Effect of manganese on calcification in the growing rat. *J. Nutr.* **23:** 445.
5. Clifford, P. A. (1945). Report on fluorine. *J. Assoc. Offic. Agr. Chemists* **28:** 277.
6. Dahl, L. K., L. M. Tassinair, and N. Gillespie (1958). Sodium in foods for a 100-mg sodium diet. *J. Am. Dietet. Assoc.* **34:** 717.
7. Danowski, T. S. (1958). Low-sodium diets—physiological adaptation and clinical usefulness. Council on Foods and Nutrition. *J. Am. Med. Assoc.* **168:** 1886.
8. Davis, J. E., and J. P. Fields (1955). Cobalt polycythemia in humans. *Federation Proc.* **14:** 331.
9. de Langen, C. D. (1954). Sodium chloride in geographical pathology and its influence on the capillary system. *Acta Med. Scand.* **149:** 75.
10. de Langen, C. D. (1954). Basal metabolism and sodium chloride. *Acta Med. Scand.* **150:** 257.
11. Electrolyte metabolism in kwashiorkor (1957). *Nutr. Rev.* **15:** 101.
12. Flink, E. B., F. L. Stutzman, A. R. Anderson, T. Konig, and R. Fraser (1954). Magnesium deficiency after prolonged parenteral fluid administration and after chronic alcoholism complicated by delirium tremens. *J. Lab. Clin. Med.* **43:** 169.
13. Franz, M., C. Kiecker, and M. Phelan (1959). Composition of 95 foods—calcium, phosphorus, magnesium, sodium, and potassium. *J. Am. Dietet. Assoc.* **35:** 1170.
14. Hadjimarkos, D. M., and C. W. Bomhorst (1958). The trace element selenium and its influence on dental caries susceptibility. *J. Pediat.* **52:** 275.

15. Kahlenberg, O. J., A. Black, and E. B. Forbes (1937). The utilization of energy producing nutriment and protein as affected by sodium deficiency. *J. Nutr.* **13:** 97.
16. Lans, H. S., I. F. Stein, Jr., and K. A. Meyer (1952). Diagnosis, treatment, and prophylaxis of potassium deficiency in surgical patients. *Surg., Gynecol., Obstet.* **95:** 321.
17. Largent, E. J., and F. F. Heyroth (1949). The absorption and excretion of fluorides. III. Further observations on metabolism of fluorides at high levels of intake. *J. Ind. Hyg. Toxicol.* **31:** 134.
18. Leverton, R. M., J. M. Leichsenring, H. Linkswiler, and F. Meyer (1961). Magnesium requirement of young women receiving controlled intakes. *J. Nutr.* **74:** 33.
19. McClure, F. J., H. H. Mitchell, T. S. Hamilton, and C. A. Kinser (1945). Balances of fluorine ingested from various sources in food and water by five young men. *J. Ind. Hyg. Toxicol.* **27:** 159.
20. McKey, B. V., F. M. La Font, G. L. Borchers, D. A. Navarrete, and J. O. Holmes (1962). Magnesium studies in adult men. *Federation Proc.* **21:** 310.
21. Magee, A. C., and G. Matrone (1960). Studies on growth, copper metabolism, and iron metabolism of rats fed high levels of zinc. *J. Nutr.* **72:** 233.
22. Malhotra, M. S., B. K. Sharma, and R. Sivaraman (1959). Requirements of sodium chloride during summer in the tropics. *J. Appl. Physiol.* **14:** 823.
23. Maurer, R. L., and H. G. Day (1957). The non-essentiality of fluorine in nutrition. *J. Nutr.* **62:** 561.
24. Moore, T. (1962). The history of selenium-vitamin E interrelationships. *Proc. Nutr. Soc. (London)* **21:** 179.
25. Nelson, G. Y., and M. R. Gram (1961). Magnesium content of accessory foods. *J. Am. Dietet. Assoc.* **38:** 437.
26. North, B. B., J. M. Leichsenring, and L. M. Norris (1960). Manganese metabolism in college women. *J. Nutr.* **72:** 217.
27. Pearson, E., H. S. Soroff, G. K. Arney, and C. P. Artz (1961). An estimate of the potassium requirements for equilibrium in burned patients. *Surg., Gynecol., Obstet.* **112:** 263.
28. *Recommended Dietary Allowances Sixth Revised Edition* (1964). Natl. Acad. Sci.—Natl. Res. Council, Publ. 1146, Washington, D.C.
29. Robinson, C. H. (1955). Planning the sodium-restricted diet. *J. Am. Dietet. Assoc.* **31:** 28.
30. Robinson, C. H. (1955). The sodium-restricted diet. Dietotherapy. *Am. J. Clin. Nutr.* **3:** 339.
31. Rodier, J. (1955). Manganese poisoning in Moroccan miners. *Brit. J. Ind. Med.* **12:** 21.
32. Rourke, M. H. (1960). Sodium in special-purpose foods and in water. *J. Am. Dietet. Assoc.* **36:** 216.
33. Schroeder, H. A., W. H. Vinton, Jr., and J. A. Balassa (1963). Effect of chromium, cadmium, and other trace metals on the growth and survival of mice. *J. Nutr.* **80:** 39.
34. Schroeder, H. A., W. H. Vinton, Jr., and J. J. Balassa (1963). Effects of chromium, cadmium, and lead on the growth and survival of rats. *J. Nutr.* **80:** 48.
35. Schultze, M. O. (1960). Nutrition. *Ann. Rev. Biochem.* **29:** 391.
36. Schwarz, K., and C. M. Foltz (1957). Selenium as an integral part of Factor 3 against dietary necrotic liver degeneration. *J. Am. Chem. Soc.* **79:** 3292.
37. Schwarz, K., and W. Mertz (1959). Chromium (III) and the glucose tolerance factor. *Arch. Biochem. Biophys.* **85:** 292.
38. Sharman, G. A. M. (1960). Selenium in animal health. *Proc. Nutr. Soc. (London)* **19:** 169.
39. Singer, L., and W. D. Armstrong (1960). Regulation of human plasma fluoride concentration. *J. Appl. Physiol.* **15:** 508.
40. Smith, A. J., and J. F. Hammarsten (1959). Intracellular magnesium in delirium tremens and uremia. *Am. J. Med. Sci.* **237:** 413.

41. Sturgeon, P., and C. Brubaker (1956). Copper deficiency in infants. *AMA J. Diseases Children* **92:** 254.

42. Tank, G., and C. A. Storvick (1960). Effect of naturally occurring selenium and vanadium on dental caries. *J. Dental Res.* **39:** 473.

43. Underwood, E. J. (1959). Mineral metabolism. *Ann. Rev. Biochem.* **28:** 499.

44. Vallee, B. L., E. E. C. Wacker, and D. D. Ulmer (1960). The magnesium deficiency tetany syndrome in man. *New Engl. J. Med.* **262:** 155.

45. Vitale, J. J., M. D. Hegsted, M. Nakamura, and P. Connors (1957). The effect of thyroxine on magnesium requirement. *J. Biol. Chem.* **266:** 597.

46. Watt, B. K., and A. L. Merrill (1963). *Composition of Foods—Raw, Processed, Prepared.* U.S. Dept. Agr., Agr. Handbook 8, revised, Washington, D.C.

47. Weidman, S. M., J. A. Weatherell, and D. Jackson (1963). The effect of fluoride on bone. *Proc. Nutr. Soc. (London)* **22:** 105.

48. Wilson, H. T., and F. H. Sink (1953). Hypopotassemia in human starvation and gastric resection. *J. Clin. Nutr.* **1:** 430.

SUPPLEMENTARY REFERENCES

Aikaina, J. K. (1963). *The Role of Magnesium in Biologic Processes.* Charles C Thomas, Springfield, Ill.

Comar, C. L., and F. Bronner (eds.) (1961). *Mineral Metabolism an Advanced Treatise.* Vol. II, The Elements. Academic Press, New York.

Davis, G. K. (1964). Magnesium. In *Nutrition, a Comprehensive Treatise.* Vol. I (G. H. Beaton and E. W. McHenry, eds.) Academic Press, New York.

Hathaway, M. L. (1962). *Magnesium in Human Nutrition.* U.S. Dept. Agr., Home Econ. Res. Rept. 19, Washington, D.C.

Hawkins, W. W. (1964). Iron, cobalt, and copper. In *Nutrition, a Comprehensive Treatise.* Vol. I. (G. H. Beaton and E. W. McHenry, eds.) Academic Press, New York.

Leverton, R. M. (1959). Sodium, potassium, and magnesium. In *Food. The Yearbook of Agriculture 1959.* (A. Stefferud, ed.) U.S. Dept. Agr., Washington, D.C.

Monty, K. J., and W. D. McElroy (1959). The trace elements. In *Food. The Yearbook of Agriculture 1959.* (A. Stefferud, ed.) U.S. Dept. Agr., Washington, D.C.

Nikiforuk, G., and R. M. Grainger (1964). Fluorine. In *Nutrition, a Comprehensive Treatise.* Vol. I. (G. H. Beaton and E. W. McHenry, eds.) Academic Press, New York.

Underwood, E. J. (1962). *Trace Elements.* 2nd ed. Academic Press, New York.

CHAPTER 13

Water

Water is an essential nutrient, yet one that is often overlooked when the nutrient needs of the body are enumerated. Actually it is possible to survive a longer time without food than without water. The survival time depends on the rate of water loss; one can live without food for over a month, but without water for only a few days. The necessity of water in maintaining life was demonstrated by the German physiologist, Rubner, who found that during starvation, an animal can live if he loses nearly all of his glycogen and fat as well as one-half of his body protein, but a loss of 20 per cent of the water in his body results in death.

Water makes up approximately 65 per cent of the body weight; about 78 lb of a 120-lb individual is water. It is difficult to establish mean values for body water, because the total volume is related to the mass of lean tissues of the body rather than to the body weight. Fat tissue contains less water than lean tissue.

Approximately two-thirds of the water content of the body is contained within the cells (intracellular fluid), and the remaining one-third is found in spaces outside the cell (extracellular fluid). The extracellular fluid consists of the fluid between tissues and cells (interstitial fluid) and the water present in the blood plasma. Between 3 to 4 qt of water circulates in the blood stream (3).

Functions of Water

Water is used in the body in a variety of ways: as a building material, as a solvent, as a lubricant, and as a temperature regulator.

As a building material water is used in the construction of every cell. The cells and tissues of the body, however, vary in their water content. For example, dentin contains 10 per cent water, fatty tissue 20 per cent, bone 25 per cent, and striated muscle 80 per cent.

As a solvent, water is essential for the normal functioning of the body cells. It is the means by which nutriment is carried to the cells and waste products of metabolism removed. However, before food can be carried to the cells it must first be digested. Water is used in digestive processes where it aids in the mastication and softening of food, supplies fluid for the digestive juices, and facilitates the movement of the food mass along the digestive tract. After digestion the nutrients, in a state of solution or suspension, pass through the intestinal wall and are carried away by either the blood or lymph. In the cells water is the fluid medium in which the many intracellular chemical reactions take place (2). After metabolism the blood, which is about 92 per cent water, picks up the waste products from the cells and carries them either to the lungs or kidneys for excretion.

Water serves as a lubricant in the joints and between internal organs. It bathes the body cells, keeping them moist and permitting the passage of substances between the cells and the blood vessels.

As a regulator of body temperature water aids in the removal of heat from the body. The evaporation of water on the skin surface is an effective way of eliminating generated body heat. It has been estimated that 1 qt of perspiration dissipates 580 Cal. of heat. However, during strenuous physical activity or in a hot dry atmosphere the loss of moisture by skin evaporation may be markedly increased. It has been reported that football players have lost 10 to 12 lb in body weight during a game caused chiefly by a loss of water through sweating.

Sources of Water for the Body

The source of water for the body comes from the fluids of the diet, the solid foods of the diet, and the water produced by the metabolism of the energy nutrients within the tissues.

The largest amount of the body water comes from ingested fluids. The average person consumes approximately 1 to 1½ qt of fluid as water, coffee, tea, soup, and other liquids each day (2).

The water content of foods varies widely, with most foods in the average diet containing more than 70 per cent moisture. Figure 13.1 shows the percentage of water in some commonly used foods. An interesting comparison to make is that between green beans, a solid food that contains 92 per cent water, and milk, a fluid food with 87 per cent water. The similarity in water content is concealed by a portion of the carbohydrates, one of the constituents contributing to the solids of both foods, being present in green beans in an insoluble form, cellulose. The main carbohydrate in milk is lactose, which is water soluble. The amount of water obtained from solid foods in the diet may vary from ½ to 1 quart per day, depending on the kind of solid foods consumed.

In the metabolism of the energy nutrients carbohydrates, fats, and proteins, water is formed. Water obtained from metabolism is a constant

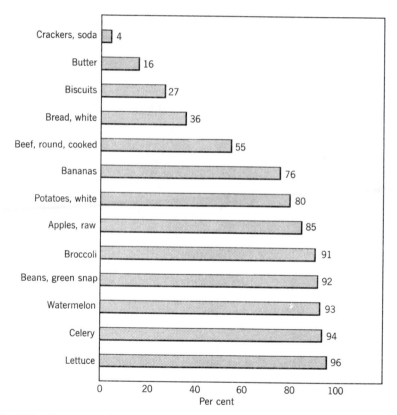

Fig. 13.1. Percentage of water in some commonly used foods. (From *Nutritive Value of Foods*, U.S. Dept. Agr., Home Garden Bull. 72, revised 1964.)

source arising from the continuous process of oxidation of food in the body for energy. However, the amount of water produced by the different food substances varies. The estimated amounts are 0.6 gm of water per gm of carbohydrate, 1.07 gm of water per gm of fat, and 0.41 gm of water per gm of protein (1). For example, the water of oxidation produced by the metabolism of a day's dietary might be as follows:

Carbohydrate	275 gm × 0.60 = 165.0 gm of water of oxidation
Fat	90 gm × 1.07 = 96.3 gm of water of oxidation
Protein	75 gm × 0.41 = 30.8 gm of water of oxidation
Total	292.1 gm (1¼ cups)

Excretion of Water from the Body

Water is lost from the body by way of the kidneys (urine), skin (perspiration), lungs (expired air), intestinal canal (feces), and eyes (tears). The amount of water lost by the body is influenced by water intake, body conditions, and environmental conditions. The largest amount of water is lost through the kidneys in the urine. The excretion of urine is greatly influenced by fluid intake. Water is lost from the skin through insensible perspiration and by sweating. The amount excreted by the skin varies according to the need for the body to lose heat to regulate body temperature.

When an individual is physically active or the environmental temperature is high, proportionately more water will be lost through the skin than under normal conditions. Insensible perspiration is usually not noticed because each area gives off such a small amount; however, a pint a day is usually lost by this means.

An example of the water balance of an individual is given in Table 13.1.

Dehydration results when the output of body water exceeds the intake. This may be due to simple deprivation of water or water loss due to conditions such as excessive diarrhea, vomiting, or sweating. Symptoms of dehydration may occur when 5 to 10 per cent of body water has been lost. These symptoms are thirst, dryness of mouth, feeling of weakness, and increased pulse rate. Dehydration may be overcome by the use of water, water and salt, or special attention to water plus minerals. Medical attention may be necessary depending on the severity and nature of the dehydration.

Recommended Allowances for Water

The National Research Council (4) states that a reasonable standard for calculating the daily water allowances is 1 ml per Cal. of food. In the average diet a large proportion of this intake comes from solid foods. For the young adult, activity and environmental conditions are the two most important variables which determine the body's need for water. During study, rest, and sleep, the loss of water from the body is small in comparison to that during active exercise such as tennis, basketball, and football. In the summer, or when the temperature is high and the humidity low, more water evaporates from the body surface. In most individuals satisfying the thirst or the desire for water is the only criterion necessary to meet the body's need. Under conditions of extreme heat where there is excessive sweating, the thirst mechanism may not allow for the drinking of sufficient water, making it necessary to supplement the natural intake. Five or six glasses of fluids should be consumed daily as water or in beverage. The habit of drinking water should be encouraged because water is important to normal functioning of the body. Water consumption at meal time is advised if the food is properly masticated, and if water is not used to wash down the food. Water is thought to aid digestion by promoting the flow of digestive juices.

Few studies have been made to determine the daily water consumption of man. The estimates of daily total tap water and other fluids consumed by 797 normal children in four dissimilar geographic areas in the United States are given in Table 13.2. Total fluid intake increased with age, but relatively speaking, tap water consumption decreased with age. It was found that even older children rarely drank as much as 1 pint (about 500 ml) of tap water daily. Information concerning the daily consumption of tap water is of importance in planning fluoridation programs.

Table 13.1. Water Balance

(Average Individual)	
Water Intake	Milliliters
Liquid food (water, coffee, milk, soup)	1100
Solid food (moisture)	500–900
Water of oxidation	400
	2000–2400
Water Output	
Vaporization (400 ml expired as moist air— lung, and 600 ml skin sweat)	920–1000
Feces	80–100
Urine	1000–1300
	2000–2400

From C. Alper Fluid and Electrolyte Balance, In *Modern Nutrition in Health and Disease,* (M. G. Wohl and R. S. Goodhart, eds.). Lea and Febiger, Philadelphia, p. 468, 1964.

Table 13.2. Fluid and Tap Water Consumption of Children Ranging in Age from Birth to Twelve Years

Age	Fluid per Day, milliliters		Tap Water per Day, milliliters	
	Mean	SE of Mean	Mean	SE of Mean
0– 2 mo	740	77	342	26
2– 4 mo	707	43	314	54
4– 6 mo	783	29	238	75
6– 9 mo	754	58	120	26
9–12 mo	793	43	160	59
12–18 mo	737	41	208	34
18–24 mo	799	30	267	56
24–30 mo	907	95	283	24
30–36 mo	894	47	312	22
3– 5 yr	926	33	349	27
5– 8 yr	1102	40	389	38
8–12 yr	1290	116	493	191

Adapted from J. S. Walker et al. Water intake of normal children. *Science* **140:** 890, 1963.

Water Supply

In the future the problem of water supply will command greater attention. The withdrawals of water for agriculture, industry, and municipal use are expected to double by 1980 and triple by 2000 (5). Irrigation will be important in increasing crop production to meet future food and fiber needs. Industrial development is contingent on a reliable water supply. In the Western river valleys streamflow is already completely allocated under water appropriation laws. The importance of water is clearly stated in the following inscription on a mural in the Colorado state capital: "Here is a land where life is written in water." Efficient use of water will be essential in the years ahead.

REFERENCES

1. Alper, C. (1960). Fluid and electrolyte balance. In *Modern Nutrition in Health and Disease*. (M. G. Wohl and R. S. Goodhart, eds.) Lea and Febiger, Philadelphia, p. 408.
2. McLester, J. S., and W. J. Darby (1952). *Nutrition and Diet in Health and Disease*. 6th ed. W. B. Saunders Co., Philadelphia, p. 121.
3. Newburgh, L. H., M. W. Johnson, and J. D. Newburgh (1948). *Some Fundamental Principles of Metabolism*. 3rd revised ed. J. W. Edwards, Ann Arbor, Mich. p. 25.
4. *Recommended Dietary Allowances Sixth Revised Edition* (1964). Natl. Acad. Sci.—Natl. Res. Council, Publ. 1146, Washington, D.C., p. 31.

5. Williams, D. A., G. E. Young, and B. Osborn (1962). Conservation and change. In *After a Hundred Years. The Yearbook of Agriculture 1962*. (A. Stefferud, ed.) U.S. Dept. Agr., Washington, D.C., p. 582.

SUPPLEMENTARY REFERENCES

Mickelsen, O. (1959). Water. In *Food. The Yearbook of Agriculture 1959*. (A. Stefferud, ed.) U.S. Dept. Agr., Washington, D.C.

CHAPTER 14

Introduction to the vitamins
and the fat-soluble vitamins

The discovery of the vitamins ushered in a new era in nutrition. It was one in which *small* things in the diet assumed *great* importance. The percentage of body weight attributable to vitamins is minute. Nevertheless, the amount, even though small, is indispensable for normal functioning.

Early evidence of the existence of vitamins came from the search for treatments of certain human diseases that persistently plagued people. One of these diseases was scurvy. It was one of the hazards explorers and sea voyagers encountered. In the year 1747 relief from scurvy was enjoyed by a few of the British navy. Freedom from the illness came about in this way. Limited amounts of lemons and oranges were aboard ship and were given to some of the sailors; the recovery was remarkable. In another part of the world, another disease was making the sailors of the Japanese navy ill. This disease was beriberi. The diet of the men consisted mainly of white rice. With the addition of vegetables, meat, and fish, a change instituted in 1884, the incidence of beriberi decreased.

Despite the improvement in health brought about by changes in the diet, the realization that a lack in the diet was responsible for scurvy and beriberi was slow. In fact, it was almost 150 years after the experiment at sea with lemons and oranges before there was acceptance of scurvy as being caused by a nutritional deficiency; and it was not until the early 1900's that scientists and physicians accepted beriberi as the result of a deficiency in the diet. That deficiencies in the diet could be responsible for disease was a new concept, which was adopted with reluctance.

Another avenue of approach to the study of the dietary deficiency diseases was the use of animals in the experimental laboratory. In the final analysis, it was the well-controlled laboratory experiments that eventually gave conclusive evidence that certain diseases are caused by the lack of dietary nutrients.

In the experimental studies a diet of pure chemical compounds was fed, pure protein (such as casein or albumen), pure fat (such as lard), pure carbohydrate (such as dextrin), and minerals. The purified diet was really the crux of the experiment, for the natural food more than likely would have provided some of the unknown factors. As it was young animals on the purified diet failed to grow; mature animals failed to maintain body weight.

McCollum (1) in his study of the history of nutrition found Jean Dumas (1800–1884) to be the earliest man of science to question the adequacy of a diet composed only of protein, carbohydrate, fat, and salts. The experience that led Dumas to such a prophetic belief was not with experimental animals, however, but with citizens of France. At the time of the siege of France by the Germans (1870–1871) food was scarce; there was no milk for children. Scientists attempted to prepare artificial milk using protein, fat, carbohydrates, and salts. The combination was disastrous to the young. It led Dumas to conclude that there was something lacking in a combination of the then known nutrients essential for life.

Animal experiments that led to the discovery of vitamins included those of Pekelharing in 1905 at the University of Utrecht, who made the important observation that a diet of casein, egg albumen, rice flour, lard, and salts kept his mice alive only four weeks. When he added milk to the mixture the mice remained healthy.

Sir Frederick Hopkins of England was the most advanced thinker of his time on animal nutrition. He said in 1906 that " . . . no animal can live on a mixture of proteins, carbohydrates, and fats, and even when the necessary inorganic material is carefully supplied, the animal still cannot flourish." Others of the era were feeding purified diets and supplementing them with natural foods to keep their animals alive. McCollum in 1907, although aware that animals could not survive on purified rations of protein, fat, carbohydrate, and mineral salts, believed with many others of his time that the failure to survive was due to the unpalatability of the mixture and the consequent refusal to eat a sufficient amount of the ration. He tried to improve the flavor by adding sugars and other variations in the ration, but the animals still failed to survive. Even though this experiment appeared to be a failure, it was successful in that it led to his discovery of vitamin A a few years later.

McCollum and Davis discovered that there was a substance present in butterfat or egg-yolk fat that made the difference between moderate success in the nutrition of young rats on certain diets and prompt failure in its absence. Osborne and Mendel at the Connecticut Experiment Station found cod liver oil also to contain this essential substance. Thus the first vitamin was discovered and called fat-soluble vitamin A.

There seemed to be only one factor needed to supplement the purified diet at the time of the discovery of vitamin A. In a couple of years, however, it was recognized that not one, but two factors were lacking in the purified diet for normal growth, one soluble in fat, the other soluble in water. Later of course, numerous new fat-soluble and many additional water-soluble factors were identified. Each is discussed in the chapters that follow. A chronological summary of the isolation and syntheses of the various vitamins follows (2).

Year	Isolation or Identification	Synthesis or Structure
1925	Vitamin D by irradiation	
1926	Vitamin B_1	
1928	Inositol	
1931	Vitamin A	
1932	Vitamin C	
1933	Riboflavin	Vitamin C
	Pantothenate	
1935	Biotin	Riboflavin
1936	Anti-egg-white factor	Vitamin D
	Vitamin E	Thiamine
1937		Vitamin A
		α-tocopherol
1938	Nicotinic acid identified as pellagra-preventing	dl-α-tocopherol
	Pyridoxine	
1939	Vitamin K	Vitamin K
		Pyridoxine
1940	P-Aminobenzoic acid	Pantothenate
1942		Biotin structure
1945	Folic acid	Folic acid
1948	Vitamin B_{12}	Folionic acid
1955–56		Vitamin B_{12} structure

There was a need for a name for the new factors in nutrition. The name which became *vitamin* originated in this way. Funk, a Polish biochemist, coined the term "vitamine" in 1911 to designate the anti-beriberi factor that he was investigating at the time. He combined *vita*, to designate "essential for life," and *amine* to indicate the chemical structure. The term was accepted and used for all of the unknown factors. In 1919 the final "e" was dropped, for by then it was abundantly clear that there were several unknown dietary nutrients, and that the known ones did not all have the amine structure. The change in spelling avoided any implication of chemical structure for the as yet unidentified dietary factors.

As a preface to the discussion of individual vitamins an explanation of the general meaning of the term should be made. Vitamins are organic compounds, necessary for growth and maintenance of life, which must be provided in the diet. The body is not able to synthesize them, at least in amounts sufficient to meet its needs. An exception is vitamin D; exposure to ultraviolet rays develops the vitamin from its precursor present in the skin. Vitamins are regulatory substances, each performing a specific function. They are carried in the blood stream to all parts of the body.

▶ VITAMIN A

In two laboratories experiments were in progress that led to the discovery of vitamin A in 1913. McCollum and Davis (7) at the University of Wisconsin fed young rats a purified diet believed to be adequate at that time. It contained protein, carbohydrate, mineral salts, and fat (lard), all of the nutrients then recognized. They used milk sugar in this experiment, which added enough impurities of nutritional value for the young to grow fairly well for a while. However, after a period the animals ceased growing. Adjustments were made in the relative amounts of the nutrients in the diet in an effort to prevent the cessation of growth but to no avail. When butterfat or egg yolk was added to the diet, growth was resumed. The addition of olive oil, on the other hand, had no effect. It was apparent that there was a difference in the nutritive value of olive oil and lard, and butterfat and egg yolk. At the Connecticut Experiment Station in the same year, Osborne and Mendel (11) fed young rats a purified diet consisting of protein, lard, starch, and protein-free, fat-free milk that provided the minerals, some lactose, and other water-soluble substances. As in the Wisconsin experiments, after a period growth failed. With replacement of lard by butter, the rats grew and matured normally. Egg yolk and cod liver oil in the diet gave the same response as butter; these fats provided the *something* that was lacking in the purified diet.

It was evident from the studies of McCollum, and Osborne and

Mendel, that the essential nutrient missing in the purified diets was soluble in fat. Knowing the solubility of the substance helped to speed the discovery of vitamin A; many compounds were thus excluded from consideration. Further help came from Steenbock's studies (1919) at the University of Wisconsin in which root vegetables were fed as a source of the fat-soluble vitamin. Yellow sweet potatoes and carrots supported normal growth and even supplied enough of the unknown substance for reproduction. Rutabagas, red beets, parsnips, potatoes, and sugar beets failed completely to provide the needed nutrient. Steenbock tested many plant materials, among them yellow corn and white corn. The animals fed yellow corn as a supplement to the purified ration grew normally and were able to reproduce; animals fed white corn failed to grow and developed deficiency symptoms (14). It is interesting that McCollum, in 1908, heard Wisconsin farmers who were attending a meeting at the University maintain that yellow corn was better feed for hogs than white corn; that was eleven years before Steenbock's studies confirming their contention. Thus in addition to solubility in fat, another characteristic of the nutrient was recognized, the association with yellow color. It had been demonstrated that animals were unable to synthesize the yellow pigment carotene. This gave a lead that it must be provided in the diet. The question still remained, however, as to the relationship between the yellow plant materials and the animal fat substances, both of which supplied the fat-soluble vitamin. Ten years later, in 1929, crystalline carotene was demonstrated to have vitamin A value by a German scientist Hans von Euler-Chelpin.

The Properties of Vitamin A and Carotene

Vitamin A is an organic compound found only in the animal kingdom. It is believed to be present in all species of fish, birds, and mammals. Yellow plant pigments of the carotenoid group, *alpha-*, *beta-*, and *gamma*-carotene, and cryptoxanthin are precursors of vitamin A. The body has the capacity of converting these carotenoid compounds contained in the diet into vitamin A. Actually the origin of all vitamin A in animal products comes directly or indirectly from the carotenoids of plants. Fish consume marine plankton; herbivorous land animals eat vegetable foods; and the carnivorous animals depend indirectly on herbivorous sources.

Two forms of vitamin A have been identified: vitamin A_1, which occurs in the livers of salt-water fish, and vitamin A_2 found in the livers of fresh water fish. Although the two vitamins differ slightly in chemical structure they are alike in physiological functions (12). Vitamin A_2 contains an additional double bond in its ring structure. In the present discussion they will be treated as one, only the term vitamin A will be used.

Vitamin A is a pale yellow substance composed of carbon, hydrogen, and oxygen. The chemical formula for vitamin A_1 is given in Fig. 14.1. It is soluble in fat, not soluble in water, stable to heat, that is, to ordinary cooking temperatures, and destroyed by both oxidation and ultraviolet irradiation.

The carotenoid pigments are compounds composed only of carbon and hydrogen. The crystals of the carotenoid pigments are a deep red color but in solution intensely yellow. Their properties of solubility and stability are like those of vitamin A. Beta-carotene is more efficiently converted to vitamin A than alpha- or gamma-carotene, or cryptoxanthin. The chemical structure of beta-carotene is such that it oxidizes to form two molecules of vitamin A; the other provitamins form only one. However, for the sake of clarity, the carotenoid group will be spoken of as *carotene*, as though it were one substance.

Unit of Measurement of Vitamin A

Vitamin A is measured in International Units (IU). The term itself indicates the universality of the unit of measurement. The Health

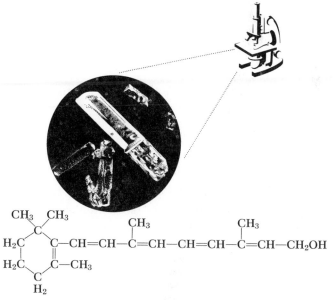

Fig. 14.1. Chemical formula of vitamin A_1, and crystalline vitamin A acetate. (Photomicrograph courtesy of Hoffman-LaRoche, Inc.)

Organization of the League of Nations proposed the universal unit for vitamin A to replace the many different units in use at that time. The International Unit of vitamin A activity as adopted by the current official body, the Subcommittee on Fat-Soluble Vitamins of the World Health Organization is equivalent to 0.3 µg of vitamin A alcohol. Equal biologic activity is afforded by 0.6 µg of the provitamin beta-carotene.

In the United States pharmaceutical companies use the United States Pharmacopeia (USP) Unit to express the vitamin A potency of their products. The USP Unit is exactly the same as the International Unit. The U.S. Pharmacopeia is a book describing drugs, chemicals, and medicinal preparations published under the official authority of the Food and Drug Administration.

Functions of Vitamin A and the Effect of a Deficiency

Growth. Failure of young rats to grow when deprived of certain foods was the initial symptom that led to the discovery of vitamin A. In the early studies before vitamin A had been isolated and chemical methods devised for its determination, growth rate was the criterion of measurement of the vitamin A potency in a food. Animals maintained on a vitamin-A-free diet will cease growing when the body is depleted of its vitamin stores. Materials to be assessed for vitamin content were then fed in known amounts for a prescribed period of time and the growth response noted. Better growth was associated with higher vitamin potency in the food.

If adequate vitamin A is not provided for normal growth, the bony structure will suffer a growth failure before the soft tissues manifest the stunting effect. The cessation of bone growth may result in overcrowding of the brain and central nervous system. It now seems clear that the paralysis sometimes accompanying vitamin A deficiency in very young animals is a result of failure of bone growth, which causes cranial pressure with consequent brain and nerve injury. In some instances there is pinching of the optic nerve, resulting in blindness.

Health of the Epithelial Tissues of the Body. The outer surface of the body is covered with epithelial tissue, the internal cavities of the body lined with it. The tissues are differentiated to better serve their individual functions; the external covering is the resistant, protective epidermis; the internal tissue is a secretory mucous membrane. Deficiency of vitamin A causes an abnormal condition of the epithelial tissues. The specialized functions of the tissue are suppressed, and it is transformed to a keratinized (dry, horny) type of epithelium. Excessive dryness of the skin may result from an insufficient intake; the mucous membrane may fail to secrete normally and becomes less resistant to bacterial invasion.

Xerophthalmia (also known as keratomalacia) is a condition of the eye resulting from severe deprivation of vitamin A (Fig. 14.2). The tear glands cease to function, the eye is dry, the cells of the *cornea* (the transparent outer covering of the iris and pupil) become dry and in serious cases ulcerated. If the condition is not arrested by provision of vitamin A, blindness ensues. The cornea, the part of the eye suffering the severe damage in xerophthalmia, is an epithelial tissue. The condition occurs in both man and animal. Xerophthalmia rarely occurs in the United States. It is, however, not an uncommon occurrence among the young in China. It is a cause of blindness among the rice and cassava-eating people of the southern part of India and Ceylon and is found in Indonesia, Malaya, the Philippines, and in parts of Central and South America (6). The majority of the cases occurs in children two to six years of age. In 1914–1918 children in Denmark were afflicted; butterfat was shipped from the country, and skimmed milk containing little vitamin A used. The condition can be developed in experimental animals deprived of vitamin A.

Composition and Functioning of Visual Pigments. The retina of the eye contains visual pigments that are a combination of vitamin A and a protein. The retina is the light-sensitive inside layer at the back of the eye; it may be likened to the sensitive film of a camera on which the image appears. Two kinds of receptor cells are in the retina—the rods that function in vision in dim light, and the cones that function in bright light and color vision. The terms "rods" and "cones" arise from the shape of the cells. Rhodopsin is a vitamin A-containing pigment in rods, iodopsin in cones (16).

The visual cycle of rhodopsin and iodopsin are believed to be similar; the cycle for rhodopsin (visual purple) is shown in Fig. 14.3. In bright light rhodopsin changes to retinene plus protein with a possible loss of some vitamin A. To resynthesize rhodopsin, vitamin A must be reoxidized to retinene and combined with a special protein opsin (Fig. 14.3). If sufficient vitamin A is not available, night blindness may occur. Night blindness is characterized by inability to see in dim light (nyctalopia) and the necessity of a prolonged time to adjust to dim light after exposure to bright light.

Metabolism of Vitamin A and Carotene

Conversion of Carotene to Vitamin A. After it was established that carotene is a source of vitamin A, the next step was to ascertain where

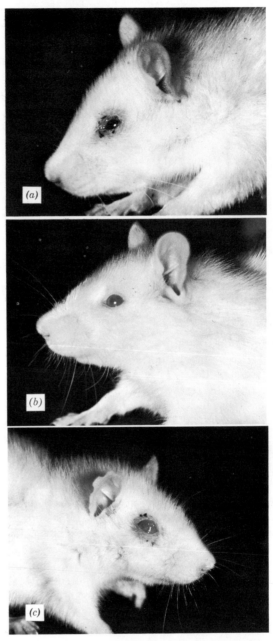

Fig. 14.2. (a) Beginning stages of xerophthalmia or dryness of the cornea and conjunctiva, both of which are curable. (b) The same rat as in (a) after 8 days of vitamin A therapy. (c) Another rat with late stages of xerophthalmia, which is incurable. (Courtesy of The Upjohn Company.)

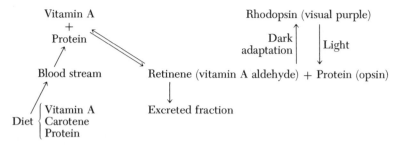

Fig. 14.3.   Schematic diagram of the formation of rhodopsin. [Adapted from Eddy and Dall-dorf (1944) *The Avitaminoses*. The Williams and Wilkins Co., Baltimore, p. 66.]

in the body the conversion of the pigment to the vitamin takes place. It was first believed that the conversion took place in the liver. It was naturally suspected because of the high vitamin A content of the organ. The hypothesis was questioned, however, when the provitamin administered intravenously was not converted to the vitamin. Further doubt was cast on that belief when blood vitamin A was elevated after feeding carotene to rats, with the liver taken out of circulation. The liver was cut off from all connections by tying off the veins, arteries, and common bile duct. It was under the conditions of this experiment, together with other evidence, that the intestinal wall was found to be the main site of the transformation in the rat.

The liver and other tissues have been shown to be alternative sites for the conversion of some carotene to vitamin A. Since man is capable of absorbing carotene from the intestine, other sites for transformation may be of importance. Elucidation is needed concerning the site and the conversion mechanism of the carotenoids to vitamin A (1, 4).

The amount of conversion of carotene to vitamin A is variable depending on the dietary source and efficiency of absorption. Pure crystalline beta-carotene was found to be more efficiently utilized than beta-carotene from green vegetables in studies with adults (13). In average diets carotene is estimated to be one-half as well utilized as preformed vitamin A; 3000 IU of carotene in the diet would be expected to yield only 1500 IU of vitamin A in the body.

Absorption. Vitamin A and carotene are absorbed from the small intestine into the lymph system. The maximum absorption is reached three to five hours after consumption. The rate of absorption of vitamin A is more rapid than that of carotene (10).

The absorption of both vitamin A and carotene is influenced by other substances in the small intestine. Bile, dietary fat, antioxidants, and detergents enhance absorption. Bile is essential for the absorption of carotene. Mineral oil may interfere with absorption, particularly if taken simultaneously with food, or if a large amount of oil is fed with a less than adequate intake of the vitamin. Both vitamin A and carotene are soluble in mineral oil; since the oil is not absorbed, some of the vitamin A and provitamin A are eliminated with it. Under certain conditions, however, the oil is found not to have a deleterious effect. In a study with adults one ounce of mineral oil taken at bed time was found not to impair the absorption of either vitamin A or carotene (5).

Storage and Excretion. In the human being about 95 per cent of the vitamin A stored in the body is found in the liver with small amounts in the lungs, body fat, and kidneys. The amount is least at birth and increases with age. The store of vitamin A in the liver depends on the quantity in the diet and the amount absorbed. It has been estimated that a normal liver may contain as much as 600,000 IU of vitamin A, enough to supply vitamin needs for one year.

Vitamin A is excreted by way of the intestine. In discussions of the vitamins to follow it will be noted that the fat-soluble vitamins are excreted by the fecal pathway, the water-soluble vitamins by the urinary pathway.

Assessment of Vitamin A Status

One of the early symptoms of vitamin A deficiency is night blindness or subnormal dark adaptation. Numerous instruments similar in principle are used for the quantitative measurement. Among them is the photometer (adaptometer) (Fig. 14.4), which measures the amount of light (intensity) required for the subject to perceive objects before and after his exposure to bright light. The intensity of light and the time required to regain vision after bleaching of the visual purple are indicative of vitamin A status. Symptoms of deficiency are recognized by the need for a greater intensity of light and a longer period of time required for the regeneration of the visual purple.

Various sources of error are present in the photometer procedure, both in the instrument and in the subjective response of the person being tested. Conditions other than that of vitamin A deficiency may impair dark adaptation. If rapid and distinct improvement follows the ingestion of vitamin A, it is evident that a shortage of the vitamin was a causative factor.

The blood level of vitamin A and carotene bear a relationship to intake and are indicative of vitamin A status within certain limits. Adults placed on a vitamin-A-free diet are found to show no change in the level for several weeks, followed by an ultimate lowering in the concentration. A carotene-free diet results in prompt reduction of the blood carotene

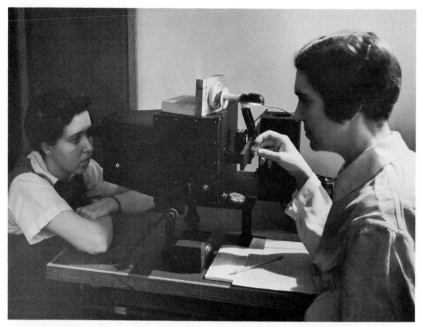

Fig. 14.4. Measuring speed of adjustment from bright to dim light using an adaptometer. (Courtesy of the U.S. Department of Agriculture, Agricultural Research Service.)

content. The body has stores of vitamin A that can be mobilized for use, whereas carotene is not stored.

Vitamin A deficiency in the population of this country appears to be relatively rare. The capacity of the body to store vitamin A provides for an effective emergency supply.

Hypervitaminosis A

Excessive consumption of vitamin A may result in toxic symptoms in both man and animal. Hypervitaminosis A is being reported increasingly in both children and adults who have taken excessive dosages of concentrates of the vitamin for varying lengths of time (3, 8, 17). A case report of a 39-year-old woman who was taking approximately 150,000 IU of vitamin A daily in hopes of improving her vision was recently described (15). The symptoms were swelling of the feet and ankles, fatigue, lassitude, weight loss, and intermittent pains in the shoulders, wrists, and knees. Discrete superficial hemorrhages in the retinae of both eyes in a 17-year-old boy who had been taking 200,000 IU of vitamin A daily for 18 months for acne was reported (9). Arctic travelers who have consumed polar bear liver, which is extremely high in vitamin A content, have manifested symptoms of acute hypervitaminosis A.

The symptoms of acute toxicity are not identical in all cases; most commonly observed are skin lesions, an itching rash in some instances, in others a coarsening of the skin, thinning of the hair, and frequently pain in the joints, with hemorrhage between the bone and its covering. These same symptoms may arise from other causes. A history of consumption of excessive amounts of the vitamin and improvement in physical condition with the discontinuance of its use led to conclusive evidence that hypervitaminosis A was the cause of the trouble in recognized cases. *Acute* toxicity may occur as an end stage of prolonged chronic toxicity resulting from overdosage over a period of time. The toxic dose is highly variable among individuals, especially infants and young children, but is believed to be over 100,000 IU daily. Ill effects from lesser amounts administered over a period of time have been reported. The Council on Foods and Nutrition of the American Medical Association state that "there is definite possibility of harm from the prolonged ingestion of vitamin A in excess of 50,000 USP units daily" (17). The use of vitamin concentrates that require only a few drops for a dose afford an easy means of giving more than is desirable. For example, around 50 drops of several of the common concentrates were found to yield one-half teaspoon, providing in that small measure 15,000 IU of vitamin A. Concentrates of the vitamin are incorporated in multiple vitamin capsules in varying amounts, some contain 5000 IU per capsule, some 15,000 IU and others 25,000 IU and 30,000 IU.

Recommended Allowances for Vitamin A

The Food and Nutrition Board Recommend Daily Allowances of vitamin A at levels believed to be "adequate to meet the needs of health." They are estimated to be about twice the minimal need. The recommendation for young men and women 18 to 35 years of age is 5000 IU; the same daily allowance is recommended for older adults. The allowance is made on the basis that 4000 IU are produced in the average diet by carotene and 1000 IU by vitamin A. Since carotene is only about one-half as well utilized by the body as is preformed vitamin A, if all the vitamin A activity in the diet were from carotene the allowance would be 6000 IU instead of 5000 IU. On the other hand, if all the vitamin were provided by the preformed vitamin the allowance would be 3000 IU instead of 5000 IU.

Food Sources of Vitamin A

Preformed vitamin A occurs only in foods of animal origin; carotene is found in both plant and animal products. The most potent sources of vitamin A are fish-liver oils, liver, butterfat, fortified margarine, and egg yolk. The concentration of vitamin A in the liver increases with age and varies with the species. The potency of butterfat and egg yolk are influenced by the diet of the cow and the hen, respectively. In the spring and summer when green grass becomes more available, the vitamin A content of the milk and eggs produced by the animals is higher. However, the improved and enriched livestock feed used today makes possible the provision of an ample source of vitamin A in animal rations the year round.

The most important sources of the provitamin are the yellow, yellowish-red, and green vegetables and fruits. The yellow carotene in the green products is masked by the presence of chlorophyll. Among the excellent sources of carotene are carrots, sweet potatoes, apricots, spinach, tomatoes, and kale. Some vegetables and fruits deviate from the general color rule; even though yellow in color, oranges, rutabagas, and yellow wax beans are not good sources of carotene. Head lettuce and avocados, two green-colored foods, provide small amounts of carotene. Foods containing little vitamin A are nuts, grains, vegetable oils, muscle meats, and light-colored fruits and vegetables. In most foods one-half or less of the carotene is converted to vitamin A. As a consequence, the carotene content of a food is divided by two in most instances to obtain the biological activity in terms of vitamin A.

The vitamin A values of some common foods are given in Table 14.1. The term vitamin A *value* of foods is used instead of vitamin A *content*. It would be incorrect to indicate that carrots, for example, contain 12,000 units of vitamin A per 100 gm; actually they contain no vitamin A at all; they are merely rich in carotene content.

In compiling the tables of food composition published as Agriculture Handbook 8, Watt and Merrill converted μg of carotene in foods to IU of vitamin A activity on the basis that 0.6 μg of beta-carotene, and 1.2 μg of the sum of the other carotenes with vitamin A activity or of cryptoxanthin are equivalent to 1 IU of vitamin A value.

Stability of Vitamin A and Carotene in Foods. Since both vitamin A and carotene are insoluble in water and stable to ordinary cooking temperatures, there is little loss in food preparation. Canning and freezing

Table 14.1. Vitamin A Value of Some Typical Foods

Food	Portion	IU/Portion
Liver, beef, fried	2 oz	30,280
Potatoes, sweet, baked	1 med	8,910
Carrots, cooked	½ c	7,610
Spinach, cooked	½ c	7,290
Kale, cooked	½ c	4,070
Mustard greens, cooked	½ c	4,060
Apricots, canned	4 med hf	2,120
Broccoli, cooked	½ c	1,875
Peaches, raw	1 med	1,320
Eggs, whole	1 med	590
Ice cream, plain	⅛ qt	370
Milk, whole	1 c	350
Cheese, process	1 oz	350
Orange juice, fresh	½ c	245
Butter (average)	1 pat	230
Margarine, fortified	1 pat	230
Bananas	1 med	190
Apples, raw	1 med	50
Pecans	1 tbsp	10
Bread, whole wheat	1 sl	trace
Oatmeal	½ c	0

From *Nutritive Value of Foods*. U.S. Dept. Agr., Home Garden Bull. No. 72, revised 1964.

cause little loss, but drying and dehydration result in considerable destruction through oxidation.

The development of rancidity in fats causes destruction of both vitamin A and carotene. Storage of fats in a cool, dry place delays the onset of rancidity and thus helps to preserve the vitamin. Margarines were found to lose less than 25 per cent of the original vitamin A content when stored at 14°F for a period as long as 2 years, but when stored at 64°F, 75 per cent of the original vitamin A content was lost in only 17 weeks (2).

Meeting the Daily Need for Vitamin A

Dietary records of college students often indicate an intake of vitamin A below the Recommended Allowance. An evaluation of these dietaries usually shows a low intake of dark green and yellow vegetables. It is estimated that vegetables and fruits provide about 60 per cent of the available supply of the vitamin A value in the United States. The inclusion daily or three to four times a week of a serving of a dark-green or yellow vegetable is an easy way to lay the foundation for an adequate intake of vitamin A. Table 14.2 shows groups of foods for meeting the daily vitamin A need.

Individuals vary in their ability to absorb carotene and in its conversion to vitamin A. Therefore, there should be sufficient intake of carotene to allow for any discrepancy. Foods providing vitamin A, such as eggs, liver, and cheese, should be included.

▶ VITAMIN D

Vitamin D will prevent and cure rickets, a disease in which bones fail to calcify. Children were afflicted with rickets for many centuries before the cause of the disease and the cure for it were known. In Central Europe rickets was known as "The English Disease" because of its prevalence in England. In that country around 1900 it reached almost epidemic proportions when industrialization resulted in both parents

Table 14.2. Foods Providing the Day's Recommended Allowance of Vitamin A for College Men and Women

Food	Portion		Vitamin A Value, IU
Liver, beef, fried	2 oz		30,280
Spinach, cooked	½ c		7,290
Broccoli, cooked	⅔ c		2,500
Eggs, whole	2 med		1,180
Peach, raw	1 med		1,320
		Total	5,000
Apricots, canned	4 med hf		2,130
Milk, whole	1 pt		700
Beans, green	¾ c		510
Egg, whole	1 med		590
Butter	1 tbsp		460
Ice cream, plain	⅛ qt		370
Orange juice, fresh	½ c		245
		Total	5,005

From *Nutritive Value of Foods*. U.S. Dept. Agr., Home Garden Bull. No. 72, revised 1964.

working in shops, leaving little time for taking babies out of doors. However, rickets was not just confined to England. It was common in most of the countries of Northern Europe and in the larger cities of the United States, where as recently as 35 years ago the disease was still common. The discovery of vitamin D and subsequently its widespread use has spared children the crippling effects of rickets.

A combination of clinical observations of children afflicted with rickets and of experimental animals in which rickets had been developed under controlled laboratory conditions led to the identification of vitamin D as the *antiricketic vitamin.* An early (1890) significant observation, made by Palm an English physician, was that the incidence of rickets is related to the amount of sunshine available; where sunshine was abundant, rickets was rare; where the sun seldom shone, rickets abounded. A few years later the concept developed that rickets, like scurvy and beriberi, might be a dietary deficiency disease. With that possibility in mind, the expected next step was to produce the deficiency in experimental animals. In 1921 Mellanby in England produced rickets in puppies by using a mixture of natural foods; then he induced recovery by giving them cod liver oil. At that time cod liver oil was known to contain only vitamin A, so the cure was attributed to it (8). Later it was discovered that even after the vitamin A content of cod liver oil was destroyed by oxidation, the antiricketic potency still remained. It was then that it became evident that cod liver oil contained two vitamins, vitamin A and the antiricketic factor (6). In the meantime, the association of rickets with calcium and phosphorus metabolism, and the favorable influence of cod liver oil on the utilization of calcium were recognized.

By 1922 the mystery of the effectiveness of sunlight in preventing rickets was on the way to solution. Rats fed a rickets-producing diet failed to develop rickets if exposed to sunlight (2). Furthermore, rats fed a rickets-producing diet that had been irradiated in the laboratory, given the same effect as exposure to the sun, also failed to develop rickets (13). After the discovery of the effectiveness of irradiating the diet as a whole, each item was removed, one at a time, and treated separately, then incorporated into the diet in an effort to determine which nutrient was responsible for the antiricketic effect. Fat was the only nutrient that on irradiation imparted antiricketic potency to the diet. With fats established as potential antiricketic factors, the next question to be solved was which portion of the fats, the alcohol or fatty acid fractions, became *activated* on exposure to the ultraviolet rays. It was found to be the alcohol portion. Intensive research soon disclosed that numerous alcohols, all of which belonged to the sterol group of alcohols, acquired antiricketic activity on irradiation. The sterols are much more complex in chemical structure than the common medicinal and beverage alcohols.

By the late 1920's it had been established that rickets could be prevented and cured by exposure to direct sunlight, by irradiation with ultraviolet light, by feeding irradiated food, and by feeding cod liver oil. Then followed the identification of the *natural* vitamin D of fish-liver oils as the same substance produced in human skin on irradiation of 7-dehydrocholesterol. The vitamin D formed from 7-dehydrocholesterol is designated as vitamin D_3. The irradiation of ergosterol, a provitamin D in plant foods, produces a different substance, designated as vitamin D_2.

The Properties of Vitamin D

The sterols that are potential sources of vitamin D are known as provitamins. There are many of them, but only two of importance, 7-dehydrocholesterol and ergosterol. The provitamin in higher animals and invertebrates is 7-dehydrocholesterol; ergosterol is present in the plant kingdom, in yeasts, and certain molds.

The pure vitamins D are white, crystalline, odorless substances that are soluble in fats and fat solvents such as ether, chloroform, acetone, and alcohol. They are resistant to heat, oxidation, acid, and alkali. The vitamins are comprised of carbon, hydrogen, and oxygen combined in chemical structures that are much alike. Crystals of vitamin D_2 and its chemical formula are shown in Fig. 14.5. The relative antiricketic potency of vitamin D_2 and D_3 appear to be no different for the human being; consequently, in the present discussion the term *vitamin D* will be used.

The Unit of Measurement of Vitamin D

Vitamin D potency, like that of vitamin A, is expressed in International and USP Units. (Other vitamins are measured in units of weight.) The amount of antiricketic activity brought about by 0.025 μg of the International Standard, pure crystalline vitamin D_3 is an International Unit. The unit was adopted by the World Health Organization in 1949 and has been used ever since. The USP Unit is the same as the International Unit.

In order to measure the *amount of antiricketic activity*, rats are usually employed as the experimental animal. Under standardized conditions of feeding and care, and by using standardized procedures for determining bone change, the potency of vitamin D in terms of International Units is determined.

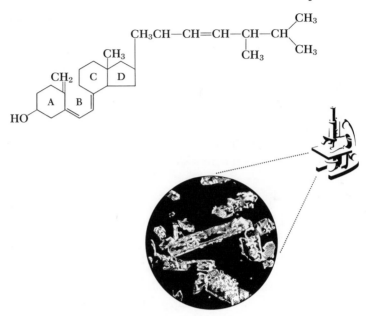

Fig. 14.5.   Chemical formula for vitamin D_2 and crystalline vitamin D_2 (calciferol). (Photomicrograph courtesy of Distillation Products Industries, Division of Kodak, Rochester, New York.)

Conversion of Provitamin D to the Vitamin

The conversion of provitamin D to the vitamin by irradiation is accomplished by a change in the structure of the compound; the second ring in the provitamin D structure opens (note ring B, Fig. 14.5). The conversion process has been studied in the laboratory with the finding that a series of intermediary products are formed before vitamin D is obtained; further irradiation beyond the vitamin D stage produces toxic products lacking antiricketic potency.

Functions of Vitamin D and the Effect of a Deficiency

Bone Formation. One of the chief functions of vitamin D is the maintenance of the normal processes of bone formation (5). A deficiency of the vitamin in the growing young results in rickets. The disease will develop in infants even though the diet provides an ample intake of calcium and phosphorus unless vitamin D is provided in the diet or adequate exposure to sunlight is possible. Late rickets (osteomalacia), a condition similar to rickets in children, occurs in adults.

In rickets the bones are susceptible to deformity when exposed to ordinary stresses. A common and severe change in the skeletal structure is enlargement of the ends of the long bones in the legs and arms. If mineral is not deposited in the developing bone cells, the weight of the body causes the noncalcified portion to flatten and mushroom outward, giving the appearance of enlarged joints. Other bone changes include the *ricketic rosary,* a row of beadlike protuberances on each side of the chest at the juncture of the rib bones and joining (costal) cartilage (Fig. 14.6), bowed legs, and knocked knees—all caused by failure of the bones to calcify normally.

The mode of action of vitamin D in relation to bone calcification remains relatively obscure. Intramuscularly injected radioactive calcium was deposited in the bones of ricketic chicks with no vitamin D in the diet. This indicated to the investigators that the primary function of vitamin D might be that of facilitating absorption of calcium from the intestine since calcium deposition in bones could proceed without it (9).

Calcium Absorption and Metabolism. That vitamin D exerts a favorable influence on the absorption of calcium is evidenced in studies

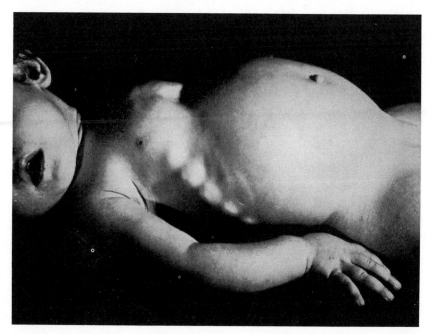

Fig. 14.6. Ricketic rosary showing enlargement of costochondral junctions. (From Wolbach, Jolliffe, Tisdall, and Cannon, *Clinical Nutrition,* Paul B. Hoeber, Inc., New York, p. 113, 1950.)

with animals and human beings (2). Figure 14.7 illustrates the decrease in calcium excretion in children with rickets after the administration of vitamin D; the fecal excretion is markedly reduced. With children 1 to 12 years of age, Jeans and Stearns found that some utilized calcium efficiently without added vitamin D; others required a supplement. Stearns (11) pointed out that there is no way of discerning from outward appearances which children need the additional vitamin, which do not, hence recommended that vitamin D be given to all children. Numerous balance studies with normal adults show no improvement in the utilization of calcium with additions of sources of vitamin D (7) except during pregnancy and lactation.

The absorption of phosphorus appears not to be influenced by vitamin D. For example, vitamin-D-deficient animals absorb phosphorus equally well, with and without an additional supplement of the vitamin.

Growth. Rickets causes a slowing of growth. Animals in which experimental rickets has been induced grow more slowly than their normal controls with an adequate vitamin D intake. Infants also fail to grow normally without a sufficient amount of the vitamin. Infants given 340 to 400 IU daily of vitamin D were found to grow more in length than those receiving 60 to 135 IU. Giving more than 600 IU daily did not increase the growth rate further (10, 12); increasing the vitamin D intake beyond 1800 IU daily decreased growth (12).

Incidence of Vitamin D Deficiency

Clinically detectable rickets is uncommon in the United States today. The widespread preventive (prophylactic) use of sources of vitamin D

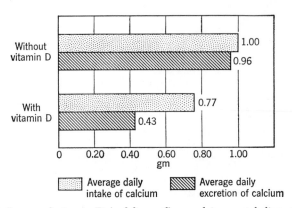

Fig. 14.7. Influence of vitamin D (cod liver oil) on calcium metabolism of infant with rickets. (Adapted from Hess, *Rickets,* Lea and Febiger, Philadelphia, p. 161, 1929.)

has all but eradicated this once common scourge of infancy. Fortification of all evaporated milk and much of the fresh milk with vitamin D almost controls rickets automatically in the United States. Osteomalacia, too, is rare in this country. It is reported to be common among women in the Orient and parts of the Near East during pregnancy and lactation, increasing in severity with each reproductive cycle.

Metabolism of Vitamin D

Vitamin D can be made available to the body through food sources or concentrates and by activation of the provitamin, 7-dehydrocholesterol, in the skin. The vitamin taken by mouth is absorbed from the small intestine chiefly by way of the lymph system. The process is facilitated by the presence of fat. Bile is necessary for normal absorption of the vitamin from the intestine. The chief site of storage of vitamin D is the liver with smaller amounts stored in the skin, brain, lungs, spleen, and bones. Excretion of vitamin D is by way of the bowel, with no excretion through the kidney.

During lactation there is some transmission of vitamin D into the milk. The amount increases with a more ample intake of vitamin D in the diet or exposure to sunlight. Summer milk contains more of the vitamin than winter milk. The laying hen, with vitamin D in the ration, transmits a portion of it to the egg yolk.

Hypervitaminosis D

Massive dosages of vitamin D may have toxic effects if continued for a period of time. Giving only two massive doses a year is used by some physicians as an acceptable means of providing vitamin D. The level at which deleterious effects result from continued high dosages varies with individuals. Some show symptoms with an intake of 50,000 IU per day for a few weeks, others tolerate as much as ten times that amount for longer periods of time. An intake of 1800 IU daily may be mildly toxic in children if continued over a period of time. The early symptoms include loss of appetite, thirst, lassitude, followed by nausea, vomiting, diarrhea, abdominal discomfort, and loss of weight. The blood calcium and phosphorus levels are elevated with increased excretion of calcium in the urine, which may cause deposits in the kidney with consequent damage to the organ and impaired function. In hypervitaminosis D, cells in various organs of the body, as well as the arteries and arterioles, become susceptible to abnormal deposition of calcium. Severe intoxication with widespread calcification of soft tissues ultimately may prove fatal if massive dosages are continued. Acute toxicity may result from a chronic condition that has been present for some time becoming acute only when a high degree of toxicity is reached.

Vitamin D preparations on the market are of such potency that dosages are expressed in drops, making it easy to give more than is desirable (1). In commonly used preparations around 50 drops measure one-half teaspoon with a potency of 3000 IU. Most multiple vitamin capsules provide 500 IU or more per capsule.

Recommended Allowances for Vitamin D

The Recommended Allowance for vitamin D for late adolescence is 400 IU daily, the same as is recommended throughout childhood. Normal adults seem to need little, if any, supplemental vitamin D. It is generally believed, nevertheless, that for adults with little exposure to the direct sunlight some vitamin D in the diet may be advisable, despite the lack of direct proof to substantiate the presumption. During pregnancy and lactation, when the calcium need is increased, the Recommended Allowance is 400 IU daily. The requirements of infants and children, and further discussion of the needs during pregnancy and lactation appear in those respective subsequent chapters.

Sources of Vitamin D

Vitamin D is not widely distributed in nature. The best sources are fish oils, especially liver oils, the concentration of which varies with the species as shown in Table 14.3. Milk, butter, and egg yolk are the only

Table 14.3. Vitamin D Content of Selected Sources

Source	Measure	Vitamin D, IU
Oil, swordfish liver[1]	1 gm	10,000
Oil, halibut liver[1]	1 gm	1,200
Oil, cod liver[1]	1 gm	100
Milk, whole[2]	8 oz	100
Liver, chicken[2]	2 oz	40
Liver, beef[2]	2 oz	38
Egg yolk[2]	1 med	27
Butter[2]	1 tbsp	4
Oil, corn[2]	1 tbsp	0

[1] From Bills, *Physiol. Revs.* **15:** 13, 1935.
[2] From Church and Church, *Food Values of Portions Commonly Used,* *Bowes and Church,* 9th ed. J. B. Lippincott, 1963.

foods in the ordinary diet that contain vitamin D, and in these the amount is small and variable. Vitamin D present in food is stable in ordinary cooking, heat-processing treatments, and storage. Milk is selected for enrichment with vitamin D because it is a rich source of calcium and phosphorus, the minerals that require vitamin D for absorption and use. It is consumed by the young, who especially need the vitamin for skeletal development.

There are fish liver oils on the market and concentrates of irradiated ergosterol; also vitamin D is included in many multiple-vitamin combinations. Some of the preparations of vitamin D are in oily solution, some are aqueous preparations. The potency as indicated on the label is assured of accuracy by the reliability of the pharmaceutical house manufacturing the product and the surveillance of the Federal Food and Drug Administration over the authenticity of labels.

Exposure to sunshine or ultraviolet irradiation results in the synthesis of the vitamin; the provitamin, 7-dehydrocholesterol, which occurs in the skin and in the blood (4), is transformed into vitamin D. The amount that can be synthesized by man by this method is not known. Smoke, haze, and fog in the atmosphere, the glass in the windows, the clothing worn, the pigmentation of the skin, all intervene to limit the ultraviolet light exposure of the skin. In the summer time, the vitamin D value of sunlight in the United States reaches the greatest intensity of the year; in December it is least. The rays of the rising and setting sun are less effective than the sun at midday.

▶ VITAMIN E

Research which eventually led to the discovery of vitamin E was conducted in the early 1920's by Mattill, Evans, and Sure. During an investigation of the influence of diet on the reproductive cycle of the rat, it was found that rats became sterile when reared on a purified diet which contained all the then-known nutrients. Even though the experimental animals fed this ration appeared to be quite healthy, they were not able to produce young. When fresh green leaves or dried alfalfa were fed to these sterile animals, reproductivity was restored in the female but not in the male of the species. The unknown factor, which prevented sterility, was first called substance X and later was named vitamin E.

Properties of Vitamin E

The chemical name for vitamin E is tocopherol (from Greek *tokos*, childbirth; *perhos*, to bear; and the chemical suffix -*ol*, signifying an alcohol). Actually there are six different tocopherols, which collectively are called vitamin E. The biological activity of the tocopherols varies, with alpha being the most potent (Fig. 14.8). The number and position of the methyl (CH_3) groups within the molecule seem to influence biological activity. This conclusion is reached because the only difference among the tocopherols is in the structure of the molecule.

Vitamin E occurs as a yellow viscous oil that is insoluble in water but soluble in all the fat solvents. Although it is quite stable to acids and heat (in the absence of oxygen), it is readily destroyed by ultraviolet light, alkalies, and oxygen.

Function of Vitamin E

It has long been believed that the function of vitamin E in the animal organism is directly related to its antioxidant property. Besides its possible function as an activator in certain enzymatic reactions, vitamin E plays an important role in the protection of vitamin A, carotene, and ascorbic acid from oxidation both in the digestive tract and in the body cells. Because of the protective property of vitamin E more efficient use can be made by the body of vitamin A and ascorbic acid.

The Effects of a Vitamin E deficiency

In Animals and Birds. Vitamin E has been shown to be essential for animals and birds, including the rat, rabbit, dog, guinea pig, chick, and duck. The most characteristic deficiency symptoms, however, occur in the rat and in the rabbit.

When rats are fed rations deficient in vitamin E, permanent sterility in the male and temporary sterility in the female result. The permanent sterility of the male rat, which is caused by a degeneration of the cellular material of the testes, cannot be relieved by vitamin E therapy. In contrast to this, conception does occur in the deficient female rat, but about the eighth day of pregnancy the fetuses, or unborn animals, die and are resorbed. However, if vitamin E is added to the rations of these

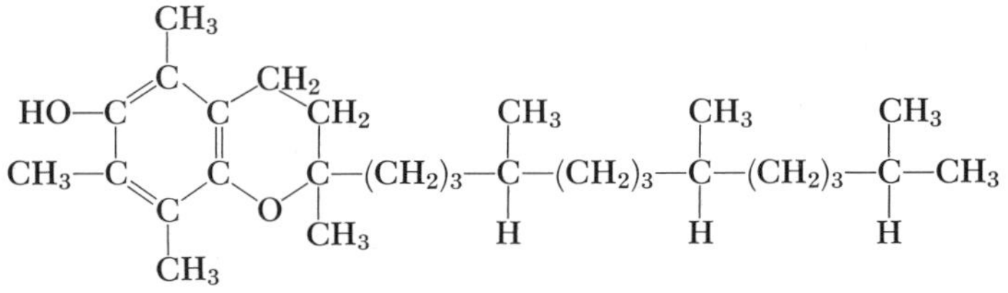

Fig. 14.8.   Alpha-tocopherol.

sterile females, their next pregnancy will be normal and they will produce living, healthy young. One of the reasons postulated for the death of the unborn young is the lack of an adequate blood supply to the fetus because of a change in the permeability of the reproductive tissues.

Young rabbits develop a condition called muscular dystrophy when they are fed a ration deficient in vitamin E. This disorder, which is characterized by a loss of muscle tone and a general weakening of the muscles, is quickly relieved when vitamin E is added back to the ration.

In Man. At this time there is no conclusive evidence to indicate that vitamin E is essential to man. It should be noted, however, that the plasma level of alpha tocopherol is lowered in normal adults after maintenance on a limited intake (2 mg daily in contrast to an estimated average of 15 mg daily for the supplemental group) for a period from 10 to 22 months. No clinical or physiological effects accompanied the lowered plasma level during the period of observation. Vitamin E seems to have no effect on the relief of sterility in human beings or on the cure of human muscular dystrophy. Horwitt (1) reported a relationship between serum levels of vitamin E and hemolysis of the red cells (erythrocytes) in the presence of hydrogen peroxide. Subjects who received the smallest amounts of vitamin E showed the greatest degree of red cell hemolysis.

Recommended Allowances for Vitamin E

The Food and Nutrition Board (4) states that until more is known about the antioxidant needs of the body and the role that selenium and other nutrients play in decreasing vitamin E needs, it is difficult to make any recommendation other than the vitamin E requirement will vary between 10 and 30 mg daily for adults. Because vitamin E is so widely distributed in the foods of the diet, it is doubtful that a vitamin E deficiency would ever develop in the human being. It is estimated that the average daily adult diet contains about 14 mg of vitamin E.

Horwitt and associates are conducting a long-term study of the human requirement for tocopherol. Some of the conclusions from their work are (2, 3):

(1) The tocopherol requirement is a function of the amounts of polyunsaturated lipids in the diet and in the tissues.
(2) When polyunsaturated fatty acids in the diet are low, the need for tocopherol decreases to very low levels, but past dietary habits which have affected tissue composition must be taken into consideration in evaluating tocopherol needs.
(3) The time of erythrocyte survival is shortened in man when a diet with a relatively low tocopherol to linoleic acid ratio is fed for prolonged periods.

Food Sources of Vitamin E

Inasmuch as vitamin E occurs mainly in plant materials, the richest sources of the vitamin are found in vegetable oils (such as wheat germ oil and cottonseed oil), leafy-green plants and vegetables, as well as whole-grain cereals. Although animal products contain little of the vitamin, liver, heart, kidney, milk, and eggs are the best animal sources of vitamin E.

▶ VITAMIN K

In 1929 Dam, a Danish scientist, reported that chicks raised on a synthetic diet developed hemorrhages under the skin that could not be relieved with the addition of ascorbic acid to the ration. This disorder, which was characterized by a prolonged blood clotting time, disappeared when a mixture of cereals or natural foods was given to the birds. Later Dam found that this antihemorrhagic factor was present in the fat-soluble fraction of certain foods. He suggested it be called vitamin K, derived from the Danish term "Koagulation Faktor." ·

Properties of Vitamin K

Two forms of vitamin K are found in nature: K_1 occurs in green leaves, and K_2 is produced by bacterial synthesis. These yellow-colored vitamins are stable to heat, unstable to alkalies, strong acids, oxidation, and light. Many structural modifications of vitamin K have been synthesized; one water-soluble form, menadione, is more potent and more widely used than the natural vitamin K (Fig. 14.9).

Function of Vitamin K

Vitamin K is essential for the synthesis of prothrombin which is a precursor of thrombin, one of the factors needed for normal blood coagulation. Even though the production of prothrombin apparently occurs in the liver, the exact function of the vitamin in this synthesis is not known. It has been suggested, however, that vitamin K may be an essential part of the enzyme system involved in the production of this blood clotting factor.

The Effects of a Vitamin K Deficiency

In Birds and Animals. Chicks fed a ration deficient in vitamin K develop a fatal bleeding disorder which is characterized by a prolonged

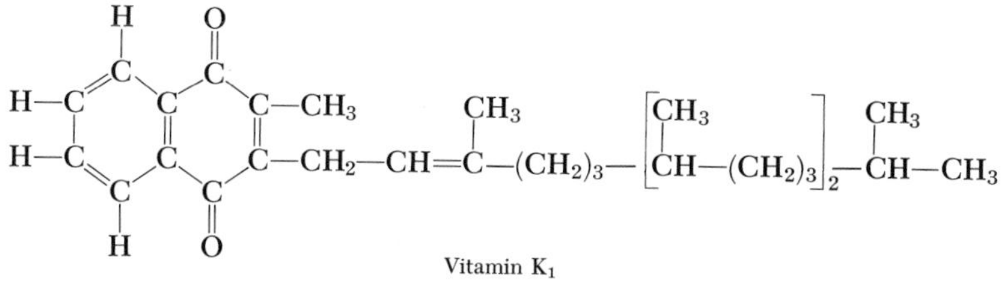

Vitamin K$_1$

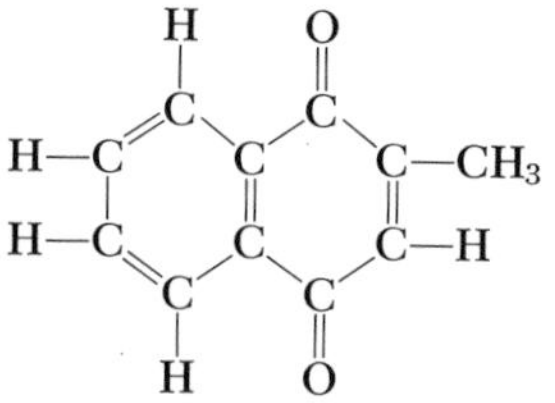

Menadione

Fig. 14.9.

clotting time of the blood. This disorder, however, may be relieved by the administration of vitamin K. It is commonly believed that vitamin K deficiency is an avian characteristic. In some studies with rats maintained on a vitamin-K-free diet, when access to their feces was completely prevented, a bleeding tendency developed (1). Some vitamin K is synthesized in the small intestine by bacteria.

In Man. Vitamin K deficiencies in man result most often from either a faulty absorption of the vitamin or liver disorders that interfere with the synthesis of prothrombin, rather than from a dietary lack of the nutrient. Inasmuch as vitamin K is supplied to the body by the food intake plus the synthesis by microorganisms in the intestinal tract, there usually is an adequate supply of the vitamin available to the body. Sometimes, however, the intake of large amounts of sulfa drugs or other antibiotics may destroy the microorganisms which synthesize the vitamin and the supply then may become low.

Because vitamin K is fat soluble, the presence of bile is necessary for its absorption as is true with the absorption of fats and other fat-soluble vitamins. Therefore, when disorders of the liver or gall bladder interfere with the secretion of the bile fluid, a vitamin K deficiency may occur. For example, in cases of obstructive jaundice, where a blockage of the bile duct prevents bile from flowing normally into the intestine, vitamin K is not adequately absorbed. On the other hand, in certain liver disorders, such as cirrhosis, adequate vitamin K may be absorbed, but the synthesis of prothrombin does not occur because of the damage to the liver cells themselves.

Newborn infants may have inadequate vitamin K supplies because microorganisms of the right type may not have had time to become established in the intestinal tract.

Recommended Allowances for Vitamin K

The Food and Nutrition Board (2) states that "with the exception of newborn infants, the average diet plus synthesis by intestinal bacteria provide adequate amounts of vitamin K."

The newborn infant has low blood serum levels of prothrombin, which decrease further during the first week of life, but spontaneously return toward the adult level in subsequent weeks. As a consequence, it has been a fairly common practice to routinely administer vitamin K to the mother prior to delivery or to the newborn shortly after delivery. The practice has been questioned—it has been difficult to demonstrate that decreased levels of coagulation factors are a direct cause of hemorrhage of the newborn (neonatal), and there is not complete agreement that routine administration of vitamin K in pregnancy affects the incidence. So the Board has recommended that (2):

Vitamin K may be administered to the normal newborn infant, routinely, but is especially indicated for infants with increased susceptibility to neonatal hemorrhage (prematurity, anoxia). . . . A single parenteral dose of 0.5–1.0 mg or an oral dose of 1.0–2.0 mg is considered adequate for prophylaxis. . . . Infants born to mothers receiving anticoagulant therapy should be given 2.0–4.0 mg of vitamin K immediately after birth.

Food Sources of Vitamin K

Vitamin K occurs in plants; good sources are alfalfa, cauliflower, cabbage, spinach, kale, and soybean. In contrast, fruits, cereals, and animal products contain little vitamin K. The occurrence of vitamin K in a wide variety of commonly eaten plant foods, its synthesis by bacteria in the intestinal tract, its stability, and its insolubility in water make a deficiency of this vitamin in the normal person quite improbable.

Antivitamins K

There are two antivitamins K, dicoumarol and hydrocoumarol, that are used therapeutically for the relief of human thrombosis, a disorder in which clots are formed abnormally in the blood stream. These antivitamins or antagonists have similar chemical structures to vitamin K but do not perform the physiological function of prothrombin formation. Thus dicoumarol acts as an anticoagulant by interfering with prothrombin synthesis.

REFERENCES

INTRODUCTION TO THE VITAMINS

1. McCollum, E. V. (1957). *A History of Nutrition.* Houghton Mifflin Co., Boston.
2. Williams, R. R. (1958). Values in the American Institute of Nutrition: background and foreground. *Federation Proc.* **17:** 726.

VITAMIN A

1. Bieri, J. G., and C. J. Pollard (1954). Studies of the site of conversion of B-carotene injected intravenously into rats. *Brit. J. Nutr.* **8:** 32.
2. Deuel, H. J., Jr., and S. M. Greenberg (1953). A comparison of the retention of vitamin A in margarines and in butters based upon bioassays. *Food Res.* **18:** 497.
3. Gerber, A., A. P. Raab, and A. E. Sobel (1954). Vitamin A poisoning in adults. *Am. J. Med.* **16:** 729.
4. Mattson, F. H., J. W. Mehl, and H. J. Deuel Jr. (1947). Studies on carotinoid metabolism. VII. The site of conversion of carotene to vitamin A in the rat. *Arch. Biochem.* **15:** 65.
5. Mineral oil dosage and vitamin A absorption (1952). *Nutr. Rev.* **10:** 265.
6. McLaren, D. S. (1963). *Malnutrition and the Eye.* Academic Press, New York, p. 218.
7. McCollum, E. V., and M. Davis (1913). The necessity of certain lipins in the diet during growth. *J. Biol. Chem.* **15:** 167.
8. Nieman, C., and H. J. K. Obbink (1954). The biochemistry and pathology of hypervitaminosis A. In *Vitamins and Hormones.* Vol. XII, Academic Press, New York, p. 69.
9. Nutritional disease and the eye (1964). *Borden's Rev. Nutr. Res.* Vol. 25.
10. Olson, J. A. (1961). The absorption of beta-carotene and its conversion into vitamin A. *The Metabolism and Function of the Fat-Soluble Vitamins, A, E & K. Am. J. Clin. Nutr.* **9,** No. 4, pt II: 1.
11. Osborne, T. B., and L. B. Mendel (1913). The relation of growth to the chemical constituents of the diet. *J. Biol. Chem.* **15:** 311.
12. *Present Knowledge of Nutrition* (1956). 2nd ed., The Nutrition Foundation, New York, p. 66.
13. *Recommended Dietary Allowances Revised* 1958. Natl. Acad. Sci.—Natl. Res. Council, Publ. 589, Washington, D.C., p. 11.
14. Steenbock, H. (1919). White corn versus yellow corn and a probable relation between the fat soluble vitamin and yellow plant pigments. *Science* **50:** 352.
15. Toxic reactions of vitamin A (1964). *Nutrition Rev.* **22:** 109.
16. Wald, G. (1960). The visual function of the vitamin A, In *Vitamins and Hormones.* Vol. XVIII, Academic Press, New York, pp. 417–430.
17. White, P. L. (1959). Vitamin preparations as dietary supplements and as therapeutic agents. *J. Am. Med. Assoc.* **169:** 41.

VITAMIN D

1. Forbes, G. B. (1957). Overnutrition for the child: blessing or curse? *Nutr. Rev.* **15:** 193.
2. Harrison, H. E., and H. C. Harrison (1963). Theories of vitamin D action. *In the Transfer of Calcium and Strontium Across Biological Membranes.* (R. B. Wasserman, ed.) Academic Press, New York, p. 229.
3. Hess, A. F., L. J. Unger, and A. M. Pappenheimer (1922). Experimental rickets in rats. III. The prevention of rickets in rats by exposure to sunlight. *J. Biol. Chem.* **50:** 77.
4. Koehler, A. E. and E. Hill (1953). 7-Dehydrocholesterol in human serum. *Federation Proc.* **12:** 232.

5. Kramer, B., and A. Kanof (1954). Vitamin D group. B. In pathology of human beings. In *The Vitamins.* Vol. II. (W. H. Sebrell, Jr. and Robert S. Harris, eds.) Academic Press, New York, p. 232.
6. McCollum, E. V., N. Simmonds, P. G. Shipley, and E. A. Park (1922). Studies on experimental rickets. XII. Is there a substance other than fat-soluble A associated with certain fats which play an important role in bone development? *J. Biol. Chem.* **50:** 5.
7. McKay, H., M. B. Patton, M. S. Pittman, G. Stearns, and N. Edelblute (1943). The effect of vitamin D on calcium retentions. *J. Nutr.* **26:** 153.
8. Mellanby, E. (1921). *Experimental Rickets.* Medical Research Council (British) Special Report Series 61, London.
9. Migicovsky, B. B., and J. W. S. Jamieson (1955). Calcium absorption and vitamin D. *Can. J. Biochem. Physiol.* **33:** 202.
10. Slyker, F., B. M. Hamil, M. W. Poole, T. B. Cooley, and I. G. Macy (1937). Relationship between vitamin D intake and linear growth in infants. *Proc. Soc. Exptl. Biol. Med.* **37:** 499.
11. Stearns, G. (1954). Early experiences with vitamin D in the nutrition of infants and children—a retrospect. *Nutr. Rev.* **12:** 193.
12. Stearns, G., P. C. Jeans, and V. Vandecar (1936). The effect of vitamin D on linear growth in infancy. *J. Pediat.* **9:** 1.
13. Steenbock, H., and A. Black (1924). Fat-soluble vitamins. XVII. The induction of growth-promoting and calcifying properties in a ration by exposure to ultra-violet light. *J. Biol. Chem.* **61:** 405.
14. Wiss, O., and F. Weber, (1944). The liver and vitamins. In *The liver,* Vol. II. (C. H. Rouiller, ed.) Academic Press, New York, p. 137.

VITAMIN E

1. Horwitt, M. K., C. C. Harvey, G. D. Duncan, and W. C. Wilson (1956). Effects of limited tocopherol intake in man with relationships to erythrocyte hemolysis and lipid oxidations. *Am. J. Clin. Nutr.* **4:** 408.
2. Horwitt, M. K., C. C. Harvey, B. Century, and L. A. Witting (1961). Polyunsaturated lipids and tocopherol requirements. *J. Am. Dietet. Assoc.* **38:** 234.
3. Horwitt, M. K., B. Century, and A. A. Zeman (1963). Erythrocyte survival time and reticulocyte levels after tocopherol depletion in man. *Am. J. Clin. Nutrition* **12:** 99.
4. *Recommended Dietary Allowances Sixth Revised Edition* (1964). Natl. Acad. Sci.—Natl. Res. Council, Publ. 1146, Washington, D.C., p. 44.

VITAMIN K

1. Barnes, R. H., and G. Fiala (1958). Uncomplicated vitamin K deficiency in the rat. *Federation Proc.* **17:** 470.
2. *Recommended Dietary Allowances Sixth Revised Edition* (1964). Natl. Acad. Sci.—Natl. Res. Council, Publ. 1146, Washington, D.C., p. 45.

SUPPLEMENTARY REFERENCES

Smith, R. W., J. Rizck, and B. Frame (1964). Determinants of serum antirachitic activity. *Am. J. Clin. Nutr.* **14:** 98.
Symposium—The metabolism and function of the fat-soluble vitamins A, E, and K (1961). *Am. J. Clin. Nutr.* **9:** 1.
Wolf, G. (1962). Some thoughts on the metabolic role of vitamin A. *Nutr. Rev.* **20:** 161.

CHAPTER 15

Ascorbic acid

The early explorers of both land and sea were menaced by outbreaks of a disorder called *scurvy*, which is a nutritional disease caused by a severe deficiency of ascorbic acid. The exploration of the world during the fifteenth and sixteenth centuries was hindered by the outbreaks of this malady. On Vasco de Gama's famous voyage around the Cape of Good Hope in 1497, as many as two-thirds of his crew died of scurvy. All the members of Jacques Cartier's second voyage to Newfoundland in 1553 suffered from this disorder when they were forced to spend the winter in Quebec. Because fresh foods were not available, some of the crew died from scurvy before the Indians taught them to prepare a tea of the bark and leaves of the spruce tree which acted both as a remedy and a preventative for the disorder.

James Lind, a ship's surgeon in the English Navy, had the genius to observe, record, and experiment with scurvy patients on board the H. M. S. Salisbury in 1747, and his classical work led to the elimination of scurvy among the crews of ships. He made the following report of his experiences in relieving scurvy on this now famous voyage (9):

On the 20th of May 1747, I took twelve patients in the scurvy. . . . Their cases were as similar as I could have them. . . . They lay together in one place and had one diet common to all. . . . Two of these were ordered each a quart of cyder a-day. . . . Two others took twenty-five gutts of elixir vitriol° three times a-day. . . .

° A strong solution of sulfuric acid combined with aromatics.

Two others took two spoonfuls of vinegar three times a-day. . . . Two of the worse patients were put under a course of sea-water. . . . Two of the others had each two oranges and one lemon given them every day. . . . The two remaining patients took the bigness of a nutmeg three times a-day of a electuary† recommended by a hospital surgeon. . . . The consequence was, that the most sudden and visible good effects were perceived from the use of the oranges and lemons; one of these who had taken them, being at the end of six days fit for duty. . . . The other was the best recovered of any in his condition; and being now pretty well, was appointed nurse to the rest of the sick. . . .

Not only did Lind show that scurvy could be cured by the intake of orange and lemon juice, but also he developed a method for the concentration and preservation of the juices from citrus fruit for use at sea. In 1795 the Royal Navy began to provide a regular daily ration of lime or lemon juice to all its men, and the name "limey," which is still used to designate an English sailor, refers to this practice.

Throughout the nineteenth century there are records of scurvy epidemics in different parts of the world. The most famous epidemic was the potato famine of 1845–1848, which killed many people in Ireland where potatoes were the main food of the diet. Even the settlers of this country suffered from scurvy in their march westward. In 1846–1848 the Mormons, on their way to Utah, were forced to spend the winter near Omaha, Nebraska. Here they lived on a diet that consisted primarily of mush with the result that 300 children and adults died, most of them of scurvy.

Although man has known for years that the use of certain kinds of foods in his diet would prevent the occurrence of scurvy, it was not until 1933 that Waugh and King at the University of Pittsburgh and Szent-Gyorgyi in Hungary identified the antiscurvy factor as ascorbic acid. Since that time, the vitamin has been manufactured in the synthetic form and today can be purchased at a very low cost.

Properties of Ascorbic Acid

Ascorbic acid is the chemical name for vitamin C; it occurs in white crystals that are easily dissolved in water (Fig. 15.1). Although the crystals of the vitamin are quite stable in the dry form, a water solution of ascorbic acid will undergo destruction when exposed to air, heat, light, or metals like copper and iron. It is unstable in alkali but relatively stable in an acid medium.

Until the last decade, just one form of the vitamin, L-ascorbic acid (also called *reduced* ascorbic acid) was recognized as giving vitamin

† Made of garlic, mustard seed, *rad-raphan*, balsam of Peru, and gum myrrh.

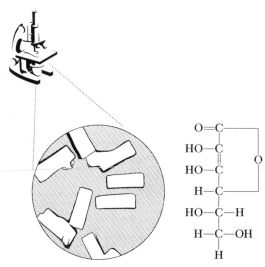

Fig. 15.1.   Crystalline ascorbic acid and the chemical formula for L-ascorbic acid. (Photomicrograph courtesy of Merck and Co., Rahway, New Jersey.)

protection to man. Now, however, another form of the vitamin has been found that can be used as well as the reduced form. It has been named *dehydroascorbic* acid. The sum of the vitamin effect from both reduced and dehydroascorbic acids is referred to as *total* ascorbic acid. Experiments, conducted to determine how efficiently college students were able to utilize the total ascorbic acid from twenty-four different fruits and vegetables, have shown that the dehydroascorbic acid was used as well as the reduced form (5). Another chemical form of the vitamin, *erythorbic acid* (D-araboascorbic acid) is sometimes used as an antioxidant in food processing. This form, however, is only slightly antiscorbutic as compared to L-ascorbic acid (12).

Functions of Ascorbic Acid

The exact biochemical function of ascorbic acid in man and animals is not yet established. It is known that the vitamin is important in the formation and maintenance of *collagen*, the cementing material that holds the cells of the body together. Also, it has been suggested that ascorbic acid plays a role in the normal metabolism of the amino acid, tyrosine, and in the function of the adrenal gland.

The role of ascorbic acid in the formation and maintenance of this collagen was first observed in a study using guinea pigs that was conducted at Harvard University (15). When the tissues of these scorbutic animals were examined under the microscope, it was found that the collagen material between the cells had disappeared. Similar examinations of the teeth and bones of the animals revealed that the cells of the dentin, the interior part of the tooth, and those at the end of the long bones were affected.

Collagen is also an important factor in the healing of cuts or wounds. In wound healing when the intake of ascorbic acid is below normal, it has been demonstrated tha wounds do not heal normally. It has been demonstrated in connective tissue studies that ascorbic acid is essential for the production of tissue to enhance immediate postoperative healing and for the maintenance of previously formed scar tissue. Furthermore, the vitamin accumulates in scar tissue immediately following wounding and persists for a long period of time (1).

Three of the symptoms of scurvy that we can directly relate to the loss of the cementing action of collagen are the hemorrhages that occur throughout the body, the loosening of the teeth, and the changes in the cells that occur in the extremities of the long bones of children and young animals. There is no doubt at the present time that a deficiency of ascorbic acid is directly related to poor collagen formation in the body, but the biochemical function of the vitamin in this reaction is still unknown.

A relationship between ascorbic acid and the oxidation of the amino acid, tyrosine, has been observed in guinea pigs and infants but not in adult man. In scorbutic guinea pigs and infants it has been demonstrated that tyrosine is not metabolized normally unless sufficient ascorbic acid is available. In adults, however, this relationship was not observed when subjects were fed small amounts of the vitamin and large amounts of the amino acid (8). The role that ascorbic acid may play in the metabolism of tyrosine appears to be that of a coenzyme.

The cortical tissue of the adrenal glands contains a high concentration of ascorbic acid. Here, too, are found large amounts of cholesterol, the proposed parent substance of the cortical hormones. Tracer studies suggest that the vitamin may be involved in the conversion of acetate to cholesterol. However, the relationship of ascorbic acid to the cortical function of the adrenals has not yet been fully explained.

At this time there is no conclusive evidence that the common cold, hay fever, and other related disorders can be prevented by high doses of ascorbic acid.

The Effects of an Ascorbic Acid Deficiency

In Animals. The only animals other than man that have a dietary need for ascorbic acid are guinea pigs and primates (monkeys, apes, chimpanzees). Other animals need the vitamin but they are able to synthesize enough ascorbic acid in their body tissues to meet the requirement.

When guinea pigs are placed on an ascorbic acid-free diet, they begin to lose weight rapidly after 16 days, and between 25 and 28 days they will die if the vitamin is not restored to the ration. Loss of appetite as well as dull and rough hair are the characteristic gross symptoms of this disorder. There are also signs of marked hemorrhages throughout the tissues and organs of the body when the animals are autopsied.

In Man. Human scurvy is rarely found in the United States today. The few cases that do occur are found in infants between the ages of 6 and 12 months who have not received adequate amounts of the vitamin in their diets and in aged or older adults who have poor food habits.

Adult Scurvy. The first symptoms of scurvy that precede the clinical lesions of the disorder are weakness, loss of weight, and fleeting pains in the arms and legs. Usually the first noticeable clinical symptom is the formation of a horny growth in the hair follicles called *follicular keratosis*, which may occur on the legs, buttocks, arms, and back. This is followed by the appearance of redness (hemorrhages) around the hair follicle. Soon the scorbutic changes in the gums become apparent. It has been observed in cases of experimentally induced scurvy that the gum lesions begin to appear after 26 weeks of ascorbic acid deprivation. At first the gums are red and swollen, and as the disorder progresses, the swelling increases, hemorrhages occur, and the gum tissues take on a blue-red color. If the condition persists, the teeth may become loosened.

The failure of new wounds to heal and the tendency of old wounds to become red and break open have been observed in scurvy patients for centuries. This incapacity for wound healing, however, was first demonstrated in 1940 when Crandon used himself as an experimental subject and ate an ascorbic acid-free diet for a period of six months (4). At the end of this dietary restricted period a wound was made in the mid-area of his back to observe the effect of the vitamin deprivation on the formation of collagen tissue during healing. Ten days after the wound was made an examination showed that only the surface cells had knitted together and that the inside of the wound had not healed (Fig. 15.2). Yet ten days after ascorbic acid had been put back in his diet, normal healing was observed upon the examination of the same wound.

An interesting study on the serum cholesterol levels before, during, and after recovery from scurvy among Bantu men has been reported (3). It was found that the scorbutic subjects had significantly lower mean serum cholesterol values than a group of healthy controls. Furthermore,

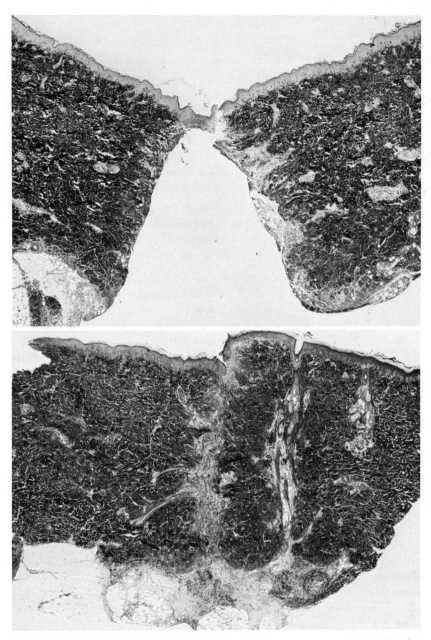

Fig. 15.2. First satisfactorily controlled experiment in human scurvy was when Crandon placed himself on an ascorbic-acid-free diet, supplemented by all other known vitamins. After 6 months on the diet a wound was made in the midback region. Biopsy 10 days after wound (top) shows no healing except of epithelium (gap in tissue was filled with blood clot). After 10 days of ascorbic acid treatment (bottom) another biopsy shows healing with abundant collagen formation. (Courtesy of J. H. Crandon and The Upjohn Company.)

the serum cholesterols of these men with scurvy failed to respond to the ingestion of fats known to elevate blood cholesterols in healthy subjects. When ascorbic acid was given to those afflicted with scurvy, there was an immediate rise in the serum cholesterol, more rapid when the vitamin was given orally than intramuscularly. Healthy subjects, however, showed no significant change in cholesterol levels when given either high-fat or low-fat diets supplemented with ascorbic acid. This relationship between ascorbic acid and cholesterol metabolism apparently is only evident in man during the stage of marked depletion of the vitamin.

Subclinical Scurvy. In this country some people who have low intakes of ascorbic acid in their diets undoubtedly suffer from subclinical or mild cases of scurvy. Nevertheless, it is impossible to describe lesions which might occur in these mild cases because of the nonspecific nature of the symptoms of scurvy. Crandon, in his classic self-induced scurvy investigation, showed the symptoms of great weakness by his inability to perform work in addition to the inability to heal wounds. However, one of the characteristic symptoms of scurvy, the changes in the gums, did not occur even after six months of ascorbic acid deprivation. In contrast to this, hemorrhagic gingivitis that responded to ascorbic acid therapy has been observed among Navajo children in Utah (14). Arctic travelers, trappers, and Eskimos are known to live on a daily ascorbic acid intake of less than 15 mg without showing any clinical symptoms of scurvy. A study from England (11) on long-time deprivation of the vitamin in human beings demonstrated that an intake of as little as 10 mg of ascorbic acid each day was sufficient to relieve the clinical symptoms of scurvy. In view of these observations, it is easy to see why mild scurvy might be hard to detect.

Recommended Allowances for Ascorbic Acid

The Recommended Allowances for ascorbic acid are higher in this country than in either Canada or the United Kingdom (Tables A-2 and A-3, appendix). A daily allowance of 30 mg has been recommended for the English people in view of the report that the clinical symptoms of scurvy were relieved when 10 mg of the vitamin was ingested. In spite of this suggestion, there is adequate evidence that higher intakes of ascorbic acid are beneficial to individuals of all ages (10).

In the past, somewhat higher ascorbic acid allowances have been proposed for men than for women. The 1963 revision of the Recommended Daily Dietary Allowances suggests, however, that all individuals over the age of 18 years need about 70 mg of the vitamin. An additional

30 mg of ascorbic acid has been proposed for the periods of pregnancy and lactation. The recommended amount of the vitamin needed for the period of growth varies (Table A-1, appendix).

Food Sources of Ascorbic Acid

Fruits and vegetables are the main sources of ascorbic acid in diets. Citrus fruits (oranges, grapefruit, lemons, and limes), berries, melons, tropical fruits (pineapple, guava, and others), leafygreen vegetables, broccoli, green pepper, cabbage, and tomatoes are all good sources of ascorbic acid (Table 15.1). The large amounts of potatoes used in low-income diets make this vegetable an important ascorbic acid food for many people.

The best natural sources of ascorbic acid have been found in the rose hip, the acerola fruit (West Indian cherry), and the *camu-camu* (a tropical fruit). Rose hips, which constitute the base of the rose bloom, are not eaten as such but in some countries are made into a sirup or extract for human consumption. During the wartime rationing of food in England, rose hip sirup was issued by the British Ministry of Food to help fortify the ascorbic acid intake of the English people. There is much interest today in the acerola fruit because of its high ascorbic acid potency. It has been reported that the ascorbic acid content of juice from ripe fruit averaged 1100 mg per 100 ml and 1250 mg per 100 ml from half-ripe fruit (6). Acerola juice, which has little effect upon the color or flavor of other juices, is used commercially to fortify low-ascorbic-acid fruit juices. The *camu-camu*, a burgandy-red tropical fruit that grows on bush-like trees along the rivers of the Amazon River Basin, has been reported to contain 2415 mg of ascorbic acid per 100 gm pulp (2). This fruit is used in the preparation of a sweetened fruit drink and in jelly.

Many of the values that were once listed in food tables for the ascorbic acid content of foods were based only on reduced ascorbic acid measurements. Because of the newer knowledge of man's ability to use dehydroascorbic acid, food table values for ascorbic acid are being revised to include the total ascorbic acid contribution of a food (7, 13).

Ascorbic Acid Losses during the Processing and Preparation of Foods

It is known that a food may lose much of its original ascorbic acid from the time it is harvested until it is eaten because of the many stages of processing and storage it may undergo. Because ascorbic acid is soluble in water and in solution is so easily destroyed by other factors, it has come to be known as the most *labile* or easily destroyed of the vitamins.

Table 15.1. Ascorbic Acid Values of Some Typical Foods

Food	mg/100 gm[1]	Portion	mg/Serving[2]
Acerola, pulp + jc, raw	1300	—	—
Green pepper, raw	128	1 med	79
Broccoli, cooked	90	⅔ c	89
Brussel sprouts, cooked	87	⅔ c	75
Turnip greens, cooked	69	⅔ c	66
Kale, cooked	62	⅔ c	45
Strawberries, raw	59	⅔ c	58
Orange	50	1 med	70
Mustard greens, cooked	48	⅔ c	45
Orange juice, frozen	45	1 c	112
Lemon juice	46	1 c	113
Grapefruit	38	½ med	52
Grapefruit juice, canned	38	1 c	84
Cabbage, cooked	33	⅔ c	37
Cantaloupe	33	¼ melon	32
Lime juice	32	1 c	80
Coleslaw	29	⅔ c	23
Spinach, cooked	28	⅔ c	33
Liver, beef, cooked	27	2 oz	15
Tomato, raw	23	1 med	34
Sweet potato, baked	22	1 med	24
Peas, green, cooked	20	⅔ c	22
Potato, baked	20	1 med	20
Tomato juice, canned	16	1 c	39
Pineapple, canned	7	2 sm sl	8
Milk, whole	1	1 c	2
Beef, ground, cooked	0	3 oz	0
Bread, white, enriched	0	1 sl	tr
Butter	0	1 tbsp	0
Egg	0	1 med	0
Sugar, white	0	1 tsp	0

[1] From *Composition of Foods—Raw, Processed, Prepared.* U.S. Dept. Agr., Agr. Handbook 8, revised, 1963.
[2] From *Nutritive Value of Foods.* U.S. Dept. Agr., Home Garden Bull. *No.* 72, revised 1964.

Therefore, in order for one to prepare and serve foods which are appetizing as well as nutritious, it is important to know how this vitamin can be conserved.

The environment in which a plant food is grown may have a significant effect on its ascorbic acid content. Temperature, amount of rainfall, type of soil, and sunlight appear to be factors directly related to the formation of plant ascorbic acid. In addition to these factors, the stage of maturity at which a food is harvested is important in order to obtain the maximum amount of this nutrient. For example, immature Lima beans and white potatoes contain more ascorbic acid than do mature ones, whereas ripe tomatoes have a much higher vitamin content than do green ones.

The Effect of Food Preservation. The manner in which a food is preserved, by freezing, by canning, or by drying (dehydration) has a significant effect on its ascorbic acid content. This fact can be well illustrated by comparing the vitamin values of fresh, frozen, canned, and dried Lima beans, all commonly used foods in the American diet. An edible portion of Lima beans weighing 100 gm has an average ascorbic acid value of 29 mg in the raw form, 22 mg when frozen, 6 mg when canned, and none when dried.

Students often ask if the amount of ascorbic acid in orange juice is in any way affected by the kind of processing it undergoes. This question can best be answered by the report of a study made at the University of Illinois where they compared the reduced ascorbic acid values as well as the cost of an average serving of fresh, frozen concentrated, canned concentrated, and canned juices from oranges. All of the orange juice analyzed in this work, regardless of processing procedures, was quite similar in ascorbic acid content, but the frozen concentrate cost less per average serving at the time of that investigation than did either the fresh or the canned.

The Effect of Storage. Two other factors that are important in conserving the ascorbic acid content of a food are the time interval between the processing and consumption of a food, and the kind of storage facilities available. From the University of Massachusetts it has been reported that pasteurized milk losses about two-thirds of the reduced ascorbic acid content after four days under refrigeration. However, if the milk was consumed within the first day after processing, about 80 per cent of the original reduced ascorbic acid would have been available. Orange juice and other citrus juices lose negligible amounts of ascorbic acid when stored in the refrigerator; the acid of the juice helps to preserve the vitamin.

The vitamin content of frozen fruits and vegetables has been observed to be affected by changes in storage time and storage temperature. Frozen cherries, peaches, and strawberries were found, by a group at the Pennsylvania State University, to have lost marked amounts of ascorbic acid when stored longer than 4 months at $+10°F$. However, when the same fruits were stored at a lower temperature, $0°F$ to $-20°F$, there was no appreciable loss of the vitamin within the same period of time. Asparagus, green beans, wax beans, broccoli, cauliflower,

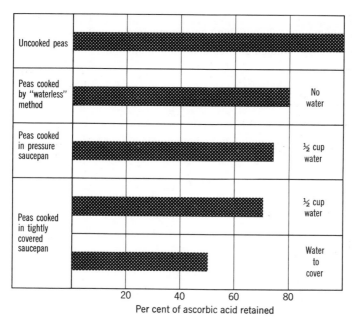

Fig. 15.3. The reduced ascorbic acid content of green peas as affected by three widely used home cooking practices. (Adapted from Krehl and Winters, *J. Am. Dietet. Assoc.*, **26:** 966, 1950.)

corn, and spinach stored at $+10°F$ lost 50 per cent of the reduced ascorbic acid content after four months storage, but when stored at $0°F$ most of the vitamin was retained. It is evident from this work that both frozen fruits and vegetables conserve the ascorbic acid value best by storage at lower temperatures.

Canned foods are also subject to marked losses in ascorbic acid when stored at elevated temperatures for long periods of time. Canned tomato juice after eight months of storage, has been shown to retain only about one-half of the reduced ascorbic acid content when held at room temperature ($68°$ to $77°F$) and only about one-third when the temperature was increased to $99°F$.

The Effect of Food Preparation. The amount of ascorbic acid in a food to be eaten is directly related to the kind of food preparation practices used. A raw food that one eats will have more of the vitamin than will one that has been cooked or baked. The removal of the natural skin of a vegetable will increase the loss of the vitamin from the food due to the leaching of the nutrient into the soaking or cooking water. Further losses of the vitamin will occur when a peeled vegetable

Table 15.2. Approximate Contribution of Some Foods to the Day's Recommended Allowances of Ascorbic Acid for College Men and Women over 18 Years

Food	Measure	Per cent/day
Apple, raw	1 med	4
Banana, raw	1 med	14
Beans, green, cooked	⅔ c	16
Beets, cooked	⅔ c	10
Broccoli, cooked	⅔ c	127
Carbonated beverage	8 oz	0
Carrot, raw	1 med	6
Catsup	1 tbsp	4
Coleslaw	½ c	26
Corn, cooked	⅔ c	13
Grapefruit	½ med	74
Hamburger in roll	1 av	0
Kale, cooked	⅔ c	65
Lettuce	2 lg lv	13
Milk, whole	1 c	3
Orange juice, frozen	½ c	80
Peaches, canned	1 c	10
Peas, green, cooked	⅔ c	31
Pineapple juice, canned	½ c	16
Potatoes, French fried	10 pieces	17
Potatoes, mashed	1 c	27
Pizza, cheese	5½ in. sector	6
Raisins	½ c	1
Tomato juice, canned	1 c	56

Adapted from *Nutritive Value of Foods*. U.S. Dept. Agr., Home Garden Bull. 72, revised 1964.

is subdivided into smaller sections; for example, when potatoes are diced, the surface area exposed to the soaking or cooking water is increased. The use of copper cooking utensils will decrease the ascorbic acid content in a food because of the destructive nature of the copper ion to the vitamin.

The method used in cooking a food will determine the amount of ascorbic acid retained by it. In order to illustrate the amounts of the vitamin that may be lost in vegetable cookery, data from Yale University have been adapted to show the retention of reduced ascorbic acid in fresh green peas cooked by three commonly used home cooking methods (Fig. 15.3). The peas retained more of the vitamin when cooked in the waterless cooker or in the pressure saucepan than when cooked in the tightly covered saucepan. In the tightly covered saucepan method, reducing the amount of water used from enough water to cover the vegetables to only one-half cup increased the amount of ascorbic acid in the cooked peas by about one-third.

A Guide to the Selection of Foods to Meet the Ascorbic Acid Needs of College Men and Women

Surveys from many areas of the United States have shown that ascorbic acid is one of the nutrients most often found to be deficient in the diets of college men and women. Because of the important role of this vitamin in the maintenance of good health and the fact that it is one of the nutrients ingested in suboptimal amounts, it is important that students know the approximate contribution of the foods eaten in relation to their daily needs.

The contribution of some foods to the day's Recommended Allowances of ascorbic acid for college men and women, over 18 years, has been tabulated (Table 15.2). An average serving of a citrus fruit or an ascorbic-acid-rich vegetable supplies 50 per cent or more of the daily allowance for the vitamin. Other fruits and vegetables supply lesser but important amounts of ascorbic acid. As can be readily seen from the table, without a serving each day of either a citrus fruit or an ascorbic-acid-rich vegetable, the Recommended Daily Dietary Allowance for ascorbic acid may not be met.

REFERENCES

1. Abt, A. F., S. von Schuching, and J. H. Roe (1960). Connective tissue studies III. Ascorbic acid, collagen, and hexosamine distribution and histology of connective tissue in scars produced in guinea pigs on various vitamin C dietary levels following wounding by abdominal incision. *J. Nutr.* **70:** 427.
2. Bradford, R. B., and A. Roca (1964). Camu-Camu—a fruit high in ascorbic acid. *J. Am. Dietet. Assoc.* **44:** 28.
3. Bronte-Stewart, B., B. Roberts, and V. M. Wells (1963). Serum cholesterol in vitamin C deficiency in men. *Brit. J. Nutr.* **17:** 61.
4. Crandon, J. H., C. Lund, and D. Dill (1940). Experimental human scurvy. *New Eng. J. Med.* **223:** 353.
5. Davey, B. L., K. H. Fisher, and S. D. Chen (1956). Utilization of ascorbic acid in fruits and vegetables. II. Utilization of 24 fruits and vegetables. *J. Am. Dietet. Assoc.* **32:** 1069.
6. Fitting, K. O., and C. D. Miller (1960). The stability of ascorbic acid in frozen and bottled acerola juice alone and combined with other fruit juices. *Food Res.* **25:** 203.
7. *Nutritive Value of Foods* (1964). U.S. Dept. Agr., Home Garden Bull. No. 72, revised. Washington, D.C.
8. Steele, B. F., C. Hsu, Z. H. Pierce, and H. H. Williams (1952). Ascorbic acid nutriture

in the human. I. Tyrosine metabolism and blood levels of ascorbic acid during ascorbic acid depletion and repletion. *J. Nutr.* **48:** 49.

9. Stewart, C. P., and D. Guthrie (1953). *Lind's Treatise on Scurvy. A Bicentenary Volume with Additional Notes.* Edinburgh University Press, Edinburgh, Scotland.

10. Uhl, E. (1958). Ascorbic acid requirements of adults: 30 mg or 75 mg? *Am. J. Clin. Nutr.* **6:** 146.

11. Vitamin C Subcommittee of the Accessory Food Factors Committee, and A. E. Barnes, W. Bartley, I. M. Frankau, G. A. Higgins, J. Pemberton, G. L. Roberts, and H. R. Vichers (1953). *Vitamin C Requirements of Human Adults.* Med. Res. Council Special Rept. Series No. 280, Her Majesty's Stationery Office, London, p. 179.

12. Wang, M. M., K. H. Fisher, and M. L. Dodds (1962). Comparative metabolic response to erythorbic acid and ascorbic acid by the human. *J. Nutr.* **77:** 443.

13. Watt, B. K., and A. L. Merrill (1963). *Composition of Foods—Raw, Processed, Prepared.* U.S. Dept. Agr., Agr. Handbook 8, revised, Washington, D.C.

14. Wilcox, E. B., and M. Grimes (1961). Gingivitis-ascorbic acid deficiency in the Navajo. I. Ascorbic acid in white cell-platelet fraction of blood. *J. Nutr.* **74:** 352.

15. Wolbach, S. B. (1933). Controlled formation of collagen and reticulum. A study of the source of intercellular substance in recovery from experimental scorbutus. *Am. J. Pathol.* **9:** 689.

SUPPLEMENTARY REFERENCES

Burch, H. B. (1961). Methods for detecting and evaluating ascorbic acid deficiency in man and animals. *Ann. N.Y. Acad. Sci.* 92.

Dodds, M. L. (1959). Vitamin C. In *Food. The Yearbook of Agriculture 1959.* (A. Stefferud, ed.) U.S. Dept. Agr., Washington, D.C.

Woodruff, C. (1964). Ascorbic acid. In *Nutrition A Comprehensive Treatise,* Vol. II. (G. H. Beaton and E. W. McHenry, eds.) Academic Press, New York.

CHAPTER 16

The B-complex vitamins
I. thiamine, riboflavin, and niacin

The B-complex vitamins are a group of related nutrients that are important for the well-being of every cell in the body. Because these factors are a part of the human enzyme systems, they are essential for the normal metabolism of food. When any of these vitamins are missing, in an otherwise adequate diet, characteristic deficiency symptoms are produced in both man and animals. At this time, the ten vitamins included in the B-complex family are thiamine, riboflavin, niacin, vitamin B_6, pantothenic acid, biotin, folacin, vitamin B_{12}, choline, and inositol. The first three of these vitamins are discussed in this chapter, the other seven are presented in the following chapter.

▶ THIAMINE

Beriberi, a nervous system disease that is caused by a lack of thiamine in the diet, has occurred in the Far East for centuries and has resulted in a high morbidity and mortality rate among the peoples of these countries. Not until 1882 was it shown by Takaki, at that time Director-General of the Medical Department of the Japanese Navy, that beriberi could be prevented in man by the intake of a good diet. A decade later the observations of Christiaan Eijkman, a Dutch medical scientist in Java, initiated the research that finally led to the identification of thiamine as the anti-beriberi vitamin. Eijkman noted that the chickens housed in the hospital yard near his laboratory developed a disorder similar to human beriberi when fed a ration solely of polished rice. Because of the general paralysis and head retractions which occurred in the birds, he called this disease *polyneuritis*. He found that the symptoms of the polyneuritis disappeared when rice polishings, the outer layers and embryo of the rice kernel, were fed to the birds. In 1911 the Polish biochemist, Funk, prepared a small amount of a crystalline material from a rice bran extract which he found cured experimental beriberi in birds. Because he called this substance *beriberi vitamine*, he is credited with coining the word vitamin. Four years later McCollum confirmed the existence of a single substance which not only cured polyneuritis but also promoted growth and he named this factor *water-soluble B*. Jansen and Donath, at Eijkman's laboratory in Java, demonstrated the vitamin's curative effect in human beriberi in 1926, after they had prepared sufficient crystals of the vitamin from rice bran. Ten years later R. R. Williams and his group in this country identified the chemical structure of thiamine and then developed the first method for its synthesis.

Properties of Thiamine

Although the term *vitamin B_1* has been used for many years to identify this factor, thiamine is now the official accepted name for the vitamin in the United States. The colorless crystals of the vitamin (Fig. 16.1), which have a yeastlike smell and a salty taste, are very soluble in water. Thiamine is quite stable in acid solutions, but in a neutral or slightly alkaline solution it is easily destroyed by heat. Commercially the vitamin is sold in the form of thiamine hydrochloride.

Function of Thiamine

Thiamine is important to the body as one of the keys in the release of energy during the metabolism of carbohydrates where, as thiamine pyrophosphate, it functions in the enzyme system. Carbohydrate metabolism may proceed to the formation of pyruvic acid, an intermediate compound; thiamine is essential for the breakdown of pyruvic acid. It is believed that the enzyme systems containing the vitamins of the B-complex family, along with other vitamins and certain minerals, work cooperatively in the utilization and storage of energy and in the normal functioning of body processes that involve growth and body maintenance.

Experimental work (9) has suggested that in addition to its function in general metabolism, thiamine also may have a specific role in the functioning of peripheral nerves.

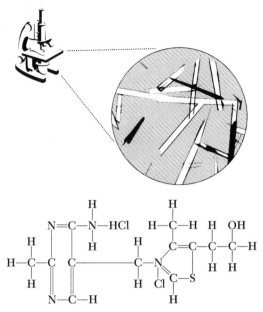

Fig. 16.1. Crystalline thiamine hydrochloride and its chemical formula. (Photomicrograph courtesy of Merck and Co., Rahway, New Jersey.)

Thiamine appears to have several indirect functions in the body because of its role in energy metabolism. The maintenance of the appetite, the tone of the muscles, and a healthy mental attitude are all related to thiamine nutrition.

One of the earliest symptoms of a thiamine deficiency in man is the loss of appetite or *anorexia*. In several human studies involving thiamine deprivation (3, 4, 10), anorexia was observed as early as the fourth day and became so severe as the deficiency progressed that the subjects had to force themselves to eat food. With the restoration of the vitamin to the diet, however, the loss of appetite disappeared very quickly. Indirectly thiamine will promote growth because the stimulation of the appetite results in an increased consumption of food.

Constipation and tenderness of the muscles of the leg calf are two symptoms frequently found in experimental thiamine deficiencies. The sluggishness of the intestinal muscles associated with constipation may be a result of insufficient thiamine in the diet. Very soon after the vitamin is restored to the food intake after periods of thiamine deprivation, subjects have reported relief from both of these symptoms.

Thiamine is often called the *morale* vitamin because of its ability to restore a healthy mental state in man following periods of experimental deprivation. When human subjects are fed restricted amounts of thiamine in their diets, changes in the emotional stability of normal subjects have been observed. Williams (10) found that his subjects on restricted intakes of thiamine became irritable, quarrelsome, and moody; they failed to cooperate; and at times they suffered periods of mental depression. Although thiamine is not beneficial in the treatment of mental disorders, it has been observed that dietary restriction of the vitamin in mental patients appears to intensify the psychiatric symptoms of their mental state (2). The interest, ambition, attention, and sociability of these patients have been observed to be definitely affected by sub-optimal intakes of the vitamin as shown by a decrease in talking and a slowing of body movement.

The Effects of a Thiamine Deficiency

In Animals. All species of animals need thiamine for normal energy metabolism. Although the ruminants (cattle and sheep) are able to synthesize adequate amounts of the vitamin in their rumens, other animals must obtain a supply of thiamine in their daily food ration in order to meet their needs.

Regardless of species, the symptoms of a thiamine deficiency in animals are quite similar. It is believed that the symptoms are related to the disturbances in carbohydrate metabolism accompanying thiamine deficiency, although the precise relationship is not known as yet. The albino rat, which may be used in the classroom to demonstrate the effects of this vitamin deficiency, develops anorexia and soon begins to lose weight when fed a ration low in thiamine. As the deficiency progresses, the animal develops a spastic gait due to a partial paralysis caused by affectation of the nerves; shows signs of a slowing of the heartbeat; regains its equilibrium with much difficulty after being rotated; and suffers from convulsions. The condition is known as polyneuritis. It is interesting to observe the dramatic recovery of these thiamine-deficient rats within eight hours after receiving supplements of the vitamin (Fig. 16.2).

In Man. Beriberi is the name of the disorder in man that results from a severe deficiency of thiamine. Although beriberi occurs very rarely in the Western countries, it is a common disease in the countries of the world where polished rice is the main item of the diet. During the period from 1954 to 1958, beriberi ranked fourth as the cause of death among the people of the Philippine Islands (8).

The three general symptoms of beriberi are polyneuritis, either edema or emaciation of the body tissues, and disturbances of the heart. The polyneuritis begins with a soreness in the muscles of the legs and is soon

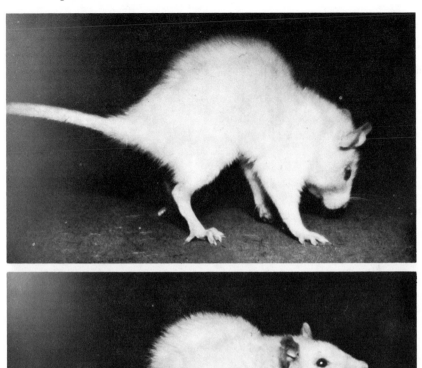

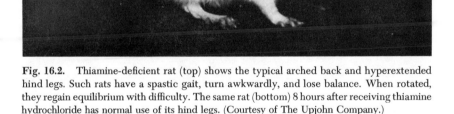

Fig. 16.2.   Thiamine-deficient rat (top) shows the typical arched back and hyperextended hind legs. Such rats have a spastic gait, turn awkwardly, and lose balance. When rotated, they regain equilibrium with difficulty. The same rat (bottom) 8 hours after receiving thiamine hydrochloride has normal use of its hind legs. (Courtesy of The Upjohn Company.)

followed by a decrease in the reflex of the knee and a drop in the muscles that support the toes and foot. This latter symptom of the disorder accounts for the high-stepping gait observed in beriberi patients (Fig. 16.3). As the disorder advances, however, the arms and other parts of the body become affected because of a degeneration and lack of coordination of the body muscles. When edema occurs in beriberi, the body tissues become swollen because of the accumulation of fluid in the body cells (Fig. 16.4). This condition is referred to as *wet beriberi* and

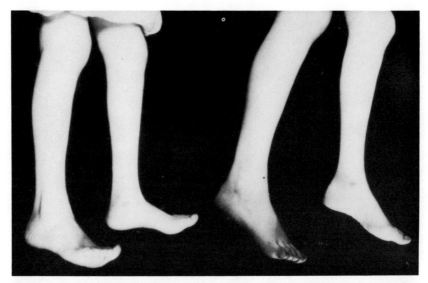

Fig. 16.3. The foot drop of beriberi. (*a*) Patient with peripheral neuritis of nutritional origin shows limit of flexion of ankles. (*b*) Moderate flexion is possible after 2½ weeks of thiamine therapy. (Courtesy of H. Field, Jr., and The Upjohn Company.)

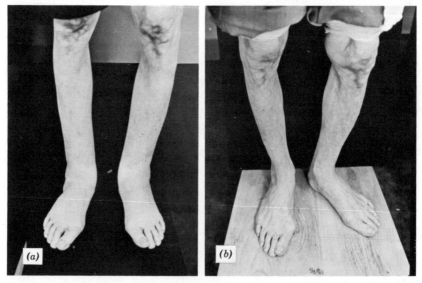

Fig. 16.4. Pitting edema. (*a*) Swelling of legs with pitting in ankle region marks beginning of so-called wet beriberi. (*b*) Same patient is shown 4 days after a single intravenous injection of 50 mg of thiamine. During this period the patient's excretion of fluid exceeded intake by 10½ lb. (Courtesy of Spies, Hillman Hospital, Birmingham, Alabama, and The Upjohn Company.)

260

is noticed first in the legs and thighs of the patient. Sometimes there is a reverse condition in which edema does not occur but rather emaciation exists; this is diagnosed as *dry beriberi*. Inasmuch as the beriberi sufferer breathes with great difficulty and his heart beats rapidly and becomes enlarged (Fig. 16.5), death in beriberi is due to these cardiac impairments. In this country beriberi heart disease has been found among some elderly hospitalized persons (1).

Cases of mild thiamine deficiency are quite common throughout the

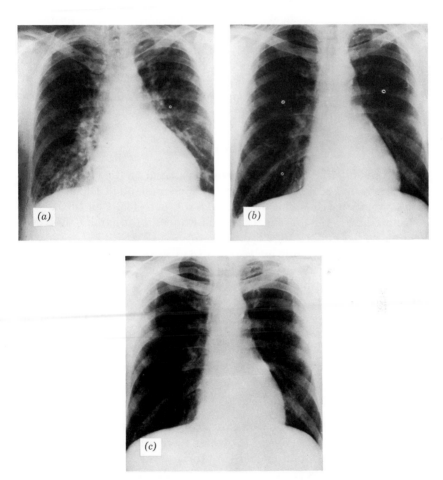

Fig. 16.5. Beriberi heart. Thiamine deficiency leads to impaired function and enlargement of the heart, particularly of the right auricle and ventricle, as shown by x-ray in (*a*). This patient was a chronic alcoholic whose diet had been poor for a long time. Polyneuritis and congestive heart failure accompanied cardiac dilation. (*b*) After 1 week of thiamine therapy, and (*c*) after 3 weeks of treatment. (Courtesy of H. Field, Jr., and The Upjohn Company.)

world. R. R. Williams (11) has written ". . . there are scores of millions, perhaps hundreds of millions, in Asia, who are suffering from mild beriberi and have done so for years and they still do not know they have it. . . ." In this country, cases of extreme deprivation of the vitamin are rare, but suboptimal intakes of thiamine have been reported to exist among people of all age groups as shown by nutrition surveys from various regions of the United States (5). From human studies of the effects of mild thiamine deprivation in the diet, one is able to recognize some of the typical symptoms which accompany subclinical cases. Fatigue, anorexia, constipation, labored breathing, lassitude (weariness), nausea, tenderness of the leg calf, depression, changes in the electrocardiogram measurement, low excretion of thiamine in the urine, and an increase of pyruvic acid in the blood are the symptoms which accompany a thiamine deficiency. Although some of these symptoms are specific for thiamine, others may result from other nutrient deficiencies.

Recommended Allowances for Thiamine

The human requirement for thiamine is based on the energy need of an individual. The 1958 revision of the Recommended Dietary Allowances proposed a thiamine value of 0.5 mg per 1000 Cal. In the 1963 revision, however, the suggested allowance for thiamine has been lowered to 0.4 mg per 1000 Cal. (7).

College men and young male adults, 18 to 35 years of age, need 1.2 mg of thiamine each day. A slightly lower allowance, 0.8 mg per day, has been suggested for the college and young adult woman of the same age group. In the stress periods of life (growth, pregnancy, and lactation) the thiamine need is increased. As one grows older, the need for the vitamin decreases with the decrease in caloric requirement. However, new experimental findings indicate that the minimum need for thiamine may be greater for the older person than for the younger one (6).

Food sources of Thiamine

All the foods of the diet with the exception of fats, oils, and refined sugars contain some thiamine. However, there are no foods particularly high in thiamine content as there are for ascorbic acid and vitamin A.

Although brewer's yeast and wheat germ head the list of the thiamine-containing foods (Table 16.1), they are not very important in the typical food intake because relatively few people eat either one of these in large amounts. The best sources of the vitamin in the average diet are pork products, legumes, and whole-grain and enriched cereals. Nuts vary

Table 16.1. Thiamine Values of Some Typical Foods

Food	mg/100 gm[1]	Portion	mg/Serving[2]
Brewer's yeast	15.61	1 tbsp	1.25
Wheat germ	2.01	1 c	1.36
Pork chop, cooked	0.96	3½ oz	0.63
Brazil nuts, shelled	0.96	1 c	1.34
Pecan nuts, shelled	0.86	1 c	0.93
Ham, smoked, cooked	0.47	3 oz	0.40
Bran flakes, 40 per cent	0.40	1 oz	0.11
Green peas, fresh, cooked	0.28	⅔ c	0.30
Bread, whole-wheat	0.26	1 sl	0.06
Bread, white, enriched	0.25	1 sl	0.06
Lima beans, fresh, cooked	0.18	⅔ c	0.20
Peanut butter	0.13	1 tbsp	0.02
Rice, white, parboiled, cooked	0.11	1 c	0.19
Beef, ground, cooked	0.09	3 oz	0.08
Egg	0.09	1 med	0.05
Orange juice, frozen	0.09	1 c	0.21
Milk, whole	0.03	1 c	0.08
Sugar, white	0	1 tsp	0
Butter	0	1 tbsp	0

[1] From *Composition of Foods—Raw, Processed, Prepared.* U.S. Dept. Agr., Agr. Handbook 8, revised 1963.

[2] From *Nutritive Value of Foods.* U.S. Dept. Agr., Home Garden Bull. *No.* 72, revised 1964.

in their thiamine content but when they are used in large amounts, prove to be rich contributors of the vitamin. The thiamine in the egg is confined to the yolk. A quart of milk each day will contribute a good share of the thiamine need.

The use of enriched cereal grains in this country has bolstered the thiamine value of the American diet. Data from the U.S. Department of Agriculture show that the national food supply contributed about 12 per cent more of the vitamin in 1962 than it did for the period prior to the adoption of cereal enrichment (1935–1939).

Thiamine Losses during Food Processing and Preparation

Vegetables. The amount of thiamine retained in a vegetable during freezing or canning is apparently related to the nature of the food used. Peas have shown no significant loss of the vitamin during the freezing procedures, but spinach and asparagus have been reported to lose about 51 per cent and 28 per cent, respectively. In a study to determine the effect of canning procedures on the vitamin retention of vegetables, it was concluded that the thiamine retention was excellent in tomatoes, good in tomato juice, only fair in asparagus, and relatively poor in snapbeans, Lima beans, corn, peas, and spinach.

Under ordinary conditions of home cooking, most of the thiamine lost in a food is due to the leaching of the vitamin into the cooking water rather than to heat destruction. This fact was observed when twelve different vegetables were processed in family-size amounts by four different cooking methods. The retention of thiamine in the vegetables averaged 91.0 per cent (waterless cooker), 84.1 per cent (tightly covered saucepan with ½ cup water), 78.9 per cent (pressure cooker), and 62.6 per cent (tightly covered saucepan with water to cover). In view of this report, it appears that the thiamine content of a vegetable can be conserved if it is cooked in the least amount of water compatible with good palatability.

Because thiamine is highly soluble in water, the liquid fraction of a canned vegetable as well as the soaking or cooking water from a vegetable will contain an appreciable amount of the vitamin lost from the vegetable solid during processing or food preparation. In order to utilize all the thiamine contained in the foods of the diet, this liquid fraction should be used and not discarded.

Meats. Because pork and its products are excellent sources of thiamine in the American diets, it is important to know the effect that cooking methods have on the retention of the vitamin in these foods.

Studies have been made on the retention of the vitamin in fresh hams and pork loins, fresh-ground pork, as well as in cured hams before and after cooking by standardized procedures. Although the thiamine content of different cuts from the same pork loin or ham may vary considerably, the retention of the nutrient after cooking is quite uniform. Pork loins and fresh hams have been shown to retain about 70 per cent of their thiamine after roasting and broiling and about 50 per cent after braising. When the vitamin content of the drippings from these pork products is added to the thiamine value of the cooked meat, there is about 70 per cent retention for all three methods of preparation. As much as 85 per cent of the vitamin was retained in ground pork patties when they were cooked by pan-broiling, oven-broiling, or electronic cookery. In the curing of ham, almost three-fourths of the original thiamine of the fresh meat has been reported to be retained. Fried cured ham has a higher thiamine content than cured ham that has been roasted, braised, or broiled. Regardless of the processing procedure or the method of cookery, it appears that cooked pork products are worthwhile contributors of thiamine to the diets.

A Guide to the Selection of Foods to Meet the Thiamine Need of College Men and Women

Servings of commonly used foods, some rich in thiamine, have been used to show their contribution to a college student's need for this nutrient. Two sets of values are presented in Table 16.2 because of the difference in the need for thiamine between college men (1.2 mg) and college women (0.8 mg).

That pork products are good food sources of the vitamin is evident

Table 16.2. Approximate Contribution of Some Foods to the Day's Recommended Allowances of Thiamine for College Men and Women over 18 Years

Food	Measure	College Men, per cent/day	College Women, per cent/day
Apple	1 med	3	5
Beans, Lima, cooked	⅔ c	17	25
Beef, ground, cooked	3 oz	7	10
Bran flakes, 40 per cent	1 oz	9	14
Bread, white, enriched	2 sl	10	15
Butter	1 tbsp	0	0
Carbonated beverage	8 oz	0	0
Chicken, leg, fried	2 oz	3	4
Chocolate bar	1 oz	2	3
Egg	1 med	4	6
Frankfurter	1	7	10
Ham, smoked, cooked	3 oz	33	50
Ice cream	⅛ qt	3	4
Milk, whole	1 pt	13	20
Oatmeal, cooked	1 c	16	24
Orange juice, frozen	½ c	9	13
Peanuts, shelled	½ c	19	29
Peanut butter	1 tbsp	2	3
Peas, green, cooked	⅔ c	25	37
Pizza, cheese	5½ in. sector	3	5
Pork chop, cooked	3½ oz	53	79
Potato chips	10 med	3	5
Potatoes, mashed	1 c	14	20
Shrimp, canned	3 oz	1	1
Sugar, white	1 tsp	0	0
Tomato juice	½ c	5	8

Adapted from *Nutritive Value of Foods*. U.S. Dept. Agr., Home Garden Bull. 72, revised 1964.

from the data presented. However, common food items that are less rich in thiamine than pork products are the main carriers of the vitamin on a daily basis. The bread, breakfast cereals, milk, etc., eaten by college students all carry thiamine. Here again, the importance of milk in the college-age diet is evident.

▶ RIBOFLAVIN

As early as 1920 some workers began to question the belief that *water-soluble B* was a single nutritive factor. Studies had shown that after a food containing this dietary essential had been autoclaved, it still had the ability to promote growth in animals even though its antineuritic powers were destroyed. This observation indicated that the water-soluble B was not a single factor but rather a mixture of factors, one that was destroyed by heat and the other that heat did not affect. About 1928 the fact had definitely been established that there were at least two different vitamins contained in this complex, an antineuritic factor (vitamin B_1, now called thiamine) and a growth-promoting factor (vitamin G or B_2, now called riboflavin).

The first steps in the isolation of riboflavin began in Germany about 1930 when a yellowish-green fluorescent material, which stimulated growth in animals, was isolated from egg white. Soon it was found that similar fluorescent substances were present in milk, liver, yeast, muscle, and certain plant materials. The fluorescent materials all proved to belong to a chemical family called the *flavins* and so were named after the foodstuff from which they were isolated, such as *ovoflavin* from egg and *lactoflavin* from milk. Later chemical studies showed that all of these fluorescent materials were identical with one another and the name, riboflavin, was the general term adopted to identify them. Riboflavin has been produced synthetically since 1935.

Properties of Riboflavin

Riboflavin occurs in yellow-orange crystals (Fig. 16.6), which are only slightly soluble in water; solutions of the vitamin have a yellowish-green fluorescence. The presence of acids, air, or heat have no destructive effect upon the vitamin, but riboflavin is easily destroyed by alkalies and light.

Function of Riboflavin

Like thiamine, riboflavin serves as a coenzyme in several of the enzyme systems of the body that are involved in the metabolism of the energy nutrients.

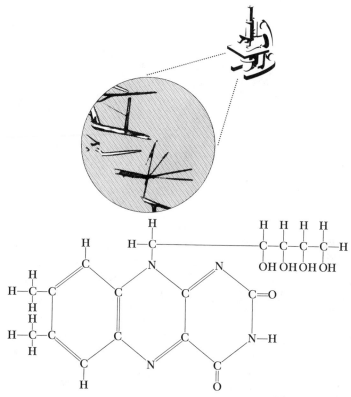

Fig. 16.6.   Crystalline riboflavin and its chemical formula. (Photomicrograph courtesy of Merck and Co., Rahway, New Jersey.)

The Effects of a Riboflavin Deficiency

In Animals. Because the rat was used as the experimental animal in the early studies of this vitamin, there is available a wealth of information on the effect of a riboflavin deficiency in this species. Growth failure, which occurs even though the animal is ingesting a sufficient quantity of food, is one of the early symptoms of riboflavin deprivation in the rat. Soon changes in the condition of the skin and eyes become apparent. At first there is *alopecia* around the nose and on the paws, and then a *dermatitis* develops in these areas (Fig. 16.7). The eye lesions in a riboflavin deficient rat vary in severity and may range from *conjunctivitis* to the formation of a permanent cataract. Digestive and nervous disturbances are also observed as the deficiency becomes more pronounced, and death will occur if the vitamin is not restored to the animal's ration. All animals need riboflavin for normal growth and body maintenance.

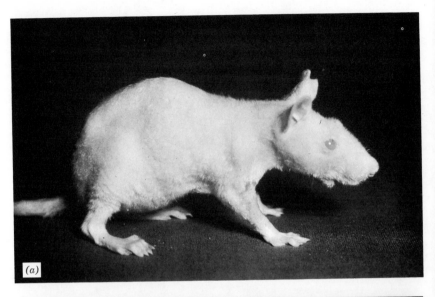

(a)

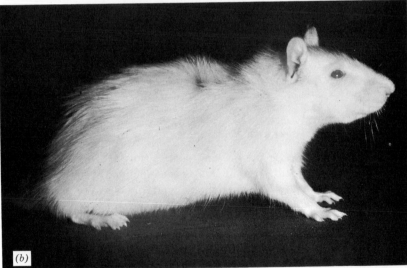

(b)

Fig. 16.7. (a) Generalized dermatitis and growth failure in riboflavin-deficient rat. (b) After two months of treatment with riboflavin the rat shows no signs of the original deficiency. (Courtesy of The Upjohn Company.)

In Man. Riboflavin deficiency in man may be complicated by a deficiency of other vitamins of the B-complex family, and for this reason the clinical symptoms of human riboflavin deprivation are not as clear-cut as are those of thiamine. The first experimentally induced riboflavin deficiency in man was reported in 1938 by Sebrell and Butler (5). They found that the women subjects of their study developed *cheilosis,* a reddening of the mucous membranes of the lips, and *seborrhea.* All of these lesions disappeared when riboflavin was restored to the diet. In a more recent study of induced human *ariboflavinosis* (1), the same kind of skin lesions were found to develop in the male subjects maintained on suboptimal intakes of the vitamin for a period of 9 to 17 months. Another lesion reported by these workers was scrotal dermititis. The changes in the tissues of the eyes due to riboflavin deprivation in humans are not as specific as the lesions of the skin. It is believed that *conjunctivitis* as well as *lacrimation* (a watering of the eye) are the ocular lesions which can be attributed to human ariboflavinosis. The condition involving the *vascularization of the cornea* (where the capillaries invade the cornea tissue) has not been proven as yet to be a specific lesion of riboflavin insufficiency in man.

Factors That May Affect Riboflavin Metabolism

The excretion of riboflavin in the urine has been designated a useful index to reflect the state of the metabolism of the vitamin in the animal organism. It is assumed that a marked increase in urinary riboflavin indicates a loss of the nutrient from the tissues whereas a decrease reflects a conservation of tissue riboflavin. Recent studies with animals and man suggest that environmental, nutritional, and/or physiological factors may affect the normal metabolism of riboflavin.

The effects of exposure to sunlight (ultraviolet irradiation) for varying periods of time on the riboflavin metabolism of the rat has been investigated at the Institute of Nutrition, USSR Academy of Medical Sciences (2). Moderate exposure of the animals to these rays apparently increased the capacity of the tissues to retain the vitamin, but there was a marked loss of tissue riboflavin during prolonged exposure. An adequate supply of dietary riboflavin, however, increased the animal's tolerance to ultraviolet light.

The influence of sleep, bed rest, work, diuresis, heat, acute starvation, and thiamine intake on the riboflavin excretion in man has been studied (6). Sleep retarded the excretion of the nutrient whereas the rate of excretion was increased in the subjects during enforced bed rest. There was a decreased excretion of riboflavin during short periods of hard physical work. Diuresis, induced by water, did not affect the excretion rate of the vitamin. Both heat stress and acute starvation increased the excretion of riboflavin in the subjects. There was an immediate increase in riboflavin excretion when thiamine was eliminated from the diet but with a combined deficiency of thiamine and ribo-flavin, the increase in the loss of riboflavin was delayed.

Recommended Allowances for Riboflavin

The need for riboflavin is related to the allowance for energy, as are those for thiamine and niacin (4).

The daily riboflavin need of college and young adult men, 18 to 35 years of age, has been suggested to be 1.7 mg whereas college and young adult women of the same age group have been assigned 1.3 mg of the vitamin each day. Middle-aged men, 35 to 55 years, need 1.6 mg and older men, over 55 years, need 1.3 mg of riboflavin each day. After the age of 35, the daily need for women has been proposed to be 1.2 mg per day. Here again, the need for this vitamin is increased during growth, pregnancy, or lactation.

Food Sources of Riboflavin

Because the best food sources of riboflavin, brewer's yeast and glandular meats, are not used to any great extent in an average diet, their value as dietary contributors is not very significant (Table 16.3). However, because it is so widely used as a dietary food, milk is prob-ably the chief source of the vitamin in most American diets. The ingestion of 3 cups of whole milk per day contributes approximately 1.26 mg of the nutrient, whch is about 74 per cent and 97 per cent, respectively, of the daily riboflavin requirement of college men and women over 18 years of age. Cheese, eggs, veal, beef, leafy green vegetables, and salmon are other foods that are good sources of the vitamin. In addition, the use of whole-grain or enriched cereal products rather than those that are unenriched will bolster the amount of the vitamin ingested. According to statistics from the U.S. Department of Agriculture, the national food supply in 1962 contributed about 12 per cent more riboflavin than it did in the period (1935–1939) prior to the adoption of cereal enrichment. Students often wonder why a 100 gm portion of whole wheat bread (0.12 mg) has less riboflavin than an equal amount of white enriched bread (0.21 mg). The answer to this is that more of the nutrient is added to the wheat flour during the enrichment process than was originally present in the whole wheat grain.

Table 16.3. Riboflavin Values of Some Typical Foods

Food	mg/100 gm[1]	Portion	mg/Serving[2]
Brewer's yeast	4.28	1 tbsp	0.34
Liver, beef, cooked	4.19	2 oz	2.37
Heart, beef, cooked	1.22	3 oz	1.04
Cheese, Cheddar	0.46	1 oz	0.08
Egg	0.28	1 med	0.14
Veal roast, cooked	0.25	3 oz	0.26
Turnip greens, cooked	0.24	⅔ c	0.24
Beef, ground, cooked	0.21	3 oz	0.18
Bread, white, enriched	0.21	1 sl	0.04
Broccoli, cooked	0.20	⅔ c	0.20
Asparagus, cooked	0.18	⅔ c	0.21
Milk, whole	0.17	1 c	0.42
Salmon, canned	0.16	3 oz	0.16
Spinach, cooked	0.14	⅔ c	0.17
Bread, whole-wheat	0.12	1 sl	0.03
Bread, white, unenriched	0.09	1 sl	0.02
Orange juice, frozen	0.01	1 c	0.03
Butter	0	1 tbsp	0
Sugar, white	0	1 tsp	0

[1] From *Composition of Foods—Raw, Processed, Prepared.* U.S. Dept. Agr., Agr. Handbook 8, revised 1963.
[2] From *Nutritive Value of Foods.* U.S. Dept. Agr., Home Garden Bull. 72, revised 1964.

Riboflavin Losses during Food Processing, Storage, and Cooking

The two factors in the processing, storage, or cooking of a food that may cause a loss of riboflavin are the leaching of the vitamin into the processing or cooking water and the destruction of the vitamin by light.

The loss of riboflavin during food preservation and preparation occurs mostly during the blanching (boiling for a short period prior to preservation by freezing or canning) or cooking process. It has been reported that peas lost 20 per cent of their riboflavin content while being blanched, but relatively no further loss of the vitamin occurred in the subsequent stages of freezing or canning. Losses of the vitamin due to varying amounts of cooking water have been observed. There appears to be about a 20 per cent loss of riboflavin from vegetables cooked in a small amount of water (one-half cup), and when the water is increased the retention of the vitamin is decreased. However, very little riboflavin is destroyed in the range of temperatures used in common cooking practices because of the heat-stable nature of the vitamin. Although the solubility of this vitamin is not as great as was found either for ascorbic acid or for thiamine, the liquid fraction from a processed food should be used in order to reclaim that part of the vitamin that has leached out into the processing water.

The destruction of riboflavin by light is a serious problem in view of the fact that one of the important dietary sources of the vitamin, milk, is often exposed to it. When a bottle of milk is allowed to stand on the doorstep on a bright sunny day for a period of two hours, as much as 85 per cent of its riboflavin value may be destroyed. In contrast to this, the exposure of a bottle of milk for one hour on a rainy, dark day may result in only about 10 per cent of the vitamin being lost. Most dairies recognize this problem and have made a constructive effort to preserve the riboflavin quantity of this food product. Both paper cartons and amber-colored bottles have been introduced to eliminate light destruction of milk riboflavin. In some localities where clear bottles are used, home storage boxes, in which the milk is placed on delivery, have been provided.

A Guide to the Selection of Foods to Meet the Riboflavin Need of College Men and Women

Like ascorbic acid, riboflavin is another of the vitamins that is often low in the food intake of college men and women (3). The contribution of some commonly used foods to the college student's need for riboflavin have been expressed in percentages of daily needs and are shown in Table 16.4.

The daily college-age need for the vitamin will be more than satisfied with as little as 2 oz of cooked beef liver. A pint of milk supplies approximately one-half of the riboflavin needed by college students. The college student who does not drink milk and rejects leafy-green vegetables and liver cannot hope to meet his need for this important nutrient by dietary means.

▶ NIACIN

The disease, *pellagra*, which is now known to be prevented by an adequate body supply of niacin, has been known for centuries. Although it was once an endemic disease caused by the intake of a diet referred to as the "Three M's" (meat—salt pork, which was almost all fat and no lean—maize, and molasses) and was found to occur in the southern part of the United States. Pellagra is still prevalent in certain sections of Italy, Spain, and Rumania where corn products are a staple part of the diet. The characteristic symptoms of pellagra involve the skin, the gastrointestinal tract, and the nervous system. Because of its specific

Table 16.4. Approximate Contribution of Some Foods to the Day's Recommended Allowances of Riboflavin for College Men and Women over 18 Years

Food	Measure	College Men, per cent/day	College Women, per cent/day
Apple	1 med	1	2
Beans, green, cooked	⅔ c	5	6
Beef, ground, cooked	3 oz	12	15
Bread, white, enriched	2 sl	5	6
Broccoli, cooked	⅔ c	11	15
Butter	1 tbsp	0	0
Carbonated beverage	8 oz	0	0
Carrot	1 med	1	2
Cheese, American	1 oz	5	6
Chocolate bar	1 oz	5	7
Egg	1 med	9	12
Frankfurter	1	6	8
Ice cream	⅛ qt	8	10
Liver, beef, cooked	2 oz	139	182
Milk, whole	1 pt	49	65
Orange juice, frozen	½ c	1	1
Pizza, cheese	5½ in. sector	7	9
Potato chips	10 med	1	1
Potatoes, mashed	1 c	6	8
Shrimp, canned	3 oz	2	2
Spinach, cooked	⅔ c	10	13
Sugar, white	1 tsp	0	0
Tuna fish, canned	3 oz	6	8

Adapted from *Nutritive Value of Foods*. U.S. Dept. Agr., Home Garden Bull. 72, revised 1964.

lesions, pellagra has often been referred to as the disease of the "Three D's" (dermatitis, diarrhea, and dementia). The characteristic dermatitis of pellagra, which is aggravated by sunlight and heat, is bilaterally symmetrical and occurs on the hands, feet, face, forearms, and other parts of the body (Fig. 16.8). The skin becomes red and the lesions itch and burn. When the mucous membranes of the gastro-intestinal tract become affected, the early symptoms include *glossitis*, anorexia, and abdominal pains. As the disorder becomes more severe, diarrhea occurs. Insomnia, irritability, fear, depression, and forgetfulness are the first neurological changes observed but as the disorder advances, dementia and paralysis may occur. If pellagra remains untreated, it may prove fatal.

Active work to determine the cause of pellagra began in this country in 1914 when the disease was very prevalent in our southern states.

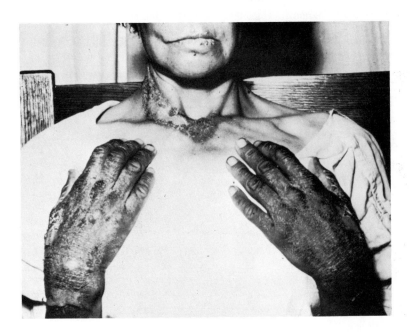

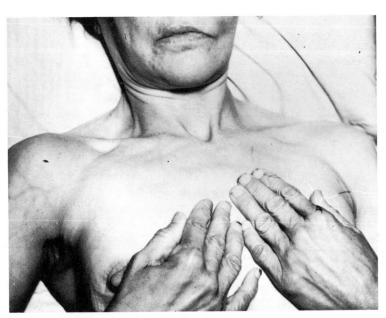

Fig. 16.8. Advanced pellagra (top) showing dermatitis outlining the exposed area of the neck as well as the lesions on the back of the hands. The same patient (bottom) after nicotinamide therapy. (Courtesy of Jolliffe and The Upjohn Company.)

Although it had been suggested that pellagra was related to the intake of a poor diet, there were many people who believed it was an infectious disease. Goldberger and his coworkers, under the auspices of the U.S. Public Health Service, were the first to induce and then cure pellagra in healthy men by dietary means. Soon after this classic experiment it was found that brewer's yeast eaten in sufficient amounts would protect a human against developing pellagra. In the meantime, the discovery of a disorder in dogs called *blacktongue*, which is analogous to human pellagra, was the symptom in the test animal that led to the final identification of this dietary factor. At the University of Wisconsin in 1937, Elvehjem and his group isolated a compound called nicotinamide from a liver concentrate and then demonstrated its effect and that of a related compound, nicotinic acid, in curing and preventing blacktongue in dogs. Although the chemical nature of nicotinamide had been known since 1870, its biological value was not recognized until this time. The first successful treatment of human pellagra with either nicotinic acid or nicotinamide was reported the same year. In order to avoid confusion with the name of the tobacco extract, nicotine, the name of the vitamin, nicotinic acid, was changed to niacin soon after its discovery. It was Cowgill at Yale who coined the name, niacin, from the letters of the three words—*ni*cotinic, *ac*id, and vitam*in*.

Properties of Niacin

Niacin occurs in colorless needles (Fig. 16.9) that have a very bitter taste. Although the vitamin is soluble in water, it is not destroyed by acids, alkalies, light, air, or heat.

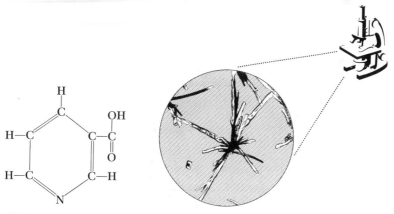

Fig. 16.9. Crystalline niacin and its chemical formula. (Photomicrograph courtesy of Merck and Co., Rahway, New Jersey.)

Function of Niacin

The principal role of niacin, as with thiamine and riboflavin, is as a constituent in coenzymes. Niacin is a constituent of two coenzymes that are essential for certain oxidation reactions to take place in the body. One of the chief functions of the coenzymes is the removal of hydrogen (dehydrogenation) from certain compounds and the transfer of it to others in a series of complex reactions.

The Tryptophan-Niacin Relationship. It has been demonstrated that one of the essential amino acids, tryptophan, can be converted into niacin in the animal body. This relationship between tryptophan and niacin was first reported in 1945 by Krehl and others (9) at the University of Wisconsin, and since that time reports have shown that human beings as well as most animals are able to change the amino acid to the vitamin. Because of this biological phenomenon, workers until 1945 had been unable to produce a human niacin deficiency by the deprivation of niacin alone in an otherwise adequate diet.

The conversion ratio of tryptophan to niacin in the human has been investigated. Horwitt and his group (7, 8) at Elgin State Hospital found the conversion ratio of tryptophan to niacin in adult men to be about 60 to 1. Using adult women as subjects, Goldsmith and co-workers (6) at Tulane University have reported similar values to confirm the validity of this conversion ratio. Studies with pregnant and non-pregnant women (13) indicate that the conversion of tryptophan to niacin is more efficient in the pregnant than in the nonpregnant state.

The Effects of a Niacin Deficiency

In Animals. Only the dog develops characteristic deficiency symptoms due to a lack of niacin. Although other animals show symptoms such as reduced growth, loss of appetite, and weight loss, these conditions are only the standard symptoms observed in most vitamin deficiencies. Blacktongue, the term used to describe a niacin deficiency in a dog, manifests itself in severe lesions of the mouth, a characteristic halitosis, diarrhea, emaciation, and a lack of appetite for both food and water.

In Man. The first report of experimentally induced pellagra in man by dietary means was made by Goldberger and Wheeler in 1915 (1). However, after the identification in 1937 of niacin as the antipellagra factor, numerous workers tried without success to produce experimental pellagra in man by niacin deprivation. It was not until 1952 that Gold-smith and her associates (2) at Tulane University were successful in inducing human pellagra by the use of corn diets low in niacin and tryptophan. Now it is known that these other workers who had failed to produce a human niacin deficiency had used experimental diets adequate in all known nutrients except niacin, and that the stumbling block was the presence of adequate tryptophan, which indirectly supplied niacin to the body.

The subjects of Goldsmith's study developed pellagra during the fifty days they were ingesting a corn diet that was low in niacin and low in tryptophan. At the end of the study they were cured of the disorder with tryptophan, which further proved the importance of this amino acid in niacin metabolism. Prior to this work the intake of vitamins of the B-complex group other than niacin was recommended to improve the multiple lesions of pellagra. In this study, however, even though added amounts of these vitamins were present in the diet, the typical lesions of the disorder were produced. This observation indicates that pellagra is caused by a deficiency of one specific factor, niacin, and not by a group of factors.

In 1955 the same group of workers (3) conducted a similar human experiment using a wheat diet instead of the typical corn diet that is associated with pellagra. It was found that the niacin deficiency took longer to develop and was less severe on the wheat diet than when the corn diet was used, even though the diets were comparable in niacin and tryptophan content. The authors point out that the low tryptophan content of the corn may not be the only explanation for the pellagragenic effect of this cereal. It may be that the relatively low digesibility of corn and the low availability of niacin in corn contribute to the earlier development of pellagra on corn diets (4).

Recommended Allowances for Niacin

The Food and Nutrition Board (NRC) has expressed the allowances for niacin in terms of *niacin equivalents* (10). Equivalents of niacin include the dietary sources of the preformed vitamin as well as the precursor, tryptophan; conversion ratio is 60 mg tryptophan equals 1 mg niacin.

The daily food intake of a college or young adult man (18 to 35 years of age) should provide 19 mg equivalents of niacin; a middle-aged man (35 to 55 years) should have 17 mg equivalents; and 15 mg equivalents have been proposed for the older man (55 years and older). College and young adult women (18 to 35 years) need about 14 mg equivalents of niacin; those over 35 years have an allowance of 13 mg equivalents of the vitamin each day. Niacin allowances for other age and stress groups are given in Table A-1, appendix.

Food Sources of Niacin

Data on the pellagra-preventing potency of foods was reported by Goldberger and others long before the recognition of niacin as a vitamin. This information was based on studies of humans suffering from pellagra and of blacktongue in dogs. Foods were rated as *good, fair,* and *little or none,* depending upon their curative effect of pellagra and blacktongue. Today, with the extensive information on the occurrence of niacin in foods, it has been shown that this early rating system corresponds well to the niacin values measured by present-day procedures.

Although niacin occurs both in plant and animal products, brewer's yeast and peanut butter are the best food sources of the vitamin (Table 16.5). Glandular meats, muscle meat, poultry, and fish are rated as excellent niacin foods, whereas eggs are rated as niacin-poor. Milk, although low in actual niacin content, must be classed as a good antipel-

Table 16.5. Niacin Values of Some Typical Foods

Food	mg/100 gm[1]	Portion	mg/Serving[2]
Brewer's yeast	37.9	1 tbsp	3.0
Liver, beef, cooked	16.5	2 oz	9.4
Peanut butter	15.7	1 tbsp	2.4
Chicken, broiler, cooked	8.8	3 oz	7.4
Heart, beef, cooked	7.6	3 oz	6.5
Bran flakes, 40 per cent	6.2	1 oz	1.7
Beef, ground, cooked	5.4	3 oz	5.1
Almonds, shelled	3.5	1 c	5.0
Cornmeal, enriched, dry	3.5	1 c	5.1
Haddock, cooked	3.2	3 oz	2.7
Bread, whole-wheat	2.8	1 sl	0.7
Bread, white, enriched	2.4	1 sl	0.5
Peas, green, cooked	2.3	⅔ c	2.5
Potatoes, mashed	1.0	1 c	2.0
Tomato juice	0.8	1 c	1.8
Orange juice, frozen	0.3	1 c	0.8
Egg	0.1	1 med	trace
Milk, whole	0.1	1 c	0.1
Butter	0.0	1 tbsp	0
Sugar, white	0.0	1 tsp	0

[1] From *Composition of Foods—Raw, Processed, Prepared.* U.S. Dept. Agr., Agr. Handbook 8, revised 1963.
[2] From *Nutritive Value of Foods,* U.S. Dept. Agr., Home Garden Bull. 72, revised 1964.

lagra food because of its high tryptophan content. Fruits and vegetables vary in their content of niacin. Whole-grain cereals contain more of the vitamin than do highly refined cereals even though cereals are low in niacin. The enrichment of corn and wheat flours in this country has done much to increase the niacin content of our diets. A report from the U.S. Department of Agriculture has shown that the national food supply in 1962 contributed about 28 per cent more niacin than it did for the period (1935–1939) prior to the adoption of cereal enrichment.

Coffee is a new item to be added to the list of niacin-contributors to the human diet (5). It has been reported that ordinary retail coffee contains about 10 mg niacin per 100 gm (11) and instant powdered coffee about 30.6 mg per 100 gm (12). Apparently the niacin level is dependent on the degree of roasting of the coffee beans: light roast equals about 1 mg niacin per cup, and dark roast equals 2.4 to 3.4 mg niacin per cup (5). In certain areas of the world where the diet is low in niacin and tryptophan, the high consumption of coffee may explain the low incidence of pellagra among these groups of people.

Niacin Equivalents of Some Typical Foods

At this time the niacin values in food tables are expressed in terms of the preformed vitamin, milligrams of niacin, not in niacin equivalents. It is not yet realistic to express food values in equivalents of niacin because of the lack of sufficient data for the tryptophan content of various foods under different conditions of processing, storage, and preparation. In the 1963 edition of *Composition of Foods—Raw, Processed, Prepared* (12) niacin values of foods are given in terms of the preformed vitamin.

To illustrate the contribution of the tryptophan precursor in foods, the niacin equivalents of some commonly used foods have been calculated (Table 16.6). The niacin assay of a cup of milk is listed as 0.1 mg. This same portion of milk contains about 120 mg of tryptophan. Using the conversion factor, 60 mg tryptophan equals 1 mg niacin, a cup of milk contributes 2.0 mg of the vitamin from its tryptophan source. Thus a cup of milk contributes 2.1 mg equivalents of niacin to the diet, not 0.1 mg.

Niacin Losses During Food Processing and Preparation

Niacin, which is the most stable vitamin of the B-complex group, is not affected by the common factors encountered in food processing or storage. Because of its water-soluble nature, however, a food may lose some of its niacin during food processing or preparation. The use of a

Table 16.6. Approximate Niacin Equivalents of Some Typical Foods

Food	Measure[1] Serving	gm (A)	Tryptophan Content[2] mg/100 gm (B)	Niacin Equivalents from Tryptophan[3] mg/Serving (C)	Niacin Content[1] mg/Serving (D)	Niacin Equivalents mg/Serving (C + D)
Beans, green, canned	1 c	239	14	0.6	0.7	1.3
Beef, ground	3 oz	85	187	2.7	5.1	7.8
Bread, white, enriched	1 sl	23	91	0.4	0.5	0.9
Carrot	1 med	50	10	0.1	0.3	0.4
Cheese, Cheddar	1 oz	28	341	1.6	trace	1.6
Chicken, broiler	3 oz	85	250	3.5	7.4	10.9
Corn, canned	1 c	256	12	0.5	2.3	2.8
Egg	1 med	50	211	1.8	trace	1.8
Lettuce	2 lg lv	50	12	0.1	0.2	0.3
Milk, whole	1 c	244	49	2.0	0.1	2.1
Orange juice	1 c	249	3	0.1	0.8	0.9
Peanut butter	1 tbsp	16	330	0.9	2.4	3.3
Peas, green, canned	1 c	249	28	1.2	2.2	3.4
Potatoes, white	1 med	136	18	0.4	2.0	2.4
Salmon, canned	3 oz	85	200	2.8	6.8	9.6
Tomato	1 med	150	9	0.2	1.0	1.2
Yeast, brewer's	1 tbsp	8	710	0.9	3.0	3.9

[1] From *Nutritive Value of Foods.* U.S. Dept. Agr., Home Garden Bull. 72, revised 1964.
[2] From *Amino Acid Content of Foods.* U.S. Dept. Agr., Home Econ. Res. Rept. 4, 1957.
[3] Calculation: $\left(\dfrac{A \times B}{100} \div 60\right)$.

280

small amount of water in cooking niacin-containing foods will minimize the loss of the vitamin during the cooking process. The liquid fraction from the processing or preparation of a food should be used in order to reclaim any of the original niacin that was lost from the food by leaching.

A Guide to the Selection of Foods to Meet the Niacin Need of College Men and Women

The approximate contribution of some typical foods to the day's recommended allowances of niacin equivalents for college students over 18 years is presented in Table 16.7. The importance of high-protein foods in the college diet as carriers of the precursor of the vitamin is evident from the contribution listed for beef, chicken, milk, and

Table 16.7. Approximate Contribution of Some Foods to the Day's Recommended Allowances of Niacin Equivalents for College Men and Women over 18 Years[1]

Food	Measure	College Men, per cent/day	College Women, per cent/day
Banana	1 med	6	8
Beans, green, canned	⅔ c	5	6
Beef, ground	3 oz	41	56
Bread, white, enriched	2 sl	9	13
Butter	1 tbsp	0	0
Carrot	1 med	2	3
Cheese, Cheddar	1 oz	8	11
Chicken, broiler	3 oz	57	78
Corn, canned	⅔ c	10	14
Cornflakes	1 oz	5	6
Egg	1 med	9	13
Frankfurter	1	12	16
Lettuce	2 lg lv	1	2
Milk, whole	1 pt	22	30
Orange juice	½ c	3	4
Peanut butter	1 tbsp	18	24
Peas, green, canned	⅔ c	12	16
Potatoes, white	1 med	13	17
Shrimp, canned	3 oz	22	30
Sugar, white	1 tsp	0	0
Tomato	1 med	6	8

[1] Contribution of foods expressed in mg niacin equivalents.

Adapted from *Nutritive Value of Foods*, U.S. Dept. Agr., Home Garden Bull. 72, revised 1964 and *Amino Acid Content of Foods*, U.S. Dept. Agr., Home Econ. Res. Rept. 4, 1957.

shrimp. A 3-oz hamburger in a roll (equivalent to about 2 slices of bread) will provide over 50 per cent of the mg niacin equivalents suggested for college-age students. Peanut butter, a favorite snack food of students, is another rich source of niacin equivalents.

▶ THE ENRICHMENT OF CEREAL GRAINS

Nearly 72 per cent of the Calories consumed by the people of the world come from rice, wheat, corn, and other grains. Wheat and rice, however, because of consumer preference and a better keeping quality, are milled to a highly refined form causing a loss of the nutrients that are important in regulating the body's use of this food energy. Moreover, diets rich in corn products may be pellagra-producing because of the insufficient amounts of niacin and tryptophan in this cereal food. In order to combat the clinical and subclinical deficiency diseases which may result from inadequate amounts of the B-complex vitamins in cereal-rich diets, the enrichment of wheat, corn, and rice products has been adopted.

The Committee on Food and Nutrition of the National Research Council, now known as the Food and Nutrition Board, deserves much credit for the adoption of cereal enrichment in this country. Although the enrichment of white flour and bread began in 1941 under a War Food Order of the Federal Government, South Carolina in 1942 became the first state to enact legislation which demanded enrichment of all wheat products sold within its boundaries. After the Second World War, when wartime directives ceased to exist, the idea of enrichment was well established as nineteen states had passed legislation requiring it. In 1962 thirty states and Puerto Rico had passed enrichment laws, and in the other states approximately 92 per cent of the white bread sold was enriched (3). In five southern states, where cornmeal and grits are used in large amounts, legislation has been extended to include the enrichment of these products. Only one state, South Carolina, has enacted legislation to include the enrichment of rice.

Thiamine, riboflavin, niacin, and iron are the four nutrients that must be added to white flour or bread under the enrichment law. The addition of vitamin D and calcium are optional but not mandatory. In order for one to see the value of the enrichment of wheat flours, a comparison of the vitamin and iron content of whole wheat, enriched white, and unenriched white flours is presented in Fig. 16.10. Enriched white flour contains about twice as much riboflavin but only four-fifths as much thiamine, niacin, and iron as is found in whole wheat flour. On the other hand, enriched flour contains nine times as much thiamine, six

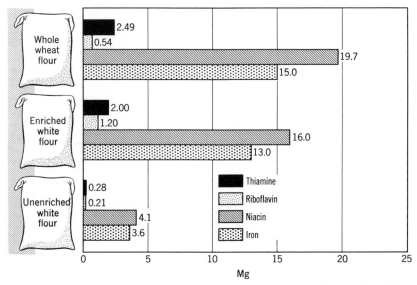

Fig. 16.10. The vitamin and iron content of one pound of wheat flours. (Adapted from *Composition of Foods—Raw, Processed, Prepared,* U.S. Dept. Agr., Agr. Handbook 8, revised 1963.)

times as much riboflavin, and about four times as much niacin and iron as does unenriched flour. The addition of these nutrients to white flour causes no change in taste, color, or cooking quality. The present cost to enrich wheat flour is about 3.6 cents per hundred pounds (3).

The value of white flour enrichment to the nutritional well-being of a population has been shown in the famous Newfoundland surveys (1, 2). Prior to the introduction of white enriched flour into Newfoundland in 1944, medical surveys were conducted in two areas of the country. Four years later a resurvey was made in the same areas to determine the benefits derived from such a program. The clinical signs of malnutrition, following the period of the addition of thiamine, riboflavin, and niacin to the diet through the enriched flour, had decreased. By 1948 the general health of the people had improved, but there was no improvement in the lesions related to ascorbic acid malnutrition where no dietary supplement of that nutrient had been provided.

The diets of the people of the United States were improved notably by enrichment of bread and flour. As shown in Table 16.8, lower income families benefited relatively more than higher income families because of a greater consumption of flour and bread.

Rice can be enriched by coating it with a mixture of thiamine, niacin, and iron, and this mixture is called *Premix*. When Premix is used

Table 16.8.   Effect of Flour and Bread Enrichment on the Thiamine, Riboflavin, Niacin, and Iron Content of Urban Diets, Spring 1948

Annual Income Class (dollars)	Per Cent of Total Nutrient in Diet Added by Enrichment With:			
	Thiamine	Riboflavin	Niacin	Iron
All income classes	16	3	13	12
1000 to 2000	20	5	15	14
5000 to 7500	13	2	9	10

From *Bread*, U.S. Dept. Agr. AIB No. 142, 1955.

in amounts of 1 part to 200 parts of rice, the enriched product has a nutritive value comparable to brown rice. In the past riboflavin was not used in rice fortification because it discolored the grains. Now a new process has been developed that overcomes this yellow spotting of the rice grains (6).

The peoples of Asia, who constitute almost one-half of the world's population, eat about 80 to 90 per cent of their Calories in the form of rice. The nutritional shortcomings of rice as a staple food are evident in the high incidence of beriberi among the peoples of this continent. The solution for the control of beriberi in the Far East appears to be in the enrichment of rice—demonstrated by studies conducted in the Bataan Province of the Philippine Islands (4, 5). Nine months after the introduction of enriched rice to the seven experimental towns it was found that nearly 90 per cent of the people who had previously shown mild to definite beriberi symptoms were greatly improved. The incidence of death due to beriberi was reduced by 67 per cent during the first year of rice enrichment, and not one death due to this disease was reported during the latter quarter of the second year. Through the efforts of Dr. R. R. Williams of the Williams-Waterman Fund (8, 9) and other scientific and civic leaders, both in the United States and in the Philippines, a plan was adopted in 1955 that brought the entire Philippines under rice enrichment by law late in 1956.

Countries or areas other than the United States, Newfoundland, and the Philippines have flour enrichment programs (7). Flour enrichment is mandatory in the State of Sao Paulo (Brazil), Chili, Denmark, El Salvador, Guatemala, Honduras, Israel, Panama, and the United Kingdom. In Australia, Belgium, Canada, Germany, Hong Kong, Italy, Japan, Portugal, Singapore, Sweden, and Switzerland, the enrichment of wheat flour is a voluntary practice.

REFERENCES

THIAMINE

1. Henderson, F. W. (1960). Beriberi heart disease in the elderly patient. *Geriatrics* **15:** 398.
2. Horwitt, M. K., E. Liebert, O. Kresler, and P. Wittman (1948). *Investigations of Human Requirements for B-complex Vitamins.* Natl. Acad. Sci.—Natl. Res. Council, Bull. 116, Washington, D.C.
3. Jolliffe, N., R. Goodhart, J. Gennis, and J. K. Cline (1939). The experimental production of vitamin B_1 deficiency in normal subjects. The dependence of urinary excretion of thiamine on the dietary intake of B_1. *Am. J. Med. Sci.* **198:** 198.
4. Keys, A., A. Henschel, H. L. Taylor, O. Mickelsen, and J. Brozek (1945). Experimental studies on man with restricted intake of B vitamins. *Am. J. Physiol.* **144:** 5.
5. Morgan, A. F., (ed.) (1959). *Nutritional Status U.S.A.* Univ. Calif. Agr. Expt. Sta., Bull. 769, Berkeley.
6. Oldham, H. G. (1962).Thiamine requirements of women. *Ann. N.Y. Acad. Sci.* **98:** 542.
7. *Recommended Dietary Allowances Sixth Revised Edition* (1964). Natl. Acad. Sci.—Natl. Res. Council, Publ. 1146, Washington, D.C.
8. Salcedo, J., Jr. (1962). Experience in the etiology and prevention of thiamine deficiency in the Philippine Islands. *Ann. N. Y. Acad. Sci.* **98:** 568.
9. von Muralt, A. (1962). The role of thiamine in neurophysiology. *Ann. N.Y. Acad. Sci.* **98:** 499.
10. Williams, R. R., H. L. Mason, B. F. Smith, and R. M. Wilder (1942). Induced thiamine (vitamin B_1) deficiency and the thiamine requirement of man. *Arch. Int. Med.* **69:** 721.
11. Williams, R. R. (1961). The classical deficiency diseases. *Federation Proc.* **20:** suppl. 7, 323.

RIBOFLAVIN

1. Hills, O. W., E. Liebert, D. L. Steinberg, and M. K. Horwitt (1951). Clinical aspects of dietary depletion of riboflavin. *Arch. Int. Med.* **87:** 682.
2. Maslenikova, E. M. (1962). Effect of light on riboflavin metabolism. *Vopr. Pitaniya* (U.S.S.R.) **21:** 65; cf. *Federation Proc. Translation Suppl.* **22:** T605 (1963).
3. Morgan, A. F. (ed.) (1959). *Nutritional Status U.S.A.* Univ. Calif. Agr. Expt. Sta. Bull. 769, Berkeley.
4. *Recommended Dietary Allowances Sixth Revised Edition* (1964). Natl. Acad. Sci.—Natl. Res. Council, Publ. 1146, Washington, D.C.
5. Sebrell, W. H., and R. E. Butler (1938). Riboflavin deficiency in man. A preliminary note. *Public Health Repts.* (U.S.) **53:** 2282.
6. Tucker, R. G., O. Mickelsen, and A. Keys (1960). The influence of sleep, work, diuresis, heat, acute starvation, thiamine intake, and bed rest on human riboflavin excretion. *J. Nutr.* **72:** 251.

NIACIN

1. Goldberger, J., and G. A. Wheeler (1915). Experimental pellagra in the human subject brought about by a restricted diet. *Public Health Repts.* (U.S.) **30:** 3336.
2. Goldsmith, G. A., H. P. Sarett, U. D. Register, and J. Gibbens (1952). Studies of niacin requirement in man. I. Experimental pellagra in subjects on corn diets low in niacin and tryptophan. *J. Clin. Invest.* **31:** 533.

3. Goldsmith, G. A., H. L. Rosenthal, J. Gibbens, and W. G. Unglaub (1955). Studies of niacin requirement in man. II. Requirement on wheat and corn diets low in tryptophan. *J. Nutr.* **56:** 371.

4. Goldsmith, G. A., J. Gibbens, W. G. Unglaub, and O. N. Miller (1956). Studies of niacin requirement in man. III. Comparative effects of diets containing lime-treated and untreated corn in the production of experimental pellagra. *Am. J. Clin. Nutr.* **4:** 151.

5. Goldsmith, G. A., O. N. Miller, W. G. Unglaub, and K. Kercheval (1959). Human studies of biologic availability of niacin in coffee. *Proc. Soc. Exptl. Biol. Med.* **102:** 579.

6. Goldsmith, G. A., O. N. Miller, and W. G. Unglaub (1961). Efficiency of tryptophan as a niacin precursor in man. *J. Nutr.* **73:** 172.

7. Horwitt, M. K. (1955). Niacin-tryptophan relationships in the development of pellagra. *Am. J. Clin. Nutr.* **3:** 244.

8. Horwitt, M. K., C. C. Harvey, W. S. Rothwell, J. L. Cutler, and D. Haffron (1956). Tryptophan-niacin relationships in man. Studies with diets deficient in riboflavin and niacin together with observations on the excretion of nitrogen and niacin metabolites. *J. Nutr.* **60:** suppl. 1.

9. Krehl, W. A., L. J. Teply, P. S. Sarma, and C. A. Elvehjem (1945). Growth-retarding effect of corn in nicotinic acid-low rations and its counteraction by tryptophane. *Science* **101:** 489.

10. *Recommended Dietary Allowances Sixth Revised Edition* (1964). Natl. Acad. Sci.—Natl. Res. Council, Publ. 1146, Washington, D.C.

11. Teply, L. J., and R. F. Prier (1957). Nutritional evaluation of coffee, including niacin bioassay. *J. Agr. Food Chem.* **5:** 375.

12. Watt B. K., and A. L. Merrill (1963). *Composition of Foods—Raw, Processed, Prepared.* U.S. Dept. Agr., Agr. Handbook 8, revised, Washington, D.C.

13. Wertz, A. W., M. E. Lojkin, B. S. Bouchard, and M. B. Derby (1958). Tryptophan-niacin relationship in pregnancy. *J. Nutr.* **64:** 339.

THE ENRICHMENT OF CEREAL GRAINS

1. Adamson, J. D., N. Jolliffe, H. D. Kruse, O. H. Lowry, P. E. Moore, B. S. Platt, W. H. Sebrell, J. W. Tice, F. F. Tisdall, R. M. Wilder, and P. C. Zamecnik (1945). Medical survey of nutrition in Newfoundland. *Can. Med. Assoc. J.* **52:** 227.

2. Aykroyd, W. R., N. Jolliffe, O. H. Lowry, P. E. Moore, W. H. Sebrell, R. E. Shank, F. F. Tisdall, R. M. Wilder, and P. C. Zamecnik (1949). Medical resurvey of nutrition in Newfoundland, 1948. *Can. Med. Assoc. J.* **60:** 329.

3. Bradley, W. B. (1962). Thiamine enrichment in the United States. *Ann. N.Y. Acad. Sci.* **98:** 602.

4. Burch, H. B., J. Salcedo, Jr., E. O. Carrasco, C. L. Intengan, and A. B. Caldwell (1950). Nutrition survey and test in Bataan, Philippines. *J. Nutr.* **42:** 9.

5. Burch, H. B., J. Salcedo, Jr., E. O. Carrasco, and C. L. Intengan (1952). Nutrition resurvey in Bataan, Philippines, 1950. *J. Nutr.* **46:** 239.

6. Lease, E. J., H. White, and J. G. Lease (1962). Enrichment of rice with riboflavin. *Food Technol.* **16:** 146.

7. Parman, G. K. (1962). Vitaminization of foods outside the United States. *Ann. N.Y. Acad. Sci.* **98:** 607.

8. Williams, R. R. (1956). *Williams-Waterman Fund for the Combat of Dietary Diseases. A history of the period 1935 through 1955.* Research Corp., New York.

9. Williams, R. R., W. R. Bradley, C. N. Frey, W. F. Geddes, F. L. Gunderson, E. J. Lease, and G. C. Thomas (1958). *Cereal Enrichment in Perspective, 1958.* Natl. Acad. Sci.—Natl. Res. Council, Washington, D.C.

SUPPLEMENTARY REFERENCES

Boggs, M. M., and C. L. Rasmussen (1959). Modern food processing. In *Food. The Yearbook of Agriculture 1959*. (A. Stefferud, ed.) U.S. Dept. Agr., Washington, D.C.

Goldsmith, G. A. (1959). Vitamins of the B complex. In *Food. The Yearbook of Agriculture 1959*. (A. Stefferud, ed.) U.S. Dept. Agr., Washington, D.C.

Goldsmith, G. A. (1964). The B vitamins: thiamine, riboflavin, and niacin. In *Nutrition a Comprehensive Treatise*. Vol. II. (G. H. Beaton and E. W. McHenry, eds.) Academic Press, New York.

Wuest, H. M. (ed.) (1962). Unsolved Problems of Thiamine. *Ann. N.Y. Acad. Sci.* **98:** 383.

CHAPTER 17

The B-complex vitamins II. vitamin B_6, folacin (folic acid), vitamin B_{12}, pantothenic acid, biotin, choline, and inositol

For a substance to be classified as a vitamin at least two species of animal must need it for the maintenance of normal body function. Although there are other factors of the B-complex family in addition to thiamine, riboflavin, and niacin that qualify as vitamins according to this definition, not all of them have been shown to be essential to man. It has been more difficult to induce experimental human deficiencies with these factors than it was with the vitamins discussed in the preceding chapters. Because of this fact, investigators have not only used deficiency diets in their human studies of these factors but also have found it necessary to employ chemical substances called *antagonists*. An antagonist, which may or may not be related chemically to a specific vitamin, will counteract the beneficial effects of the vitamin and for this reason is sometimes called an *antivitamin*. For example, in the induction of experimental pantothenic acid deficiency in man the subjects were fed omega-methyl pantothenate, which is an antagonist of pantothenic acid.

Vitamin B_6, folacin, vitamin B_{12}, pantothenic acid, biotin, choline, and inositol are discussed in this chapter. The crystalline structures of four of them are shown in Fig. 17.1.

Since most of these factors act as coenzymes in the enzyme systems of the body, they may be thought of as quite similar in their function. Because these vitamins are needed in minute amounts and are found in the commonly used plants and animal foods of the diet it is not likely

288

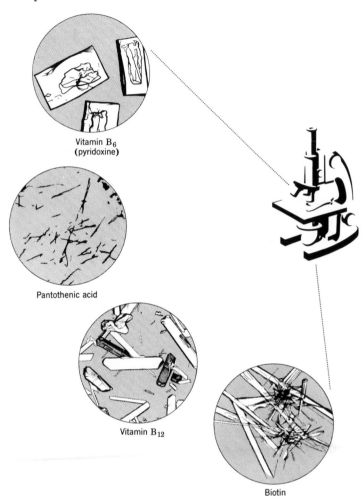

Fig. 17.1.   Crystals of vitamin B_6, pantothenic acid, vitamin B_{12}, and biotin. (Photomicrographs courtesy of Merck and Co., Rahway, N.J.)

that human beings will ever have a deficiency. In general the ordinary practices of food processing and food preparation do not significantly affect the content of any of these vitamins in the food intake.

Vitamin B_6, folacin, pantothenic acid, and vitamin B_{12} are essential in human nutrition and must be included in the daily diet. A human dietary need of biotin, choline, and inositol is questionable at this time. Choline can be synthesized in the body from several substances, and biotin is synthesized by bacteria in the intestinal tract.

▶ VITAMIN B$_6$

This factor was named pyridoxine by György in 1934. However, there are three closely related chemical compounds with potential vitamin B$_6$ activity—pyridoxine, pyridoxal, and pyridoxamine (Fig. 17.2). The pyridoxal and pyridoxamine forms occur mainly in animal products whereas pyridoxine is found largely in products of vegetable origin.

Functions of Vitamin B$_6$

Vitamin B$_6$ functions as part of coenzyme systems in the body that aid in the metabolism of amino acids, fatty acids, and in the release of energy. It occurs in tissues predominantly as pyridoxal or pyridoxamine phosphate.

Pyridoxal phosphate (vitamin B$_6$ coenzyme) functions in a number of reactions that are essential in the metabolism of amino acids: decarboxylation (removal of CO_2 group), transamination (transfer of NH_2 group), and desulfuration (removal of H_2S group). The conversion of the amino acid, tryptophan, to the vitamin, niacin, depends on the action of this coenzyme. There appears to be a relationship between vitamin B$_6$ and essential fatty acid metabolism. Witten and Holman (24) postulate that vitamin B$_6$ is responsible for the conversion of linoleic acid to arachidonic.

A pyridoxine deficiency has been shown to affect antibody formation in man and animals. Hodges and associates (13, 14) reported that an induced pyridoxine or pantothenic acid deficiency resulted in impairment of the human antigenic response to tetanus and typhoid immunizations.

The Effects of a Vitamin B$_6$ Deficiency

In Animals. All species of animals appear to need vitamin B$_6$ for normal growth, yet different kinds of symptoms result when different

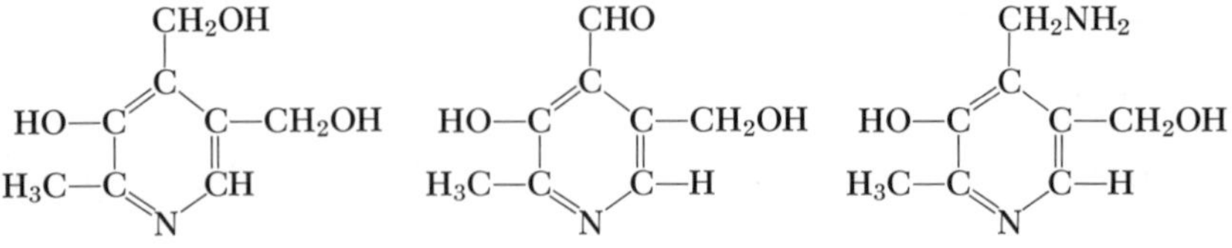

Fig. 17.2.   Chemical formulas of the vitamin B$_6$ group.

species of animals are deprived of it. Although the rat loses weight very quickly on a vitamin-B₆-deficient ration, the characteristic lesion in this species is a skin disorder called *acrodynia*, which may develop on the tail, paw, nose, mouth, or ears (Fig. 17.3). As the deficiency advances, however, the rat may suffer from muscular weakness and convulsions.

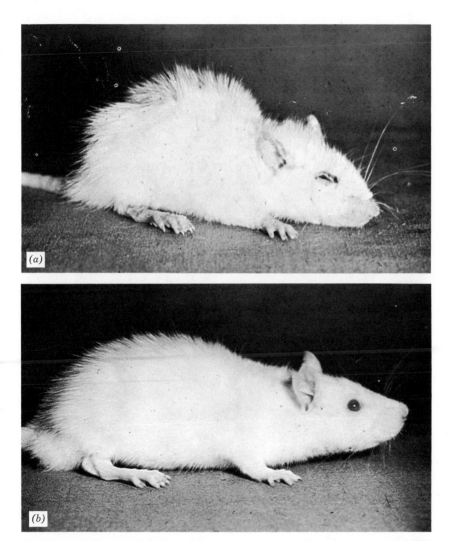

Fig. 17.3. (*a*) The acrodynia-like syndrome of pyridoxine deficiency is characterized by edema and denuding of the ears, paws, and snout. (*b*) The same rat is shown again completely recovered after three weeks of treatment with pyridoxine hydrochloride. (Courtesy of The Upjohn Company.)

Vitamin-B_6-deficient dogs, pigs, and monkeys do not show the acrodynia exhibited in rats but instead develop an anemia in which the red blood cells are small and low in hemoglobin (microcytic hypochromic anemia). Nevertheless, in the later stages of the deficiency, these animals too may suffer from convulsions. Neither the acrodynia nor the anemia is a characteristc symptom of calves deprived of vitamin B_6. These deficient animals show anorexia, listlessness, a poor coat of hair, and sometimes convulsions.

In Man. The human need for vitamin B_6 has been established from deprivation studies of both adults and infants. It was necessary to resort to experimentally induced vitamin B_6 deficiency to establish the need for the vitamin. So widespread is the occurrence of vitamin B_6 in foods that a deficiency does not occur naturally. The three symptoms observed in these human experiments where skin lesions, anemia, and convulsive seizures.

To study the effect of vitamin B_6 deprivation in adults (22), eight subjects were fed a low vitamin B_6 diet as well as desoxypyridoxine, the antagonist of the vitamin. After two to three weeks on this diet seven of the subjects developed a greasy scaliness on the skin about the nose, mouth, and eyes (Fig. 17.4). These lesions remained unchanged when

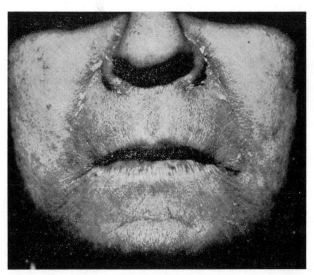

Fig. 17.4.   Dermatitis in man due to a pyridoxine deficiency induced by the antivitamin desoxypyridoxine. The skin is red and rough in the nasolabial folds and on the chin, and the greasy scales are clearly visible. (Courtesy of Vilter, *J. Lab. Clin. Med.*, **42:** 335.)

thiamine, riboflavin, and niacin were ingested but disappeared in several days after the administration of vitamin B_6.

The effect of a vitamin B_6 deprivation is more dramatic in the infant than in the adult. The two infants that were studied experimentally by Snyderman and her group (19) stopped gaining weight some weeks after being fed a diet deficient in the vitamin. Although one of the infants developed convulsive seizures after 76 days on the diet, the other one showed no convulsive activity pattern but did develop anemia after about 130 days of vitamin deprivation. Both of these conditions, however, were quickly relieved by the administration of pyridoxine. Between 1951 and 1953, reports came from various parts of the United States describing symptoms of a nervous irritability and convulsive seizures in infants less than 6 months old. It was found that all the babies affected had been fed the same commercial, canned, liquid-milk formula. A history of the symptoms and treatment of this disorder in a 2½-month-old infant, who had been fed the liquid milk formula from birth, has been described (6). At 4 weeks of age the baby appeared to be irritable and showed a stiffening of the body and after 2½ months went into convulsive seizures. Three minutes after the baby had received an intramuscular injection of 100 mg of pyridoxine hydrochloride, the convulsions had stopped and the child's pattern of activity was normal. It is now known that the cause of these convulsive seizures was a lack of vitamin B_6 in the diets of the infants fed that particular preparation because the natural vitamin B_6 of the milk formula had been destroyed by the heat processing during its manufacture.

The sole use of non-fat milk (skim) powder in infant diets might also produce a vitamin B_6 deficiency because of the destruction of the vitamin during processing. Because of this experience, processed milk formulas are now analyzed and those on the market contain a sufficient amount of the vitamin. A daily allowance of 400 μg of vitamin B_6 has been suggested for the artificially fed infant (17). Although vitamin B_6 relieves the convulsive seizures resulting from a deficiency of the nutrient, it has been shown to be of no value in the control of convulsive seizures in the treatment of epilepsy in children (15).

There are other abnormalities that may be related to a deficiency of vitamin B_6 in animals. Several studies support the finding that a deficiency of the vitamin favors the deposition of kidney stones (calcium oxalate) in animals and man (7, 8, 18). Certain types of human anemias have been observed that respond to pyridoxine therapy (12). That the vitamin may offer some protection against dental caries during human pregnancy has been suggested also by the study of Hillman and his associates (11).

Recommended Allowances for Vitamin B$_6$

The human allowance for this vitamin has not been definitely established but at this time a daily intake of 1.5 to 2.0 mg per day has been suggested as a reasonable allowance for the adult (17). Because vitamin B$_6$ is widespread in both plant and animal foods, this amount will be provided in the average mixed diet (Table 17.1). It has been reported that in high- and low-cost adequate diets and even in poor diets in the United States, the vitamin B$_6$ content is about 2 mg, 2.7 mg, and 1 mg, respectively, per day (Table 17.2).

Food Sources of Vitamin B$_6$

Vitamin B$_6$ is widely distributed among the plant and animal foods of the diet. Although the best sources of the nutrient are found in muscle meats, liver, vegetables, and whole-grain cereals, few foods can be classified as poor sources of vitamin B$_6$. For example, a slice of whole-wheat bread (0.096 mg) contains about four times as much of the vitamin as does a slice of white bread (0.023 mg). Milk, a widely used food in the American diet, contributes about 0.175 mg of vitamin B$_6$ per pint. The pyridoxine content of selected foods is given in Table 17.1.

▶ FOLACIN° (FOLIC ACID)

Long before folacin was either isolated or synthesized, its deficiency symptoms had been described in man, animals, and microorganisms. Many laboratories had independently studied the effect of a folacin deficiency in a variety of species, and different names for this nutrient such as vitamin M, vitamin B$_c$, and L. *casei* factor had been reported. Now it is known that there is a series of biologically active derivatives of folacin (pteroylglutamic acid) that make up the folic acid group of vitamins. Members of this group include folacin, pteroyltriglutamic acid, pteroylheptaglutamic acid, and folinic acid or citrovorum factor, a derivative of folic acid (9). It appears that folinic acid is the biologically active form of the vitamin.

Function of Folacin

The folic acid group functions as coenzymes in the transfer of one carbon unit which is important in the metabolism of many body

° The term adopted in 1949 by the American Institute of Nutrition to replace the name folic acid.

Table 17.1. Vitamin B6, Pantothenic Acid, Biotin, Folic Acid, and Choline Content of Selected Foods[1]

Food	Portion Amt	Wt, gm	Vit B6, µg	Pantothenic Acid, mg	Biotin, µg	Folic Acid, µg	Choline, mg
Bread, white	1 sl	23	23.0	0.101	0.3	3.4	—
Bread, whole wheat	1 sl	23	96.0	0.182	0.4	6.9	—
Cheese, Cheddar	1 oz	30	18.7	0.114	1.0	4.5	13.6
Egg	1	50	126.0	0.795	11.2	2.5	252.0
Milk, whole	1 c	244	87.8	0.756	11.5	1.5	36.6
Apple	1	130	39.0	0.130	1.2	2.6	—
Banana	1	100	320.0	0.310	4.4	9.7	—
Orange	1	100	31.0	0.220	1.9	5.1	—
Apricots, canned	½ c	125	67.5	0.125	—	0.6	—
Pineapple, canned	½ c	125	88.7	—	—	1.0	—
Beef, liver	2 oz	57	378.5	5.324	54.7	167.6	290.7
Beef, round	3 oz	100	495.0	0.520	2.6	10.5	68.0
Ham	3½ oz	100	440.0	0.640	5.0	10.6	122.0
Chicken, dark	3½ oz	100	25.0	0.692	10.0	2.8	—
Chicken, white	3½ oz	100	130.0	0.804	11.3	3.0	—
Tuna, canned	3½ oz	100	670.0	0.420	3.0	1.8	—
Beans, Lima	3½ oz	100	170.0	0.450	—	34.0	—
Beans, snap, green	3½ oz	100	63.0	0.200	—	27.5	42.0
Broccoli	⅔ c	100	171.0	1.290	—	53.5	—
Carrots	½ c	55	66.0	0.150	1.4	4.4	7.0
Peas, green	3½ oz	100	150.0	0.820	9.4	25.0	75.0
Spinach	3½ oz	100	198.0	0.310	6.9	75.0	22.0

[1] Dashes in the table indicate that no representative value was found in the literature.

From Hardinge and Crooks. *J. Am. Dietet. Assoc.* **38:** 240, 1961.

Table 17.2. Average Content of Selected Nutrients in High-Cost, Low-Cost Adequate, and Poor Diets as Calculated from Food Composition Tables and Determined by Microbiologic Assays

Nutrients per Day	High-Cost		Low-Cost		Poor	
	Calculated	Analyzed	Calculated	Analyzed	Calculated	Analyzed
Calories	3013		2439		1117	
Protein, gm	126	130	112	116	32	31
Folic acid, μg	120.4	193.4	117.0	157.4	30.8	47.3
B_6, mg	—	2.0	—	2.7	—	1.0
Pantothenic acid, mg	11.0	16.3	8.9	14.2	4.1	6.0
B_{12}, μg	—	31.6	—	16.0	—	2.7

Adapted from Mangay Chung et al. *Am. J. Clin. Nutr.* 9: 578, 1961.

compounds. Purines and pyrimidines, examples of these types of compounds, are utilized in the building of nucleoproteins and are found in the nucleus of every cell. Folacin is necessary for normal blood formation (hematopoiesis) because of its presumed function in the formation of purines and pyrimidines. In a study of megaloblastic anemias Vilter (23) reported that "all evidence points toward a dominant chemical role for the folic acid coenzymes in hematopoiesis, with vitamin B_{12} and ascorbic acid playing dependent parts."

The Effects of a Folacin Deficiency

In Birds and Animals. Although all animals have a need for folacin, the amount required in the daily ration varies from species to species, because some of them can produce the vitamin by intestinal synthesis. The dog, rabbit, and rat meet their need for the vitamin by intestinal synthesis, but chicks and monkeys must have folacin in their feed, otherwise a deficiency will occur (Fig. 17.5).

In Man. Folacin is effective in the relief of certain types of human macrocytic anemias. In order to show better the cause and effects of this type of anemia, a brief description is given of the development and growth of the red blood cells. After the red blood cells are produced in the marrow of the bone, they must undergo a process of growth and development called *maturation* before the cells are discharged into the blood stream ready to carry on their function in the body. In the first stages of their development, the immature red blood cells are large, nucleated, and contain little or no hemoglobin. A *megaloblast* is an example of this type of immature cell. As maturation proceeds, the

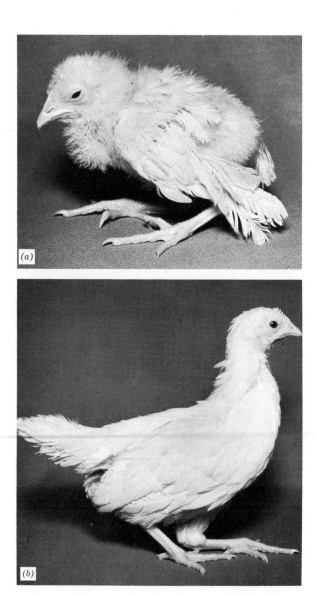

Fig. 17.5. (*a*) Folic-acid-deficient chick is stunted, poorly feathered, and severely anemic. (*b*) The chick taken from the same batch and fed the same ration supplemented with 100 μg of folic acid per 100 gm ration shows approximately normal growth rate, feathering, and blood values. The chicks are 4 weeks old. (Courtesy of The Upjohn Company.)

nucleus becomes smaller, more and more hemoglobin is formed, and the size of the cell is reduced. The mature red blood cell is called an *erythrocyte*. The process of maturation is dependent on the action of certain enzyme systems, and it is believed that it is in this role, as part of a coenzyme, that folacin functions in hematopoiesis.

A person suffering from a macrocytic anemia caused by a folacin deficiency shows a characteristic blood pattern as well as other typical symptoms of the disorder. In the blood stream there are many large, immature megaloblasts and relatively few mature erythrocytes. Because of this condition, the oxygen-carrying capacity of the cells, which have not formed adequate amounts of hemoglobin, is greatly reduced and results in symptoms of weakness, rapid breathing, and a slowing down of the body processes. The normal growth and development of other blood factors, the white blood cells (*leucocytes*) and blood platelets (*thrombocytes*) are also altered during a folacin deficiency. A decrease in the leucocytes, which are the body's chief defense against micro-organisms, will result in less resistance to disease on the part of the anemia patient, and his normal process of blood coagulation may be affected by the lowered number of thrombocytes. Besides the effects caused by an alteration of certain blood constituents, the macrocytic anemia patient may show weight loss, inflammation of the tongue, and disturbances of the intestinal tract.

Folacin has been demonstrated to be effective in relieving the symptoms in patients with tropical and nontropical sprue, nutritional macrocytic anemia, macrocytic anemia of pellagra, megaloblastic anemia of pregnancy, and megaloblastic anemia of infancy (4, 20). Also, this nutrient has been shown to improve hematopoiesis in pernicious anemia but "it is an incomplete treatment for this disease" (20). Folacin has no effect whatsoever in relieving the neurological manifestations characteristic of pernicious anemia; actually it appears to aggravate the neurological lesions which involve the degeneration of the nerve cord (see section on vitamin B_{12} in this chapter). The microcytic type of anemia does not respond to folacin therapy (see Chapter 11).

That combined deficiencies of folacin, vitamin B_{12}, and ascorbic acid are much more common than a single deficiency of any one of these nutrients has been proposed. Vilter et al. (23) believe that "the usual defect responsible for a megaloblast is an abnormality in folic acid metabolism which reduces the amount or the activity of the folic acid coenzymes. Deficiencies of vitamin B_{12} and ascorbic acid adversely influence formation of these coenzymes. . . ."

A variety of antagonists of folacin has been identified. When these antivitamins, such as aminopterin, are fed to animals, one of the early alterations in the process of hematopoiesis is a reduction in the number of leucocytes or white blood cells produced. As a result of this finding, the administration of folacin antagonists has brought temporary relief, but not a cure, in cases of human leukemia, a disease in which there is a marked increase in the production of leucocytes.

Recommended Allowances for Folacin

At this time the National Research Council has not suggested a folacin allowance for man. However, based on the folacin analysis of adequate diets (0.193 and 0.157 mg per day) and inadequate diets (0.047 mg per day) in the United States (Table 17.2), it has been stated that a "... diet containing 0.15 mg total folic acid activity should supply at least 0.05 mg folic acid which is active for human beings" (17).

Because folic acid in amounts greater than 0.1 mg per day may mask the neurological symptoms of pernicious anemia, the sale of the vitamin without prescription in amounts recommending doses greater than 0.1 mg per day is prohibited in the United States (*Federal Register*, July 20, 1963) (17).

Food Sources of Folacin

Folacin is widely distributed in nature, especially in the green foliage of plants; hence the name folacin. The richest food sources are found in chicken livers and vegetables such as asparagus, broccoli, endive, leaf lettuce, and spinach. Liver, legumes, and other leafy-green vegetables are good contributors of the vitamin (see Table 17.1).

▶ VITAMIN B_{12}

Ever since 1926, when Minot and Murphy found that pernicious anemia (Addison's anemia) could be controlled by the ingestion of whole liver, many laboratories have been searching for the factor responsible for this therapeutic action. But it was not until 1948 that scientists isolated a red crystalline material that in very small amounts was beneficial in the relief of this form of anemia. The substance, which is the most recently discovered vitamin, was named vitamin B_{12}. It is a red crystalline compound with a complex formula ($C_{63}H_{88}N_{14}O_{14}PCo$) containing two minerals, cobalt and phosphorus. Vitamin B_{12} is not a single substance but may exist in several different forms, which have been given the generic name cobalamin. The two active members of this group are vitamin B_{12} (cyanocobalamin) and vitamin B_{12a} (hydroxocobalamin).

Function of Vitamin B_{12}

Vitamin B_{12} functions as a coenzyme in the metabolism of the body cells, particularly for cells of the bone marrow, the nervous system, and the gastrointestinal tract. Its role in metabolism is not yet completely understood. In the past the function of vitamin B_{12} had been related to the effectiveness in relieving the abnormal blood pattern and neurologic symptoms of pernicious anemia, because of its initial use in the relief of this disorder. From the hematologic viewpoint, vitamin B_{12} seems to be a factor without which the reduced folic acid coenzymes cannot be formed or function effectively to assist in the production of normal red blood cells in the bone marrow (23).

The existence of the B_{12} coenzymes was first reported by Barker in 1958 (1). Since then data have accumulated on the biological role of these factors, and at the present time the B_{12} coenzymes have been related to seven different enzymatic reactions or processes (2).

Soon after the discovery of vitamin B_{12}, it was suggested that this nutrient might function to promote growth in animals and man. Although a few isolated studies have been reported on the growth-promoting effect of vitamin B_{12} in small numbers of underweight children, further work is necessary before the role of the vitamin as a human growth stimulant can be established.

Vitamin B_{12} and Pernicious Anemia

Pernicious anemia is a chronic disease of genetic origin characterized by a macrocytic anemia, glossitis, and neurological disturbance. Stiffness of the limbs, irritability, drowsiness, and depression are some of the typical neurological symptoms. When liver was effective in treatment of the disease, Castle postulated that a substance in food (extrinsic factor) combined with a substance in the gastric juice (intrinsic factor) to form the antipernicious anemia factor. Vitamin B_{12} is now recognized as the extrinsic factor. The intrinsic factor is a mucoprotein formed in the gastric juice. Pernicious anemia patients lack the intrinsic factor that functions in the body to remove vitamin B_{12} from the material to which it is bound and with the help of calcium to attach vitamin B_{12} to the intestinal wall. Thereafter, by enzymatic action, the intrinsic factor facilitates the passage of vitamin B_{12} through the mucosal cells into the blood stream (23). Very minute doses of the vitamin, 10 to 15 μg per day given by injection (intramuscularly), are effective in relieving the disorder and larger amounts given every three or four weeks, prevent the recurrence of pernicious anemia in patients (Fig. 17.6).

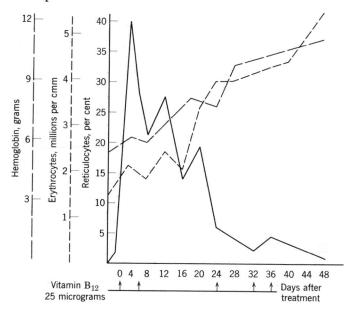

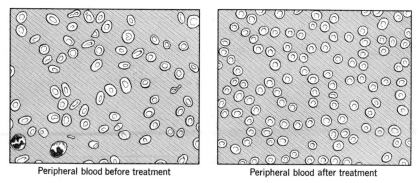

Peripheral blood before treatment   Peripheral blood after treatment

Fig. 17.6.   Patient with pernicious anemia in relapse, typical hematologic response to treatment with vitamin B_{12}. (Courtesy of Merck, Sharpe, and Dohme Research Laboratories.)

It is of interest to mention the observations of Herbert and Sullivan (10) on the relative effectiveness of vitamin B_{12} (cyanocobalamin) and coenzyme B_{12} in the treatment of pernicious anemia in a limited number of subjects. In the case of the deficiency with only hematologic damage, small doses of coenzyme B_{12} appear to be more effective in relieving the blood symptoms than do equal portions of cyanocobalamin. However, when both hematologic and neurologic symptoms were present, cyanocobalamin rather than coenzyme B_{12} was more effective in relieving the blood symptoms. From these limited data, these workers speculate that ". . . although coenzyme B_{12} seems more potent than cyanocobalamin when only the hematopoietic system is damaged, a *very small* dose of coenzyme B_{12} may go preferentially to the nervous system when that system is damaged, and thus be less hematopoietically potent in patients with both hematologic and neurologic damage."

Vitamin B_{12} Deficiency in Man

The first documented case of pernicious anemia in man caused by an actual lack of dietary vitamin B_{12} was reported in 1956 (16). The characteristic blood pattern was found in this patient who had existed on an animal-food-free diet for about eight years. The administration of vitamin B_{12}, however, brought about complete relief from the anemia. Deficiency manifestations may occur in persons infested by the fish tape worm, sprue, and other malabsorption syndromes (17).

Recommended Allowances for Vitamin B_{12}

The human allowance for vitamin B_{12}, under normal conditions of health, is unknown, but it has been suggested that a diet containing 3 to 5 μg per day should satisfy man's need (17). A diet containing adequate amounts of meat, eggs, and milk will more than satisfy this need.

In a study by Chung and associates (5) of high-cost, low-cost, and poor diets, the daily vitamin B_{12} contents were 31.6, 16.0, and 2.7 μg, respectively (Table 17.2).

Food Sources of Vitamin B_{12}

Animal proteins are the chief source of vitamin B_{12} in the food intake. A summary of many assay reports of the vitamin B_{12} value of foods shows liver, kidney, oysters, and clams to be excellent sources of the nutrient. Lean beef, milk, veal, lamb, poultry meat, and salt water fish are considered good vitamin B_{12} foods whereas cereal grains, vegetables, and legumes are poor carriers of the vitamin.

▶ PANTOTHENIC ACID

About 1940, pantothenic acid received a great deal of publicity because of its possible use as a remedy to overcome the graying of hair in human beings. Based on the observation that the fur of a black-haired rat would gray when it was deprived of the vitamin, studies were undertaken to observe the effects of adequate intakes of pantothenic acid on individuals with prematurely graying hair and on elderly people with gray hair. The findings from these studies indicated, however, that the vitamin had no consistent effect on relieving the process of graying hair in man.

Functions of Pantothenic Acid

Pantothenic acid functions in the body as a part of the coenzyme called coenzyme A. This coenzyme mediates acetylation, the transfer or acceptance of the acetyl group (CH_3CO). Certain fats and amino acids can be formed from the intermediate products of carbohydrate metabolism by splitting off or adding an acetyl group(s). Coenzyme A is one of the enzymes involved in the series of chemical reactions that are necessary to break down carbohydrates and fats for the production of energy. The formation of the porphyrin part of the hemoglobin molecule requires coenzyme A. Pantothenic acid, a part of coenzyme A, is thus of importance in many phrases of cellular metabolism.

The Effects of a Pantothenic Acid Deficiency

In Animals and Birds. The symptoms of a pantothenic acid deficiency in birds and animals vary from species to species. The chick shows growth failure and then develops a characteristic type of skin lesion which involves the eyelids and the mouth, whereas the fur of a black-haired rat will turn gray when the animal's ration is low or deficient in this nutrient (Fig. 17.7). Other characteristic symptoms that have been observed when rats are deprived of the vitamin, are the failure to grow and the degeneration of the cells of the outer layer, the cortex, of the adrenal gland.

In Man. The absence of pantothenic acid in the diet, alone, has not been effective in producing an experimental deficiency in man. Only when human subjects were fed an antagonist of the vitamin (omega-methyl pantothenate) in a diet deficient in other nutrients as well, were symptoms produced (3). Symptoms developed early in the experiment with the men showing signs of rapid heart beat on exertion, dizziness, and a lowered blood pressure. Because they became fatigued easily, the men slept more during the day than was normal. During the third week of vitamin deprivation, both anorexia and constipation developed, while in the following week the men became quarrelsome and discontented. As the deficiency progressed, the subjects complained of numbness and

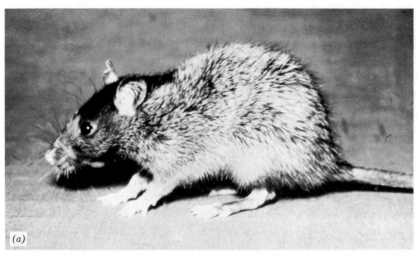

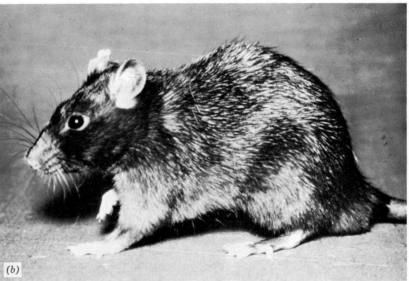

Fig. 17.7. (a) The general loss of hair color characterizes a pantothenic deficiency in black rats. (b) A diet adequate in calcium pantothenate restores much of the black pigment within a month. (Courtesy of The Upjohn Company.)

tingling in the hands and feet and showed definite signs of muscular weakness. When pantothenic acid was restored to their diets, however, it alone did not immediately improve all the symptoms of the deficiency state. Consequently, it is believed that the deficiency effects observed might have been due to the toxicity of the antagonist rather than to a complete lack of pantothenic acid; only the use of a diet supplemented with all the vitamins brought about complete recovery in all the subjects.

Recommended Allowances for Pantothenic Acid

Although the daily allowance for pantothenic acid is not yet known, it has been suggested to be about 10 mg per day (17). The average amount in the adequate American diet has been reported to be between 16.3 mg (high-cost diet) and 14.2 mg (low-cost diet) per day and about 6 mg per day in inadequate diets (Table 17.2).

Food Sources of Pantothenic Acid

Inasmuch as this vitamin is found in all plant and animal tissues its name, which was coined from the Greek and means "from everywhere," is appropriately chosen. The richest amounts of the nutrient have been found in liver, kidney, yeast, egg yolk, and fresh vegetables. Like other B-vitamins, whole-grain cereals contain appreciably more pantothenic acid than do refined cereal products. Milk, also, is an important carrier of the nutrient in the diet (1.5 mg pantothenic acid per pint, Table 17.1).

▶ BIOTIN

The studies leading to the discovery of biotin began when it was observed that rats fed a ration rich in raw or slightly cooked egg white developed a peculiar skin disorder, showed extreme loss of body hair, and finally died. This condition was referred to as "egg-white injury," and the toxic factor in the egg-white protein which was responsible for the disorder was identified and called *avidin*. Avidin is destroyed when eggs are cooked. Then, a protective factor that counteracted the toxic effect of the avidin was found in such foods as liver and yeast, but it was called by many names such as vitamin H, Factor X, and others before its identification as biotin was established. Now, it is known that the "egg-white injury" occurred when the biotin from a food combined with the avidin of the egg white to form an insoluble substance that could not be absorbed from the intestinal tract.

Function of Biotin

To date, the exact function of biotin in man is not known, but it appears that this nutrient is an essential part of certain coenzymes. There is evidence that biotin is involved in carbon dioxide fixation reactions and in the reverse of this reaction, decarboxylation (17). An example of carbon dioxide fixation occurs in the conversion of pyruvic acid to oxaloacetic acid, an important step in carbohydrate metabolism. Carboxylation reactions are involved in the synthesis of fatty acids and formation of urea. Biotin appears to be necessary for the biosynthesis of folic acid and is closely related metabolically to folic acid and pantothenic acid.

The Effects of a Biotin Deficiency

In Animals. The symptoms of biotin deficiency in animals are quite similar from species to species. In the early stages of biotin deficiency in rats, the animal loses hair around the eyes, which produces a characteristic "spectacle eye condition," and as the disorder progresses there is a general loss of hair over the entire body (Fig. 17.8). Loss of weight, abnormal posture, and a spastic gait are observed in the advanced stages of the deficiency, and death will occur if biotin is not restored to the rat's ration.

In Man. A biotin deficiency in man has been induced experimentally by feeding male subjects a low biotin diet that contained 30 per cent of the total Calories in the form of egg white (21). By the end of the first month on the experimental diet, all the subjects had developed a fine scaliness on their skin. During the ninth and tenth week of the deprivation, the men experienced mild depression, extreme weariness, sleepiness, pains in the muscles, and highly sensitive skin. Later, however, they developed anorexia and nausea. Because the symptoms of the deficiency state disappeared so quickly after the restoration of biotin to the diets of the subjects, it was concluded that this vitamin is an essential nutrient for man.

Recommended Allowances for Biotin

As yet recommended allowances for biotin have not been established, but it has been suggested that probably between 0.150 and 0.300 mg of the vitamin provide the daily needs (17). Because biotin is widely distributed in foods, with the average diet supplying the suggested daily

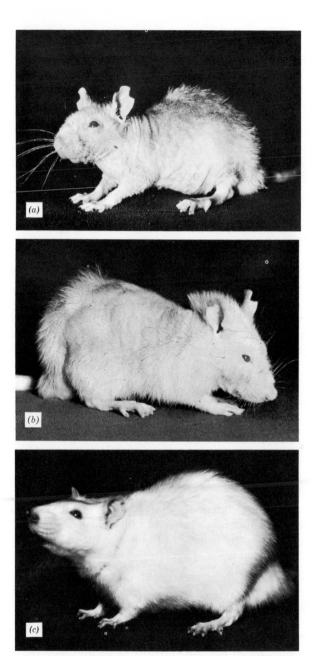

Fig. 17.8. Egg white injury is a biotin deficiency produced by feeding a rat egg white that contains a biotin antagonist avidin. The resulting dermatitis, which begins around the eyes and produces the characteristic spectacle eye, has progressed in the rat in (a) to generalized alopecia. The same rat is shown again (b) 3 weeks after adequate amounts of biotin were added to the diet. Growth has resumed and skin lesions are improved. After 3 months of treatment (c) the animal is normal. (Courtesy of The Upjohn Company.)

need besides being synthesized in the intestinal tract, it is very unlikely that a deficiency of the nutrient occurs in man.

Food Sources of Biotin

Biotin is found in many foods of both plant and animal origin. The richest food sources of the vitamin are found in kidney and liver, and good sources of biotin include eggs, milk, most fresh vegetables, and some fruits. Meat, wheat products, and corn products, however, are considered to be poor in biotin. (See Table 17.1.)

▶ CHOLINE

There is some doubt as to whether choline should be included in the list of the vitamins because it occurs in the body in very large amounts and has never been related to a deficiency in man. Beside these two reasons, it is known that choline may be synthesized in the body when sufficient amounts of the amino acid, methionine, are available. Nevertheless, choline has tentatively been included with the vitamins of the B-complex family because it does occur with them in foods. Choline is a methylated nitrogen-containing base which was first isolated from bile in 1862 (Fig. 17.9).

Functions of Choline

Choline functions in protein and fat metabolism. It is a source of labile methyl (CH_3) groups which are used in the synthesis of vital protein substances such as epinephrine, the hormone of the adrenal medulla (9). Choline is used in the formation of phospholipids such as lecithin, an important emulsifying substance. Choline apparently functions in another way by serving as the precursor of a related compound (acetylcholine) which is necessary for the transmission of nerve impulses in the nervous system.

The Effects of a Choline Deficiency

In Animals and Birds. Not all species of animals and birds need dietary choline, but it has been shown to be an essential factor in the ration of the rat, chick, and dog. A lack of choline in the diet of the rat results in a marked accumulation of fat in the liver and an enlargement and hemorrhaging of the kidney. The fatty infiltration of the liver tissue and the kidney damage can be reversed with the administration of

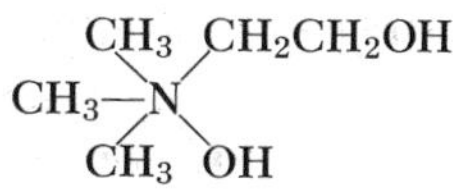

$$CH_3-N \begin{array}{c} CH_3 \quad CH_2CH_2OH \\ \diagup \\ \diagdown \\ CH_3 \quad OH \end{array}$$

Fig. 17.9.   Chemical formula of choline.

either choline or methionine to the animal. Vitamin B_{12}, however, has also been shown to be effective in relieving the symptoms of this deficiency. Although the characteristic effect of a choline deficiency in chicks is perosis or "slipped tendon disease," it is believed that both choline and manganese are necessary for the prevention of this crippling effect in the chicken (see Fig. 12.3).

Recommended Allowances and Food Sources of Choline

Since the effects of a choline deficiency have not as yet been observed in man, no human allowance for the factor has been suggested. The average American diet has been estimated to contain 250 to 600 mg of choline (9).

The richest animal sources of this factor are found in egg yolk, glandular meats, and brain; wheat germ and the legumes are the richest plant sources of choline.

▶ INOSITOL

Like choline, there has been some question as to whether inositol should be considered a member of the B-complex family of vitamins. It appears that inositol may be a component of the body tissue rather than a specific nutrient because it is found in foodstuffs and required by animals and microorganisms in far greater amounts than are any of the other members of the vitamin group. For the time being, however, inositol is included here because it does occur with the B-complex group in foods.

The Effects of an Inositol Deficiency

In animals and birds. Although the function of inositol in the animal organism is not known, it has been observed that there is a retardation of growth when the factor is missing in the ration of the mouse, rat, guinea pig, and chick. Rats also show a loss of hair that is characterized by a "spectacle eye condition" suggestive of the lesion observed in a biotin deficiency of this species.

Recommended Allowances and Food Sources of Inositol

Inasmuch as there is no evidence of the effects of inositol deprivation in man, the amount of this factor that one needs each day is not known.

Heart, liver, wheat germ, yeast, and whole grain cereals have been found to be good food sources of inositol.

REFERENCES

1. Barker, H. A. (1958). A coenzyme containing pseudovitamin B_{12}. *Proc. Natl. Acad. Sci.* 44: 1093.
2. Barker, H. A. (1964). Introduction. In *Vitamin B_{12} Coenzymes. Ann. N.Y. Acad. Sci.* 112: 550.
3. Bean, W. B., and R. E. Hodges (1954). Pantothenic acid deficiency induced in human subjects. *Proc. Soc. Exptl. Biol. Med.* 86: 693.
4. Chanarin, I., B. M. MacGibbon, W. J. O'Sullivan, and D. J. Mollin (1959). Folic acid deficiency in pregnancy. *Lancet* 2: 634.
5. Chung, A. S. M., W. N. Pearson, W. J. Darby, O. N. Miller, and G. A. Goldsmith (1961). Folic acid, vitamin B_6, pantothenic acid, and vitamin B_{12} in human dietaries. *Am. J. Clin. Nutr.* 9: 573.
6. Coursin, D. B. (1954). Convulsive seizures in infants with pyridoxine-deficient diet. *J. Am. Med. Assoc.* 154: 406.
7. Crawhill, J. C., E. F. Scowen, and R. W. E. Watts (1959). Conversion of glycine to oxalate in primary hyperoxaluria. *Lancet* 2: 806.
8. Crawhill, J. C., R. R. de Mowbray, E. F. Scowen, and R. W. E. Watts (1959). Conversion of glycine to oxalate in a normal subject. *Lancet* 2: 810.
9. Goldsmith, G. A. (1959). Vitamins of the B complex. In *Food. The Yearbook of Agriculture, 1959* (A. Stefferud, ed.) U.S. Dept. Agr., Washington, D.C., p. 143.
10. Herbert, V., and L. W. Sullivan (1964). Activity of coenzyme B_{12} in man. In *Vitamin B_{12} Coenzymes. Ann. N.Y. Acad. Sci.* 112: 855.
11. Hillman, R. W., P. G. Cabaud, and R. A. Schenone (1962). The effects of pyridoxine supplements on the dental caries experience of pregnant women. *Am. J. Clin. Nutr.* 10: 512.
12. Hines, J. D., and J. W. Harris (1964). Pyridoxine-responsive anemia. Description of three patients with megaloblastic erythropoiesis. *Am. J. Clin. Nutr.* 14: 137.
13. Hodges, R. E., W. B. Bean, M. A. Ohlson, and R. E. Bleiler (1962). Factors affecting human antibody response. IV. Pyridoxine deficiency. *Am. J. Clin. Nutr.* 11: 180.
14. Hodges, R. E., W. B. Bean, M. A. Ohlson, and R. E. Bleiler (1962). Factors affecting human antibody response. V. Combined deficiencies of pantothenic acid and pyridoxine. *Am. J. Clin. Nutr.* 11: 187.
15. Livingston, S., J. M. Hsu, and D. C. Peterson (1955). Ineffectiveness of pyridoxine (vitamin B_6) in the treatment of epilepsy. *Pediatrics* 16: 250.
16. Pollycove, M., L. Apt, and M. J. Colbert (1956). Pernicious anemia due to dietary deficiency of vitamin B_{12}. *New Engl. J. Med.* 255: 164.
17. *Recommended Dietary Allowances Sixth Revised Edition* (1964). Natl. Acad. Sci.—Natl. Res. Council, Publ. 1146, Washington, D.C.

18. Renal stones, magnesium, and vitamin B_6 in rats (1961). *Nutr. Rev.* **19:** 306.
19. Snyderman, S. E., L. E. Holt, Jr., R. Carretero, and K. Jacobs (1953). Pyridoxine deficiency in the human infant. *Am. J. Clin. Nutr.* **1:** 200.
20. Spies, T. D. (1962). The pteroylglutamites and vitamin B_{12} in nutrition. In *Clinical Nutrition.* (N. Jolliffe, ed.) Harper and Brothers, New York, p. 635.
21. Sydenstricker, V. P., S. A. Singal, A. P. Briggs, N. M. de Vaughn, and H. Isbell (1942). Observations on the "egg-white injury" in man. *J. Am. Assoc.* **118:** 1199.
22. Vilter, R. W., J. F. Mueller, H. S. Glazer, T. Harrold, J. Abraham, C. Thompson, and V. R. Hawkins (1953). The effect of vitamin B_6 deficiency induced by desoxypyridoxine in human beings. *J. Lab. Clin. Med.* **42:** 335.
23. Vilter, R. W., J. J. Will, T. Wright, and D. Rullman (1963). Interrelationships of vitamin B_{12}, folic acid, and ascorbic acid in the megaloblastic anemias. *Am. J. Clin. Nutr.* **12:** 130.
24. Witten, P. W., and R. T. Holman (1952). Polyethanoic fatty acid metabolism. Pt. 6. Effects of pyridoxine on essential fatty acid conversion. *Arch. Biochem. Biophys.* **41:** 266.

SUPPLEMENTARY REFERENCES

Chow, B. F. (1964). B. vitamins: B_6, B_{12}, folic acid, pantothenic acid, and biotin. In *Nutrition A Comprehensive Treatise,* Vol. II. (G. H. Beaton and E. W. McHenry, eds.) Academic Press, New York.
Goldsmith, G. A. (1959). *Nutritional Diagnosis.* Charles C Thomas, Springfield, Ill.
Krehl, W. A. (1962). Vitamins of undetermined clinical importance. In *Clinical Nutrition.* (N. Jolliffe, ed.) Harper and Brothers, New York.
Whipple, H. E. (ed.) (1964). Vitamin B_{12} coenzymes. *Ann. N.Y. Acad. Sci.* **112:** 547.

CHAPTER 18

Dietary interrelationships

In the living organism the chain of reactions which any one nutrient follows in its absorption and use by the body may be influenced by the kind and amount of certain other nutrients supplied in the diet. With the discovery that interrelationships do exist among some nutrients, the next logical step in research would be to ascertain by extensive exploration if there are other interrelationships among nutrients. Nutrition in 1965 is at this exploratory stage.

The following discussion illustrates some of the known interrelationships. The nutrients selected serve merely to introduce a relatively new aspect of nutrition. Some interdependencies among nutrients have been discussed in preceding chapters; however, a more complete study is reserved for advanced courses in nutrition.

Protein-energy Interrelationships. Protein, carbohydrate, and fat are the energy-providing nutrients in the diet. Because of the limitation of the world's protein supply, attention is focused sharply on the possible sparing effect of Calories from carbohydrate and fat on the need for protein (4, 10, 11). Under normal conditions the nitrogen balance is improved by either an increase in energy or an increase in protein intake (12). On a fixed *adequate* intake of protein, augmenting the energy intake is found to increase the nitrogen balance. Also, on a fixed *adequate* energy intake, adding to the amount of protein ingested increases the nitrogen balance.

Limits, however, to continuing increases in nitrogen storage on a diet constant in nitrogen content but increasing in energy value have been observed (3). Proponents of the relationship explain that most likely had the level of nitrogen intake been higher, the progression of increasing storage with increasing energy consumption would have continued (12).

The isocaloric substitution of fat in the diet for all carbohydrate on a constant nitrogen intake causes an increase in nitrogen excretion. When an almost complete shift to fat from carbohydrate occurs in the diet of man, nitrogen excretion increases notably in the first two to five days, declining in the succeeding days. If fat is only partially substituted for dietary carbohydrate, the rise in nitrogen output is less, and the elevation is for a shorter period than if the substitution had been total. The nitrogen loss may not be detected if observations are delayed for a few days after the shift from carbohydrate to fat (12, 15). It is noteworthy that the loss of nitrogen is transient, and in a few days there is an adjustment to fat as the major source of Calories.

Amino Acid Interrelationships. Relationships have been demonstrated among some of the amino acids. The amount of certain essential amino acids needed in the diet is reduced by the presence of certain nonessential acids. For example, tyrosine, a nonessential amino acid with a chemical formula similar to that of phenylalanine, exerts a sparing effect on the need for phenylalanine (16). Cystine, a nonessential amino acid spares methionine, an essential amino acid; both are sulfur-containing (18).

Adverse effects of an excess of one amino acid on the utilization of another occur. An excess of leucine depresses the utilization of isoleucine and valine (7). An excess of lysine depresses the use of arginine (4, 9). The bases for the unfavorable effects have not been established.

Amino Acid-Vitamin Interrelationships. Three amino acid-vitamin interrelationships are cited here, but there are many others, particularly in the vitamin B group. It is recognized that methionine contributes methyl groups ($-CH_3$) for the synthesis of vitamin B_{12} (13). In a study of chicks that were fed diets lacking in vitamin B_{12} and methionine and containing 0, 4, and 24 per cent fat, there was loss of weight as the fat content of the diet was increased (6). With the addition of vitamin B_{12}, growth increased. With the addition of methionine to the vitamin B_{12}-deficient ration, the growth rate was equal to that when vitamin B_{12} was provided, with the exception of the fat-free ration when growth was less.

An important amino acid-vitamin relationship is the sparing action of the amino acid tryptophan for the vitamin niacin. This relationship is discussed in Chapter 16. Studies indicate that the percentage of conversion of tryptophan to niacin in the human being is approximately the same regardless of the status of the protein nutrition (17).

The relationship of pyridoxine (in the form of pyridoxal phosphate) to amino acid metabolism is discussed in Chapter 17.

Vitamin Interrelationships. Interrelationships among vitamins have been studied extensively, but only a few of the investigations are discussed here. Most of the observations are with experimental animals.

Functions of vitamin B_{12} are interrelated with those of many of the other B vitamins. Folacin will relieve the symptoms of macrocytic anemia caused by an inadequacy of vitamin B_{12} but not the neurological symptoms.

The absorption of vitamin B_{12} is influenced by some members of the vitamin B complex. Deficiency of vitamin B_6 in the rat was found by Hsu (8) to depress absorption of vitamin B_{12}. On the other hand, folic acid deficiency in rats increased the absorption of vitamin B_{12}. Deficiency of thiamine, riboflavin, pantothenic acid, niacin, biotin, or choline caused no significant change in absorption.

Interrelationships among the fat-soluble vitamins have been under study for many years. One of the established relationships is the decreased storage of vitamin A in animals on a diet deficient in vitamin E.

Vitamin-Mineral Interrelationships. The vitamin D-calcium-phosphorus interrelationship was one of the first associations between vitamins and minerals to be recognized in nutrition. This relationship is discussed in Chapters 10 and 14. Ascorbic acid and the absorption of iron is discussed in Chapter 11.

Vitamin E and selenium have an interrelationship which has now been recognized. In the absence of vitamin E, selenium can replace the vitamin completely or partially in a number of vitamin E-deficiency diseases, including liver necrosis in rats, exudative diathesis in chicks, and muscular dystrophy in lambs and calves (2, 14). (See also Chapter 12.)

Mineral Interrelationships. Among the interrelationships in minerals is that of copper and zinc. For 30 years it had been known that excess dietary zinc was a cause of anemia in rats. Later (1946) it was found that copper could partially reverse the anemia, and copper, iron, and cobalt together could restore the hemoglobin concentration to normal (1).

Selenium is an antagonist of sulfur metabolism. One of the mechanisms by which selenium causes toxic effects in animals is by replacing sulfur in certain sites vital to metabolism. Although not clearly indicated, it is thought that selenium may replace sulfur in the major body sulfur compounds, methionine and cystine. It is also possible that selenium may substitute for sulfur in enzyme systems containing the sulfhydryl groups (—SH) or other sulfur linkages (14).

From the early studies of mineral interrelationships, low-calcium rations were found to inhibit phosphorus balances. Magnesium too was found to be involved. Studies with rats show that the addition of calcium and phosphorus to a magnesium-low diet will precipitate symptoms of magnesium deficiency. The major interference is a reduction in magnesium absorption leading to a high ratio of calcium to magnesium in tissue (5).

Knowledge of interrelationships is an important phase of nutrition. Now that concentrates of nutrients are available and can be used in varying amounts, to know how the consumption of one affects the body's use of another or others is essential.

REFERENCES

1. Adelstein, F. J., and B. L. Vallee (1962). Copper. In *Mineral Metabolism*. Vol. II, Pt. B. (C. L. Comar and F. Bronner, eds.) Academic Press, New York, p. 383.
2. Bieri, J. G. (1961). The nature of the action of selenium in replacing vitamin E. *Am. J. Clin. Nutr.* 9: 89.
3. Clark, H. E., S. P. Yang, L. L. Reitz, and E. T. Mertz (1960). The effect of certain factors on nitrogen retention and lysine requirements of adult human subjects. 1. Total caloric intake. *J. Nutr.* 72: 87.
4. *Evaluation of Protein Quality* (1963). Natl. Acad. Sci.—Natl. Res. Council, Publ. 1100, Washington, D.C., p. 21.
5. Forbes, R. M. (1963). Mineral utilization in the rat. I. Effects of varying dietary ratios of calcium, magnesium, and phosphorus. *J. Nutr.* 80: 321.
6. Fox, M. R. S., L. O. Ortiz, and G. M. Briggs (1959). The effect of dietary fat on vitamin B-methionine relationship. *J. Nutr.* 68: 371.
7. Harper, A. E., D. A. Benton, and C. A. Elvehjem (1955). L-leucine, an isoleucine antagonist in the rat. *Arch. Biochem. Biophys.* 57: 1.
8. Hsu, J. M. (1963). Effect of deficiencies of certain B vitamins and ascorbic acid on absorption of vitamin B_{12}. *Am. J. Clin. Nutr.* 12: 170.
9. Jones, J. D. (1962). Observations on the toxicity of lysine. *Federation Proc.* 21: 1.
10. *Malnutrition and Disease* (1963). World Health Organ., Basic Study No. 12, Geneva.
11. *Meeting Protein Needs of Infants and Preschool Children* (1961). Natl. Acad. Sci.—Natl. Res. Council, Publ. 843, Washington, D.C.
12. Munro, H. W. (1964). General aspects of regulation of protein metabolism by diet and hormones. In *Mammalian Protein Metabolism*. Vol. I. (H. W. Munro and J. B. Allison, eds.) Academic Press, New York.
13. Plaut, G. W. E. (1961). Water-soluble vitamins, Pt. II. *Ann. Rev. Biochem.* 30: 409.
14. Scott, M. L. (1962). Selenium. In *Mineral Metabolism*. Vol. II, Pt. B. (C. L. Comar and F. Bronner, eds.) Academic Press, New York, p. 543.
15. Swift, R. W., G. P. Barron, K. H. Fisher, R. L. Cowan, E. W. Hartsook et al. (1959). The utilization of dietary protein and energy as affected by fat and carbohydrate. *J. Nutr.* 68: 281.
16. Tolbert, B., and J. H. Watts (1963). Phenylalanine requirements of women consuming minimal tyrosine diet and the sparing effect of tyrosine on the phenylalanine requirement. *J. Nutr.* 80: 111.
17. Vivian, V. M. (1964). Relationship between tryptophan-niacin metabolism and changes in nitrogen balance. *J. Nutr.* 82: 395.
18. Wretlind, K. A. J., and W. C. Rose (1950). Methionine requirement for growth and utilization of its optical isomers. *J. Biol. Chem.* 187: 697.

CHAPTER 19

Selection of an adequate diet

An adequate diet is one that provides all the essential nutrients in sufficient quantities to meet the needs of the body. Thus far, the energy and nutrient needs, including carbohydrates, fats, proteins, minerals, vitamins, and water, have been discussed in some detail. The information concerning each of the nutrients in terms of the day's food is now brought together in this chapter. Easy rule-of-thumb methods for knowing which foods and how much of each one are needed to provide an adequate diet have been developed on the basis of *food groups;* for this purpose, foods similar in nutritive value are considered together as a group. The pattern for the adequate diet is developed by recommending sufficient food servings from the various groups.

▶ GUIDES FOR PLANNING AN ADEQUATE DIET

A plan for selecting an adequate diet developed around *4 food groups* will be discussed. There are other plans, developed on the same principle as the 4-group plan, differing only in number of groups. All of the plans are developed in accordance with food habits of the people of the United States and the foods available to them. In other countries where the habits of eating and the food supply are different, the food patterns are of necessity also different.

The 4-group plan is flexible, allowing for a wide choice of foods within most of the groups. Meals planned in one home are likely

316

to differ from those in another, even though the meals in each home follow the same food pattern. Foods selected by persons eating out may vary widely, and still at the same time each is in complete accordance with the recommendations of the same food pattern.

The Four-Food Group Plan

The 4-group plan (milk, meat, vegetable-fruit, cereal) was developed in 1958 and is a simplified version of the 7-group plan that originated during wartime 1943 (Fig. 19.1) (2). In this 4-group plan the citrus

The 7 food groups	Daily amounts	Main nutritive contributions
Green and yellow vegetables	1 or more servings	Vitamin A value Ascorbic acid Iron
Oranges, grapefruit, tomatoes . . . or raw cabbage or salad greens	1 serving	Ascorbic acid
Potatoes, other vegetables and fruits	2 or more servings	Vitamins and minerals in general Cellulose
Milk and milk products	Children ¾ to 1 quart Adults 1 pint	Calcium Riboflavin Protein Phosphorus
Meat, poultry, fish and eggs	1 serving meat, fish or poultry 1 egg (at least 4 a week)	Protein Phosphorus Iron B–vitamins
Bread, flour and cereal (whole grain enriched or restored)	3 or more servings	Thiamine Niacin Riboflavin Iron Carbohydrate Cellulose
Butter or fortified margarine	2–3 tbsp.	Vitamin A Fat

Fig. 19.1. The basic 7 food groups. (From *Natl. Wartime Nutrition Guide*, U.S. Dept. Agr.)

The 4 food groups	Daily amounts		Main nutritive contributions
Milk group: Milk, cheese, ice cream (cheese and ice cream can replace part of the milk)	Children Teen agers Adults Pregnant women Nursing mothers	3-4 cups 4 or more cups 2 or more cups 4 or more cups 6 or more cups	Calcium Riboflavin Protein Phosphorus
Meat group: Beef, veal, pork, lamb, poultry, fish, eggs, with dry beans and peas as alternates	2 or more servings		Protein Phosphorus Iron B-vitamins
Vegetable—fruit group	4 or more serv., including a dark green or deep yellow vegetable at least every other day. A citrus fruit or other fruit or vegetable rich in ascorbic acid—daily Other fruits and vegetables including potatoes		Vitamins Minerals Cellulose
Bread—cereals group: (Whole grain, enriched, restored)	4 or more servings		Thiamine Niacin Riboflavin Iron Carbohydrates Cellulose

Fig. 19.2.   The 4-food group plan. (Adapted from *Essentials of An Adequate Diet.* U.S. Dept. Agr., Agr. Inf. Bull. 160, 1956.)

fruits, green and yellow vegetables, and other vegetables and fruits are combined into one group, and the butter and fortified margarine group omitted. In Fig. 19.2 the daily quantities of each group recommended to provide the *foundation* of an adequate diet and the main nutritive contribution of each group are given. Calories are the least well supplied by this pattern. However, as a usual practice, fats and sugars, which are not listed, are eaten as such or combined in baked goods and desserts, with a result that the energy intake is increased. Also in order to satisfy the appetite, additional servings from the food groups may be expected, which will contribute both to the energy and nutrient intake.

The percentages of the Daily Recommended Allowances provided by the foundation pattern will vary with individual needs. The person with a greater requirement will have those needs less well satisfied, of course, than the person with a lesser daily need. A day's dietary planned with the use of the 4-food groups is illustrated in Table 19.1. This menu contains more than the minimum number of servings in three of the four groups of the plan (see Fig. 19.2). The nutrients contributed by foods in the four foundations groups in this dietary are shown in Table 19.2. Butter, jelly, mayonnaise, lemon pie, and sugar are not included in the calculations. A comparison of the percentage of the Daily Recommended Allowances provided by foods in the 4-group plan is made (Fig. 19.3). Young men obtained a lower percentage of their allowance from the foundation groups simply because the recommendations for men are higher for some nutrients than for women. However, the young man, in satisfying his energy need and promoted by a natural urge to eat, selects more of all food groups. The result is that in actual practice the diets of young men are, as a rule, more nearly adequate than those of young women.

The 4-group plan is useful as an educational tool to show the foundation for an adequate diet. Because it is such a simple plan, some may not realize its importance. For the most efficient use of the 4-group plan, one should know the main nutrients contributed by the various foods in each group.

► THE NUTRITIVE VALUE OF FOOD COMMODITIES

Each food group, and each food within the group, makes a particular contribution to the nutrient content of the diet. Some foods supply many more of the nutrients and in much greater concentration than do others. The nutritional contribution of the major food commodities, milk and milk products; meat, fish, and poultry; vegetables and fruits; and cereal and cereal products, will be discussed in the following paragraphs.

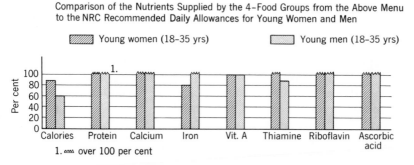

Comparison of the Nutrients Supplied by the 4-Food Groups from the Above Menu to the NRC Recommended Daily Allowances for Young Women and Men

Fig. 19.3. A day's dietary showing the nutrient contributions of the 4-food groups in meeting the NRC Recommended Daily Allowances for young women and men.

Table 19.1.   Menu with the Four-Group Plan as a Guide

Breakfast		Lunch		Dinner	
Orange juice	4 oz	Swedish meat balls	3 oz	Veal cutlet	3 oz
Egg, soft-cooked	1	Green beans	½ c	Baked potato	1 med
w.w. toast	2 sl	Waldorf salad	⅔ c	Broccoli	⅔ c
Butter	1 pat	Pan roll	1	Hard roll	1
Jelly	1 tbsp	Cup custard	6 oz	Butter	1 pat
Milk, whole	8 oz	Iced tea	8 oz	Lemon pie	1 sl
		Snack—1 milk shake		Iced tea	8 oz

Milk and Milk Products

Milk is described as nature's "most nearly perfect food." Some of all of the known essential nutrients are found in milk, but it is a much better source of some than others. Milk and milk products are excellent sources of calcium, protein, and riboflavin. Vitamin A, phosphorus, and thiamine are also supplied in good amounts. Milk and milk products are poor sources of iron and of ascorbic acid (Table 19.3).

The importance of including milk or milk products in the diet in order to obtain sufficient calcium was discussed in Chapter 10. For students, or anyone for that matter, drinking milk is one of the best ways of assuring an adequate calcium intake. Each gram of milk contains about 1 mg of calcium, with a glass of milk supplying about one-third of the recommended calcium intake for the college student.

Milk contains protein of high biological value; it complements the incomplete proteins of cereal products, fruits, and vegetables. As milk can very well be served as a beverage at each meal of the day, a source of complete protein can thus be assured. An easy way to remember the protein value of milk is that each ounce contains about 1 gm of protein. With a quart of milk costing about 25 cents (a variable factor, of course) and supplying 36 gm of protein, a gram of milk protein costs less than one cent.

Evaporated milk contains the same nutrients as whole milk. The process of evaporation, and pasteurization also, reduces the thiamine and ascorbic acid content by about one-fifth to one-fourth. Evaporated milk is convenient to use and economical.

The fortification of milk with vitamin D is a good public health measure. By adding vitamin D to milk the essential nutrients for bone formation, calcium, phosphorus, protein, and vitamin D, are brought together in one food.

The popularity of nonfat milk solids is increasing with the American

Table 19.2. Nutrients Supplied by Foods in the Four-Group Plan from the Menu of Table 19.1

Food	Measure	Energy, Cal.	Protein, gm	Calcium, mg	Iron, mg	Vit. A, IU	Thiamine, mg	Ribo-flavin, mg	Ascorbic Acid, mg
Milk group									
Milk (beverage, custard, milk shake)	2½ c	400	22.5	720	0.3	875	0.2	1.05	5
Ice cream (shake)	⅛ qt	145	3	87	0.1	370	0.03	0.13	1/6
Total		545	25.5	807	0.4	1245	0.23	1.18	6
Meat group									
Egg, soft, ck.	1	80	6	27	1.1	590	0.05	0.15	—
Egg (custard)	1	80	6	27	1.1	590	0.05	0.15	—
Meat balls	3 oz	245	21	9	2.7	30	0.07	0.18	—
Veal cutlet	3 oz	185	23	9	2.7	—	0.06	0.21	—
Total		590	56	72	7.6	1210	0.23	0.69	—
Vegetable-fruit group									
Orange juice	4 oz	50	0.5	13	0.3	245	0.11	0.03	64
Green beans	½ c	15	1.0	31	0.4	340	0.04	0.06	8
Apples	½ c	35	tr	4	0.2	25	0.02	0.01	1
Celery	¼ c	4	tr	10	0.1	60	0.01	0.01	2
Potato, baked	1 med	90	3	9	0.7	tr	0.10	0.04	20
Broccoli	½ c	20	2.5	66	0.6	1875	0.07	0.15	68
Total		219	7.0	124	2.1	2435	0.32	0.28	150
Bread-cereal group									
Bread, w. w.	2 sl	110	4	44	1.0	tr	0.10	0.06	tr
Roll, pan	1	115	3	28	0.7	tr	0.11	0.07	tr
Roll, hard	1	160	5	24	0.4	tr	0.03	0.05	tr
Total		385	12	96	2.1	tr	0.24	0.18	tr
Grand total		1734	100.5	1108	12.4	5000	1.05	2.35	169

From *Nutritive Value of Foods*. U.S. Dept. Agr., Home Garden Bull. 72, revised 1964.

Table 19.3. Nutritive Value of Milk and Some Milk Products

Milk and Milk Products	Energy, Cal.	Protein, gm	Calcium, mg	Iron, mg	Vitamin A, IU	Thiamine, mg	Ribo-flavin, mg	Ascorbic Acid, mg
Milk, whole (1 c)	160	9.0	288	0.1	350	0.08	0.42	2
Buttermilk, cultured, skim (1 c)	90	9.0	298	0.1	10	0.09	0.44	2
Evaporated, water added (1 c)	173	9.0	318	0.2	410	0.05	0.42	1
Cheese, process (1 oz)	105	7.0	219	0.3	350	trace	0.12	0
Cheese, cottage, creamed, skim milk (½ c)	120	15.5	106	0.3	190	0.03	0.28	0
Ice cream (⅛ qt)	145	3.0	87	0.1	370	0.03	0.13	1

From *Nutritive Value of Foods*. U.S. Dept. Agr., Home Garden Bull. 72, revised 1964.

Table 19.4. Nutritive Value of Some Meat, Fish, Poultry, and Egg

Food	Energy, Cal.	Protein, gm	Calcium, mg	Iron, mg	Vitamin A, IU	Thiamine, mg	Ribo-flavin, mg	Ascorbic Acid, mg
Beef, round (3 oz)	165	25.0	11	3.2	10	0.06	0.19	0
Beef liver, fried (3 oz)	195	22.5	9	7.5	45,420	0.22	3.55	23
Pork, lean and fat, loin, roast (3 oz)	310	21.0	9	2.7	—	0.78	0.22	0
Chicken (3 oz)	170	18.0	18	1.3	200	0.03	0.11	3
Salmon (3 oz)	120	17.0	°	0.7	60	0.03	0.16	0
Egg (1)	80	6.0	27	1.1	590	0.05	0.15	0

° Value depends on amount of bone consumed.

From *Nutritive Value of Foods*. U.S. Dept. Agr., Home Garden Bull. 72, revised 1964.

homemaker. She seems to appreciate the lower cost, ease of storage, and lower Calorie intake. With the removal of cream from the milk, which is done prior to drying, the caloric value is reduced by about one-half. In addition, vitamin A and the other fat-soluble vitamins are removed. If nonfat milk solids are used to replace the whole milk, care must be taken to provide for additional vitamin A value from other sources such as green and yellow vegetables and liver because milk is depended on to provide some of the vitamin A need.

An ounce of Cheddar-type cheese provides about the same nutritive value as a glass of milk. In the manufacture of cheese some of the whey is removed, taking with it some of the water-soluble nutrients including lactose, the water-soluble vitamins (B-group), and minerals. Cottage cheese made with rennet has a higher calcium content than that made entirely by the souring of the milk (acid coagulation). In this process calcium, which is soluble in an acid medium, is carried into the whey.

Meat, Fish, Poultry, and Eggs

Meat, fish, and poultry are somewhat similar in nutritive value. Their outstanding nutrient contributions are protein and iron, with some phosphorus, thiamine, riboflavin, and niacin.

The protein in this group of foods, as in milk, is of high biological value. A 3-oz serving of meat supplies approximately 20 gm of protein, which is about one-third the Recommended Allowances for young adult women and over one-fourth for young adult men.

Iron is present in relatively high concentration in the organ meats, especially liver and kidney, and in somewhat lesser amounts in muscle tissues. Meat is a poor source of calcium. Some fish products, chiefly shell fish and canned salmon, in which a portion of the bone is edible, are somewhat better than meat as a source of calcium.

Pork muscle is high in thiamine content whereas other muscle meats contain only moderate amounts. The glandular organs, liver, kidney, heart, and tongue are higher than muscle meats in riboflavin content. Liver, the storage place for vitamin A, is the only edible animal tissue containing any appreciable amount of this vitamin.

Eggs are important for their protein, iron, phosphorus, vitamin A, and riboflavin contributions to the diet. The protein in egg, which is located both in the yolk and the white, is of good biological value. One egg contains about 6 gm of protein, approximately two-thirds the amount in one glass of milk. Phosphorus is distributed in both the white and the yolk. Iron and vitamin A are contained only in the yolk. Table 19.4 gives the nutritive value of some kinds of meat, fish, poultry, and eggs.

Vegetables and Fruits

As a group, vegetables and fruits contribute minerals, vitamins, and cellulose to the diet. Not to be disregarded is the interest they add because of their variety in color, flavor, and texture. The great number of fruits and vegetables available for use differ markedly in nutrient content. For the sake of clarity they are grouped according to their contribution of nutrients to the diet.

In general the green and yellow vegetables and fruits are outstanding in their vitamin A values. One serving of sweet potatoes, carrots, kale, or cantaloup furnishes sufficient vitamin A to meet the Recommended Allowance for vitamin A for persons of all ages. In addition leafy-green vegetables are higher in calcium, iron, ascorbic acid, and the B-vitamins than other vegetables. Some of the green vegetables, spinach, chard, sorrel, and beet greens contain oxalic acid, which combines with calcium during digestion forming an insoluble salt that cannot be absorbed, and makes the calcium in those vegetables of no use to the body. However, these green vegetables, even though not supplying calcium, are invaluable in the diet for the generous amounts of iron, ascorbic acid, and vitamin A value they provide. The ascorbic acid content of broccoli, Brussels sprouts, kale, and similar vegetables is particularly high.

Head lettuce, celery, cabbage, and other light green vegetables are important for their cellulose content. Raw cabbage is a good source of ascorbic acid. The light green vegetables are low in vitamin A value; attention is called to this because of the association of the green color with vitamin A value.

Citrus fruits and tomatoes are dependable sources of ascorbic acid. Tomato juice contains about one-third as much as the citrus fruits. Because they are available in some form the year round and are well liked, it is customary to include citrus fruits in most dietary plans. Other foods such as strawberries, cantaloups, kale, and green peppers are about as rich in ascorbic acid as citrus fruits, but because of cost, unavailability, or lack of acceptance, do not fit into the diet as a routine item as well as citrus fruits. Ascorbic acid is easily destroyed during storage, freezing, and cooking. Citrus fruits retain their ascorbic acid content better than other foods due to the preserving action of the acids they contain.

Vegetables of the seed, root, and tuber classes, like Lima beans, corn, green peas, sweet potatoes, and white potatoes are higher in carbohydrate content than other varieties. Starch is stored in these areas of the plant's structure.

Vegetables and fruits as a rule are low in protein, fat, and total Calories. Table 19.5 shows the contribution of some fruits and vegetables to the diet.

Cereals and Cereal Products

Cereals are seeds of the grass family—wheat, corn, rice, oats, rye, and barley. From these cereal grains flours (whole wheat, white, rye, barley, etc.) are manufactured for the preparation of the many varieties of breads, cakes, pastries, breakfast cereals, macaroni products, hominy, corn sirup, corn meal, and other products. Figure 19.4 shows the parts of a wheat kernel; other cereal grains are similar in structure. Whole wheat has the following composition in terms of grams of the constituent per 100 gm of whole wheat: 72 carbohydrate, 2 fiber, 12 protein, 2 fat, 2 ash, and 10 moisture.

In many of our neighboring countries cereals are the main food of the diet, furnishing 50 to 90 per cent of the total Calories; in the United States about one-third of our Calories is from cereal or cereal products. More wheat and corn is grown in this country than other cereals; most of the wheat is used for human consumption, a large part of the corn is fed to livestock.

The cereal grains are easy to grow, easy to store, and have good keeping qualities. Whole grain cereals contribute Calories (mainly in the form of carbohydrate), thiamine, iron, riboflavin, and partially incomplete protein. Cereals are easy to digest, have a bland flavor, and supply roughage or cellulose.

In the preparation of cereal products for the market, parts of the cereal grain are removed. In the case of brown rice only the outer husk is removed whereas in the preparation of white rice all of the outer coats are removed, leaving mainly the endosperm (center) portion. Whole wheat flour is made from the entire grain except for the husk; white flour is just the endosperm portion. Most of the cellulose, minerals, and B vitamins are in the outer layers or coats of the grain. The endosperm portion contains the carbohydrate and incomplete protein. The germ contains most of the fat of the grain and some of the thiamine. Because the fat tends to become rancid during storage and also seems to hold a great attraction for insects, the germ is usually removed in milling. Furthermore, the public prefers the refined product for most uses.

The protein in cereal products varies in biological efficiency but as a whole is classified as partially incomplete. However, with supplementation of protein from milk or meat or eggs, the cereal proteins make a significant contribution to the diet. About 20 per cent of the protein in

Table 19.5. Nutritive Value of Some Fruits and Vegetables

Food	Energy, Cal.	Protein, gm	Calcium, mg	Iron, mg	Vitamin A, IU	Thiamine, mg	Riboflavin, mg	Ascorbic Acid, mg
Apple (1 med)	70	tr	8	0.4	50	0.04	0.02	3
Banana (1 med)	85	1.0	8	0.7	190	0.05	0.06	10
Broccoli, ck (½ c)	20	2.5	66	0.6	1875	0.07	0.15	68
Cabbage, ck (½ c)	18	1.0	38	0.3	110	0.04	0.04	28
Carrots, ck (½ c)	23	0.5	24	0.5	7610	0.04	0.04	5
Green beans, ck (½ c)	15	1.0	31	0.4	340	0.04	0.06	8
Kale, ck (½ c)	15	2.0	74	0.7	4070	—	—	34
Lettuce, Iceberg, (50 gm)	7	0.4	10	0.2	167	0.03	0.03	3
Lima beans, ck (½ c)	90	6.0	38	2.0	225	0.15	0.08	14
Orange juice, fresh (½ c)	50	0.5	13	0.3	245	0.11	0.03	64
Peaches, cn (½ c)	100	0.5	5	0.4	550	0.01	0.03	4
Potato, white, baked (1 med)	90	3.0	9	0.7	tr	0.10	0.04	20
Tomato juice (½ c)	23	1.0	9	1.1	970	0.07	0.04	20

From *Nutritive Value of Foods.* U.S. Dept. Agr., Home Garden Bull. 72, revised 1964.

WHOLE WHEAT

This cross section of a grain of wheat shows the various nutrients in the different parts of the grain.

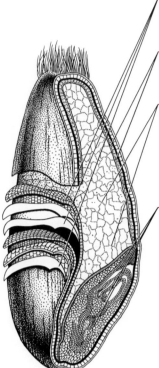

The Bran—the brown outer layers. This part contains:
1. Bulk-forming carbohydrates
2. B vitamins
3. Minerals, especially iron

The Aleuron Layers—the layers located right under the bran. They are rich in:
1. Protein
2. Phosphorus, a mineral

The Endosperm—the white center. This is mainly:
1. Carbohydrates (starches and sugars)
2. Protein

This is the part used in highly refined white flours. Less refined flours and refined cereals are made from this part and varying amounts of the aleuron layer.

The Germ—the heart of wheat (embryo). It is this part that sprouts and makes a new plant when put into the ground. It contains:
1. Thiamine (Vitamin B_1). Wheat germ is one of the best food sources of Thiamine.
2. Protein—this protein is of value comparable to the proteins of meat, milk and cheese.
3. Other B vitamins
4. Fat and the fat-soluble Vitamin E.
5. Minerals, especially iron.
6. Carbohydrates

Fig. 19.4. The whole wheat kernel, its structure, composition, and nutritive value. (Courtesy of Ralson Purina Company.)

the average American diet is from cereal sources; on low-cost dietaries the percentage is relatively higher. Milk and cereal make a good nutritional team, cereal supplying iron, thiamine, and partially complete protein, and milk providing calcium, vitamin A, and complete protein. The use of milk solids (dried milk) in bread improves the nutritive contributions of this product.

The importance of restoring to milled cereals the nutrients lost in the milling process is discussed in Chapter 16. It is important that whole grain, restored or enriched cereals, and cereal products be selected for the diet in order to benefit from their greater nutritive contributions. Table 19.6 gives the nutritive contributions of some cereal products to the diet.

Table 19.6. Nutritive Value of Some Cereals and Cereal Products

Cereal and Cereal Products	Energy, Cal.	Protein, gm	Calcium, mg	Iron, mg	Vitamin A, IU	Thiamine, mg	Ribo-flavin, mg	Niacin, mg	Ascorbic Acid, mg
Oatmeal, ck (1 c)	130	5.0	21	1.4	0	0.19	0.05	0.3	0
Rice, white, enriched ck (1 c)	185	3.0	17	1.5	0	0.19	0.12	1.6	0
Macaroni, unenriched ck (1 c)	155	5.0	11	0.6	0	0.02	0.02	0.4	0
Macaroni, enriched ck (1 c)	155	5.0	11	1.3	0	0.19	0.11	1.5	0
Cake, plain (3 x 2 x 1½)	200	2.0	35	0.2	90	0.01	0.05	0.1	0
Bread, white, unenriched (1 sl)	60	2.0	16	0.2	0	0.02	0.02	0.3	0
Bread, whole wheat (1 sl)	55	2.0	23	0.5	0	0.06	0.03	0.7	0
Muffin, enriched (1)	140	4.0	50	0.8	50	0.08	0.11	0.7	0
Biscuit, enriched (2½″ diam)	140	3.0	46	0.6	0	0.08	0.08	0.7	0
Pan roll, enriched (12 per lb)	115	3.0	28	0.7	0	0.11	0.07	0.8	0

From *Nutritive Value of Foods.* U.S. Dept. Agr., Home Garden Bull. 72, revised 1964.

▶ METHODS OF ASSESSING THE ADEQUACY OF DIETS

How does one know that a diet which has been planned or eaten is adequate in nutrient content? There are numerous procedures for assessing the nutritive value of the diet. One of the most simple is the use of a "score card." The use of a food pattern as a guide in planning an adequate diet has already been discussed, and score cards have been developed for determining how well the diet meets the suggested pattern. A more precise method of evaluating the nutritive adequacy of diets is computing the nutrient content of each food using a food composition table. The most precise method of all is actual laboratory determination of the energy, protein, mineral, and vitamin content. The choice of the procedure for evaluating the energy and nutrient content of a diet depends on the use to be made of the findings and the accuracy with which the food consumption data were collected.

Use of Dietary Score Cards

Dietary score cards set up for evaluating the diet on the basis of food groups are used chiefly as a basis for nutrition education programs (Table 19.7). A limitation of the score card is its failure to give the complete nutritive contribution of each food. On the other hand, it is a commendable educational tool in that it encourages a varied diet and provides a good "rule of thumb" for the selection of an adequate diet.

Use of Food Composition Tables

By far the most common method of determining the nutrient content of the diet is the use of food composition tables (1). From the earliest chapters in the text information from food tables has been used in the study of the energy value and content of the different nutrients of various foods. The values are obtained by laboratory analysis with each representing many determinations (see Table A-8 in Appendix).

The composition of the same food varies widely, particularly in fruits and vegetables. Growing conditions, variety, fertilizer treatment, care in handling, all make a difference. Preparation of the food for the table, preservation, and storage also have an influence on the composition of most foods. Those who have compiled food tables have had to decide on the values that they considered most representative for inclusion in the table. The necessity of exercising judgment in preparing a food table accounts for some of the differences that exist among the compilations

Table 19.7. A Dietary Score Card

Foods	Each Day You Need	Score for One Day	Your Score
Green and yellow vegetables (raw or cooked in small amount of water)	1 serving	10	
Oranges, grapefruit, tomatoes, or other vitamin-C-rich food	1 serving	10	
Potatoes and other vegetables and fruits	3 servings	5	
Milk and milk products	Children, 3–4 cups Adolescents, 3–4 cups Adults, 2 cups	20	
Meat, poultry, or fish	1 serving	15	
Meat, poultry, fish, or meat alternates (dried beans, peas, peanut butter)	1 serving	10	
Eggs	1 daily (at least 4 a week)	5	
Cereal, whole grain or enriched or 2 slices bread	1 serving	5	
Bread, whole grain or enriched	1 or 2 slices at every meal	5	
Butter or other fats	2 to 3 level tbsp butter or enriched marga-rine	5	
A good breakfast, including some form of protein, as milk or egg		10	
	Total	100	

of food composition values. As a rule the most recent food table includes new data that add to the accuracy.

Short Methods Using a Food Composition Table

Short methods for dietary calculation have been developed in which foods similar in composition are grouped together, a representative value for each of the nutrients is calculated, and the values assembled in a table. Totalling the amount of foods of like composition in a diet and computing the nutritive contribution of the group is shorter, of course, than computing each food separately (see Table A-7 in Appendix). That is the manner in which the short methods save time in calculation.

The short methods are found to agree with the long or usual method if applied to a varied diet, and if the food habits do not differ widely from the usual pattern of the dietary habits of the people of this country as a whole. In regions where there is a relatively higher intake of certain foods, such as corn meal in the southern region, a revision in the cereal and bread portion of the table becomes necessary to obtain an accuracy approaching that of calculating each food individually. For survey studies the shorter method of dietary calculation has been found satisfactory. Time required for computation can be reduced without great sacrifice to accuracy. (See Table 9.3.)

Chemical Analysis

In research studies designed to determine quantitatively the nutrient intake as part of a metabolic balance study, the composition of a food is determined by laboratory analysis rather than by use of a food composition table. Laboratory analysis is the most accurate of any procedure for determining the nutritive value of food, since the nutrient content of some foods varies widely. To illustrate, the ascorbic acid content of thirteen different varieties of potatoes ranged from 8.2 to 17.4 mg per 100 gm of fresh weight, and for thirty-five varieties of cabbage from 32.4 to 100.7 mg per 100 gm of fresh weight (3, 4). It should be recognized, however, that the ascorbic acid content of foods varies more than for most nutrients, and that fruits and vegetables vary more in composition than most other foods.

The differences between computed and analyzed values for given diets have been studied. It is generally concluded that agreement is sufficiently close to warrant the use of food tables in dietary surveys, reserving laboratory analyses for controlled studies.

▶ PLANNING A FAMILY FOOD BUDGET

Ultimately, daily menus, a market list, and a plan for purchasing food must be made by families who maintain households and by agencies who make allowances for families in need of assistance. The Consumer and Food Economics Research Division of the U.S. Department of Agriculture prepares materials that are of genuine assistance as guides in planning food budgets. The quantities and kinds of foods needed to adequately nourish different individuals are estimated at low-cost, moderate-cost, and a more expensive diet. The Research Division has prepared plans for twenty age-sex groups and for eleven food commodity groups. These groups include milk and milk products; meat, poultry, and fish; eggs; dry beans, peas, and nuts; grain products; potatoes; citrus fruits and tomatoes; dark green and dark yellow vegetables; other vegetables and fruits; fats and oils; sugars and sweets.

To plan a food budget for a family of a certain size it is necessary to add together the estimated quantities needed for each family member (Appendix Tables A-11, A-12, A-13, A-14). For example, a week's food plan for a family of a man and a woman both 33 years of age, a girl 8, and a boy 11 would be as summarized in Table 19.8.

The student of nutrition is aware that merely planning for kinds and amounts of food is not enough; the planning is made best with knowledge of the food preferences of the family and the availability and price of these foods. The budget plan allows for choice of foods within the commodity groups. Further adjustment can be made even between the groups with a knowledge of food values. For instance, potatoes could not substitute for eggs nutritionally, but another serving of meat would substitute very well.

The estimated cost of one week's food supply for a four-member family (a girl 8, a boy 11, man and woman each 33 years of age) as of January 1963 was $32.80 for the moderate-cost plan (Table 19.9).

It is gratifying that an adequate diet can be provided at different cost levels. The low-cost plan contains substantially more potatoes and grain products. The lower-cost meat cuts can be used in the limited-expense plan with the assurance that the nutritive value is equal to that of the higher-priced cuts. The moderate-cost and liberal plans include more milk, eggs, meat, fruits, and vegetables. More expensive items such as foods out of season and the more highly processed foods are allowed for in the moderate-cost and liberal plans.

Table 19.8. Quantity of Food for a Family of Four for One Week

Food Groups	Unit	Low-Cost Plan	Moderate-Cost Plan	Liberal Plan
Milk, milk products	qt	16.5	17.5	19.0
Meat, poultry, fish	lb	11.5	17.2	20.8
Eggs	no.	25.0	29.0	29.0
Dry beans, peas, nuts	lb	1.4	0.9	0.9
Grain products	lb	12.5	11.5	10.9
Potatoes	lb	10.0	8.5	7.8
Citrus fruit, tomatoes	lb	7.5	9.0	11.5
Dark green, deep yellow vegetables	lb	3.5	3.5	3.5
Other vegetables, fruits	lb	19.8	22.5	25.2
Fats, oils	lb	3.1	2.8	2.8
Sugars, sweets	lb	3.0	3.9	4.6

From *Family Economics Review*. U.S. Dept. Agr., Oct. 1964.

Table 19.9. Cost of One Week's Food at Home[1] Estimated for Food Plans at Three Cost Levels, June 1964, U.S.A. Average

(Food plans revised, October 1964)

Sex-Age Groups[2]	Low-Cost Plan, Dollars	Moderate-Cost Plan, Dollars	Liberal Plan, Dollars
Families			
Family of two, 20–35 years[3]	14.60	19.60	22.70
Family of two, 55–75 years[3]	12.20	16.50	18.70
Family of four, preschool children[4]	21.40	28.40	32.80
Family of four, school children[5]	24.60	33.00	38.30
Individuals[6]			
Children, under 1 year	2.90	3.80	4.10
1–3 years	3.70	4.80	5.50
3–6 years	4.40	5.80	6.70
6–9 years	5.20	7.00	8.30
Girls, 9–12 years	6.00	8.00	8.90
12–15 years	6.60	8.80	10.20
15–20 years	6.90	9.00	10.20
Boys, 9–12 years	6.10	8.20	9.40
12–15 years	7.10	9.70	11.00
15–20 years	8.30	10.90	12.60
Women, 20–35 years	6.20	8.30	9.40
35–55 years	6.00	7.90	9.10
55–75 years	5.10	6.90	7.80
75 years and over	4.70	6.20	7.20
Pregnant	7.50	9.60	10.80
Nursing	8.60	11.10	12.30
Men, 20–35 years	7.00	9.50	11.20
35–55 years	6.60	8.80	10.20
55–75 years	6.00	8.10	9.20
75 years and over	5.60	7.80	8.90

[1] These estimates were computed from quantities in food plans in tables 1 to 3. The costs of the food plans were first estimated by using the average price per pound of each food group paid by nonfarm survey families at three selected income levels in 1955. These prices were adjusted to current levels by use of *Retail Food Prices by Cities* released periodically by the Bureau of Labor Statistics.

[2] Age groups include the persons of the first age listed up to but not including those of the second age listed.

[3] Ten percent added for family size adjustment. For derivation of factors for adjustment, see HERR No. 20, Appendix B.

[4] Man and woman 20–35 years; children, 1–3 and 3–6 years.

[5] Man and woman 20–35 years; child, 6–9 and boy 9–12 years.

[6] The costs given are for individuals in 4-person families. For individuals in other size families, the following adjustments are suggested: 1-person, add 20 per cent; 2-persons, add 10 per cent; 3-persons, add 5 per cent; 5-persons, subtract 5 per cent; 6-or-more-persons, subtract 10 per cent.

From *Family Economics Review*. U.S. Dept. Agr., Oct. 1964.

► FOOD VALUES AND FOOD COSTS

The buying of food is the largest single expense item in the budget for most families. An average of 19 per cent per capita of disposable personal income is spent for food in the United States. With increasing income, the per cent going for food diminishes.

Economical purchase of food makes it possible to provide adequate diets at lower cost. Some nutrients are provided at less expense by one food or group of foods than by others. The approximate percentage of the food dollar spent for milk and milk products; meat, fish, poultry, eggs, dry beans, and nuts; vegetables; fruits; and grain products is shown in Fig. 19.5. Other foods not included in Fig. 19.5 are fats, sugar, and sweets, and miscellaneous items, which account for about 20 per cent of the total food expenditure. The protein group of foods is the most expensive, amounting to 37 cents of the food dollar or 37 per cent of the food expenditure. Milk and milk products account for 15 cents of the food dollar, vegetables 12 cents, grain products 11 cents, and fruits 8 cents.

Foods differ in the economy with which they provide the nutrients of the diet. Protein, calcium, vitamin A value, and thiamine were selected to illustrate this point. Using Fig. 19.5 as a guide, in each food group if the nutrient bar exceeds the cost bar in length, that food group is a good buy for providing that nutrient, because the per cent of the expenditure for that group of foods is less than the per cent of the nutrient obtained. The relative lengths of the bars will vary, of course, with price. It can be clearly seen that the milk group of foods is an excellent buy for calcium but only fair for supplying thiamine; the meat, fish, poultry, eggs, dry beans, and nuts group is a good buy for protein but a poor buy for calcium; vegetables are excellent for vitamin A, poor for protein; fruits are not a good buy for the nutrients listed, but had ascorbic acid been selected as one of the nutrients in the illustration, fruits would appear as a good buy for that nutrient. Grain products are a good buy for protein and thiamine, and it may be surprising to note, for calcium, accounted for in part by the use of bread containing nonfat milk solids. Of course, little if any vitamin A value is furnished by grain products. The protein of cereals is economical to purchase and becomes of good nutritional quality when supplemented with milk or other sources of complete protein. Grain products are a good buy for protein because, as shown in Fig. 19.5, the cost bar is shorter than the protein bar.

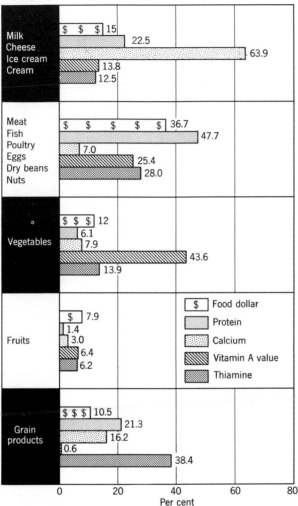

Fig. 19.5. Percentage of food dollar spent for each food group and percentage of total protein, calcium, vitamin A, and thiamine supply provided by each group. Fats and oils (4.4 per cent of money value), sugars and sweets (4.9 per cent of money value), and miscellaneous foods (7.6 per cent of money value) complete the remainder of the food groups. They were not included because of the small contributions made to the nutrients except for the fats, which account for 10 per cent of vitamin A. (Adapted from *Dietary Levels of Households in the United States,* Report 6, U.S. Department of Agriculture, p. 24, 1957.)

REFERENCES

1. Church, C. F., and H. N. Church (1963). *Food Values of Portions Commonly Used—Bowes and Church.* 9th ed. J. P. Lippincott, Philadelphia.
2. *Essentials of an Adequate Diet* (1956). U.S. Dept. Agr., Agr. Inf. Bull. No. 160, Washington, D.C.
3. Leichsenring, J. M., and L. M. Norris (1951). *Factors Influencing the Nutritive Value of Potatoes.* Univ. Minn. Agr. Expt. Sta., Tech. Bull. No. 196, Minneapolis.
4. Patton, M. B., and M. E. Green (1954). *Cabbage: Factors Affecting Vitamin Values and Palatability.* Ohio Agr. Expt. Sta., Bull. No. 742, Wooster.

SUPPLEMENTARY REFERENCES

Batjer, M. Q., and M. Atwater (1961). *Meals for the Modern Family.* John Wiley and Sons, New York.

McMasters, V. (1963). History of food composition tables of the world. *J. Am. Dietet. Assoc.* **43:** 442.

Nutrition Handbook for Family Food Counseling (1963). National Dairy Council, Chicago.

Watt, B. K., and A. L. Merrill (1963). *Composition of Foods—Raw, Processed, Prepared.* U.S. Dept. Agr., Agr. Handbook 8, revised, Washington, D.C.

CHAPTER 20

Food habits
and their significance

Thus far the nutrients necessary for an adequate diet have been discussed. Also food plans to assure an adequate daily intake of nutrients and Calories have been considered. How well do college students in the United States and the people as a whole meet the recommendations for an adequate diet? What are some of the influences on food habits? How adequate is the food supply for the people of the world?

▶ THE EATING HABITS OF COLLEGE STUDENTS

Certain general patterns of food selection characterize the diets of college students (16, 19, 29, 30, 32). Surveys (1952–1957) show that as a rule certain nutrients are more generously supplied in the diets than others. Protein and niacin are more generously supplied than any of the nutrients, reflecting an adequate intake of foods in the meat, fish, and poultry group; on the other hand, calcium, ascorbic acid, and vitamin A usually meet the Recommended Allowances the least well. Such shortcomings in the diet indicate that the students were eating less than the desirable amounts of milk and milk products, foods of the citrus fruit and tomato group, and leafy green and yellow vegetables. The thiamine intake is influenced to considerable extent by the caloric value of the diet; students whose diets contain less than the recommended energy intakes generally also have less than the recommended thiamine intakes.

Nutritionists at the University of Rhode Island wished to know why the ascorbic acid content of the diets of the coeds whom they were observing at that institution failed so frequently to meet the NRC recommendations—more often than any other nutrient except for iron. They found on investigation that the supply of ascorbic acid available to the students in the dormitory fare was adequate, if from the fruits provided for breakfast they chose a citrus rather than another fruit. Seldom did the intake of ascorbic acid meet the Recommended Allowance if citrus fruit was not eaten during the day (28).

College men eat better diets than college women in terms of meeting the Recommended Allowances. There is seldom a deviation from this pattern in all of the survey studies (19, 29, 30). Men drink more milk and eat more milk products and as a consequence, have a more satisfactory calcium and riboflavin intake than women. Ascorbic acid is less well supplied in the diets of women than of men. Most men have an acceptable intake of iron; many women do not. Diet records show as many as 36 to 42 per cent of the diets of college women provide less than two-thirds of the Recommended Allowance for iron. The unfortunate circumstance in this shortage of iron in the diets of young women is that this mineral is needed to take care of the continuing loss of iron through menstruation.

Skipping breakfast or eating an incomplete breakfast is reflected in the total nutrient intake for the day. Students at Montana State University who omitted breakfast or ate one that failed to meet the meal pattern of a fruit, a cereal, and eggs and/or meat, had a less adequate total nutrient content in the day's diet than those who did eat a complete breakfast. The missing nutrients as a result of no morning meal, or a poor one, were not made up in the later meals of the day (19). (For further discussion of breakfasts see Chapter 24.)

Between-meal eating is common practice among university students. Seven-day food records kept by eighty-five Brandeis University freshmen revealed that snacks accounted for 13 per cent of the total caloric intake. Carbohydrate provided 52 per cent of the Calories in the snacks (18).

▶ FOOD CONSUMPTION OF FAMILIES

In the spring of 1955 a nationwide survey of the food consumption of families in this country was made by the Household Economics Research Division and Market Development Branch of the U.S. Department of Agriculture (8). Families were interviewed by trained workers to obtain information on the food practices of the family. The survey was the most comprehensive to have been undertaken in this country up to that time.

The findings from the survey are representative of the national food habits at a time when there was an abundant supply of food and full employment. The markets offered a variety of products at various stages of preparation and at a wide range of prices. On the whole, the nutritive value of the diets was good. The adequacy of the food consumed reflected in some ways the general high level of purchasing power. Protein and niacin were most adequately provided, indicating a good supply of foods from the meat group of commodities. However, even with the abundance of food and the ability to buy the foods of choice in most cases, some nutrients were still inadequately supplied. Calcium and ascorbic acid were provided in less than the recommended amounts more frequently than all other constituents.

There were differences in the food consumption patterns and adequacy of the diets of families over the nation. These differences were related to place of dwelling (whether urban or farm), to family income, and to family size. How families eat is found to be related also to the home-maker's nutritional knowledge and level of education. Also sex and age of the individual make a difference in his food habits.

Influence of Urban or Rural Living

Farm families were found to have a higher energy intake than non-farm families, which may have been influenced by the family's outdoor physical labor and the abundant supply of home-produced foods. When the value of the home-produced foods was estimated at the price the family would pay for the same food on the market, it amounted on an average to around 40 per cent of the total cost of the food consumed. It should be noted that at the time of this survey, the farm family was producing less of their own food than in previous periods when surveys were made, reflecting a trend in the farm family food supply. During the depression of the thirties and the wartime of the forties, home gardens were imperative for food supply, in contrast to the abundance of food when the 1955 survey was made. Another such extensive survey is in progress now (1965). The chief differences between the urban and farm family diets in the kinds of foods consumed was the use of greater quantities of dairy products, grains, sugars, and fats by farm families and relatively less meat, as shown in Table 20.1.

Influence of Income

Surveys of food consumption practices show a definite relationship between the income of the family and the amount expended for

Table 20.1. Comparison of Urban, Rural Nonfarm, and Farm Family Diets in Quantities Per Person for One Week

		Urban	Rural Nonfarm	Rural
Meat, fish, poultry	lb	4.4	3.8	3.8
Eggs	doz	0.6	0.6	0.7
Fruits, potatoes, other vegetables	lb	10.2	9.6	9.6
Dark green and deep yellow vegetables	lb	0.6	0.4	0.4
Citrus fruit	lb	0.6	0.5	0.4
Milk, cream, ice cream, cheese	qt[1]	4.3	4.4	5.2
Sugars and sweets	lb	1.1	1.3	1.8
Flour, cereal, baked goods	lb	2.6	3.3	3.9
Fats and oils	lb	0.8	0.9	1.1

[1] milk equivalent.

From *Food Consumption and Dietary Levels.* U.S. Dept. Agr., ARS 62-6, p. 3, 1957.

food (24). As the income goes up the amount of money spent for food increases but at a proportionately slower rate so that the *per cent* of the income going for food decreases. High-income families spend a lesser per cent for food than those with lower incomes. Some of the increase in expenditure at higher income levels goes for larger quantities of foods; much of it goes for increased services in the form of foods requiring less preparation time by the homemaker, as well as buying meals away from home. Families with more money also tend to choose more costly foods within a food group. For example, in the consumption study in 1955, families with an annual income between $2000 and $3000 paid, on the average, 56 cents a pound for meat; those with incomes from $4000 to $6000 paid 62 cents; and the families with a $6000 to $8000 annual income spent 66 cents. The cheaper cuts of meat were used by low income families; steak (other than round) appeared on the menu during the week in 24 per cent of the low-income families, and in 37 and 44 per cent, respectively, of the medium- and high-income households (8).

The adequacy of the diet improves with increase in income. Vitamin A, riboflavin, and ascorbic acid, selected as representative of the diet as a whole, increased in adequacy as the income increased (Fig. 20.1). It is true that spending more money for food tends to provide a better diet, but at each income level above subsistence in this extensive survey, some families were eating diets of good quality whereas others were choosing poor diets (8). Some of the families with incomes in the top third failed to meet the NRC recommendations (Fig. 20.2). Most of the diets of these high-income families provided sufficient protein and niacin, but as many as 23 per cent of the diets failed to supply the recommended amount of calcium.

Influence of Family Size

The 1955 survey confirmed the already well-established relationship that large families spend more for food in total, but the amount expended for each family member is less than in small families. To illustrate, city families were selected in the income bracket of $4000 to $4999, with the number in the family increasing from two to six. The expenditure for food in terms of per cent of income increased, and the money value of the food per person decreased as the number in the family increased (Fig. 20.3).

There are some explanations for the smaller expenditure per person in larger families. It is possible, as a rule, to prepare food more economically for a large number of persons. Also in large families there are usually small children who require less of some of the foods. Furthermore, the quantities of foods, especially those that are higher in price,

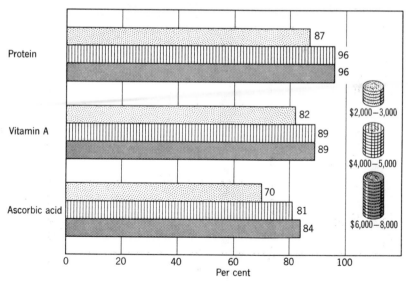

Fig. 20.1.   Income and percentage of city families meeting the NRC Recommended Allowances for selected nutrients. (Adapted from Clark, *Nutrition Education Conference*, U.S. Dept. Agr., Misc. Publ. 745, p. 15, 1957.)

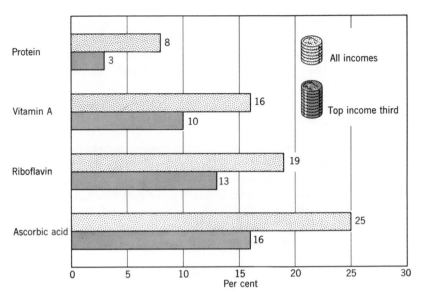

Fig. 20.2. Family diets not meeting NRC Recommended Allowances in top income third and all incomes. Money alone will not provide a good diet. (Adapted from Clark, *Nutrition Education Conference*, U.S. Dept. Agr., Misc. Publ. 745, p. 16, 1957.)

Number of family members	Percent of income spent for food	Money value of food per person (basis of 1 week)
	26	$11.54
	35	10.30
	39	8.74
	46	8.20
	48	7.10

Fig. 20.3. Influence of family size on percentage of income spent for food and money value of food per person. (Adapted from *Food Consumption and Dietary Levels*, U.S. Dept. Agr., ARS 62-6, p. 8, 1957.)

342

are used more sparingly in the larger households than in the small. This follows as a consequence of the usual smaller income per capita in large families.

Influence of Homemaker's Nutritional Knowledge, Educational Level, and Employment

In a study of "what homemakers know about nutrition," conducted by nutritionists at Cornell University (31), a higher percentage of those who had what the investigators termed a minimal knowledge of nutrition, fed their families diets that met the Recommended Allowances than the homemakers who had only some or no knowledge. Minimal knowledge was defined as the "ability to give a correct reason for the inclusion of at least three of the seven basic food groups."

Adequacy of the diets of the families was found to bear a relationship to educational level of homemakers. The majority of the homemakers whose family's diets met the NRC Recommended Allowances were high school graduates and had had some college education. When the amount of formal education of the homemaker and income of the family were examined in relation to how the family ate, both elements were observed to have an effect, but the influence of educational level was greater than that of income (Fig. 20.4). Within an income bracket better feeding of the family paralleled additional years of schooling of the homemakers.

Whether the homemaker was employed or not was found to make

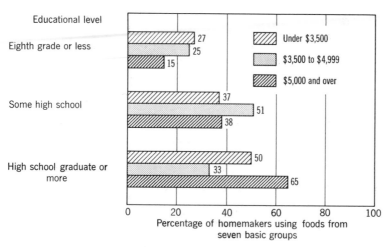

Fig. 20.4. Adequacy of feeding practices of homemakers with various levels of education as related to income. (Adapted from Young et al., *J. Am. Dietet. Assoc.*, **32**: 324, 1956.)

little difference in how well the diets of the family met the Recommended Allowances; however, more money was spent for food by the employed than non-employed homemakers (11).

Influence of Sex and Age

Within the family group some members fare better than others in the adequacy of their diets. As a general rule boys and men consume relatively better diets than the girls and women. These data from a study in Groton Township, New York, illustrate the common pattern of food selection within a family group. As a whole, the young children (age groups under 10 years) fare best, followed next by the rest of the male members of the family. The least adequate diets were among the adolescent girls and women of childbearing age (35).

Other Influences on Food Habits

Family tradition and cultural background exert an influence on food habits which is less tangible than the influences discussed in the preceding paragraphs but real none the less. Another factor, and the ultimate determining one, is availability of food. Whatever it may be that prompts people to eat as they do, whether it be sheer availability of food, religion, the practices of their forebears, or even prejudices that may have developed, their established eating customs are an intimate part of them (13). The oneness of customs of eating with the person himself gives a feeling of security, a sense of well-being, and of "rightness in the world" when he is able to follow them; on the other hand, inability to get certain foods or to prepare them as desired may engender frustration.

The following account of an Afghanistan farmer could be told of most anyone in most any country. Improved maize was introduced that yielded approximately three times as much as the local varieties. Resistance to the new crop was strong; the reason—the taste of the bread compared unfavorably with the taste of bread made using traditional maize (12).

As an aid in menu planning, the Department of the Army studied the food preferences of the men. They found the best-liked food to be fresh milk, with hot rolls, hot biscuits, strawberry shortcake, and grilled steak close seconds. The least-like foods as a group were vegetables (20). What the investigators concluded about the eating habits of the army man is not reserved for him alone, but it would seem for all: "He eats what is available, what he likes, what his culture defines as food, what his personal history dictates, and what society and his peers say he should eat."

"What the culture defines as food" notably influences choice of food. Horseflesh, an edible substance, is such an example. In ancient times horsemeat was more widely used as a human food than it is today. The origin of today's prejudice is not known; some believe it might "derive from the animal's high status and its supposed holy qualities and association with deities" (26). Another example is the case of the spotted pig; in the Chin States of Upper Burma, the small black local pig was crossed with a better meat producer. The offspring was spotted, and for that reason, by tradition unfit for eating (3).

Recognizing the fundamental nature of people's eating habits helps to understand their resistance to change. Dr. Aykroyd (2), speaking before the Third International Congress of Dietetics, clearly focused on the problem when he stated, "Each group tends to regard its food and meal patterns as the normal and natural ones." It may seem that refusing unfamiliar food by persons in need is reprehensible and unappreciative on their part, but the response is most likely deep seated and can only be changed by education and time.

The food habits most deeply entrenched are those followed by people living in isolated areas where the same food supply has prevailed for many years. On the other hand, people who travel widely learn to enjoy foods that are new to them, and familiar foods served in unfamiliar ways.

Change in Food Supply. Availability of food obviously exerts an influence on food consumption. Varied and more nearly adequate diets are found in countries where food production is high. In many newly developing countries the yield of crops per worker is low and diets are limited.

A plan in the United States known as the Food Stamp Program was instituted in mid 1961 to make agricultural products available to needy families. The effect of the program on the adequacy of the diet was assessed in selected areas. Before the Stamp Program was in effect, one-half the families who later participated in the Program had diets that met the Recommended Allowances. After they were in the Stamp Program, two-thirds of the families had diets that met the recommendations. Eligible families who did not participate showed a negligible increase in number of diets meeting the Recommended Allowances (22).

▶ **TRENDS IN FOOD HABITS IN THE UNITED STATES**

The food consumption in this country, from 1910 when the first official records were kept to the present time, show certain general trends in eating habits (Fig. 20.5). The change has been toward an improved diet.

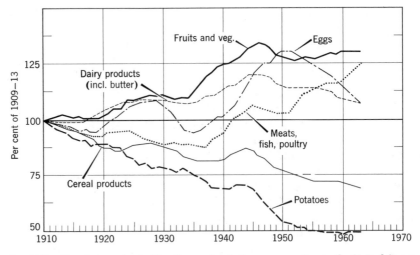

Fig. 20.5. Trends in eating habits. Per capita civilian consumption in the United States. The five-year moving average is centered for plotting. The year 1963 is shown by symbols. (From *Handbook of Agricultural Charts*, U.S. Dept. Agr., Handbook 258, p. 27, 1963.)

The commodities that have shown a general upward trend in per capita consumption are fruits and vegetables, and until something over a decade ago, dairy products. The lessened consumption of some items, including cream, butter, evaporated, and to a lesser extent whole fluid milk, turned the trend in the use of dairy products downward. It is the increased consumption of citrus fruits, tomatoes, and green and yellow vegetables that accounts for the upward trend in the consumption of fruits and vegetables. The foods that have taken a downward trend are potatoes and cereal products. However, the 1963 records show a shift in the consumption of potatoes with an increase over the 1957–1959 period (6). The consumption of meat and eggs has been variable. Since the depression of the early thirties, the per capita use of meat, fish, and poultry has moved upward. The trend in the use of eggs has been downward over the past ten years.

▶ FOOD SUPPLY FOR PEOPLE OF THE WORLD

Through the Food and Agriculture Organization of the United Nations information is gathered on the supply of food for the people of the world. There is not enough food at the time this is being written, nor was there enough at the first meeting of the FAO in 1945. In the intervening years, the quantity of food produced has increased but the world population has also increased. However, developments are promising. In 1945 food production per capita was not increasing as fast as the population; by 1949 the relationship was reversed with food production per capita in the lead. Dr. B. R. Sen, Director-General, Food and Agriculture Organization indicated in 1962 (25), that taking the world as a whole, the rate of population growth in developing countries approached 2.5 per cent per annum, and the volume of agriculture was increasing at slightly less than 3 per cent per annum. Improved production within the countries and better global distribution of food has contributed to the more favorable supply. Much credit is due to the work of the FAO in helping the member countries to improve their farming practices (15).

The regions of population concentration and regions of large food production do not coincide. Total food production has increased in the past decade from as much as 20 per cent in some developing countries to as much as 50 per cent in others. Improvements in diets that would have been expected by the increase in food production have been, as Dr. Sen states, "largely nullified by population increase." Figure 20.6 shows the relationship between world population and agricultural production; Fig. 20.7 shows the food deficit countries. The method used for identifying food deficit countries was computation of the national average food supply per capita and comparison of the amount of food energy, animal protein, total protein, and fat provided with minimum reference standards.

The projected trend of increases in population and food supply per capita indicate that in economically advanced countries agricultural output can be expanded easily, in less-developed countries agricultural

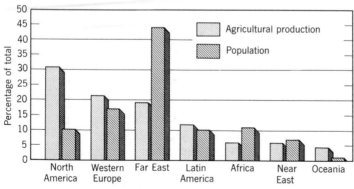

Fig. 20.6.   Regional shares of world population and agricultural production, average 1957 to 1959. Production data based on price-weighted aggregates. (From *Development Through Food*, Food Agr. Organ. U.N. Basic Study 2, p. 58, 1962.)

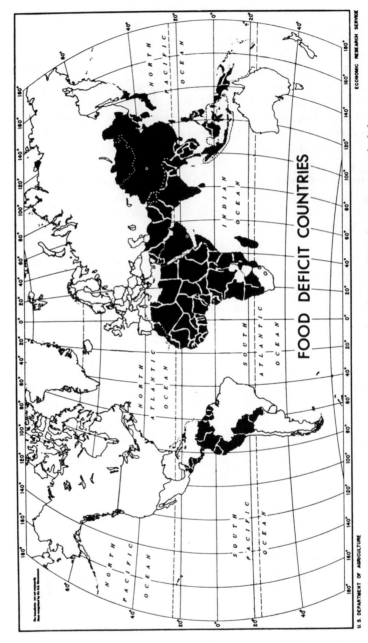

FOOD DEFICIT COUNTRIES

Fig. 20.7. Map showing food deficit countries of the world. Deficit countries are shaded on the map (Courtesy of Brown, U.S. Dept. Agr., Foreign Agr. Econ. Rept. 11, p. 37, 1963.)

production is increased with difficulty (Table 20.2). The total increase in food supply between 1958 and 1980 sufficient to provide a minimum adequate nutritional standard, it is estimated, will require an annual average rate of increase of 3.5 per cent. Over the last several years the annual rate of increase in food production has been 2.9 per cent (7).

Despite the remarkable progress that has been made, problems remain—of how to increase productivity, how to distribute the world's food supply to avoid surpluses in one area and meager supplies in another, how to know what foods are needed and how much. There is a further problem with which the FAO workers must cope, and that is breaking through years of established traditions to persuade adoption of new and better methods of production and better use of the natural resources.

The cost of food in relation to income is a barrier to attaining a diet that meets a satisfactory nutritional level. In order to compare the cost of food relative to income in different countries, the FAO has estimated the income on the basis of the number of hours required for the average factory worker to earn the cost of three diets each with a different

Table 20.2. Percentage Increases of Food Supply Needed during 1958-1980 to Meet Anticipated Requirements in Various Regions of the World

	Projected Population Growth 1958-1980, %[a]	Per capita Increase of Food Supply Presently Required to Meet Target, %	Total Increase of Food Supply, 1958-1980 Required to Meet Target and Population Growth, %	Rate of Annual Increase Needed 1958-1980, %	Recent Annual Rate of Increase in Food Supply[b], %
Underdeveloped countries	56	33	107	3.4	2.7
Latin America	85[c]	5[c]	94[c]	3.1[c]	2.5[d]
Far East	55	41	86	2.9	3.0[e]
Near East	62	17	90	3.0	3.1
Africa	36	28	55	2.0	1.3
Developed countries	28	—	28	1.2	3.6
World	48	14	69	2.4	2.9

[a] Based on United Nations "Medium" projections as shown in "The Future Growth of World Population" (United Nations Publications, Sales No. 58 XIII 2).
[b] Computed from averages of food production in 1952/53 and 1959/60, FAO, State of Food and Agriculture, 1960, and FAO Yearbook, 1959.
[c] Excluding River Plate countries. [d] Including River Plate countries. [e] Excluding mainland China.
From Population and Food Supply, The United Nations, Basic Study No. 7, 1962, p. 29.

caloric value and animal protein content. In Table 20.3 Diet A is representative of diets in economically underdeveloped countries; Diet B is representative of the diets in countries at early stages of industrialization; Diet C is representative of diets in economically advanced countries. Each set of diets contains the foods customarily used in the respective countries, and the cost is also based on prices in those countries. Even small increases in income reflect improved diets among the most deprived. It should be pointed out that whereas Diet A needs improvement, it is folly to hope or to plan for diet C for the people of the world.

It is apparent that there can be no substantial improvement in the diets of less well-developed countries until production is increased and the people as a whole have higher incomes. However, some improvement can be effected through education in nutrition, and special food distribution and welfare plans (7).

▶ DIETARY STUDIES AND THEIR USE

Dietary studies provide a means of determining the kinds and amounts of foods eaten by individuals or groups (23). The information may be a dietary history, that is, a record of foods usually eaten, or an accounting of current food selection practices. The records may be concise or they may be generalizations; they may be for a small community or on a national or worldwide scale. The use to be made of the findings

Table 20.3. Number of Hours' Work Required for Average Factory Workers to Earn the Cost of Three Representative Meals for One Person for One Day

	Diet A	Diet B	Diet C
Calorie value of diet	2100	2500	3000
Grams of animal protein	10–12	15–20	40–45
Country		*Hours of Work*	
India	2.1	2.9	4.5
Japan	1.8	2.3	3.8
Italy	1.1	1.5	3.2
Mexico	0.6	0.8	1.4
Sweden	0.4	0.6	0.9
Denmark	0.3	0.4	0.7
Canada	0.2	0.3	0.5
United States	0.2	0.2	0.4

From *The State of Food and Agriculture*. Food Agr. Organ. U.N., p. 108, 1957.

dictates to considerable extent the methods to be used in collecting the information.

Food consumption data serve widely divergent interests. For effective nutrition education programs, a knowledge of the food habits of the persons for whom the plans are being made is an essential prerequisite. Nothing can be more irritating than to be advised to follow a practice that is already in effect. In conjunction with the assessment of nutritional status, a dietary history of the usual food practices, together with current variations, permits a more advised interpretation of the findings.

The Food Intake of Individuals

For obtaining information on the food habits of individuals four different procedures or combinations thereof are in common use (1, 4, 9, 14, 17, 27, 34, 36, 37). They include 1) the dietary history, 2) the 24-hour recall, 3) the dietary record, and 4) weighed dietaries. The methods differ in the precision with which the records are obtained.

The dietary history yields information on the usual pattern of food consumption followed over a period of time. It is obtained by interview, as a rule. Burke, who developed the method and used it so successfully in the Harvard prenatal studies, has pointed out that the person doing the interview is the key to success in taking the history. The interviewer, she believes, must be a keen observer and must have a familiarity with the characteristic food habits of the group she is interviewing. The dietary history is used most commonly in research studies; long-term food habits help to explain the current nutritional status of individuals.

The 24-hour recall is the most expedient method of obtaining information on food eaten. It usually entails a brief interview in which the subject is asked to recall all food consumed during the last 24-hour period, starting with the last meal or food eaten. The most common use for information obtained by this method is as the basis for educational programs. In research studies that have involved the food habits of large numbers of individuals, the recall method has proved to be both fairly quick and sufficiently accurate to be used with confidence.

In the food record procedure the individual keeps an account of the kinds and amounts of all foods eaten for a specified period of time. The Northeast Regional Research group (36) found that a one-week record was sufficiently long to give representative information for use as the basis for an educational program. Students in college, high school students, even children in the elementary grades keep food records which serve as the basis for nutrition education with the respective groups. For those who are attempting to reduce, a record of everything eaten and a tally of the total Calorie intake has been found to be an effective curb on the appetite. The days of the week selected for the study are found to make a difference in the final results; school children, and college students also, tend to eat differently over the weekend than on other days of the week (10).

A fourth method of determining the food intake of individuals is by actually weighing all food eaten. This method is precise and accurate but time consuming and expensive. As a consequence, it is confined chiefly to research studies in which food samples representative of that eaten are analyzed quantitatively in the laboratory for nutrient content.

The Food Intake of Groups

Two methods commonly used for obtaining information on the food habits of families and other groups are the food-inventory method and the food-list method.

In the food-inventory method, all foods on hand are weighed at the beginning and close of the study period, and a record is kept of all foods added to the supply during that time. From these records it is possible to determine by weight the amount of food used by the family or institutional group. An estimate of waste must be made either by actual weight or by computing the inedible portion as indicated in food composition tables. The latter procedure does not take into account plate waste and spoilage. Corrections must also be made for food eaten by guests and for meals eaten away. Menus used during the period of study are an added check on the validity of the food records.

For the food-list method, an estimate is obtained of the quantities of food (by weight, retail unit, or household measure) used during a certain period by the family or group. This method has the advantage of requiring only a short visit by the worker, and much less of the time of the group being studied than the inventory method. It is not as accurate as the inventory procedure but it gives an acceptable estimate when an approximation is all that is desired.

The National Average Nutrient Consumption Per Capita.

Estimates of yearly per capita consumption of various foods on a national basis are derived from statistics of production, foreign trade, inventories on hand, industrial uses, feed, use and losses in distribution between farm and kitchen. Calculations on the nutrient content of the supplies available for human consumption are made, and the per capita value determined by using census population figures. These values are indicative of the relative adequacy of the national food supply. The per capita national averages are for the country as a whole and are of value in indicating trends in food habits and for estimating production needs (5).

REFERENCES

1. Adelson, S. (1961). Practical procedures for dietary surveys. *Proc. Third Intern. Congr. Dietet.*, London, p. 158.
2. Aykroyd, W. K. (1961). Reflections on human food patterns. *Nutrition* 15: 65.
3. Burgess, A., and R. F. A. Dean (eds.) (1962). *Malnutrition and Food Habits.* The Macmillan Co., New York, p. 16.
4. Burke, B. S. (1947). The dietary history as a tool in research. *J. Am. Dietet. Assoc.* 23: 1041.
5. *Consumption of Food in the United States 1909–1952. Supplement for 1962* (1963). U.S. Dept. Agr., Agr. Handbook No. 62, Washington, D.C.
6. Consumption of food (1963). *Natl. Food Situation*, U.S. Dept. Agr., Washington, D.C., August, pp. 6–7.
7. Cook, R. C. (1962). *Population and Food Supply.* Food Agr. Organ. U.N., Basic Study No. 7, Rome.
8. *Dietary Levels of Households in the United States. Household Food Consumption Survey, 1955* (1957). U.S. Dept. Agr., Rept. 6, Washington, D.C.
9. *Dietary Surveys: Their Technique and Interpretation* (1949). Food Agr. Organ. U.N., FAO Nutr. Studies No. 4, Rome.
10. Eppright, E. S., M. B. Patton, A. L. Marlatt, and M. L. Hathaway (1952). V. Some problems in collecting dietary information about groups of children. *J. Am. Dietet. Assoc.* 28: 43.
11. *Food Consumption and Dietary Levels of Households as Related to Employment of Homemaker, United States, by Regions. Household Food Consumption Survey, 1955.* (1960). U.S. Dept. Agr., Rept. 15, Washington, D.C.
12. Foster, G. M. (1962). *Traditional Cultures: and the Import of Technological Change.* Harper and Row, New York, p. 76.
13. Guthe, C. E., and M. Mead (1943). *The Problem of Changing Food Habits.* Natl. Acad. Sci.—Natl. Res. Council, Bull. 108, Washington, D.C.
14. McHenry, E. W., and G. H. Beaton (1963). *Basic Nutrition*, Revised edition. J. B. Lippincott Co., Philadelphia, p. 309.
15. *Millions Still Go Hungry* (1957). Food Agr. Organ. U.N., Rome.
16. Mirone, L., and E. L. Whitehead (1957). Milk drinking by college students. *J. Am. Dietet. Assoc.* 33: 1266.
17. Morgan, A. F. (ed.) (1959). *Nutritional Status U.S.A.* Univ. Calif. Agr. Expt. Sta., Bull. 769, Berkeley.
18. Myers, M. L., E. M. Sullivan, and F. J. Stare (1963). Foods consumed by university students. *J. Am. Dietet. Assoc.* 43: 336.
19. Odland, L. M., L. Page, and L. P. Guild (1955). Nutrient intakes and food habits of Montana students. *J. Am. Dietet. Assoc.* 31: 1134.
20. Peryam, D. R., B. W. Polemis, J. M. Kamen, J. Eindhaven, and F. J. Pilgrim (1960). *Food Preferences of Men in the U.S. Armed Forces.* Quartermaster Food and Container Institute for the Armed Forces, Chicago.
21. *Recommended Dietary Allowances Sixth Revised Edition* (1964). Natl. Acad. Sci.—Natl. Res. Council, Publ. 1146, Washington, D.C.
22. Reese, R. B., and S. F. Adelson (1962). *Food Consumption and Dietary Levels under the Pilot Food Stamp Program.* U.S. Dept. Agr., Agr. Econ. Rept. 19, Washington, D.C.
23. Reh, E. (1962). *Manual on Household Food Consumption Surveys.* Food Agr. Organ. U.N., Rome. 96 pp.

24. Rockwell, G. R. (1959). *Income and Household Size.* U.S. Dept. Agr., Marketing Res. Rept. 340, Washington, D.C.
25. Sen, B. R. (1962). The nutritional state of the world. In *The Role of Food in World Peace.* Ohio State Univ., Columbus.
26. Simoons, F. J. (1961). *Eat Not This Flesh.* University Wisconsin Press, Madison, p. 87.
27. Stevens, H. A., R. E. Bleiler, and M. A. Ohlson (1963). Dietary intake of five groups of subjects, 24-hour recall as dietary patterns. *J. Am. Dietet. Assoc.* **42:** 387.
28. Tucker, R. E., P. T. Brown, and D. I. Hedrick (1955). *Ascorbic Acid Content of Fruits and Vegetables Served College Students.* Univ. Rhode Island Agr. Expt. Sta., Bull. 331, Kingston.
29. Tucker, R. E., et al. (1952). *Cooperative Nutritional Status Studies in the Northeast Region. 4. Dietary Findings.* Univ. Rhode Island Agr. Expt. Sta., Bull. 379, Kingston.
30. Wilcox, E. B., H. L. Gillum, and M. M. Hard (1955). *Cooperative Nutritional Status Studies in the Western Region. 1 Nutrient Intake.* Utah State Univ. Agr. Expt. Sta., Bull. 383, Logan.
31. Young, C. M., K. Berresford, and B. C. Waldner (1956). What the homemaker knows about nutrition. III. Relation of knowledge to practice. *J. Am. Dietet. Assoc.* **32:** 321.
32. Young, C. M., E. Day, and H. H. Williams (1954). *Nutritional Status Studies of Students.* Cornell Univ., Ithaca, N.Y.
33. Young, C. M., B. M. Einset, E. L. Empey, and V. U. Serraon (1957). Nutrient intake of college men. *J. Am. Dietet. Assoc.* **33:** 374.
34. Young, C. M., G. C. Hagan, R. L. Tucker, and W. D. Foster (1952). A comparison of dietary study methods. II. Dietary history vs. seven-day record vs. 24-hour recall. *J. Am. Dietet. Assoc.* **28:** 218.
35. Young, C. M., and H. L. Pilcher (1950). Nutritional status survey Groton Township, New York. 2. Nutrient usage of families and individuals. *J. Am. Dietet. Assoc.* **26:** 776.
36. Young, C. M., et al. (1952). *Cooperative Nutritional Status Studies in the Northeast Region. III. Dietary Methodology Studies.* Univ. Mass. Agr. Expt. Sta., Bull. 469, Amherst.
37. Young, C. M., and M. F. Trulson (1960). Methodology for dietary studies in epidemiological surveys. II. Strengths and weaknesses of existing methods. *Am. J. Public Health* **50:** 803.

SUPPLEMENTARY REFERENCES

Anderson, L., and J. H. Browe (1960). *Nutrition and Family Health Service.* W. B. Saunders Co., Philadelphia.

Fleck, H., and E. D. Munves (1962). *Introduction to Nutrition.* The Macmillan Co., New York.

Guthe, C. E. and M. Mead (1945). *Manual for the Study of Food Habits.* Natl. Acad. Sci.—Natl. Res. Council, Bull. III, Washington, D.C.

Handbook of Household Surveys (1964), United Nations Studies in Methods Series F No. 10, New York.

Martin, E. A. (1963). *Nutrition in Action.* Holt, Rinehart, and Winston, New York.

Mead, M. (1964). Food Habits Research: Problems of the 1960's. Natl. Acad. Sci.—Natl. Res. Council, Pub. 1225, Washington, D.C.

CHAPTER 21

Nutritional status
and weight control

The physical well-being of an individual is related closely to his status of nutrition. Furnishing adequate food to a well-functioning body assures good nutrition. On the other hand, poor nutrition results from an inadequate food intake, or a failure of the body to use efficiently the nutrients supplied to it.

Malnutrition is not a simple syndrome. The poorly nourished individual, as a rule, suffers from a complexity of deficiencies. The great diversity of body functions that may be ill-affected by inadequate nutrition complicates the process of assessing nutritional status.

▶ **METHODS OF ASSESSING NUTRITIONAL STATUS**

The appearance of an individual gives some indication of his state of nutrition even to the untrained eye. Underweight and overweight individuals are readily recognized. A child who is the "picture of health" or one who is pale and listless can be easily identified (Fig. 21.1 and 21.2).

For a more refined diagnosis one or all of the following three procedures may be used: clinical observations, physical measurements, and laboratory analyses (10, 23). In assessing nutritional status, the methods to be used are determined by the purpose for which the observations are being made, and the personnel and funds available for doing the work.

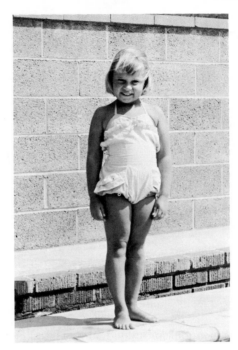

Fig. 21.1.   A well-nourished 5 year old.

In conjunction with the assessment of nutritional status, a dietary history of usual food practices, together with those currently followed, permits a more advised interpretation of findings (discussed in Chapter 20).

Clinical Signs as a Means of Assessing Nutritional Status

The appearance and behavior of an individual are useful guides in evaluating state of nutrition (24). A periodical examination by a physician helps detect incipient undernutrition in children.

Characteristics of a Well-Nourished Person

General appearance of vitality and well-being; eyes are clear and bright with no dark circles beneath them; hair is smooth and glossy.

Skeleton is sturdy; strong, straight arms and legs, well-shaped head and chest; sound, well-formed teeth, set in well-shaped jaws, good occlusion, healthy gums.

Muscles well developed and strong, with proper balance of various muscles; posture generally erect.

Subcutaneous fat sufficient to make a moderate padding over the skeleton and muscles, giving the body a well-rounded contour.

Body functions related to nutrition proceed normally; good appetite and digestion, regular elimination; sleep sound and refreshing; stable nervous system; good endurance, prompt and adequate recovery from fatigue.

Characteristics of a Poorly Nourished Person

Does not have the appearance and buoyance of physical well-being.

Lacks some or all of the characteristics of the well-nourished person.

Hyperirritable and unhappy, with a strained, tense attitude especially when underweight.

Even though lacking in physical endurance, often hyperactive when underweight.

Specific symptoms of poor nutrition due to an insufficiency of certain nutrients in the diet are described in the chapters devoted to essential dietary components.

Physical Measurements as a Means of Assessing Nutritional Status

During childhood acceptable growth is a fairly good index of nutritional status. Physical measurements of individual children to determine their growth is the most widely used method for assessing nutritional status. Body weight and height are the measurements most commonly made; children are weighed and measured at school, at home, and at the physician's office. Adults, too, tend to follow their weight closely. Weight-height measurements have the distinct advantage of being easily and quickly made. Certain precautions must be taken, however, so that the measurements are accurate. The following suggestions if followed closely will help to reduce the error in determining body weight: weigh wearing the same amount of clothing each time, after emptying the bladder and without a recent drink, and an hour or so after a meal. An accurate scale should be used.

Certain precautions should be taken in measuring height also. The stance makes a difference. For the measurement, the subject should stand

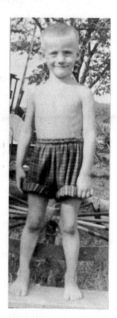

Fig. 21.2. A 5-year old showing symptoms of undernutrition.

with back against a flat surface, such as a wall or a measuring board on which a tape has been attached. With heels together and against the flat surface, the individual is asked to "stand straight." By placing a board, prepared for this purpose, on his head, parallel to the floor, the height can be read from the tape. There is a tendency for all of us, both young and old, to slump a bit with the progress of the day. It is more pronounced on some days than others and is related to a considerable degree to fatigue. As a consequence, repeated measurements taken following the reminder "to stand straight" give values that agree more closely than those taken without directions given as to stance.

Physical measurements, repeated at intervals, give a picture of the pattern of growth of the individual child. Each grows at his own rate and in a fashion peculiar to himself, influenced both by his inheritance and the environment in which he lives (13). Despite the marked differences in growth behavior among individual children, there is a common all-over pattern that most children seem to follow.

The general trend of growth in height from birth to maturity assumes an S curve, representing four different phases of growth rate. The first phase is one of rapid growth, extending from birth through the first year. This is followed by a period of slower growth covering the years from early childhood to around 12 years of age. The third phase is another period of accelerated growth, beginning with the preadolescent "spurt," reaching a peak at about the thirteenth year for girls, and the fifteenth for boys. As illustrated in Fig. 21.3, boys and girls who were taller at six years old grew faster and stopped growing earlier than those who were shorter at that age. The last phase of growth is one of decline as adulthood approaches.

Valuable as height-weight measurements are in following the growth of individual children, sometimes they are misused. When a child is expected to meet the size recorded in standard height-weight-age tables, we believe that his measurements are being misused. In the past the custom of using deviations from the tables in body weight as criteria for judging under- or overnutrition was more prevalent than it is today. It is apparent to those who really understand that it is not reasonable to expect children of the same age to be the same weight (Fig. 21.4). There are inherent factors of difference. One of the most significant is that of body build. Not only does the height of an individual make a difference in body weight but also the width of the hips, the breadth of the shoulders, and the size of the bones affect the weight.

It is now generally recognized that if the growth of a child is to be related to a standard, that standard must make allowances for differences in body build. Several such procedures have been developed, allowing for variable heights and weights at each age level. Meredith (27), at the

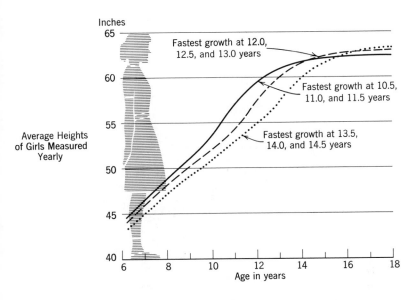

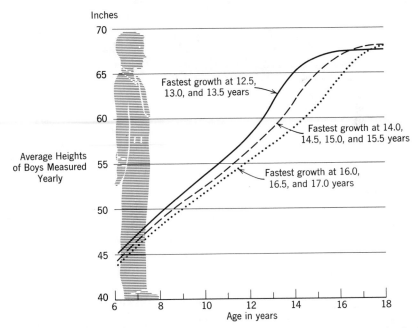

Fig. 21.3. The growth pattern of boys and girls. (Courtesy of Hathaway, *Food, Yearbook of Agriculture 1959*, p. 184, 1959.)

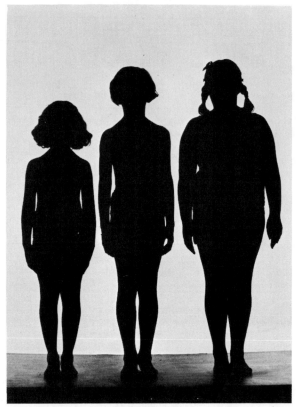

Fig. 21.4.   Three 8-year-old girls of different body builds and sizes. (Courtesy of Agriculture Research Service, U.S. Department of Agriculture.)

University of Iowa, established standards of reference from his measurements of Iowa children. He established five zones of height and five zones of weight for each age from 4 to 18 years. The descriptive terms applied to zones of height are *tall, moderately tall, average, moderately short,* and *short.* For weight they are *heavy, moderately heavy, average, moderately light,* and *light.* Charts bearing the zones of height and weight for age make it possible to plot the height and weight of individual children and then to follow visually their growth pattern (Fig. 21.5). The chart gives an indication of body build. For example, if the child's height for his age falls in the short zone, it means he is short for his age; if his weight falls in the average zone, it means he is of average body weight for his age, and so on. Meredith explains that in using the physical growth chart, "the relation of an individual's height and weight curves to the appropriate normative curves gives information on

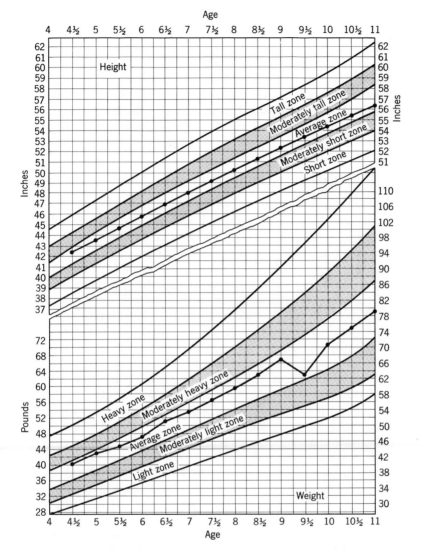

Fig. 21.5. Meredith physical growth chart for recording the growth in height and weight. The record reproduced on the chart is based on actual height and weight measurements provided by Dr. Meredith. In using the chart to plot the height, find the age across the top, the height along the upper left hand margin, locating the dot on the chart at the intersection of imaginary lines extended from those points. For weight, find the age along the lower edge of the chart, weight along the lower left hand margin, and locate the dot on the chart at the intersection of the imaginary lines. At 9½ years, Susan whose chart this is, developed allergies and infected tonsils, which apparently caused failure to gain weight until she was successfully treated. (Courtesy of Mrs. Martin and D. H. V. Meredith, permission the University of Chicago Press. From Martin, *Roberts' Nutrition Work with Children*, p. 128 and 371, 1954.)

satisfactoriness of growth. Downward dips, plateaus, or sharp upward turns indicate probable need of medical attention."

Another procedure for following the development of children was introduced by Wetzel (44). His method, too, is graphic, employing a chart known as the *Wetzel Grid*. There are three panels on the chart, one locates the child as to body build, another includes his physical development in relation to his age, and the third, designated as the energy panel, relates to the basal heat production and energy need of the child.

Laboratory Analyses as a Means of Assessing Nutritional Status

The laboratory method of assessing nutritional status is relatively more sensitive than the other two methods (recognition of clinical signs and physical measurements), particularly in detecting early evidences of poor nutrition. Chemical determinations of the composition of the blood and urine, microscopic examination of the blood, and x-ray photographs of the bones and teeth are among the laboratory procedures used in assessing nutritional status by this general method. Alterations from the accepted range of values forewarn of conditions which, if not checked, may cause a stunting of growth and other symptoms of malnutrition apparent to the naked eye (32).

There are certain limitations to the widespread use of laboratory analyses as a means of assessing nutritional status. The techniques demand trained personnel, the procedures are lengthy, and the cost almost prohibitive for routine use. As a consequence, this method is confined chiefly to use in medical clinics and in research studies.

To illustrate the use of the laboratory method a research study of the nutritional status of New Mexico adolescents is cited (18). Included in the determinations was analysis of the blood for the following constituents: hemoglobin, serum protein, ascorbic acid, riboflavin, and vitamin A. Average values for the group under study were determined for each constituent. How these values were then further used is illustrated by the example of ascorbic acid. The investigators found 51 per cent of the children to have serum ascorbic acid levels below 0.5 mg per 100 ml; levels below 0.6 mg are usually considered borderline and 0.4 mg definitely abnormal. The "generally low" ascorbic acid values of the blood were found to be accompanied by a low ascorbic acid content of the diet.

Certain of the common laboratory methods for detecting symptoms of insufficient nutrients in the diet are cited in preceding chapters devoted to the specific nutrients.

► NUTRITIONAL STATUS OF POPULATIONS

Within the last two decades the nutritional assessment of populations has been in progress around the world. Some research was supported by private, other by public funds. During the years 1947–1958 an extensive survey in the United States was sponsored by state agricultural experiment stations, the Cooperative State Research Service with funds for Regional Research, the U.S. Department of Agriculture, the Institute of Home Economics of the U.S. Department of Agriculture, and the public health departments of several states (29). International surveys have been conducted by the Interdepartmental Committee on Nutrition for National Development (ICNND), representing departments of the United States Government concerned with health, agriculture, and defense, and also by medical and health units brought together by the Food and Agriculture Organization of the United Nations.

In the survey carried out in the United States, men, women, and children were studied. The sample was comprised of 4210 men and women from 12 states, and 4394 children from 18 states. The findings from this broad national study were summarized by Agnes Fay Morgan in a bulletin entitled *Nutritional Status—USA* (29).

Certain findings were common among all groups from all regions of the country. Concerning the diets, the nutrients most frequently provided in less than the recommended amounts were vitamin A, ascorbic acid, calcium, and iron. The blood values in general, conformed with expectations from the diet record. The concentrations of vitamin A and ascorbic acid of the blood of nearly all the persons examined were described as ranging from generally fair to good; the hemoglobin level from fair to excellent. The physical symptoms such as, roughness of skin, inflammation and thickening of the mucous membrane of the eyes, swollen and reddened gums, occurred more frequently in the groups with low blood levels of vitamin A and ascorbic acid than in those with satisfactory levels.

The success of the Eskimo in adapting to his limited and uncertain food supply has puzzled nutritionists for many years. In 1958 a special study of the health and nutritional status of Alaskan Eskimos was initiated (21). Two battalions of National Guardsmen and the civilian population in selected villages in two regions of the state served as the sample. From this extensive study only the data on men have been published thus far. The findings on the habits of the villagers are reported here because they are expected to be more representative of the population as a whole. However, the investigators warn that the food pattern of the Eskimo is highly variable. The total daily energy intake for all men averaged 1855 ± 784* Calories; protein 136.0 ± 95.2* gm (25 to 30 per cent of total Calories); fat 72.9 ± 46.4* gm (35 per cent of total Calories); carbohydrate 167.6 ± 79.4* gm (35 per cent of total Calories). The diet that the 97 men who comprised the sample were consuming was lower in total Calories, higher in protein, lower in carbohydrates, and somewhat lower in fat than the common pattern for the United States which for adults is protein 10 to 15 per cent, fat 35 to 40 per cent, and carbohydrate 45 to 50 per cent of the total Calories. Contrary to popular belief, the diets of Eskimos were not high in fat content.

The average calcium, iron, and vitamin intakes are summarized in Table 21.1, together with values proposed by the Interdepartmental Committee on Nutrition for National Development (ICNND) for evaluating nutrient intake data, and the National Research Council (NRC) Recommended Daily Allowances for men 35 to 55 years of age. The average nutrient intake equaled the National Research Council recommendation for calcium, iron, and riboflavin. When using the mean as an index of intake, the wide variation among individuals, as evidenced by the large standard deviation, should be noted. Average thiamine intakes were at the lower level of the ICNND range. Vitamin A and vitamin C intakes were considerably lower than the National Research Council recommendations. The average vitamin A intake would be classified as deficient according to the ICNND guide. Biochemical findings revealed accordingly, low serum vitamin A levels and occasional Bitot spots, which are white, elevated patches on the conjunctiva of the eye. The average vitamin C level in the blood came within the ICNND acceptable range; however, the levels of some individuals were classified as deficient but scurvy was not observed. The investigators term this circumstance a dietary "riddle" and explain the paradox by pointing out that sporadically a few exceptionally rich sources of vitamin C such as willow leaves and cloudberries are included in the diet.

The nutritional status of the population of a number of developing countries of the world has been studied by teams of investigators from this country and others. Kark (16) describes three major forms of disturbed nutrition that may be found: hunger and starvation due to lack of food; protein malnutrition; and the least common of the three, classical vitamin deficiency diseases such as pellagra, beriberi, rickets, and scurvy.

At a conference on Malnutrition and Food Habits (7), malnutrition in five selected regions, Uganda, South India, Central America, Mexico,

* Standard deviation.

Table 21.1. Daily Food Consumption of Eskimo Men[1] as Compared to the ICNND Guide to Evaluation[2]; and the NRC Recommended Daily Allowance[3]

| | | Average Daily Intake | | ICNND Guide | | NRC |
		Mean	Standard Deviation	Deficient	Acceptable	RDA
Calcium	mg	1.0	1.3	<0.3	0.4–0.8	0.8
Iron	mg	10.5	7.1	6–8	9–12	10
Vitamin A	IU	1621	1449	<2000	3500–5000	5000
Thiamine	mg	0.64	0.61	<0.2 mg per 1000 Cal.	0.3–0.5 mg per 1000 Cal.	1.0
Riboflavin	mg	1.64	1.29	<0.7	1.2–1.5	1.6
Vitamin C	mg	36	36	<10	30–50	70

[1] From *Am. J. Clin. Nutr.* 11: 63, 1962.
[2] From *Manual for Nutrition Surveys*. Interdepartmental Comm. on Nutr. for Natl. Defense, p. 123, 1957.
[3] *Recommended Dietary Allowances Sixth Revised Edition.* Natl. Acad. Sci.—Natl. Res. Council. Publ. 1146, 1964.

and Indonesia were discussed. A common problem was the inadequate food of the preschool child. The nursing child fares well but not the child who has been weaned. The mortality rates in this group are up to forty times as high in developing countries as in developed countries. The mortality rates from birth to one year of age are about five times greater than in developed countries (38), owing in part to a shortage of food. A further cause is the cultural practice in some regions of requiring the child after he has been weaned to feed himself without assistance.

The prevalence of nutrition problems is disclosed through ICNND surveys. In general, a survey team is composed of the following specialists: "clinical nutritionists, dentists, and on occasion pediatricians to assess the lesions associated with nutritional deficiency; biochemists to analyze blood and urine samples; nutrition specialists and dietitians to collect data on food and nutrient intake, food patterns, taboos, customs, and food preparation; and food technologists and agricultural specialists to evaluate existing agricultural and food-processing practices and determine ways and means for improvement" (34).

Reporting on six countries in which surveys were done, the major nutrition problems identified in Ethiopia were Calorie and vitamin A deficit; in Haiti, a Calorie, protein, and riboflavin deficit; in Lybia, a Calorie, thiamine, and vitamin C deficit; in Taiwan, a riboflavin and vitamin A deficit; in Viet-nam, a riboflavin and thiamine deficit; in Ecuador, no problems were identified for the country as a whole, but in specific areas dietary deficiencies were indicated by the presence of anemia and goiter among the population.

► WEIGHT CONTROL

The Problem of Being Overweight

Obesity is the most common deviation from normal nutrition among the adult population of this country today. From the "Build and Blood Pressure Study," in which records obtained between 1935 and 1954 from twenty-six large life insurance companies were combined, the following estimates of men and women above average weight were made (20): in the 10 per cent or more above *average* weight for height and age classification were 10 per cent of the men and 25 per cent of the women; in the 20 per cent or more above *average* weight for height and age were 5 per cent of the men and 11 per cent of the women. If instead of *average* weight *desirable* weight, which is based on greatest longevity, is the standard for comparison, the overweight problem appears more serious. The *desirable* weights proposed are from 15 to 25 lb less than the *average* weight for those past 30 years of age.

Even though the incidence of obesity was found to be higher among women than men (20), the average weight of women is about 5 lb less than it was a generation ago, whereas for men the average is about 5 lb more (35). Contrast in the clothing worn by women today and a generation ago may be a contributing factor.

Factors Contributing to the Incidence of Overweight

When asked why the incidence of obesity is so high, some answer that it is simply the result of eating too much. That is true, and the answer is based on a fundamental law of science, the *Law of Conservation of Energy*. Stated in simple terms, the provisions of this law, which apply to the energy balance in any machine, are that energy cannot be created and cannot be destroyed but it can be changed from one form to another. Thus in the case of the body as a machine, if the energy value of the food exceeds the Calorie expenditure for work and for heating the body, the remainder will be stored in the tissues as potential energy. Because the body has a relatively limited capacity to store protein and carbohydrate, most of the excess is converted to fat and stored as such.

The question remains as to why people are impelled to eat more food than is needed to supply the energy requirements of the body. There are basic, underlying reasons responsible in the case of each individual. Among the contributing factors are disturbed appetite control, psychosomatic influences, lowered energy need with age, insufficient physical exercise, the role of food in social life, and the *habit* of eating more food than is needed. Obesity in any one person is the end product of a great many contributing factors.

Disturbed Appetite Control. The primary motivations for excessive eating are complex and as yet incompletely understood. We know that appetite is the factor that compels people to eat; by definition, appetite means "desire for food."

"Feeding" and "satiety" control areas have been identified in experimental animals in the hypothalmus of the brain (39). By electrical stimulation of the feeding center, hyperphagia results; destruction of it causes aphagia. Stimulation of the satiety center decreases food intake, destruction of it results in hyperphagia. Mechanisms for the control of these centers are being investigated in several research laboratories.

Increase in blood glucose has been observed in experimental animals to increase the activity of the satiety center and slightly decrease the activity of the feeding center (1). The observation is reasonable because the level of blood glucose rises after eating. Drugs have been identified that suppress appetite by way of the hypothalmus, either by stimulating the satiety center or by suppressing the feeding center (35).

Appetite allows eating when there is no need for food. The kinds of foods desired are those that have been eaten previously and enjoyed, or foods, although new, look, smell, or taste like those enjoyed. All persons have been victims of tricks of the appetite. For instance, at the end of a heavy meal all proffered food is declined on the basis of "being full" until offered a favorite delicacy which is eaten, and enjoyed.

At Cornell University twelve students whose weights normally remained constant were given a special liquid supplement of 1100 Cal. each night about 10 o'clock. The purpose of the investigation was to see if the body could control the appetite, automatically reducing the caloric intake at other times of day to make allowance for the extra Calories in the supplement. Some adjustment was made by the body, approximately 50 per cent—the intake in the usual meals was reduced by 500 Cal. The students gained weight. This practical experiment indicates that there is a regulatory mechanism in man that *helps* to maintain energy balance but it appears not to operate perfectly in all persons (11).

At one time it was thought that the contractions characteristic of an empty stomach brought about the desire to eat. Doubt was cast on this, however, when in experimental animals the desire for food continued after the contractions of the stomach were stopped by severing the nerve connections or by actually removing the stomach.

Psychological Aspects. It is believed that some persons eat excessively to compensate for distraught feelings and pent-up emotions. Idleness and boredom tend to lead to nibbling; taking a snack seems to help break the monotony.

A more fundamental emotional involvement is described by Bruch and others (5, 6, 33). Bruch believes that the weight the body stubbornly holds is the "preferred" weight for that individual. It may not be the weight the person professes to desire or the weight the doctor may have recommended. It is the weight, however, that the body "in its mysterious self-regulatory capacity, *prefers* as its pattern of adaptation."

Lowered Energy Need with Age. It is characteristic of persons past middle age to tend to gain weight. One of the contributing causes is diminishing energy need with advancing age. The basal metabolic rate is lower, and in addition there is usually a greater disinclination to exercise than in the younger years. The decreased energy need gradually creeps up on people. They fail to adjust their caloric intake and as a consequence begin to accumulate more fatty tissue than is desirable.

Insufficient Exercise. Among the general factors contributing to overweight is failure to get enough exercise. In fact Mayer and Stare of Harvard (26) have called inactivity "the most important factor explaining the frequency of 'creeping' overweight in modern Western societies." We enjoy the use of many labor-saving devices which, we are reluctant to admit, contribute to our failure to exercise. It is a genuine help to sedentary persons who have a tendency to gain weight to plan a regular schedule of physical exercise properly strenuous for their age.

Food and Friendship. Serving food is a friendly gesture and as such often results in the consumption of more food than is desirable for weight watchers. Eating together and giving gifts of food are integral parts of our social life. No one wishes to change these cordial customs, but it does mean that for persons wishing to control their weight, adjustment for the added energy must be made in other meals of the day.

Habit. Habit is responsible for overweight in many people. The practice of following certain meal patterns and selecting certain foods is continued even though the energy need may have been reduced. For example, if 60 extra Calories of energy are consumed each day (an extra slice of bread, or one small apple, or two Brazil nuts, or a specified amount of any other food), in a year this extra food consumption would amount to 21,900 Cal., which is roughly equivalent to 2433 gm fat (21,900 Cal./9 Cal. per gm fat). The amount of weight added would be about 5 lb annually, and in 10 years an approximate 50 lb.

Relation of Obesity to Health

Certain ill effects to health are attributed to obesity. Blood pressure tends to rise with increasing degree of overweight, also the mortality rate increases (Table 21.2). The increased incidence of death among the obese was greatest for persons with diabetes for both men and women, followed by nephritis and diseases of the digestive system, mainly biliary tract and liver disorders for men, and of the heart and circulatory system for women (Table 21.3).

The relationship between the incidence of obesity and heart disease is not entirely clear. Whereas life insurance statistics show obesity to be a predisposing factor to heart disease, a study of coronary heart disease among men 46 to 64 years of age living in Minneapolis showed coronary patients to have no greater tendency to obesity than men of the same age of normal health (17).

Overweight in Children

Some children are a bit overweight simply because they have a good appetite, eat food high in nutritive value, and have a good digestive system to take care of the quantity of food eaten. They are well fed. On the other hand, there are children who are overweight who are poorly nourished. Their diets have provided more than enough energy but less than enough of some or all of the nutrients for good nutrition (14).

The incidence of overweight was found to occur more frequently in girls than in boys in studies of children from the elementary grades through high school. Whether the parents are normal weight or obese makes a difference in the incidence of obesity in the child. Observations of

Table 21.2. Mortality Rate among Overweight Men and Women

Excess Mortality (per cent) for Various Degrees of Overweight

Age Group[1] (without known minor impairments)	Deviation above Average Weight		
	10%	20%	30%
Men[2] 15–69	5	15	30
15–39	3	15	30
40–69	8	16	31
Women[3] 15–69	2	11	20
15–39	1	6	12
40–69	3	15	25

[1] At issue of insurance policy.
[2] Compared with all persons insured as standard risks.
[3] Compared with all women insured as standard risks.

From *Statistical Bulletin*, Metropolitan Life Insurance Co., February–March 1960, New York. Pages 8 and 2, respectively.

Table 21.3. Causes of Death with Per Cent Mortality above Normal among Overweight Men and Women[1]

	Excess Mortality (per cent)	
Cause of Death	For Men[2]	For Women[3]
Cardiovascular-renal diseases		
Heart and circulatory diseases	43	51
Coronary artery disease	35	35
Vascular lesions of central		
nervous system	53	29
Nephritis	73	—
Malignant neoplasms	16	13
Diabetes mellitus	133	83
Pneumonia and influenza	32	27
Diseases of digestive system	68	39
Accidents and homicides	18	—

[1] All cases, with and without known minor impairments, compared with all persons insured as standard risks.

[2] Men, approximately 20 per cent or more above average weight, ages 15 to 69 at issue of insurance policy.

[3] Women, approximately 15 per cent or more above average weight, ages 15 to 69 at issue of insurance policy.

From *Statistical Bulletin*, Metropolitan Life Insurance Co., February–March 1960. New York. Pages 9 and 3, respectively.

Boston children showed an incidence of obesity of 8 to 9 per cent if the parents were of normal weight; if one of the parents was obese, the incidence was 40 per cent; 80 per cent if both parents were obese (25).

Overweight children were found by Mayer (25) to be less active than children of normal weight. They participated in active sports less than one-third as much as non-obese children. Also it was possible through exercise, without attention to the diet, for obese children to lose weight.

Body Composition and Overweight

Obesity is a condition of too much fat in the body. It is a simple matter to weigh an individual but it is not so simple a task to ascertain the proportion of fat in the total weight. For the intelligent treatment of the overweight person, information on the proportion of fat in the individual is needed.

The average content of fat in the body increases with age. At 20 years of age American males have a fat content of about 10 per cent; at age 55 years, 23 per cent. The female at age 20 years, has an average fat content of about 20 per cent; at 55 years, the amount increases to 30 per cent (35).

One method of estimating body fatness is by the skinfold measurement (4, 9, 36). It is apparent that fat is located in subcutaneous tissues; also that the thickness of a fold of skin is influenced by the amount of fat present. More fat obviously is deposited in some areas than in others. When calipers especially designed and calibrated for skinfold measurements are used and measurements are made at selected locations, values are obtained for fat content that approximate the estimates obtained by other more basic methods (42).

A basic experimental method for estimating amount of body fat involves determining the specific gravity of the individual (i.e., ratio of body weight to the weight of water which the body displaces when submerged). This method is based on the fact that the fat-free body (or lean body mass as it is also termed) is quite constant in composition with a specific gravity value of around 1.100. When "diluted" with fat, which has a lower specific gravity (in the neighborhood of 0.92), the specific gravity of the body as a whole is reduced (9). The amount of reduction in the specific gravity is an index of fatness. Actual measurement of the specific gravity of a living subject is not easily determined. The person must be weighed in air and weighed submerged in water. When measuring the body's displacement in water a correction is made for the volume of residual air in the lungs. One means of weighing in water is by using a scale from which an aluminum chair is suspended; the subject is equipped with a snorkel for breathing (41).

Other procedures have been explored as a means of predicting body fatness. Among them is the use of x-rays to record the thickness of the fat layer at specified points on the body. Another is the potassium-40 method, which involves measuring by gamma ray emission the concentration in the body of this naturally occurring isotope. The potassium-40 method is based on the assumption that potassium occurs in the lean body mass only and not in fat tissue, and that the relationship of the amount to that of lean body mass is a constant. By determining the amount of potassium-40 in the whole body, an indication of lean body mass can be estimated. Subtracting lean body mass from total weight yields the weight of body fat (2).

Avoiding Weight Gain

The time to begin curtailing caloric intake is when the first extra pounds are added. Better than reducing is avoiding the need to do so.

The diet for weight reduction is restricted in energy value, but with the protein, mineral, and vitamin content maintained at an adequate level.

The shortage of Calories in the diet is made up from the stores of body fat. The energy value of the diet should be sufficiently limited to bring about a loss of fat at a rate compatible with health; it is generally recommended that the rate not exceed around 2 lb per week.

The diet should be acceptable, insofar as possible, to the person who is reducing, containing foods that are especially enjoyed and offering a possibility of making choices among foods. Such a diet plan can then be adhered to with less feeling of deprivation. It is likely that the diet pattern, with some liberalization, will need to be followed even after normal weight has been attained. When there is a tendency to be overweight a watchful eye to the caloric intake is a good investment in prevention.

The energy level for reduction is peculiar to each individual. In general, however, the level recommended for moderate weight reduction ranges between 1000 and 1500 Cal. for women, and between 1500 and 2000 Cal. for men. These levels approximate roughly the energy need for basal metabolism per day. If the deficit is approximately 1000 Cal. per day, theoretically, about 2 lb per week can be lost.

Irregularity in weight loss of an individual who is maintained on a diet of the same caloric value day after day may be due in part to differences in water retention and also the amount of exercise. An unusually high weight loss (5 or 7 lb) in the first week or so on a reducing diet is most likely due to water loss. On the other hand, failure to lose weight even after faithful adherence to the low-energy diet for as long as two weeks may be due to water retention in the tissues. Then there may occur a considerable loss of fluid by way of the kidneys within a period of a few days, with a loss of weight approaching that which was anticipated in accordance with the caloric restriction. Thus water retention may mask for a few days the loss of fat. Those who persist on the restricted diet and do not surrender with the plea that "it makes no difference when I eat less" are rewarded often by a sudden and sizable reduction in weight. The same pattern of reduction may then be repeated, a plateau followed by sudden and considerable loss of weight (30) (Fig. 21.6).

Diet plans that are adaptations of the normal diet are most satisfactory for reduction. In average diets the distribution of energy among the three foodstuffs, carbohydrate, protein, and fat, in terms of per cent of total Calories is as follows: for the adult, carbohydrate 45 to 50, protein 10 to 15 and fat 40 to 45; for the child, carbohydrate 50, protein 15 per cent, and fat 35. In reducing diets these percentages are changed according to the type of diet fed. The relative proportion of energy from carbohydrate, protein, and fat has been varied in reducing diets in an effort to obtain a palatable food intake that allays the feeling of hunger often experienced, and to prevent the physical exhaustion often felt during reduction.

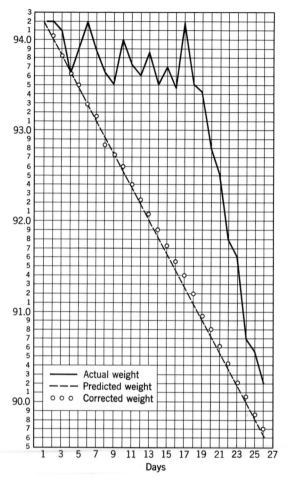

Fig. 21.6. The weight curve of an obese girl. (From Newburgh and Johnston, *The Exchange of Energy*, Charles C. Thomas Company, Springfield, Ill., p. 93, 1930.)

Diets relatively low in fat have been the usual pattern for reducing (3, 19). However, with a diet plan providing approximately 50 per cent of the total energy from fat, low in carbohydrate (20 to 25 per cent of the total Calories), and high in protein (25 to 30 per cent of the total Calories) more satisfactory weight losses in college women were obtained than with diets lower in fat content (43). A feeling of satiety accompanies the consumption of this diet; there is less hunger between meals. An unusual sense of well-being is enjoyed by those on the restricted diet.

The same diet plan can be used for weight reduction as for normal nutrition by omitting the high-energy foods, especially those which supply "Empty Calories" (Calories without food nutrients). A daily food pattern that provides an adequate intake of the essential nutrients for an adult but is restricted in caloric value follows:

Vegetable	2 servings (⅔ cup) of green or yellow vegetables
	1 serving (⅔ cup) of another vegetable
	(1 medium potato may be included to take the place of a serving of cereal or bread)
Fruit	1 serving of citrus fruit or other rich source of ascorbic acid
	1 serving (½–⅔ cup) of another fruit
Meat	3 oz lean meat, fish, or poultry
	1 other source of good protein, which may be another serving of meat, a milk product, or legumes
Egg	1 each day (or 3 to 5 per week) as such or in other foods
Milk	1 pint of milk daily as such or in other foods; the milk may be skimmed
Cereal	2 servings of whole-grain or enriched cereal; this may be 2 slices bread (no cereal) or cereal may be substituted for 1 slice of bread
Fat	2 tbsp of butter, enriched margarine, or other fat.

Using this dietary pattern as a guide, the following menu has been planned to provide almost 1200 Cal., with approximately 50 per cent coming from fat, 35 per cent from carbohydrate, and 15 per cent from protein. In actual practice foods other than those listed in the diet plan

	Energy, Cal.	Prot., gm	Fat, gm	CHO, gm
BREAKFAST				
Orange juice (½ glass)	54	1	tr	14
Egg (1)	77	6	6	tr
Toast, w.w. (1 sl) plus 1 tsp butter	88	2	4	11
Milk, skimmed (1 glass)	87	9	tr	13
(Coffee, if desired, no cream or sugar)	0	0	0	0
	306	18	10	38
LUNCH				
Broiled meat patty (2 oz)	200	13	17	0
Green beans (⅔ c) with 1 tsp butter	51	1	4	4
Celery sticks (1 c)	18	1	tr	4
Apricots (4 medium halves + 2 tbsp sirup)				
without added sugar	100	1	tr	26
	369	16	21	34
DINNER				
Pot roast of beef (3 oz)	245	22	16	0
Carrots (⅔ c) with 1 tsp butter	62	1	4	6
Head lettuce (⅙ head) with lemon juice	7	1	tr	1
Bread w.w. (1 sl)	55	2	1	11
Milk, skimmed (1 glass)	87	9	tr	13
Pineapple, fresh (⅔ c)	50	tr	tr	13
	506	35	21	44

Table 21.4. Energy Value of Selected Vegetables and Fruits

Vegetables Supplying Approximately 5 to 25 Calories per Serving (⅔ cup)

Asparagus	Cucumber	Parsley
Beans, green	Endive	Pepper
Cabbage	Escarole	Radishes
Cauliflower	Lettuce	Sauerkraut
Celery	Mustard greens	Squash, summer

Vegetables Supplying Approximately 25 to 50 Calories per Serving (⅔ cup)

Beets	Kale
Broccoli	Rutabaga
Brussels sprouts	Spinach
Carrots	Tomato

Vegetables Supplying over 50 Calories per Serving (⅔ cup)

Beans, Lima	Peas, green
Corn	Potatoes, white
Onions	Potatoes, sweet
Parsnips	Squash, winter

Fruits Supplying Approximately 100 Calories

Apple, 1 med	Orange juice, 1 cup
Apricots, 4 med halves (sirup packed)	Orange, 1 large
Banana, 1 med	Peach, raw, 2 med
Cantaloupe, 1 melon (5 in. diameter)	Peach, canned in sirup, 2 lg halves
Dates, 4	Pear, 1 raw
Grapefruit, ½ large (5 in. diameter)	Pineapple, 1 cup raw, 2 sm slices
Grapefruit juice, 1 cup	canned
Grapes, 1 cup	Raisins, ¼ cup

but of comparable energy value may be selected according to the taste of the individual. Vegetables and fruits relatively low in caloric value (Table 21.4) may be used freely.

To be omitted from a reducing diet are the extras, such as the whipped cream on the baked apple, the dressing on the salad, and the jelly on the bread. These adjuncts quickly increase the total caloric intake and contribute little to the nutrient content of the diet. In Table 21.5 some of the foods to be avoided are listed.

Table 21.5. Foods to Avoid in Reducing Diets

Candy	Jelly, jams, and similar sweets
Cream	Mayonnaise
Fatty meat	Nuts
French dressing	Pies, cakes, and rich desserts
Gravy	Rich sauces

Is There a Fast and Easy Way to Reduce? Having put on weight over a long period, a long period may be required to take it off. The understandable eagerness of the overweight person to complete the reducing project in a hurry, has prompted the concoction of "fad diets" and "proprietary mixtures" claimed to hasten the process. Such irregular means may jeopardize health. A drastic and unusual reducing diet such as the "banana and skimmilk" diet, or the diet that consists of a "special tablet," or just eggs for some of the days of the week and the usual diet the remainder, are generally low not only in energy content as they should be, but also in one or more of the nutrients, all of which should be adequate in a reducing diet. Such diets are not acceptable for a long-time program, either from the nutritional standpoint or palatability. The proprietary mixtures, pills, and tablets, some of which depress the appetite, should be taken only on the recommendation of a physician and with his continuous supervision.

A practice commonly followed by persons who wish to reduce is to skip a meal, particularly breakfast. We now have research to show that this is not a good plan. Omitting breakfast lowers an individual's efficiency in the late morning hours. Furthermore, omission of a meal usually results in a less adequate total nutrient intake. The breakfast studies are reviewed more completely in Chapter 24.

Staying Reduced

Taking off weight is only the first step; keeping it off is the second problem and often a continuing one (15). Additional Calories should be returned to the diet gradually and only to the extent that there is not an increase in weight. Restriction in food intake is apt to leave the person with a feeling of deprivation; eating is normally an enjoyable experience. Satisfaction in achieving the desired loss in weight, however, is compensation for those who are seriously intent on that goal.

The Problem of Undernutrition

Causes of Undernutrition. Undernutrition may result from a shortage of food, from an inadequacy of certain nutrients, or from an ill-functioning body that fails to utilize the nutriment supplied to it efficiently.

Insufficient food is a world problem (37). There is not enough food in some countries today to allay hunger or to prevent widespread undernutrition. In Table 21.6 the energy and animal protein supply in areas of the world as estimated by FAO are given; the available food in many countries is so meager that millions are hungry. Failure to grow

Table 21.6. Levels of Daily Per Capita Consumption of Food by Regions and Groups of Countries

	Calories			Total Protein, gms			Animal Protein, gms		
Regions	Pre-war	Immediate Post-war	Recent	Pre-war	Immediate Post-war	Recent	Pre-war	Immediate Post-war	Recent
Far East	2120	1910	2070	63	54	56	8	6	8
Near East	2320	2190	2470	76	70	76	15	14	14
Africa	2180	2100	2360	61	61	61	15	15	11
Latin America	2140	2380	2470	66	67	67	30	29	25 .
Europe	2850	2870	3040	85	91	88	27	31	36
Northern America	3140	3120	3120	89	90	93	50	60	66
Oceania	3270	3180	3250	97	95	94	65	65	62
Group I[1]	2130	1960	2150	63	56	58	10	8	9
Group II[1]	2910	2850	3060	86	91	90	33	40	44
World	2410	2260	2420	72	66	68	18	18	20

Source: Sukhatme, P. W. The World's Hunger and Future Needs in Food Supplies, *Royal Statistical Soc.*, Series A (General). **124:** 477, 1961.

[1] The Group I countries include the Far East, Near East, Africa and Latin America (except River Plate countries). The Group II countries include Europe, northern America, River Plate countries and Oceania. These groups correspond fairly closely to the underdeveloped and developed countries of the world.

Reproduced from *Population and Food Supply.* Food Agr. Organ. U.N., Basic Study No. 7. p. 24, 1962.

because of lack of food (Fig. 21.7) and the development of deficiency diseases like kwashiorkor from a lack of protein and other essential nutrients plague the children of these countries.

The Underweight Person. Undernutrition in the midst of a shortage of food is to be expected; its occurrence in the midst of plenty is an existing paradox. Some individuals, both children and adults, who are underweight fail to gain weight despite an adequate supply of available food. Status of health and habits of life influence the ability of persons to gain weight. Improvement in general health is, as a rule, accompanied by an increase in appetite, and a consequent gain in weight. Living at a rapid pace in an atmosphere of tenseness with little time for relaxation may lead to poor eating habits, faulty digestion, and, as a result, underweight. Slowing the tempo of living, relaxing for a period before meals, aids in better utilization of the food eaten.

The diet for gaining weight should have a Calorie content in excess of body needs; protein, minerals, and vitamins should be supplied in amounts equal to or above the normal levels. If there is appetite failure, foods high in concentrated carbohydrates and fats should be avoided

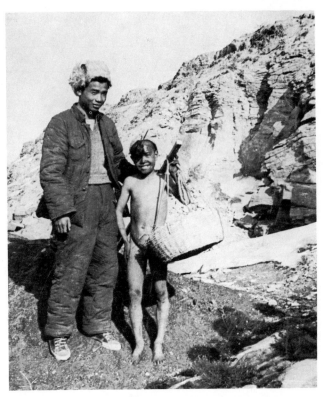

Fig. 21.7. Two boys of the same age. One worked in a coal mine eating whatever food was available. The other spent 4 years, well-nourished at a boarding school. (Courtesy of Food and Agriculture Organization of the United Nations, Rome, 1957, from *Millions Still go Hungry.*)

because of their satiety value. Eating a little more at each meal than is desired, and making a habit of eating between-meal snacks that are low in satiety value, such as Graham crackers or fruit, are means of adding to the total energy intake.

The Effects of Undernutrition. With children, and the young of other species as well, an inadequate food intake limits growth. The young are endowed with an impulse to grow; the capacity to do so is controlled by the environment. A most important factor in the environment is nutrition. In experimental animals deprived of sufficient energy intake to take care of their daily needs, the stores of fat are first called on to supply the needed energy, then protein from muscle tissue. There is little loss of weight in the brain, bone, and kidney tissues during inanition; a greater loss occurs in the heart, liver, pancreas, and the organs of the alimentary tract.

The body's normal resiliency to stresses is reduced in the severely underfed person. He is more susceptible to cold, manifesting a subnormal body temperature. There is a tendency to subnormal blood pressure, and to edema. Disease is more prevalent and recovery from illness, surgery, and injury more delayed than in the normal person. Tuberculosis and rheumatic fever are both linked with inadequate food intake as a causative factor.

Normal tissue function is dependent on adequate nutrition. The gastrointestinal tract is particularly susceptible to the effects of an inadequate diet. Limited and monotonous food supply may result in loss of appetite, gastrointestinal motility may be disturbed, and diarrhea, one of the most serious complications of severe deprivation, may develop. The liver, too, may suffer damage, particularly by a diet inadequate in protein, becoming more susceptible to injury by toxic agents.

Voluntary physical activity is altered by the degree of undernutrition. Children who are mildly undernourished show an increase in motor restlessness. Marked loss in body weight results in weakness and tiredness. The capacity to do physical work decreases with continued caloric restriction (31, 40).

The welfare of individuals and the global problem of relations among nations make the food shortage in parts of the world a matter for concern. Condon, Director-General of the World Health Organization, stated in 1963 (22) that "malnutrition is one of the most important health problems of the world. It is estimated that between one-half and two-thirds of the world's population suffers from it." The emotions and behavior of people are altered by deprivation of food. Irritability, gloominess, and an uneasy state of mind prevail. During semistarvation people are intensely preoccupied with thoughts of food. As the shortage progresses, it becomes a matter of each man for himself. Despite the state of unrest, a great apathy rests over semistarved persons (12). The effects of undernutrition vary with the severity of the deprivation and the capacity of the individual to adjust to the physical and mental stress.

Adaptation to Undernutrition. The body possesses great power of adaptation to stresses imposed upon it (8, 28). Cannon suggested that the term "homeostasis" be used to describe the ingenious mechanisms operating in the body to maintain normal conditions and to restore the physiological processes to the "steady state" after they have been disturbed.

The body adjusts to undernutrition remarkably well; evidence for this is the survival—even though at a lowered level of well-being—of deprived persons. Body weight is lowered, the basal metabolism reduced, and activity restricted with insufficient food. Each of these changes diminishes the energy need. Within limits, the body thus reduces its energy needs in accordance with the energy supply available to it.

To further illustrate the body's capacity to adjust to a lowered food intake, we may cite the more efficient use that it makes of protein and calcium. With protein, a day or two after the nitrogen intake is decreased, the nitrogen excretion in the urine begins to decrease. Thus in a week or so nitrogen equilibrium at the lower level of intake is established. Adjustment to a limited calcium intake requires a much longer time than for protein. There is evidence that calcium liberated within the tissues and body fluids can be reused thus conserving the available supply.

The capacity for nutritional adaptation is explained by Mitchell (28) in this way: "If an animal in equilibrium with its food supply (meaning a well-nourished animal) is subjected to nutritional stress, such as an inadequate (or an excessive) supply of one or more of the essential nutrients, the animal will react in such a way as to minimize, as far as possible, or to undo entirely the effects of the nutritional stress."

Rehabilitation Following Undernutrition. The severely undernourished person is found to make good progress toward recovery on a diet high in Calories and generous in protein content. Intravenous feeding has proved to be less effective than taking food by mouth. Predigested foods do not seem to hasten recovery any more rapidly than ordinary foods. It is best for emaciated persons whose stomachs have shrunk from lack of food to eat small amounts at frequent intervals.

Can refeeding completely overcome the ill effects caused by deprivation of food? The degree of emaciation, individual differences in capacity to withstand such a stress, and the duration of the deprivation are factors that make a difference. In general, recovery can be complete. This conclusion is based chiefly on studies of British and French children whose growth was retarded by wartime restrictions, but who later did attain their expected size. It is likely that adults do not suffer permanent injury unless the deficit of certain nutrients has been extreme and prolonged.

REFERENCES

1. Anand, B. K., G. S. Chhina, and B. Singh (1962). Effect of glucose on the activity of hypothalamic "feeding centers." *Science* 138: 507.
2. Barter, J., and G. B. Forbes (1963). Correlation of potassium-40 data with anthropometric measurements. *Ann. N.Y. Acad. Sci.* 110: 264.
3. Brewer, W. D., *et al.* (1952). Weight reduction on low-fat and low-carbohydrate diets. II. Utilization of nitrogen and calcium. *J. Am. Dietet. Assoc.* 28: 213.
4. Brozek, J., J. K. Kihlber, H. L. Taylor, and A. Keys (1963). Skin-fold distributions in middle-aged American men. *Ann. N.Y. Acad. Sci.* 110: 492.
5. Bruch, H. (1957). The emotional significance of the preferred weight. In *Symposium on Nutrition and Behavior.* The Natl. Vitamin Foundation, New York, p. 90.

6. Bruch, H. (1958). Psychological aspect of obesity. *Borden's Rev. Nutr. Res.* **19:** 57.

7. Burgess, A., and R. F. A. Dean (eds.) (1962). *Malnutrition and Food Habits.* The Macmillan Co., New York.

8. Cannon, W. B. (1939). *The Wisdom of the Body.* W. W. Norton and Co., New York, p. 19.

9. Cowgill, G. R. (1958). Evaluating body composition. *Borden's Rev. Nutr. Res.* **19:** 1.

10. *Expert Committee on Medical Assessment of Nutritional Status* (1963). World Health Organ., Rept. Series No. 258, Geneva.

11. Fryer, J. H. (1958). The effects of a late-night caloric supplement upon body weight and food intake in man. *Am. J. Clin. Nutr.* **6:** 354.

12. Guetzkow, H. S., and P. H. Bowman (1946). *Men and Hunger.* Brethren Publishing House, Elgin, Ill., p. 19.

13. Hathaway, M. L. (1957). *Heights and Weights of Children in the United States.* U.S. Dept. Agr., Home Econ. Res. Rept. No. 2, Washington, D.C., p. 131.

14. Hathaway, M. L., and D. W. Sargent (1962). Overweight in children. *J. Am. Dietet. Assoc.* **40:** 511.

15. Jolliffe, N. (1952). *Reduce and Stay Reduced.* Simon and Shuster, New York, p. 12.

16. Kark, R. (1962). Food and hunger in a world of turmoil. In *Food for World Peace, an International Symposium.* Ohio State University, Columbus, p. 42.

17. Keys, A. (1955). Weight changes and health of men. In *Weight Control.* Iowa State College Press, Ames, p. 108.

18. Lantz, E. L., and P. Wood (1958). Nutrition of New Mexican Spanish-American and "Anglo" adolescents. II. Blood findings, height and weight data, and physical condition. *J. Am. Dietet. Assoc.* **34:** 145.

19. Leverton, R. M., and M. R. Gram (1951). Further studies of obese young women during weight reduction. Calcium, phosphorus, and nitrogen metabolism. *J. Am. Dietet. Assoc.* **27:** 480.

20. Lew, E. A. (1961). New data on body weight. *J. Am. Dietet. Assoc.* **38:** 323.

21. Mann, C. V., E. M. Scott, L. H. Hursh, C. A. Heller, J. B. Youmans, C. F. Consolazio, E. B. Bridgforth, A. L. Russell, and M. Silverman (1962). The health and nutritional status of Alaskan Eskimos. *Am. J. Clin. Nutr.* **11:** 31.

22. *Malnutrition and Disease* (1963). World Health Organ., Basic Study No. 12, Geneva.

23. *Manual for Nutrition Surveys.* Second edition (1963). Interdepartmental Committee on Nutrition for National Defense. National Institutes of Health, Bethesda, Md.

24. Martin, E. A. (1954). *Roberts' Nutrition Work with Children.* University of Chicago Press, Chicago, p. 19.

25. Mayer, J. (1961). Obesity: Physiologic consideration. *Am. J. Clin. Nutr.* **9:** 530.

26. Mayer, J., and F. J. Stare (1953). Exercise and weight control. Frequent misconceptions. *J. Am. Dietet. Assoc.* **29:** 340.

27. Meredith, H. V. (1949). A "physical growth record" for use in elementary and high schools. *Am. J. Public Health* **39:** 878.

28. Mitchell, H. H. (1944). Adaptation to undernutrition. *Am. J. Dietet. Assoc.* **20:** 511.

29. Morgan, A. F. (ed.) (1959). *Nutritional Status U.S.A.* Univ. Calif. Agr. Expt. Sta., Bull. No. 769, Berkeley.

30. Newburgh, L. H., and M. W. Johnston (1930). *The Exchange of Energy between Man and the Environment.* Charles C Thomas, Springfield, Ill. p. 92.

31. *Nutrition and Working Efficiency* (1962). Food Agr. Organ. U.N., Basic Study No. 5, Rome.

32. Pearson, W. N. (1962). Biochemical appraisal of the vitamin nutritional status in man. *J. Am. Med. Assoc.* **180:** 49.

33. Rome, H. P. (1960). Obesity: psychiatric aspects. *Staff Meetings of the Mayo Clinic* **35:** 131.

34. Schaefer, A. E., and F. B. Berry (1960). U.S. interest in world nutrition. *Public Health Rept. (U.S.)* **75:** 677.
35. Shank, R. E. (1961). Weight reduction and its significance. *Nutr. Rev.* **19:** 289.
36. Stitt, K. R. (1962). *Skinfold Measurement: a Method of Determining Subcutaneous Fat.* Dept. Foods and Nutr., Univ. Ala., Tuscaloosa.
37. *Study in Human Starvation. Sources of Selected Foods. Diets and Deficiency Diseases* (1953). The American Geographical Society, New York.
38. Teply, L. J. (1964). Nutritional needs of the pre-school child. *Nutr. Rev.* **22:** 65.
39. Trevarthen, C. B. (1962). Alimentary responses evoked from forebrain structures in Macaca mulattos. *Science* **136:** 260.
40. Youmans, J. B. (1952). Some current aspects of nutrition. *J. Am. Dietet. Assoc.* **28:** 1029.
41. Young, C. M., B. A. Gehring, S. H. Merrill, and M. E. Kerr (1960). Metabolic responses of young women while reducing. *J. Am. Dietet. Assoc.* **36:** 447.
42. Young, C. M., McCarthy, J. H. Fryer, and R. S. Tensuan (1963). Basal oxygen consumption as a predictor of lean body mass in young women. *J. Am. Dietet. Assoc.* **43:** 125.
43. Young, C. M., I. Ringler, and B. J. Greer (1953). Reducing and post-reducing maintenance on the moderate-fat diet. *J. Am. Dietet. Assoc.* **29:** 890.
44. Wetzel, N. C. (1943). Assessing the physical condition of children. *J. Pediat.* **22:** 82, 208, 329.

SUPPLEMENTARY REFERENCES

Breckenridge, M. E., and E. L. Vincent (1960). *Child Development.* 4th ed. W. B. Saunders Co., Philadelphia.
Brock, J. F. (1961). *Recent Advances in Human Nutrition.* Little, Brown, and Co., Boston.
Martin, E. A. (1963). *Nutrition in Action.* Holt, Rinehart, and Winston, New York.

CHAPTER 22

Food fads and fallacies

Fallacious beliefs concerning foods and their usefulness to the body are not new. However, with increasing scientific knowledge and improved means of communication, it might be expected that faddism would be less prevalent. The opposite seems to be true. The purveyors of half-truths or untruths "thrive by misinterpreting scientific facts" (3).

Concern for the influence of faddism on health has prompted the American Medical Association and the Food and Drug Administration to sponsor jointly national conferences on Medical Quackery. Food and Drug Commissioner George P. Larrick stated at the 1961 conference that, "the most widespread and expensive type of quackery in the United States today is the promotion of vitamin products, special dietary foods, and food supplements." An estimate made by the Food and Drug Administration is that 10,000,000 Americans spend $500,000,000 a year or $50 per buyer on nutritional nostrums (2).

Why does nutrition quackery thrive? It seems a paradox; the food supply is abundant and most people enjoy eating. Also, the purchase of food would be less expensive than the purchase of the special products and supplements. However, the faddist makes reckless promises of beauty, youth, health, and relief from pain and disease. It would seem that the interest of the people of the United States in science, and in health and medicine, should contribute to the vulnerability of the faddist. However, if there is considerable concern about health, it may be a favorable climate for quackery to be created. Milstead (8) believes

383

overconcern to be "one of the most significant factors in the increase in medical and nutritional quackery in recent years." Also the belief that science can accomplish magic may tend to make people gullible. The public is interested to learn of advances in science; the food faddist is ready and eager to satisfy that interest, but with misinformation.

Financial gain is the chief interest of the faddist. Extravagant claims are made for a product that has been concocted or for a dietary plan or health scheme sponsored in order to realize sales. The purchase of such nostrums and notions is an economic waste. Even more serious, however, is the delay incurred in seeking sound medical attention when it is needed (1).

Aside from the propagandists who have something to sell, there are many persons who have misconceptions about food. The misconceptions might be classed as folklore or "old wives" tales. The beliefs are handed down from one generation to the next; they are traditional, unquestioned. In this category, the admonition "to feed a cold and starve a fever" might be placed.

Some unsound beliefs are due to superstitions and fears. When traced back to their origins, circumstances were usually that illness had followed the eating of a certain food or food combination. Even though the illness was coincidental, the incrimination of the food as the cause persisted. An example of such an ill-grounded belief is the fear of combining seafood and milk in the same meal. There is no basis, of course, for the fear.

On the other hand, it may be wise to stop and consider practices that vary from those to which we are accustomed, particularly the habits of persons living in isolated areas. The beliefs they hold may well have a grain of truth. Centuries ago burnt sponge was recommended for simple goiter; later it was found to contain iodine, the element which if insufficient in the diet may cause a goitrous condition. The English fed limes to their sailors suffering with scurvy; later it was found that an insufficiency of ascorbic acid was the cause of scurvy and that limes contain that vitamin.

Common Dietary Misconceptions

A survey made by a committee of the American Dietetic Association indicated the following to be among the more commonly observed dietary misconceptions.

THAT FRUITS, ESPECIALLY CITRUS AND TOMATO, ARE TOO ACID TO BE HANDLED BY THE BODY. The acids in fruits are organic acids. With few exceptions after absorption they are oxidized to carbon dioxide and water, both of which compounds are readily eliminated. The inorganic residue remaining, after oxidation of the organic portion, is basic in reaction. Fruits are base-forming with the exception of prunes, plums, and cranberries, which contain organic acids (benzoic in prunes and plums and quinic in cranberries) that the body cannot oxidize.

THAT GARLIC CURES HIGH BLOOD PRESSURE. There is no evidence to indicate that garlic possesses either remedial or curative properties for elevated blood pressure.

THAT BEETS BUILD BLOOD. Beets are not a good source of the nutrients recognized to be essential in blood formation. Protein and iron are the chief blood-building constituents. Copper also is essential for the formation of hemoglobin. Vitamins that function in the maintenance of a normal blood picture include folacin and vitamin B_{12}.

THAT FOODS COOKED IN ALUMINUM UTENSILS WILL CAUSE CANCER. There is no basis of truth for such a belief. Foods cooked in aluminum utensils are increased in aluminum content, but little, if any, of the metal is absorbed from the gastrointestinal tract by man or animal. The small amount that may be absorbed exerts no ill effect (12, 16).

THAT THE FOLLOWING COMBINATIONS OF FOODS ARE POISONOUS: MILK AND ORANGE JUICE OR OTHER CITRUS FRUIT; MILK AND FISH. The belief is entirely erroneous. Such food combinations are eaten daily by many with no ill effects.

THAT RAW CUCUMBERS WITHOUT SALT ARE POISONOUS. There is no evidence to support this belief.

THAT A GOOD WAY TO DIET IS TO SKIP BREAKFAST. Omission of breakfast results in lowered physical efficiency. Omitting some food at each of the regular mealtimes is a better plan than skipping some meals. (For discussion of overweight and for reports on studies of the effect of omitting breakfast, see Chapters 21 and 24, respectively.)

THAT HONEY IS NOT FATTENING. No particular food is fattening. Calories consumed in excess of need are deposited as fat. A tablespoon of strained honey (21 gm) is higher in caloric value than a tablespoon of sugar (12 gm), 65 and 45 Cal., respectively.

THAT MEAT GIVES YOU STRENGTH. Meat has a high satiety value. The extractives give a flavor that is enjoyed and the protein is effective in delaying the onset of hunger sensations.

THAT FRUIT JUICES DO NOT CONTRIBUTE CALORIES TO THE DIET. Fruit juices contribute Calories to the diet as follows per cup: lime, 65; lemon, 60; orange, 110; pineapple, 135; and prune, 200.

THAT TOAST HAS FEWER CALORIES THAN BREAD. The caloric value of bread is unchanged by toasting. Water is lost in the process and part of the starch is dextrinized, neither of which changes the energy value of the bread.

THAT VEGETABLE FATS AND OILS CAN BE USED IN ANY QUANTITY AND

ARE NOT FATTENING. Vegetable fats and oils are high in caloric value, and are comparable to animal fats.

THAT ADULTS NEED NO MILK. Without milk or a milk product in the diet, it is difficult to supply the recommended calcium allowance of adults. In addition, dairy products provide in significant amounts protein of high quality, phosphorus, vitamin A, and riboflavin.

THAT SKIM MILK HAS LITTLE NUTRITIVE VALUE. Skim milk is whole milk with the butterfat removed. It remains a superior food, even though low in fat and vitamin A content.

THAT PORK LIVER IS LESS NUTRITIOUS THAN BEEF OR CALVES LIVER. The composition of the three meats is similar in energy value and protein content. Pork liver is higher in iron and thiamine content and lower in vitamin A as shown below:

| | 100 Gram Edible Portion Cooked | | | |
	Iron, mg	Vitamin A, IU	Thiamine, mg	Riboflavin, mg
Beef liver	8.8	53,400	0.26	4.19
Calves liver	14.2	32,700	0.24	4.17
Pork liver	29.1	14,900	0.34	4.36

From *Composition of Foods—Raw, Processed, Prepared.* U.S. Dept. Agr., Agr. Handbook 8, revised, 1963.

THAT YOGURT IS AN AID IN RETAINING YOUTH AND BEAUTY. There is no evidence to indicate that yogurt or other fermented milks are wonder foods. Yogurt is whole milk that has been inoculated with the microorganism *Lactobacillus bulgaricus*. It is consumed by some because the flavor is enjoyed. In certain cases it has been recommended to patients as a means of lessening the incidence of the normally occurring putrefactive bacteria in the intestine.

THAT NATURAL FOODS ARE THE ONLY ONES THAT ARE SAFE FOR THE CONSUMER. The safety of additives to processed foods is guarded by the Food and Drug Administration; nutrients are added to some processed foods to enhance the nutritive value.

THAT WHITE-SHELLED EGGS ARE MORE NUTRITIOUS THAN BROWN. The nutritive value of an egg is not related to the color of the shell; that is determined by the breed of the hen.

THAT LARGE AMOUNTS OF GELATIN DISSOLVED IN WATER AND TAKEN AS A FOOD SUPPLEMENT WILL STRENGTHEN FINGERNAILS. Fingernail formation apparently is influenced by a number of factors including state of nutrition, endocrine state, disease, and environment. Gelatin is a pure protein. Whether protein of itself, in any form, will improve fingernail condition is questionable.

THAT WATER IS FATTENING. Water has no caloric value and therefore cannot be converted to body fat.

Detecting Faddism

There are certain characteristics that help the unsuspecting public to discern truth from fiction. Mitchell (9) has described the characteristics of misinformation and the perpetrators of it as follows:

Earmarks of quackery and misleading propaganda should be familiar to the layman. Extravagant claims for cure or relief of various complaints are always to be doubted. Vague labeling which offers no figures or exact information to live up to is one way by which these promoters have avoided the teeth of the law. Labels are never so extravagant as detached advertisements or literature because the laws are stricter about labels.

Promoters of most of the fad diet systems or health institutes have personality, poise, and persuasion. They are convincing speakers with a smattering of scientific knowledge. This lends an air of plausibility which masks overstatement, understatement, and sheer misinterpretation. They mix the true and the false or misleading to suit their needs, to sell their products, or to scare their victims into spending money for a course of lectures to cure them of imaginary ills. They use scientific words and phrases to cover false ideas. They accomplish most by personal appearances but they also work through the mails, the radio, the newspapers, handbills, newsstand publications, and books with arresting titles.

And it should be added, they operate door to door.

Myths about Food and Nutrition

There are four myths that the Food and Drug Administration finds to be almost universally propounded by the person with a product or a nostrum to sell (6).

The number one myth is that *all diseases are due to faulty diet*. The premise is that it is almost impossible to consume an adequate diet from foods, hence the promotion of the product to be sold. "The product in question usually contains a long list of ingredients, often including some which are supposed to possess secret benefits which nutrition scientists have not yet discovered." Janssen (6) pointed out that "the promoter with the pill that '*has* everything' will generally also claim that it can '*do* everything'—in other words, that it is a cure-all and the answer to every health problem."

The second myth is that *soil depletion causes malnutrition*. There is no scientific evidence to support this statement. An impoverished soil deminishes the quantity of the crop produced rather than the quality. Some slight variations in the nutritive value of crops have been related to soil fertility, however, of more importance is the genetic strain of the crop (15).

The only recorded instance of a relationship between human nutritional status and soil composition is that of the incidence of endemic goiter in regions of low iodine content of the soil. The deficiency of iodine is taken care of by the use of iodized salt in the United States and some other countries also.

The third myth commonly promoted is that of *overprocessing*. The fact is, that some methods cause some loss of minerals and vitamins but most of the nutritive value is retained (7). This misinformation is employed to support the sale of certain cooking utensils or food supplements. Furthermore, food consumption data indicate that the supply of nutrients per capita is at an all time high (5).

The fourth myth is concerned with so-called *subclinical deficiencies*. Janssen (6) explains the implications of this myth as follows: "According to this theory, anyone who has a tired feeling or an ache or pain in any part of the body is probably suffering from a subclinical deficiency and needs to supplement his diet with various concoctions. The food-fad promoters teach that practically everybody is in this category because of our depleted, over processed, and poisoned food supply." Such symptoms are universal and may result from many causes. Symptoms of dietary deficiencies should be diagnosed by a competent physician.

A false statement that influences old persons in particular is that, as a person grows older "he develops an increased or unusual requirement for some nutrient or food that is not supplied by the ordinary diet" (13, 14). Actually the energy requirements *decrease* with age. In fact, the Recommended Allowances for none of the nutrients increases with age. To the contrary, for women in the 55 to 75-year group, the recommendation for iron is less than for the younger adult group; for riboflavin and niacin, the recommendations are less for both men and women, and less for thiamine for men.

Means of Deception

Some of the kinds of products and practices that are avenues for deception include:

Mail Order Products. Responsible mail order companies give full value for purchases made. However, the Food and Drug Administration warns that exaggerated claims are prevalent in mail order literature on health products. The Postmaster General has warned that quackery in this field is at an all-time high. This warning applies particularly to mail promotion of nutritional products (6).

"Health Lecturers." The lecturer usually attacks well-known foods or products and has for sale a special line of health foods or special utensils.

Books and Literature. There are many good books on nutrition and health on the market. However, "any book that advocates a quick 'cure' for a serious illness such as cancer or arthritis is certainly questionable" (2). Also there are books on the market that are inaccurate in content and filled with misinterpretations written in an authoritative style (15).

Doorbell "Doctors." We are warned to beware of house-to-house salesmen of vitamin and food supplements. They may "attempt to discuss your health and dietary problems and to give advise regarding them. They are salesmen, *not* doctors" (6).

Means to Counter Misinformation and Fraud

Stronger laws, stronger law enforcement, and public information and education were suggested by Commissioner Larrick of the Food and Drug Administration (8) as three means of alleviating the influence of misinformation and fraud.

Public service groups that can lend assistance in detecting deception are: Better Business Bureau; Department of Investigation, American Medical Association, 535, No. Dearborn St., Chicago 10, Ill.; U.S. Post Office Department, Office of General Counsel, Washington 25, D.C. for queries about mail order products; Food and Drug Administration, U.S. Dept. Health, Education, and Welfare, Washington 25, D.C.

Additional sources of authoritative information about food and nutrition for the professional and lay person are: agricultural and home economics extension services located at state universities and with county offices; food and nutrition departments in home economics in colleges and universities; state departments of health; Agricultural Research Service, Human Nutrition and Consumer Use Division, U.S. Department Agriculture, Washington 25, D.C.; American Dietetic Association, 620 North Michigan Ave., Chicago 11, Illinois; American Home Economics Association, 1600 Twentieth St. N.W., Washington 9, D.C.; Council on Foods and Nutrition, The American Medical Association, 535 North Dearborn St., Chicago 10, Ill.; Food and Nutrition Board, National Academy of Science—National Research Council, 2101 Constitution Ave., Washington 25, D.C.

► PROTECTION OF THE CONSUMER

We are fortunate in this country to enjoy certain assurances by law that our food supply is wholesome. Also we may feel confident when making a purchase that the product conforms to the label description. Some of our protection is through federal laws, some by state laws, and some through local regulations. The federal regulations cover products that pass through interstate commerce, the state laws are effective within the state, and local regulations such as county and city apply to those circumscribed areas.

Important among the federal regulations as prescribed by the Food, Drug and Cosmetic Act of 1938 is that of accurate labeling of products. Foods bearing labels that are false or misleading are prohibited to be shipped from one state to another or imported from another country. The federal law in addition imposes certain specific requirements for the labels of foods intended for special dietary uses in order to inform the purchaser of the value of the food for such uses. It is required that the vitamin and mineral content and other dietary properties be declared on the label. Figure 22.1 is a copy of a label from a cereal preparation for

	Approximate Analysis
	%
Carbohydrate	44.9
Protein (N × 6.25)	35.0
Moisture	7.0
Minerals (ash)	7.3
Calcium	0.90
Phosphorus	0.90
Iron	0.30
Copper	0.001
Fat	4.0
Crude fiber	1.8
Calories per oz	105
Tablespoonfuls per oz	12

Each ounce contains not less than 0.3 mg thiamine, and 0.1 mg riboflavin and supplies the above percentages of the minimum daily requirements of nutrients.

Fig. 22.1.   Label from a special cereal preparation for babies. (Courtesy of Pablum Products, Division of Mead Johnson and Company, Evansville, Indiana.)

No Sugar Added
Typical Analysis of Food Values

Available Carbohydrates 8.2%
(total Carbohydrates minus crude fiber)
Protein 0.7%
Fat 0.1%
Minerals 0.5%
Sodium: per 100 grams, 3 mg.; per ½ cup, 3 mg.
Available Calories: per 100 grams, 37; per ½ cup, 42

For Dietary Purposes

Prepared from fully matured, carefully selected, sun-ripened Florida Grapefruit;
Grapefruit Juice; and non-nutritive Sucaryl® (Cyclamate Calcium, Abbott), 0.1%.
Cyclamate Calcium is a non-nutritive artificial sweetener which should be used by
those persons who must restrict their intake of ordinary sweets.

Fig. 22.2.   Label from a can of grapefruit for persons on diets limited in sugar content (Courtesy
of Tillie Lewis Foods, Inc. Stockton, California.)

babies. The federal law also makes a special requirement that foods
intended for the dietary management of disease or the control of body
weight carry labels stating the percentage by weight of the protein, fat,
available carbohydrate content, and the caloric value of a specified quantity
of the food (4, 10). Figure 22.2 is the label from a can of grapefruit
prepared for use by persons on special diets limited in sugar content
and persons on low-caloric diets.

The regulations of the state laws vary from state to state. Most of
them cover mislabeling of products and provide for certain sanitary
regulations of products manufactured and put on the market within the
state. Local laws apply for the most part to control of the quality and
sanitation of milk and milk products on the market and to the sanitary
condition of local eating establishments.

The Federal Trade Commission is another agency that assists in
protecting the consumer through the control of false and misleading
advertising. The Commission can take action against claims that show
a tendency to mislead or could be construed as deluding the public
through advertising by way of radio, television, public lectures, pam-
phlets, books, newspapers, form letters, and other types of communication. The Commission can act, however, only if the false or misleading
matter can be classified as commodity advertising (11).

The protection afforded the consumer by governmental agencies does
not relieve the individuals of their responsibility in attempting to discern
between fact and fiction. The authenticity of claims made and beliefs
followed can be ascertained only by seeking reliable sources of informa-

tion based on research findings. The frailty of human nature in accepting proffered nostrums without investigation encourages the spread of fallacies.

REFERENCES

1. Beeuwkes, A. M. (1954). Food faddism and the consumer. *Federation Proc.* **13**: 785.
2. Cooley, D. (1962). *Beware of "Health" Quacks.* AMA, Dept. Investigation, Chicago.
3. Cooper, L. F., E. M. Barber, H. S. Mitchell, H. J. Rynbergen, and J. C. Greene (1963). *Nutrition in Health and Disease.* J. B. Lippincott Co., Philadelphia, p. 114.
4. Day, P. L. (1960). The food and drug administration faces new responsibilities. *Nutr. Rev.* **18**: 1.
5. Friend, B. (1963). Nutritional review. *Natl. Food Situation.* U.S. Dept. Agr., Washington, D.C., **106**: 34.
6. Janssen, W. E. (1960). Food quackery—a law enforcement problem. *J. Am. Dietet. Assoc.* **36**: 110.
7. Larrick, G. P. (1961). The nutritive adequacy of our food supply. *J. Am. Dietet. Assoc.* **39**: 117.
8. Milstead, K. L. (1959). The Food and Drug Administration's attitude of food fads and nutritional quackery. In *The Role of Nutrition Education in Combatting Food Fads.* The Nutrition Foundation, New York, p. 16.
9. Mitchell, H. S. (1941). Food facts and fads. *J. Am. Dietet. Assoc.* **17**: 667.
10. Nelson, E. M. (1954). Control of nutrition claims under the Food, Drug, and Cosmetic Act. *Federation Proc.* **13**: 790.
11. *Protection of the Consumer by the Federal Trade Commission* (1945). Federal Trade Commission, Washington, D.C.
12. *A Select Annotated Bibliography on the Hygienic Aspects of Aluminum and Utensils* (1933). Mellon Institute of Industrial Research, Bibliographic Series Bull. 3, Pittsburgh, Penn.
13. Shank, R. E. (1963). Statement on frauds and quackery affecting the older citizen. In *Hearings before the Special Committee on Aging.* U.S. Senate, Eighty-eighth Congress. Pt. I, January 15, 1963. U.S. Govt. Printing Office, Washington, D.C.
14. Statement on frauds and quackery affecting the older citizen (1963). In *Hearings before the Special Committee on Aging.* U.S. Senate, Eighty-eighth Congress, Pt. III, January 17, 1963, U.S. Govt. Printing Office, Washington, D.C.
15. Trulson, M. F., M. B. McCann, and F. J. Stare (1959). Food fads versus professional and public education. In *The Role of Nutrition Education in Combatting Food Fads.* The Nutrition Foundation, New York, p. 5.
16. The use of aluminum cooking utensils in the preparation of foods (1951). *J. Am. Med. Assoc.* **146**: 477.

SUPPLEMENTARY REFERENCES

Deutsch, R. M. (1961). *The Nuts Among the Berries.* Ballentine Books, Inc., New York.
Mitchell, H. S. (1959). Don't be fooled by fads. In *Food. The Yearbook of Agriculture,* 1959. (A. Stefferud, ed.). U.S. Dept. Agr., Washington, D.C., p. 660.

CHAPTER 23

Diet and dental health

Dental caries is the most widespread chronic disease in industrialized countries. It is an affliction which invades all age groups, although at different rates. Except for a few individuals, each year brings new cavities in the teeth. This happens not only in childhood but continues in adulthood as well. Girls tend to have a higher incidence of dental decay than boys (31). Earlier eruption of teeth in girls has been cited as a causative factor for the difference. However, in a study of 2068 boys and girls in five Western states, the higher incidence in girls occurred but it was not related to earlier eruption time (43). Of course, wide individual variation in the incidence of dental caries exists at all ages.

A circumstance that might give a clue to the cause of dental caries is that ancient man, in general, had relatively little dental decay. This superior condition of the teeth of primitive man was discovered from studies of unearthed teeth. Primitive people living today in various parts of the world have relatively little tooth decay as did their ancient counterparts.

In Awo Omamma, a coastal Nigerian city, only two small dental cavities were found in a group of nearly 600 natives, despite evidence of serious malnutrition in all age groups. The fluorine content of the water was low. The diet consisted chiefly of yams and cassava, with small amounts of green vegetables and occasionally dried fish (42). However, when civilization reaches them and influences their customs and food habits, an increase in the incidence of dental caries invariably follows.

For example, the Eskimos had few carious lesions until they had had appreciable contact with traders or lived in the vicinity of trading posts. The Samoans enjoyed a relatively low incidence of tooth decay until navy personnel were located on the island, as did the Indians of Ecuador until a missionary settlement was established there (35, 36, 40, 44). Dental decay is indeed a greater affliction of civilized man than for those living under primitive circumstances.

▶ STRUCTURE AND DEVELOPMENT OF THE TOOTH

It is paradoxical that teeth, which are seemingly so carefully constructed for permanency by having the hardest tissue in the body for an outside covering, should be so susceptible to injury, that is, the formation of caries. As shown in Fig. 23.1, *enamel* covers the entire exposed portion of the tooth, or *crown. Cementum,* covers the root, the portion embedded in the gum. In the center of the tooth is the *pulp,* a soft connective tissue containing the blood vessels and nerves for nourishment and enervation. Surrounding the pulp is *dentin,* which forms the largest portion of the tooth.

Tooth formation begins before birth. Calcification of the deciduous (baby) teeth is in process as early as the fourth to sixth prenatal month. At birth all of the deciduous teeth (twenty in number) are in an advanced stage of development and calcification and the four six-year permanent molars have already begun to calcify in the jawbones. By 2½ years of age, the deciduous teeth of most children are fully erupted.

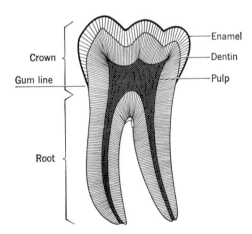

Fig. 23.1.   Cross section of tooth. (Courtesy of I. Schour. Adapted from Maximov and Bloom, *Textbook of Histology,* 4th ed., W. B. Saunders Co., Philadelphia, p. 381, 1942.)

The first permanent teeth to erupt are the incisors and the six-year molars which appear at about 6 years of age. Often the six-year molars, located sixth in line from the center of the mouth, are not recognized by the lay person as permanent teeth, and as a consequence necessary precautions are not taken to preserve them if they become defective. By the eleventh to thirteenth year the other permanent teeth, with the exception of the third molars (wisdom teeth) have erupted. The wisdom teeth usually appear between the seventeenth and twenty-first year, although they may erupt later or may remain unerupted in the jaws or never even develop.

► FACTORS INFLUENCING
 THE INCIDENCE OF DENTAL CARIES

A complete explanation of the cause of dental caries has not been established, although certain influencing factors are recognized. In general these influences fall into two classes, those having to do with the oral environment and external contact of materials with the tooth, and those having a systemic effect through materials carried internally into the tooth through the blood supply. The latter influence is of particular significance in tooth development during which the future caries-resistance of the tooth is largely determined.

The Influence of Oral Environment

Microorganisms in the Mouth. Dental caries is accepted unquestionably now to be of bacterial origin. The proof came in 1954 when Orland and his coworkers (32) found that rats raised under germ-free conditions did not develop carious lesions whereas comparable animals maintained under ordinary laboratory conditions did have tooth decay. Inoculations of the germ-free animals with bacteria (enterococci) resulted in the development of carious lesions (33). Studies are now aimed at identifying strains of organisms active in the development of caries. The question of whether or not these findings are applicable to the human is answered by MacDonald (27) in this way, "no data exist which necessitate an assumption of any fundamental differences in the mechanisms responsible for caries in different species."

That bacteria may be involved in the development of carious lesions has been under consideration for over three-quarters of a century and the mode of action sought (27). The earliest proposal, made in 1882, was that caries are initiated by acid decalcification of the enamel; an explanation which still holds true today. The acid is believed to arise from the fermentative processes of bacteria acting on carbohydrate substrates. In 1929 proteolytic organisms were suggested as initiating the development of carious lesions by modifying the protein matrix of the teeth thus permitting the loss of inorganic salts. In the lesion decalcification is caused by the acid and breakdown of organic components through proteolysis (38).

Even though dental caries is demonstrated experimentally to be an infectious disease, a characteristic in the experimental animal which places limits on the incidence is the inherited susceptibility or resistance to caries. There have been numerous studies employing a cross-fostering technique, whereby the young of caries-resistant and caries-susceptible mothers are interchanged. The young of the caries-resistant mothers, even though exposed to the strongly cariogenic microorganisms from caries-active rats, maintained high resistance. The implication is that the bacterial flora allowing for caries development is not readily established in the caries-resistant rat (17).

Carbohydrate in the Diet. There is substantial evidence from research with animals that carbohydrate in the diet is associated with the development of dental caries (41). Even in caries-susceptible rats, when no carbohydrate was fed, freedom from caries was possible; with its inclusion, caries developed. Experimentally, this study was most contributive, pointing directly to carbohydrate as a factor in caries production. For the human being it would be difficult and impractical to provide or afford such a diet as a routine measure.

The form in which carbohydrate is fed is found to make a difference in the extent of the harmful effect on the tooth. Sucrose fed in solution causes less tendency for caries to develop than when fed in granular form. An extensive study contributing information on the effect of the form of carbohydrate on the incidence of dental caries is the nine-year observation in a mental institution in Vipeholm, Sweden (16). The persons participating in the study were young adults; the average age of the control group was 34.9 years and of the experimental group 28.0 years. In one phase of the study the patients were fed a basal diet low in carbohydrate (130 gm daily) and especially low in sugar. No sugar was added as such, but the foods contained about 30 gm. The control group was given 150 gm margarine, the experimental groups were given 300 gm of sucrose either with meals, in solution or added to bread, or between meals in the form of toffees, chocolate, or caramels. In the control group the increase in dental caries during the two years of this phase of the study was almost zero; the highest incidence was in the between-meal-group. The amount of sugar was the same but the manner of feeding, whether with meals or between meals, and the form of the food were different. That between-meal consumption of sugar increases dental caries over meal feeding of a similar amount was confirmed by King and his coworkers (23) in England in a study with children.

Fat in the Diet. Several studies with animals have shown that increasing the proportion of fat in the diet reduces the incidence of caries. The mechanism of the action of fat is not known. It is suggested that since fats tend to form a film on the tooth, its effectiveness may be that it acts as a barrier helping to keep carbohydrate from the bacteria in the plaques on the teeth and also lessening the retention of foods on the surface of the tooth (21).

Pyridoxine in the Diet. It appears that there may be a relationship between pyridoxine activity and dental disease, although research concerning the question, particularly in human beings, is limited. Pyridoxine-deficient dogs and monkeys manifest an unusually high incidence of dental defects. Pregnant women receiving supplements of pyridoxine were found to have a smaller increase in number of decayed, missing, and filled teeth (DMF) over the initial incidence than did comparable persons with no pyridoxine supplement. The mechanism by which pyridoxine functions in diminishing the incidence of caries is not known. It is effective in post-development teeth, and thus would appear to exert a favorable effect on the oral flora (18).

Influence of Saliva. Normal exposure of the tooth to saliva is a deterrent to caries development. This observation was clearly demonstrated in studies with animals from whom the salivary glands were removed. Without saliva, the incidence of dental caries increased markedly and the lesions were more severe (5, 21).

Oral Hygiene. Brushing the teeth thoroughly within 10 minutes after each ingestion of food, or if that was not possible, rinsing the mouth, was found to effect a reduction in the incidence of dental caries in a study with college students. The observations covered a period of 2 years with 429 individuals in the experimental group, who either brushed their teeth or rinsed their mouths after eating, and 276 persons in the control group who followed their usual habits of mouth hygiene. The control group at the end of 2 years had developed an average of 3.87 new carious surfaces, detected through clinical and radiographic examinations; the experimental group had developed only 2.02 carious surfaces (15).

Influence of Systemic Nutriture

The adequacy of the nutrients supplied the tooth during the formative period influences its resistance to decay. Research studies amply substantiate the beneficial effects of an adequate diet in building a tooth. In the study of the incidence of caries among preschool children at the Forsyth Dental Infirmary in Boston, the diet of the mothers during pregnancy and the diet of children were found to have an influence. The mothers of children who had a low-caries incidence had drunk more milk during pregnancy than had the mothers of children in the high-caries group. In addition, more of the low-caries children had had supplements of vitamin D either throughout life or during the winter months and were found to be consuming better diets at the time of the study than the high-caries group (4). In still another experimental study, tooth decay was reduced in children living in certain institutions in New York by supplementation of their diet with sufficient foods to make the diet completely adequate (28).

Influence of Specific Dietary Nutrients—Vitamin D. Vitamin D in the diets of children is found to favor a reduction in dental caries. The most extensive observations are those reported by the Committee on the Investigation of Dental Disease in England (20.) Children 5 to 14 years old were studied over a period of 3 years in three institutions in Birmingham. Supplements of cod liver oil and vitamin D as irradiated ergosterol in olive oil, reduced the incidence of tooth decay.

Calcium and Phosphorus. Good retentions of calcium and phosphorus were found to be associated with freedom from dental decay in children (8). In a study of 98 Iowa children those with no dental caries retained an average of 17 mg of calcium and 15 mg of phosphorus per kg of body weight each day; those with dental caries, on the other hand, retained only 10 mg and 9 mg, respectively. The difference in retention of the minerals between the non-carious and carious group was sufficiently great to be statistically significant.

Ascorbic Acid. It has long been established that ascorbic acid is essential for the development of dental tissues. In scurvy, changes are observed in the pulp and the odontoblasts (tooth-forming cells) of the tooth. Caries susceptibility, however, is not known to be influenced by the level of ascorbic acid in the diet.

State of Health

Good nutrition, freedom from emotional tenseness, and compliance with good health habits, are believed to favor a reduction in tooth decay "as a corollary of other evidences of betterment of well-being" (7).

▶ THE INFLUENCE OF TOOTH STRUCTURE
ON RESISTANCE TO CARIES

Teeth that are well formed and calcified seem to have a higher resistance to decay than do teeth that are poorly formed. It was found in the microscopic examination of 1500 sectioned deciduous teeth of English children, that 78 per cent of those with well calcified enamel and dentin were free from caries, whereas only 6 per cent of the poorly developed teeth (hypoplastic) were caries-free (13). The gross structure of the teeth also bore a relationship to the caries incidence; the better the structure, the lower the incidence of dental caries (1). Although structure is a contributing factor, we must recall that there are perfectly formed teeth that decay, and imperfectly formed ones that do not. It should be noted that perfectly formed teeth in man are a great rarity.

▶ FLUORINE AND DENTAL HEALTH

The relationship between fluorine (fluoride) and tooth physiology was recognized first as a public health hazard. In certain areas of the world and in this country, it was noted that the enamel of human teeth was *mottled.* These teeth were dull and chalky in appearance, some showed evidences of pitting and corrosion, and in severe cases the teeth were stained a color ranging from yellow to black. In 1931 mottled enamel (chronic endemic fluorosis) was associated with the ingestion of an excessive amount of fluoride in the drinking water. Soon after this finding, fluoride analysis of public water supplies in many areas of the United States began. It became evident then that dental fluorosis could be prevented by avoiding waters containing excessive amounts of fluorides or by removing the toxic amounts of the mineral by chemical means. It was found, however, that water containing as little as one part per million (ppm) of a fluoride caused little or no mottling of the teeth. Dean (12) was among the first to relate the incidence of very mild fluorosis to a low rate of dental caries in children. This fact has been observed also by workers in the U.S.S.R. (34) who report that even 0.2 to 0.3 mg fluoride per liter of drinking water has significant protective value against caries in children 7 to 9 and 11 to 14 years.

That a relation between the fluoride content of drinking water and the incidence of dental caries in children exists is shown in Figure 23.2. The mechanism by which fluoride operates to increase the resistance is not known. It is proposed, however, that it may be by adsorption of minute quantities on the surface of the enamel with the formation of an

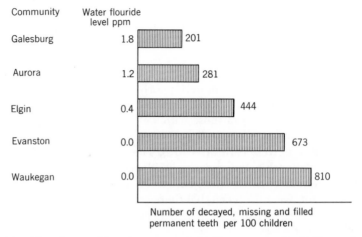

Fig. 23.2. The relation of fluoride content of drinking water to the incidence of dental caries in permanent teeth among 12- to 14-year-old children in natural fluoride areas. (From R. F. Sognnaes, *Chemistry and Prevention of Dental Caries,* Charles C. Thomas, Springfield, Ill., p. 184, 1962.)

acid-resisting protective layer, or that fluorine may be antibacterial if the concentration is sufficiently high.

Controlled Fluoridation Studies

Controlled studies of water fluoridation were begun between 1944 and 1947. Before this time, all the evidence of the role of fluoride in dental health was based on the findings of individuals who were born and continued to live in a natural fluoride area.

The study of fluoridation can be divided into three phases (6). The first, or the period of discovery, constitutes all the early work including the announcement of the relationship between very mild dental fluorosis and a low rate of dental decay in children. During 1945 the second phase, or period of controlled experimentation, began with the initiation of the famous fluoridation studies in this country (Newburgh-Kingston, New York and Grand Rapids-Muskegon, Michigan). Since that time other communities, both here and abroad, have set up similar fluoridation studies. Only two, however, the Newburgh-Kingston study and the United Kingdom study will be described here. The results of the eleventh year of the Grand Rapids-Muskegon study (2) showed a reduction in caries of the permanent teeth to be between 60 and 65 per cent in those children born and reared in Grand Rapids since fluoridation began. Because the results of these fluoridation investigations showed marked control of dental decay among children, the third phase of the fluoridation story, the period of development, began. In 1963 more than 2300 cities and towns had fluoridated water supplies, and more than fifty million people were using fluoridated drinking water in the United States (29).

The Newburgh-Kingston Study

This ten-year experiment began in May 1945 in these two New York communities, located 30 miles apart on the Hudson River. Both cities have the same source of drinking water, inhabitants of similar racial and economic backgrounds, and populations of equal proportions (about 30,000). The water supply of Newburgh, the test city, was treated with sodium fluoride so as to contain 1.0 to 1.2 ppm whereas in Kingston, the control city, no fluoride was added to the water supply. Annual dental examinations and periodic medical evaluations were made throughout the ten-year period of the selected children from these two communities.

At the end of the ten-year period the medical and dental data were evaluated in order to assess the effects of the intake of fluoridated water on the incidence of tooth decay among the children of the two towns. The medical officers reported that there was no significant difference in the height, weight, selected laboratory tests, or in x-ray studies between the children of the test and control cities (39). The report of the dental team, however, stated that the clinical and x-ray dental examinations of children between the ages of 6 and 16 years showed that the DMF (decayed plus missing plus filled teeth) of the permanent teeth was lower among the children from Newburgh than from Kingston (3) (Fig. 23.3).

The United Kingdom Study

The favorable report of a mission sent by the British government in 1953 to study and assess the effectiveness, safety, and practicability of fluoridation in the United States precipitated the fluoridation studies begun in 1955–1956 in three areas of the United Kingdom. The study areas were Watford, England; Kilmarnock, Scotland; and part of Anglesey County in North Wales.

The findings, based on the observations of several thousands of children (3 to 7 years) from the start of the study to 1961, showed good agreement with those reported from the Grand Rapids study (9). The caries reduction among 4-year-olds after fluoridation was 54 per cent in the British study and 42 per cent in the Grand Rapids study. The caries reduction among 5-year-olds in the two studies was also quite similar (47 per cent, United Kingdom and 45 per cent Grand Rapids).

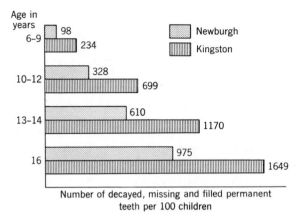

Number of decayed, missing and filled permanent
teeth per 100 children

Fig. 23.3. Comparison of the incidence of dental caries in permanent teeth of children from 6 to 16 years of age in Newburgh with 10 years of fluoridation and Kingston without fluoridation. (From R. F. Sognnaes, *Chemistry and Prevention of Dental Caries.* Charles C. Thomas, Springfield, Ill., p. 185, 1962.)

In spite of the fact that findings among American, British, and Canadian studies provide ample evidence of the value of fluoridation of drinking water as a preventive measure against dental caries, opposition to fluoridation exists. The main lines of argument against fluoridation are that it is ineffective, dangerous, and unethical. To counteract this opposition, a special public relations policy is needed. The reader is referred to a paper by Dalzell-Ward (11) for more information on fluoridation and public relations.

Other Methods of Fluoride Administration

Throughout the world people live in areas where public water supplies are not available and it would be impossible to fluoridate safely the individual water sources. This situation has initiated the search for methods of fluoride administration other than the fluoridation of drinking water.

The four methods of systematic fluoride administration that are being used in various parts of the world to counteract tooth decay are the intake of sodium fluoride tablets, fluoride enrichment of table salt, local application of fluoride solutions to the enamel surfaces of the teeth (topical application), and the use of toothpaste containing fluorides (37).

A sodium fluoride tablet which contains 1 mg of fluoride is being given each day to some children. The effectiveness of this type of program bears further study, however.

In Switzerland sodium fluoride has been added to table salt as a therapeutic measure. This method of fluoride administration would appear to be difficult to control because of the variation in salt consumption among individuals and the fact that salt should not be given to infants. Procedures for topical application of fluoride have been studied and developed. This technique involves the swabbing of the teeth with a fluoride solution at prescribed intervals of time. Although the incidence of dental caries has been reported to have been reduced by 40 per cent when a 2 per cent solution of sodium fluoride was applied topically to the teeth of large numbers of children (24), salts of fluoride other than sodium have been investigated. Workers from the Dental School at Indiana University (19) have found that children received greater protection from topically applied stannous chlorofluoride than from sodium fluoride.

The use of toothpaste as a means for fluoride application is an outgrowth of topical fluoride application studies. The results from a supervised toothbrushing study (22) conducted among more than 500 children in the fourth and fifth grades have shown that after one year, the children who used a stannous fluoride dentifrice had about 35 per cent fewer new decayed, missing, and filled teeth (DMF) than those who used a fluoride-free dentifrice. More recently Kyes and his coworkers (25) have conducted clinical trials on fluoridated toothpastes, and have found that they are not universally successful in combating tooth decay. Several factors that interfere with the development of a satisfactory stannous fluoride toothpaste appear to be the decrease of available fluoride and stannous ions upon storage of the paste, and a reduction of the fluoride available to the teeth due to the reaction of the saliva with the fluoridated paste (37).

Effect of Fluorides on Dental Caries in Adults

Most of the data available on fluoridation and fluoride administration at this time concern children up to 14 years of age. Although data on the effects of fluorides on the reduction of dental caries for older age groups are too few to draw conclusions, the reports of some recent studies are cited here.

Adults appear to benefit from the topical application of stannous fluoride. Muhler (30) has reported that a year after a single topical application of 10 per cent stannous fluoride, 200 university students showed a 24 per cent reduction in the increment of DMF teeth.

The relationship between maternal ingestion of fluorides during pregnancy and the incidence of caries in the deciduous teeth of the child has been studied. Comparisons have been made of the caries in deciduous teeth of groups of children born prior to and after the fluoridation of the water supply in Newburgh, New York (10). Although the findings from this study show little difference in the average number of dental caries between the groups, fluoride metabolism during pregnancy warrants further study.

The incidence of dental caries among adults who have consumed naturally fluoridated water almost continuously throughout life has been reported (14). The dental caries experience of almost 1000 native residents of Aurora, Illinois, between the ages of 18 and 59, who had consumed 1.2 ppm of natural fluoride almost continuously throughout life has been found to be between 40 and 50 per cent less than of a similar group from Rockford, Illinois, who had ingested fluoride-free water throughout their lifetime.

▶ **DIET AND HEALTH OF PERIODONTAL TISSUES**

The periodontium (periodontal tissues), which includes the bone, connective tissue, and epithelium that hold the teeth in the jaws, is notably susceptible to poor nutrition. Particularly important in the maintenance of these tissues is ascorbic acid. In a study of adult men whose gums had been treated previously for gingivitis, less likelihood of its return existed among those ingesting 75 mg of ascorbic acid daily than those who consumed only 25 mg daily (26).

The physical character of the diet may also affect the health of the periodontium. A diet containing foods that require vigorous chewing may be better for the health of the gums than the soft, sticky foods that tend to cling to the teeth, particularly at the gum line, contributing to the development of gingival disease.

REFERENCES

1. Allen, I. (1941). A survey of nutrition and dental caries in 120 London elementary school children. *Brit. Med. J.* **1**: 44.
2. Arnold, F. A. (1957). Grand Rapids fluoridation study—results pertaining to the eleventh year of fluoridation. *Am. J. Public Health* **47**: 539.
3. Ast, D. B., D. J. Smith, B. Wachs, and K. T. Cantwell (1956). Newburgh-Kingston caries-fluorine study. XIV. Combined clinical and roentgenographic dental findings after ten years of fluoride experience. *J. Am. Dental Assoc.* **52**: 314.
4. Berk, H. (1943). Some factors concerned with the incidence of dental caries in children; multiple pregnancy, and nutrition during prenatal, postnatal, and childhood periods. *J. Am. Dental Assoc.* **30**: 1749.
5. Bixler, D., J. C. Muhler, and W. G. Shafer (1954). Experimental dental caries. V. The effects of desalivation and castration on caries and fluorine storage in the rat. *J. Nutr.* **52**: 345.

6. Black, A. P. (1955). Facts in refutation of claims by opponents of fluoridation. *J. Am. Dental Assoc.* **50:** 655.

7. Boyd, J. D. (1954). Epidemiologic studies in dental caries. VI. A review of intrinsic factors as they may affect caries progression. *J. Pediat.* **44:** 578.

8. Boyd, J. D., C. L. Drain, and G. Stearns (1933). Metabolic studies of children with dental caries. *J. Biol. Chem.* **103:** 327.

9. Bransby, E. R., and J. R. Forrest (1963). Dental effects of fluoridation of water with particular reference to a study in the United Kingdom. *Proc. Nutr. Soc. (London)* **22:** 84.

10. Carlos, J. P., A. M. Gittelsohn, and W. Haddon, Jr. (1962). Caries in deciduous teeth in relation to maternal ingestion of fluoride. *Public Health Rept. (U.S.)* **77:** 658.

11. Dalzell-Ward, A. J. (1963). Fluoridation and public relations. *Proc. Nutr. Soc. (London)* **22:** 91.

12. Dean, H. T. (1938). Endemic fluorosis and its relation to dental caries. *Public Health Rept. (U.S.)* **53:** 1443.

13. *Diet and the Teeth. An Experimental Study. Pt. III. The Effect of Diet on Dental Structure and Disease in Man* (1934). Med. Res. Council, Special Rept. Series 191, London.

14. Englander, H. R., and D. A. Wallace (1962). Effect of naturally fluoridate water on dental caries in adults. Aurora-Rockford, Illinois, Study III. *Public Health Rept. (U.S.)* **77:** 887.

15. Fosdick, L. S. (1950). The reduction of the incidence of dental caries. I. Immediate tooth-brushing with a neutral dentrifice. *J. Am. Dental Assoc.* **40:** 133.

16. Gustaffson, B. E., et al. (1954). The Vipeholm dental caries study. The effect of different levels of carbohydrate intake on caries activity in 436 individuals observed for five years. *Acta Odontol. Scand.* **11:** 232.

17. Heredity and infectious components of tooth decay (1961). *Nutr. Rev.* **19:** 105.

18. Hillman, R. W., P. G. Cabaud, and R. A. Schenone (1962). The effects of pyridoxine supplements on dental caries experience of pregnant women. *Am. J. Clin. Nutr.* **10:** 512.

19. Howell, C. L., and J. C. Muhler (1954). Effect of topically applied stannous chlorofluoride on the dental caries experience in children. *Science* **120:** 316.

20. *The Influence of Diet on Caries in Children's Teeth* (1936). Med. Res. Council, Special Rept. Series 211, London.

21. Jenkins, G. N. (1962). Chemistry of food and saliva in relation to caries. In *Chemistry and Prevention of Caries.* (R. F. Sognnaes, ed.) Charles C Thomas, Springfield, Ill., p. 126.

22. Jordan, W. A., and J. K. Peterson (1957). Caries-inhibitory value of a dentifrice containing stannous fluoride. First year report of a supervised toothbrushing study. *J. Am. Dental Assoc.* **54:** 589.

23. King, J. D., M. Mellanby, H. H. Stones, and H. N. Green (1955). *Effect of Sugar Supplements on Dental Caries in Children.* Med. Res. Council, Special Rept. Series 288, London.

24. Knutson, J. W., and W. D. Armstrong (1943). The effect of topically applied sodium fluoride on dental caries experience. *Public Health Rept. (U.S.)* **58:** 1701.

25. Kyes, F. M., N. J. Overton, and T. W. McKean (1961). Clinical trial of caries inhibitory dentrifices. *J. Am. Dental Assoc.* **63:** 189.

26. Linghorne, W. J., et al. (1946). The relationship of ascorbic acid intake and gingivitis. *Can. Med. Assoc. J.* **54:** 106.

27. MacDonald, J. B. (1962). Microbiology of caries. In *Chemistry and Prevention of Caries.* (R. F. Sognnaes, ed.) Charles C Thomas, Springfield, Ill., p. 89.

28. McBeath, E. C. (1952). Experiments on the dietary control of dental caries in children. *J. Dental Res.* **12:** 723.

29. McClure, F. J. (1963). Personal communication.

30. Muhler, J. C. (1958). The effect of a single application of stannous fluoride on the incidence of dental caries in adults. *J. Dental Res.* **37:** 415.

31. Odland, L. M., L. Page, and S. T. Dohrman (1955). Dental caries experience of Montana students. *J. Am. Dietet. Assoc.* **31:** 1218.

32. Orland, F. J., et al. (1954). Use of the germfree animal technic in the study of experimental dental caries. I. Basic observations on rats reared free of all microorganisms. *J. Dental Res.* **33:** 147.

33. Orland, F. J., et al. (1955). Experimental caries in germfree rats inoculated with enterococci. *J. Am. Dental Assoc.* **50:** 259.

34. Ovrucky, G. D. (1959). Caries-preventing effect of drinking water containing minimum amounts of fluorine. *Gigiena i Sanit. (USSR)* **2:** 75.

35. Restarki, J. S. (1943). Incidence of dental caries among pure-blooded Samoans. *U.S. Naval Med. Bull.* **41:** 1713.

36. Rosebury, T., and M. Karshan (1937). Dietary habits of Kuskokwim Eskimos, with varying degrees of dental caries. *J. Dental Res.* **16:** 307.

37. Rushton, M. A. (1963). Fluoridation. *Proc. Nutr. Soc. (London)* **22:** 79.

38. Schatz, A., and J. J. Martin (1960). Destruction of bone and teeth by proteolysis-chelation: Its inhibition by fluoride and application to dental caries. *N. Y. J. Dentistry* **30:** 124.

39. Schlesinger, E. R., D. E. Overton, H. C. Chase, and K. T. Cantwell (1956). Newburgh-Kingston caries-fluorine study. XIII. Pediatric findings after ten years. *J. Am. Dental Assoc.* **52:** 296.

40. Shaw, J. H. (1952). Nutrition and dental caries. In *A Survey of Literature of Dental Caries.* (P. C. Jeans, ed.) Natl. Acad. Sci.—Natl. Res. Council, Publ. 225, Washington, D.C., p. 415.

41. Shaw, J. H. (1954). The effect of carbohydrate-free and carbohydrate-low diets on the incidence of dental caries in white rats. *J. Nutr.* **53:** 151.

42. Tabrah, F. L. (1962). Absence of dental caries in a Nigerian bush village. *Science* **138:** 38.

43. Tank, G., N. C. Esselbaugh, K. P. Warnick, and C. A. Storvick (1959). *Cooperative Nutritional Status Studies in the Western Region. III. Variation in Dental Caries Experience Among Children of Five Western States.* Oregon State Coll. Agr. Expt. Sta., Tech. Bull. 45, Corvallis, p. 35.

44. Wright, H. B. (1941). A frequent variation of the maxillary central incisors with some observations on dental caries among the Jivare (Shuara) Indians of Ecuador. *Am J. Orthodontics Oral Surg.* **27:** 249.

SUPPLEMENTARY REFERENCES

Hodge, H. C. (1963). Safety factors in water fluoridation based on the toxicology of fluorides. *Proc. Nutrition Soc. (London)* **22:** 111.

Symposium in tooth formation and dental caries (1961). *J. Am. Med. Assoc.* **177:** 304.

CHAPTER 24

Nutrition needs of children

Nutritional life really does not begin with birth. It actually begins during the prenatal period and is subjected to influences even earlier. The well-being of the infant is influenced not only by the diet of the mother during pregnancy but also by her status of nutrition prior to that period. Although she may serve to some extent as a factor of safety for the unborn child, the mother who is poorly nourished tends to give her baby a poor start in life nutritionally. Nutrition during pregnancy is discussed in Chapter 25.

▶ THE FIRST YEAR

At no other time of life is food so important as in the first year. The kind, amount, and sanitation of the food as well as the manner of feeding require particular attention, which pays dividends in the form of a healthy, happy baby. The nutrient requirements are high per unit of body weight because of rapid growth; never again after birth is growth so rapid. Furthermore, a baby has had little time to build reserves of needed nutrients and must rely on his daily food to supply them for the most part.

A well-nourished baby is usually round and chubby in appearance. After birth he progressively accumulates subcutaneous fat for about nine months, after which the amount diminishes. However, by one year he may still be quite chubby or he may be equally healthy but slender

(Fig. 24.1). In the well-nourished infant the muscle tissue feels firm, which is a good index of his status of nutrition. The pattern of growth varies during the first year; it is most rapid during the first months after birth. An ounce a day (2 lb a month) may be added to the body weight during the first three months. Then the pace slows to a gain of about a pound a month. Increase in length follows a similar pattern; babies increase about 20 per cent in height in the first three months, then they slow down so that by one year the total increase is about 50 per cent of the length at birth.

In the following paragraphs research and practical findings related to successful feeding of infants will be recounted. This general information is presented to give an understanding of the fundamentals. So important is this phase of the infant's life that specific directions and supervision of the feeding should come from a physician.

Breast Feeding Versus Artificial Feeding

The natural food provided for the human infant is human milk. Even so, either by choice or by necessity, it is not the universal infant food (1).

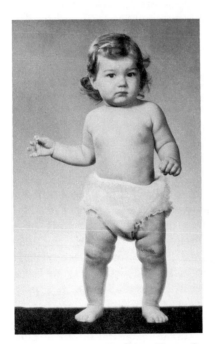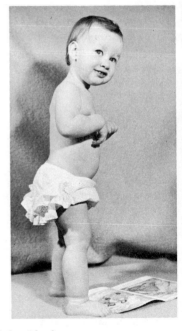

Fig. 24.1.   Two well-nourished baby girls of one year.

There has been a trend toward less breast feeding in this country over the last two decades. In 1946 (3) a survey of hospitals in the United States indicated that as nearly as could be estimated, only 38 per cent of the infants in this country were entirely breast fed even through the new-born period. In 1956 a similar survey showed a reduction to 21 per cent in total breast feeding with an additional 16 per cent partially breast fed on discharge from the hospital. In 1961 a nationwide survey by mail indicated 24 per cent of the infants to be completely breast fed during the first week with an additional 6 per cent who were breast fed but received in addition supplemental or complemental feedings (21).

In this country more women of the "upper" economic-educational class breast feed their infants than women of the middle class (21). The reverse is true in India; fewer women of higher socio-economic status than those less well off economically breast feed their infants (11). The trend observed in India is also characteristic of other developing countries.

A comparison of the welfare of 263 infants, some of whom were breast fed and others artificially fed, was made by the Harvard School of Public Health (27). There was little difference between the progress of the two groups. During the second six months of life the artificially fed infants had a slightly higher incidence of respiratory infections. The mothers of the artificially fed infants were carefully instructed in the method of preparation of the formula and of feeding the baby, which was doubtless a factor in the success.

With improvement in the formulas for artificial feeding there may be no longer any nutritional advantage in prescribing human milk; however, there are advantages still in breast feeding. Important among them are that it is free from bacterial contamination, it requires no preparation, and it is less likely to be associated with infant eczema and other allergic manifestations (8). Economy has been listed as an advantage, but actually the mother requires additional milk and a more abundant diet during lactation.

The choice between breast and artificial feeding is a matter for the mother to decide with her physician. In the judgment of Aldrich and his Committee on Maternal and Child Feeding of the National Research Council, breast feeding has the advantage of preventing or decreasing the severity of many gastrointestinal disturbances, especially in environments where sanitation and health measures are not adequate (2).

Whether or not breast feeding improves the parent-child relationship is controversial. Results from a recent study indicate that "warmth and nervous stability of the mother" are more important than whether the child is breast fed or fed by bottle (14).

Supplying the Needed Nutrients

A discussion of supplying the needed nutrients for infants must of necessity focus on milk. The composition varies somewhat with different species. Our chief interest is with human and cows' milk, although goats' milk is sometimes fed to infants. In comparison to cows' milk, human milk contains more lactose, iron, ascorbic acid, and vitamin A per unit of volume, and less of protein, calcium, phosphorus, riboflavin, and thiamine (Figs. 24.2 and 24.3). It is believed that each milk is adapted for the best nourishment of the young of the respective species.

Carbohydrate. Lactose is the carbohydrate in all milks. The quantity in cows' milk is about two-thirds that found in human milk, with the concentration further decreased in the artificial feeding by the addition of water in making the formula. Consequently some form of carbohydrate is usually added in preparing artificial feedings. The kind and amount should be at the discretion of the physician; sucrose and corn sirup are commonly used. The only disadvantage to these sugars is that they taste sweet. Lactose, the sugar that nature has placed in milk for use of the young, is the least sweet tasting of all the common sugars. However, lactose is not used because it is expensive and there is no evidence that

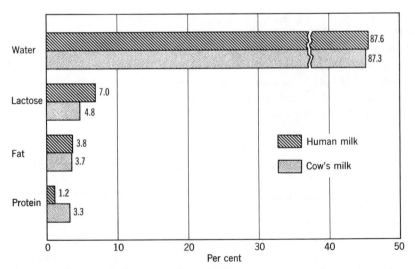

Fig. 24.2. Composition of human and cows' milk in grams of water, lactose, fat, and protein in 100 ml of milk. (Adapted from *Composition of Milks,* Natl. Res. Council, Publ. 254, p. 62, 1953.)

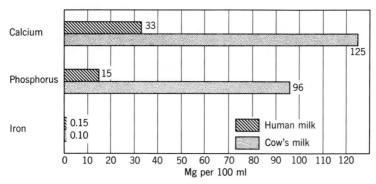

Fig. 24.3. Calcium, phosphorus, and iron content of human and cows' milk. (Adapted from *Composition of Milks*, Natl. Res. Council, Bull. 254, p. 63, 1953.)

it is more satisfactory than other products. Combinations of maltose and dextrins taste less sweet than sugar and sirup and have been used successfully in infant formulas.

It should be pointed out that artificial feeding with fresh whole milk and evaporated milk formulas with no added carbohydrate whatsoever has been used by some physicians with success. Some infants thrive on such formulas, others do less well. Mothers seemed to like the omission; the feedings are simpler to prepare.

Protein. The protein content of cows' milk is approximately triple that of human milk. The casein content of each milk is higher than the content of lactalbumin; however in cows' milk the casein is relatively higher, the lactalbumin lower than in human milk.

Raw cows' milk tends to form large, firm curds in the stomach of the infant. Dilution of the milk contributes to the formation of softer curds as does heat treatment, acidification, and homogenization.

The quantitative requirement of infants for the essential amino acids has been studied. A combination of pure amino acids in the proportions found in human milk was used to supply the protein in the formula. The amino acid under study was removed from the diet or reduced in amount. When as a result of the lack of the amino acid the gain in weight or nitrogen retention decreased considerably, it was restored to the diet in a stepwise manner until the level at which satisfactory weight gain and nitrogen storage were restored. The amino acid requirements determined by this method are compared in Table 24.1 with the intakes of breast fed infants and those fed cows' milk in quantities that supported normal health and growth (15).

The amino acid needs of the infant for growth and of the adult for

Table 24.1. Essential Amino Acid Requirements of Infants Compared with Intake in Human Milk and Cow's Milk

Amino Acid	Minimum Requirement[1] (mg/kg/Day)	Human Milk[2] (150 ml/kg/Day)	Cows' Milk[2] (2.0 gm Protein per kg per Day)
Histidine	34 (16–34)	35	45
Isoleucine	126 (80–126)	102	122
Leucine	150 (76–229)	162	216
Lysine	103 (88–103)	114	156
Methionine (in presence of cystine)	45 (33–45)	50	58
Phenylalanine (in presence of tyrosine)	90 (47–90)	104	110
Threonine	87 (45–87)	81	87
Tryptophan	22 (15–22)	27	24
Valine	105 (85–105)	107	132

[1] Observations made by Holt and Snyderman. Variations are shown in parentheses.
[2] Figures calculated from data in *The Composition of Milks*. Natl. Res. Council, Publ. 254, 1953.

Adapted from Holt et al., *Protein and Amino Acid Requirements in Early Life*. New York University Press, New York, p. 33, 1960.

maintenance of nitrogen equilibrium are quite different. The estimated need of the infant is much greater on the basis of unit of body weight than the adult need. Another difference is that histidine is essential for the infant but not the adult. These comparisons are summarized in Table 24.2.

The Recommended Allowance for daily protein intake of the infant up to one year is 2.5 ± 0.5 gm per kg. The allowance per kilogram decreases progressively from birth. The Food and Nutrition Board state that they found it "difficult to reach agreement on appropriate recommendations for the very young infant." They point out that:

Human breast milk contains a rather low level of protein, approximately 7 per cent of the total calories, but it is generally accepted that the breast-fed infant is adequately nourished with regard to protein. On the other hand, cow's milk and formulas prepared from it which have been widely used in the past for infant feeding supply much greater quantities of protein than does breast milk. These formulas are known to be reasonably successful. Thus, it is probable that the protein requirement is not higher than the amount supplied by human milk, but there has been reluctance to lower the recommended allowance until there is evidence that artificial formulas containing lower levels of protein are equally successful (20).

Breast feeding provides the infant an intake of about 1.5 to 2.5 gm of protein per kg body weight during the first six months of life.

Fat. The total quantity of fat in human and cows' milk is about the same, approximately 3.5 to 4.0 gm per 100 ml. However, the kinds of fatty acids of the fats in the two milks differ. Cows' milk contains proportionately more of the saturated fatty acids; human milk, on the other hand, is proportionately higher in the content of unsaturated fatty acids. The occurrence of some of the fatty acids in human and cows' milk is given in Table 24.3. The amount of linoleic acid, an unsaturated fatty acid, in human milk is about five times that in cows' milk. Arachidonic acid, also an unsaturated fatty acid, occurs in about equal amounts in the two milks. Arachidonic acid was considered an essential fatty acid at one time, but it is now known that it can be derived from linoleic acid.

Evidence of linoleic acid deficiency was observed in young infants who were fed in one instance a diet practically devoid of fat, or in another, a diet that provided an average amount of fat (42 per cent of

Table 24.2. Essential Amino Acid Requirements of Infants and Adults, mg/kg/day

Amino Acid	Infant Requirement	Adult Requirement		
		Men	Women	Average
Histidine	34	—	—	—
Isoleucine	126	10.4	5.2	7.8
Leucine	150	9.9	7.1	8.5
Lysine	103	8.8	3.3	6.1
Methionine (in presence of cystine)	45	—	3.9	3.9
Phenylalanine (in presence of tyrosine)	90	4.3	3.1	3.7
Threonine	87	6.5	3.5	5.0
Tryptophan	22	2.9	2.1	2.5
Valine	105	8.8	9.2	9.0

Adapted from Holt et al., *Protein and Amino Acid Requirements in Early Life,* New York University Press, New York, p. 34, 1960.

Table 24.3. Distribution of Some of the Lipid Components in Human and Cows' Milk

| | gm/100 gm Milk Fat Mature Milk | |
	Human	Cow
Total fat	3.8	3.7
Fatty acid distribution		
Saturated fatty acids		
Butyric	0.4	3.1
Caproic	0.1	1.0
Caprylic	0.3	1.2
Capric	1.7	2.6
Unsaturated fatty acids		
Linoleic (octadecadienoic)	8.3	1.6
Arachidonic	0.8	1.0

From *The Composition of Milks*. Natl. Res. Council, Publ. 254, p. 65, 1953.

the Calories) but was extremely low in linoleic acid content (less than 0.1 per cent of the Calories). The characteristic symptom of the deficiency was dryness of the skin with desquamation, thickening, and later chafing. Rate of growth was slow for most of the infants on low linoleic acid intakes. Symptoms disappeared promptly when linoleic acid was provided at the level of 1 per cent or more of the Calories (13).

Minerals: Calcium. Cows' milk contains over three times as much calcium as human milk per unit of volume. A thriving breast-fed baby receives about 60 mg calcium per kg body weight whereas the infant fed a standard-type cows' milk formula will receive about 160 mg calcium per kg. The per cent of the calcium retained is higher for human than cows' milk, 66 per cent and 35 to 50 per cent, respectively. Because of the higher intake, the actual amount of calcium retained is greater from cows' milk feedings. The retention from human milk must be adequate, however, because breast-fed babies manifest excellent growth.

The Recommended Allowance of 0.7 gm daily is intended for the artificially fed infant during the first year of life (20).

Iron. Both human and cows' milk contain very little iron. The infant is born with a store of iron that the body holds tenaciously, using it throughout infancy. The capacity of the infant to retain fetal iron would not have been known had not the use of radioactive iron in metabolism studies been possible. One such study was done in this way:

women were given transfusions of blood during pregnancy in which the red cells contained radioactive iron, which made it possible to follow the iron on its course and to locate it in the infant.

At birth the infant contains about 80 mg iron per kg body weight (19). Of this total 50 mg per kg is in the blood as circulating hemoglobin, 25 mg per kg is present as storage iron, divided equally between the liver and other body tissues. The remaining 5 mg per kg is found in bone marrow, myoglobin, and intracellular enzymes.

The hemoglobin level is high at birth (around 22 gm per 100 ml) decreasing to a minimum (around 10.5 to 11.5 gm per 100 ml) at about three months of age, the time that iron-containing foods need to be added if they have not already been included in the diet. Providing dietary iron much earlier is apparently wasted effort for very little, if any, is used for hemoglobin formation prior to three to four months after birth. The iron that is used for this function during the first months of life enters the body during fetal development (transplacental iron). Even at one year 70 per cent of the iron in hemoglobin is transplacental in origin (25). Iron-rich foods used with success at the third to fourth month include egg yolk, green vegetables, meats, and enriched cereals.

In the United States a study of hospitalized infants indicated iron deficiency anemia to be characteristic of this group of infants (22). In developing countries iron deficiency anemia is common among infants (16). The fortification of a prepared milk formula with iron (12 mg per reconstructed quart) was found in experimental studies with infants to maintain hemoglobin and serum iron concentrations at normal levels in both full-term and premature infants (17). Beal and her coworkers (6) have warned against large-scale fortification of infant foods in the United States. They believe that the potential danger of storing iron in excess is a greater hazard than iron deficiency. (See Chapter 11 for discussion of iron overload.)

The extent to which maternal iron deficiency predisposes the infant to anemia is controversial at the time this review is being written (1965). A British study in which the maternal diet was supplemented with iron had no effect on the red cell values of children at 6, 12, and 18 months as compared with a control group (7).

It is now believed that the source of fetal iron is maternal plasma. For many years it was considered to be maternal red cells; evidence to the contrary is chiefly from experimental studies with the rabbit using radioactive iron. It was observed that as pregnancy progressed, relatively less of the plasma iron entered the maternal bone marrow and more was directed to the fetus. Near the end of the prenatal period the fetus was getting around 90 per cent of the total iron carried in the maternal plasma (7). Moore and Dubach (19) comment that "the changes in plasma iron turnover that occur in the human during pregnancy are probably less dramatic; pregnancy in the rabbit places a relatively greater demand for iron on the mother."

The intake of iron recommended by the National Research Council for infants from 3 to 12 months is 1.0 mg per kg body weight. A representative weight suggested by the Council for the first year is 8 kg, thus making around 8 mg daily the suggested intake.

Consumption studies show the mean intake of iron during the first year to be at an acceptable level for the most part; however, the intake is variable. There are many infants who are fed less and many who are fed more than the recommended amount. A survey of one-day records of 4000 six-month-old infants indicated an intake of 9.4 ± 6.7 mg for infants in urban areas and 7.9 ± 6.6 mg for infants in rural areas (10). The Denver longitudinal studies of 59 infants showed that the median intake over the first year was 0.83 mg per kg body weight daily or approximately 6.6 mg daily. The blood picture and rate of growth indicated to the investigators that the intake was sufficient (6). In another study of 40 infants, 9 to 11 months of age, the average intake of iron was 7.7 mg daily (12).

The Vitamins: Vitamin A. Total vitamin A in milk is comprised of preformed vitamin A and the carotinoid pigments. The proportion of the preformed vitamin is greater than that of carotinoids in human milk; in cows' milk the two portions are approximately equal (Table 24.4).

The Food and Nutrition Board recommend 1500 IU of vitamin A daily for the infant through the first year. This is approximately the amount in one quart of cows' milk of average composition. A quart of milk is more than the infant consumes in a day during his early months,

Table 24.4. Vitamin Content of Human and Cows' Milk

(per 100 ml Whole Milk)		
Vitamin	Human	Cow
A, μg	53	34
Carotenoids, μg	27	38
D, IU	0.42	2.36
Ascorbic acid, mg	4.3	1.6
Niacin, μg	172	85
Riboflavin, μg	42.6	157
Thiamine, μg	16	42

Adapted from *Composition of Milks.* Natl. Res. Council, Publ. 254, Washington D.C. 1953.

which makes it understandable that some physicians recommend a supplement of vitamin A during that period.

Thiamine. The amount of thiamine in the diet of the mother during lactation seems to be the major influence on the quantity secreted into the milk. If the diet of the mother included pork, the thiamine content of the milk was increased. If the intake of thiamine remained fairly constant from day to day, the milk thiamine remained fairly constant also.

The National Research Council recommendation is 0.4 mg per day to one year of age. Neither breast milk nor the modified-cows'-milk formulas provide the recommended amounts. The average thiamine content of human milk is about 0.21 mg per 100 Calories; the average whole milk dilution formula provides not more than 0.24 mg per 1000 Calories, and is most likely less by 20 per cent or more because of the heat treatment it receives. However, supplements to the diet during the first year (enriched cereals, egg, meat, and vegetables) provide additional thiamine.

Riboflavin. The riboflavin content of cows' milk varies somewhat with the breed of cow. The most serious cause of loss of this vitamin in market milk is exposure to light; it is stable to heat and to the processes of evaporation, drying, and homogenization.

The amount of riboflavin in human milk is found to bear a definite relationship to the riboflavin content of the maternal diet. For instance, on days when liver was an item in the mother's diet, a higher concentration of riboflavin appeared in the milk. The average concentration is about 0.6 mg per 1000 Calories in human milk, three to four times the amount in cows' milk. The relative utilization of riboflavin from the two milks is not known.

The recommendation for daily intake of riboflavin for infants is 0.6 mg during the first year.

Niacin. Human milk contains about twice as much niacin as does cows' milk whereas the reverse is true for tryptophan, the amino acid precursor. The concentration of niacin equivalent per 1000 Calories of human milk is 7.5 mg. The allowance recommended is 6.0 mg niacin equivalent per 1000 Calories.

Ascorbic Acid. The ascorbic acid content of human milk varies with the diet of the mother but generally exceeds that of cows' milk. Commercial processes, including pasteurization, evaporation, and drying, are destructive of ascorbic acid so that little is left by the time the cows' milk formula reaches the infant. Ascorbic acid is fed to the formula baby as a matter of course today, beginning shortly after birth. For safety it is usually recommended for the breast-fed infant also. Orange juice is commonly used as the source, although some young infants do not tolerate it well. As a consequence, pediatricians often replace it with ascorbic acid preparations.

The amount of ascorbic acid recommended by the Food and Nutrition Board is 30 mg daily during the first year. That amount is available in approximately one-fourth cup of orange juice.

Vitamin D. The amount of vitamin in milk is influenced by the diet. However, despite adding a source of the vitamin to the maternal diet, an insufficient amount is transmitted to the milk to cure rickets in infants. Physicians routinely recommend a supplemental source of vitamin D for both breast-fed and artificially fed infants, beginning soon after birth and continuing throughout the period of growth.

The requirements for vitamin D for infants and children have been defined by Jeans and Stearns (18) as the amounts that, with ample intakes of calcium and phosphorus and a diet otherwise adequate, will insure sufficient retention of minerals to permit normal growth and mineralization of the skeleton and teeth. The infant and young child who are growing rapidly have a proportionately greater need for the vitamin than the older child. A daily intake of 135 IU is sufficient to prevent rickets in infants, but better growth is obtained with 300 to 400 IU daily. Increasing the intake to 600 IU is found to accrue no additional benefits to the infant in rate of growth or calcium utilization (18, 23). The Recommended Allowance is 400 IU daily.

There are a number of commercial preparations on the market for supplying vitamin D; some are in combination with vitamin A. The preparation may be in oil or aqueous solution; the latter is preferred by many physicians to avoid the possibility of aspirating oil droplets into the lungs.

The Use of Vitamin Preparations. It is easy to exceed the recommended level of vitamin intake by the use of vitamin concentrates. A study of the vitamin A intake of 64 Denver children showed that after the first three months, three-fourths of the children met the Recommended Allowance by diet alone. Then, in addition, a concentrate of vitamin A was given 64 per cent of the time, which gave a median intake of 10,000 IU of vitamin A from all sources. The Recommended Allowance is only 1500 IU for children of that age (Fig. 24.4).

The intakes of vitamin D and ascorbic acid of the same group of Denver children that were observed for the vitamin A content of the diet, showed the median intake of vitamin D to be 1000 IU daily at 4 to 6 months; 840 IU daily at the end of the first year (5). In a survey in State College, Pennsylvania, of the nutritive intake of 40 infants, it

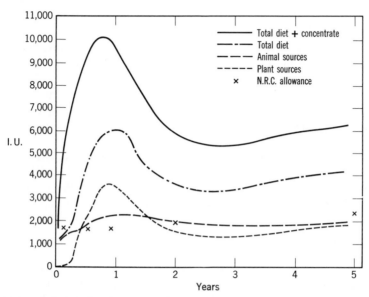

Fig. 24.4. Median intake of vitamin A from various sources contrasted with the Recommended Dietary Allowance in the first 5 years of life. (Courtesy of Beal, *J. Nutr.*, **60:** 340, 1956.)

was found that all were given vitamin supplements, none of which contained vitamin D at a potency of less than 1000 IU per daily dosage (12).

In the Denver study the ascorbic acid intake was from preparations of the vitamin rather than from food sources during the first 6 to 9 months, after which the diet was the major source. The median intake of ascorbic acid increased from 20 mg daily at one month to 53 mg at one year (5).

The long-term effects of moderately high intakes of vitamins have not been determined but warrant attention. It is of concern that children have the amount of necessary nutrients for their best health—neither too little nor too much.

Adding "Solid" Foods

Some babies are given solids as early as the first 4 weeks of life; others not until 3 months or later. A comparison of the response of two groups of infants, one with early feeding of solids, the other with later, revealed little difference in growth rate, number of illnesses, incidence of digestive disturbances, and food refusals (9). Spock and Lowenberg (26) give the general recommendations that babies should be having some variety of solid foods by the time they are 5 to 6 months old; in some cases earlier than that; in others, later. The time of adding solid foods is an individual matter, influenced by maturity of the infant, appetite, digestion, and tendency of the infant toward allergies (4). There seems to be no physiological need for these foods until the third or fourth month; at that time they are needed particularly to supply iron and thiamine but make valuable contributions to the intake of other nutrients as well.

Enriched cereals are commonly added first to supply extra energy, iron, thiamine and other nutrients. Pureed fruits are tolerated well as a rule and are frequently added next. The pureed vegetables then become a part of the expanding diet, as do egg yolk and strained meats.

Feeding the Baby

Greater emphasis is now being directed toward early feeding experiences of the infant in relation to his emotional development. During the first months of his life he learns whether or not he can trust the people on whom he is dependent. He experiences hunger, and with the satisfaction of that need he has a feeling of trust for the person who feeds him. Being hungry is one of his first frustrations, being fed one of his first satisfactions. The understanding of the fundamental importance of these first experiences of the infant has resulted in a departure from the rigid feeding schedule whereby the infant was fed at regular intervals, whether it meant awakening him from a sound sleep or letting him cry until the appointed hour for the feeding. The inflexible schedule has been replaced by the self-regulation schedule, in which the baby determines his own feeding schedule to a considerable extent. Mothers as a rule learn to know when the cry is a hungry one or for some other need. On occasion too much permissiveness, that is, feeding the baby at each cry, is as bad as too rigid discipline. During the first weeks of life, infants on self-regulation schedules tend to choose a feeding interval of less than 4 hours, with the interval lengthening so that by one year of age the general regimen of three meals a day is satisfactory to them.

▶ THE PRESCHOOL YEARS

During the years from 2 to 6, which are commonly designated as the preschool years, growth proceeds at a slower rate than during the first year. Within this period the baby leaves behind babyhood and develops into childhood. The gain in weight may be only 4 or 5 lb in a year during the preschool period whereas the infant may gain that much in a couple of months when he is very young. The preschool child grows relatively more in height and takes on an appearance of being taller and thinner. The round, chubby look of babyhood is gone; the arms and legs grow longer in proportion to the trunk; the short neck of infancy grows longer, and the head, which at birth accounted for about one-fourth of his total length, grows more slowly and assumes less of the total stature. The preschool child is streamlined in comparison to the chubby infant (Fig. 24.5).

The well-nourished preschool child is sturdily built. He gradually overcomes his infantile lordosis (sway-back) and uncertain waddle to become more like the adult in posture and stride. The well, normal child is alert

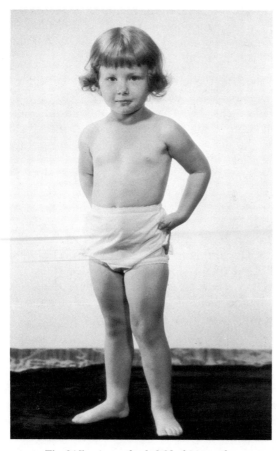

Fig. 24.5.   A preschool child of 34 months.

and busy exploring his environment, establishing himself as an individual in it.

The nutrient needs of children is an individual matter influenced by the rate of growth, activity, and status of nutrition of the child. Hence, the following discussion of food requirements sets forth general principles as guides to be adapted to each child.

Nutrient Needs of Children One to Six

Energy. The Food and Nutrition Board, with emphasis on individual variation, suggests 1300 Cal. daily for the child 1 to 3, and 1600 Cal. for the child 3 to 6 years of age (Table 24.5). The best measure of adequacy of energy intake is gain in body weight. That does not mean growth in reference to standard tables, but that each child is gaining at his own individual rate. Ideal supplements to increase the caloric intake are foods high in nutrient content such as milk, fruits, vegetables, and cereals (whole-grain or enriched). Foods to be avoided are concentrated sweets and foods high in fat.

Protein. Protein in the diet of the preschool child is of particular importance, because these years are marked by notable increase in muscular development (11). The Recommended Allowance for protein in early childhood is 32 gm for the years 1 to 3, and 40 gm for the child of 3 to 6 years. The allowances for protein provides approximately 10 per cent of the Calories.

Foods that provide protein in the diet of the preschool child are: milk, a glass at each meal would add approximately 20 to 24 gm protein daily; an egg providing 6 gm; and one serving of meat, fish, or poultry providing 8 to 10 gm.

The protein intake of preschool children of middle class families observed in the Harvard longitudinal studies (4, 5) ranged from 13.0 to 13.7 per cent of the total Calories, and provided 40 to 50 gm of protein daily. In an Ohio study of children attending day care centers and nursery schools, the diets of all the children met the Recommended Allowance for protein of 32 to 40 gm daily (10).

Calcium. In a study of calcium utilization preschool children were found to retain as much calcium from a pint of milk as from one and one-half pints or one and one-half quarts (Fig. 24.6). The Food and Nutrition Board, however, recommend 0.8 gm daily. During the first to ninth year of life the daily retention of calcium for skeletal growth has been estimated to be between 75 and 150 mg daily. The Food and Nutrition Board pointed out that the need will be more than adequately met by the 0.8 gm recommendation.

Table 24.5. Recommended Daily Dietary Allowances. Designed for the Maintenance of good Nutrition of Practically All Healthy Persons in the U.S.A.

	Age[1], Years	Weight kg	Weight (lb)	Height cm	Height (in.)	Energy, Cal.	Protein, gm	Calcium, gm	Iron, mg	Vitamin A Value, IU	Thiamine, mg	Riboflavin, mg	Niacin Equiv.,[2] mg	Ascorbic Acid, mg	Vitamin D, IU
Children	1-3	13	(29)	87	(34)	1300	32	0.8	8	2000	0.5	0.8	9	40	400
	3-6	18	(40)	107	(42)	1600	40	0.8	10	2500	0.6	1.0	11	50	400
	6-9	24	(53)	124	(49)	2100	52	0.8	12	3500	0.8	1.3	14	60	400
Boys	9-12	33	(72)	140	(55)	2400	60	1.1	15	4500	1.0	1.4	16	70	400
	12-15	45	(98)	156	(61)	3000	75	1.4	15	5000	1.2	1.8	20	80	400
	15-18	61	(134)	172	(68)	3400	85	1.4	15	5000	1.4	2.0	22	80	400
Girls	9-12	33	(72)	140	(55)	2200	55	1.1	15	4500	0.9	1.3	15	80	400
	12-15	47	(103)	158	(62)	2500	62	1.3	15	5000	1.0	1.5	17	80	400
	15-18	53	(117)	163	(64)	2300	58	1.3	15	5000	0.9	1.3	15	70	400

[1] Allowances are for the midpoint of the specified age periods; the line for children 1–3 is for age 2 years (24 months); 3–6 is for age 4½ years (54 months), etc.

[2] Niacin equivalents include dietary sources of preformed vitamin and the precursor, tryptophan. 60 mg tryptophan represents 1 mg niacin.

From Recommended Dietary Allowances Sixth Revised Edition. Natl. Acad. Sci.—Natl. Res. Council Publ. 1146, 1964.

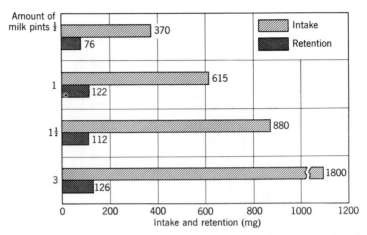

Fig. 24.6.   Daily calcium retention by preschool children on different levels of intake from milk. (Adapted from Outhouse et al., *J. Nutr.*, 17: 205, 1939.)

How well in actual practice do diets provide the recommended 0.8 gm daily of calcium? Surveys of food habits indicate that many children do not get that much. The nutrition histories of 58 Denver children between age 1 and 5 years showed one-half the children to have less than ¾ gm of calcium daily; half the children were drinking less than a pint of milk each day, which is the chief source of calcium in the diet (1, 2). In an Ohio study about two-thirds of the 100 children observed consumed diets containing at least 1 gm calcium daily. The children ate their noon meal at a nursery (10).

Iron. The Recommended Allowance for iron for the preschool child is 8 mg daily for children one to 3 years of age, and 10 mg for those 3 to 6 years of age.

The amount of iron needed has been determined for the most part by balance studies. Another approach is that of adding together the estimated amounts of the mineral used for growth, maintenance, and storage. Johnston at Cornell University computed the iron requirement of children in that way, using as a basis findings from her studies and others in the literature (Table 24.6). Growth needs were predicted from increases in body weight and blood volume; requirement for maintenance was estimated from day-to-day losses in body excretions. The storage needs were computed by subtracting from the estimated store of iron in the adult (about 1300 mg), the estimated store of the 2 year old (about 100 mg), and assuming the difference (1200 mg) to be the amount to be stored between 2 years of age and adulthood. It was presumed that smaller children would be able to contribute less to the total needed accumulation of iron than those who are older. Accordingly, it was assumed that one-eighth of the total amount would be stored between the ages of 2 and 6 years, leaving seven-eighths for the time between 6 years and adulthood. In order to retain 0.1 mg daily, which was the estimated allotment to the preschool years, an iron intake of 6 to 7 mg daily was estimated to be necessary, making allowance for poor absorption of iron from food (approximately 10 per cent).

It is not easy to supply the 8 to 10 mg of iron recommended daily unless some iron-rich foods are included in the day's menu. Eggs, meats, particularly liver, and green vegetables each can be counted on to provide 1 mg or more of iron in a child's serving. Enriched and whole-grain bread supply approximately 0.5 mg per slice, and enriched cereals from 0.5 to 1 mg per serving. One and one-half pints of milk provide 0.3 mg. Fruits provide some iron, most of them less than 0.5 mg per serving. Summing the rough estimate of iron from foods that would likely be in a *good* diet for a day, it amounts to around 7 to 8 mg.

Do children's diets meet the Recommended Allowance? In the study of the Denver children frequently referred to already, 75 per cent of the children between 2½ and 5 years had intakes of iron that were less than the Recommended Allowance. This is a contrast to the first 2½ years when the intake, bolstered by specially prepared baby foods, particularly cereals, adequately provided the recommended amount. Hemoglobin and erythrocyte values were within the limits recognized as normal for healthy preschool children despite an intake of iron less than the Recommended Allowance by a majority of the children (1). We need not interpret this finding to suggest that the Recommended Allowance be lowered. The children studied had had a generous intake

Table 24.6. Iron Requirement of Children

Function	5 Years of Age		10 Years of Age	
	Boys mg/Day	Girls mg/Day	Boys mg/Day	Girls mg/Day
Growth	0.2	0.3	0.4	0.5
Maintenance	0.3	0.3	0.4	0.4
Storage	0.1	0.1	0.2	0.4
Total to absorb	0.6	0.7	1.0	1.3
Food-iron required	6.0	7.0	7.0	9.0
National Research Council allowance	8.0	8.0	12.0	12.0

Adapted from Johnston, *J. Am. Dietet. Assoc.* 29: 760, 1953.

of iron in the years preceding this period. Also, we are well aware of the adjustment capacity of the body in maintaining a normal state despite nutrient intakes that are less than desirable.

The Eating Habits of the Preschool Child

It is natural for children of this age to vary in their eating habits from day to day and from meal to meal. Their preferences for kind as well as amount of food may be quite unpredictable. Such vacillations are recognized as part of developing childhood.

Allowing some choice of food by nursery school children has met with good success. Children were found to increase their food intake and to have fewer eating problems when some departure from a set menu was allowed. A choice as simple as the selection between two vegetables was found to bring about better habits of eating and enjoyment of food.

The unusual experiments of Davis must be mentioned in connection with children making their own food selections (6). She allowed newly weaned infants ranging in age from 7 to 9 months to select their own diet from a variety of natural foods, placed within their reach. All foods available to the children were excellent in nutritive value. They were provided from ten groups of foods including meats (muscles cuts), glandular organs, sea food (haddock), cereals (whole-grain wheat and barley, oatmeal, yellow corn meal, and rye wafers), bone products (bone marrow and bone jelly, containing soluble bone substances, made by boiling veal bones in water), eggs, milk, fruits, vegetables, and sea salt. During the year-long observations it was noted that the children had a tendency to select certain foods in "waves," eating large quantities of a favored food at one time, very little if any at all at another time. The children nourished themselves well. This study and subsequent ones that Davis did with older children reveal that children, with full responsibility for their own selection of amount and kind of food from a variety set before them, vary their preferences in unpredictable ways.

During the preschool years children have definite food likes and dislikes. There are certain characteristics of foods that tend to influence a child's reaction to them. Of course, there are marked individual differences but in general as Lowenberg (8) has pointed out, preschool children prefer mild-flavored foods; those with a soft, jellylike texture; and those that are lukewarm in temperature. Finger foods are popular with them; fresh carrots and rutabagas prepared as raw sticks were preferred to the cooked products (7). Colorful foods hold a special appeal.

The food likes and dislikes of parents affect the eating habits of the child. The effect may come about indirectly as observed by Bryan and Lowenberg (3) in that the foods disliked by the parents were not served the family. Similarly in an Ohio study (10), foods disliked by both parents were, with few exceptions, either unfamiliar to the child or disliked by him.

Factors in the environment contribute to the good eating habits of children. An attitude of expecting the child to eat and recognizing *that the child himself has something to contribute to his nutrition program* makes for good progress. Foods are more acceptable to the child if served in amounts suitable to him, with an awareness of his food preferences, his appetite, and his physical and emotional well-being at the time. The atmosphere during meal time should be pleasant; the chair on which he sits, the table from which he eats, and the utensils which he uses should be the right size to make eating easy and comfortable for him.

The preschool child is much interested in his environment, more so than in his food, a contrast from the babyhood he has just outgrown. The mother who is forewarned of this lagging interest is not alarmed at the change but recognizes it as a natural occurrence.

Refusing to eat is a weapon of strength for the child who is permitted to use it. The attention commanded from concerned adults contributes to the power of the tool. Refusals sometimes are initiated by the child when he is forced to eat when ill or overtired.

Foods for the Day

A general pattern of foods for a good daily diet for the preschool child is presented in Table (24.7) (9).

► THE SCHOOL CHILD AND THE ADOLESCENT

To be well nourished is one of the rights of childhood. The responsibility of turning this right into a reality rests with the parents, shared by teachers, school nurses, scout and recreation leaders, in fact, all who are interested in the welfare of children.

Measurements repeated generation after generation reveal that children in the United States are growing taller and in most instances heavier in each succeeding generation. Figure 24.7 shows the height and weight of boys and girls in Boston and vicinity at two periods about 50 years apart. Figure 24.8 shows the height and weight of children in Iowa and Ohio at periods 12 years apart. One of the factors responsible

Table 24.7. Food for the Day for the Preschool Child

Food	Amounts	Comments
Milk	2 to 3 cup	Some children do not have this capacity at the preschool age. If your child does not, let him drink what he wants and try to get in more by using it in cooking.
Meat or fish or poultry	1 serving	Beef, lamb, pork, poultry, fish, or liver may be used. Occasionally cheese may be substituted for a serving of meat. (For an average serving at this age, nutritionists sometimes estimate about one level tablespoon of meat or vegetables per year of age. But this is no hard and fast rule. In serving food to a young child, put on his plate only what you think he will eat.)
Egg	1	
Potatoes	1 average serving	
Vegetables	1 or 2 average servings of green or yellow	Suggestions: Carrots Cabbage Lettuce Spinach Squash Green peas Green beans Broccoli Green peppers Tomatoes Celery
Fruits	2 average servings	One of these to be orange or grapefruit for vitamin C
Cereal	1 average serving	Whole-grain or enriched
Bread	3 slices	Whole-grain or enriched
Butter or fortified margarine	2 tbsp	
Vitamin D supplement	As recommended by physician	

for increased growth is most likely nutrition. In addition, improved housing and sanitary conditions, increased immunization against disease, and better medical care have also contributed to making it possible for children to be "free to grow" unhampered by limiting environmental factors.

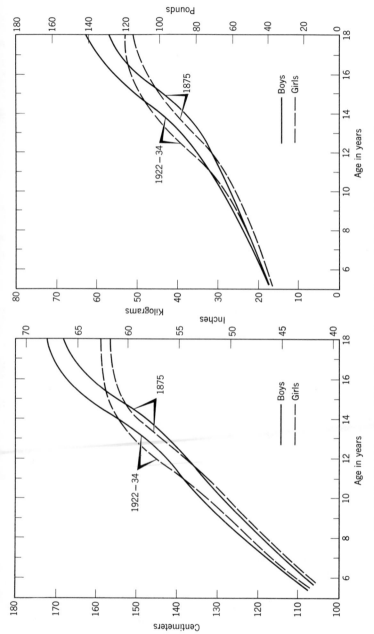

Fig. 24.7. Heights and weights of boys and girls in two periods about 50 years apart, Boston and vicinity. (Courtesy of Hathaway, U.S. Dept. Agr., Home Econ. Res. Rept. 2, 1957.)

429

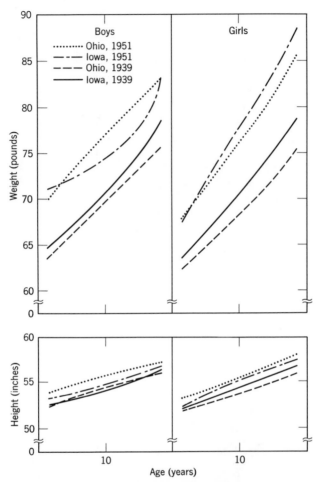

Fig. 24.8. Changes in height and weight of children in Ohio and Iowa between 1939 and 1951. (Courtesy of Patton and Hunt, *J. Am. Diet. Assoc.*, **35**: 459, 1959.)

Nutritional Needs

For adequate nutrition in childhood, the diet must provide sufficient nutrients for building new tissue (26). The rate of growth determines the amount needed for this purpose. The nutrient need for growth is in addition to the needs for energy, regulating body functions, and repair of tissue already formed. Children who are well-nourished reflect their state of well-being in their general appearance of vitality and fitness, their good posture, and well-developed musculature (Fig. 24.9).

In the years from 7 to 10 growth continues at a steady pace, followed by marked acceleration during the preadolescent period. The growth spurt in boys begins around 13 to 15 years and in girls around 10 to 11 years. Both boys and girls continue to grow rapidly for 4 or 5 years during the adolescent period. The rate then tapers off to the relatively small gains characteristic of early adulthood as final body size is approached.

During the span of years from 7 to 18, the total daily nutrient needs increase with each advance in age for the boys, and to age 15 for the girls. (Table 24.5). As teenagers, boys have higher nutritional requirements than at any other time in their life. Girls have a higher requirement than at any earlier time but less than the recommendations for women during pregnancy and lactation. The needs of the adolescent are influenced greatly by their rapid growth (Fig. 24.10).

The adequacy of the energy intake of individual children can be judged most readily by observing their patterns of growth and the amount of muscle and fat they have. If the growth rate seems to be normal

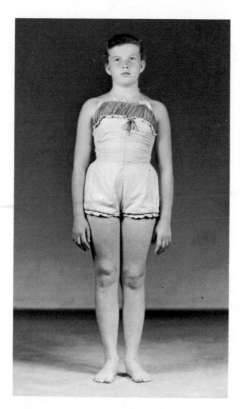

Fig. 24.9.   A well-nourished 12-year-old girl.

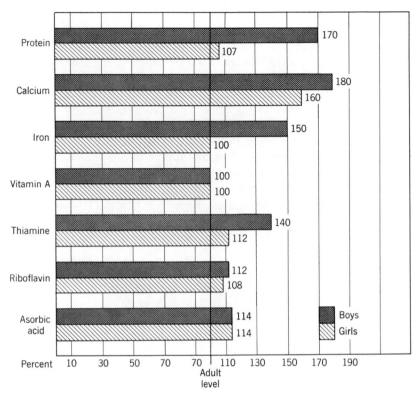

Fig. 24.10. Comparison of Recommended Allowances for the adolescent with those for the adult. Recommendations for boys 15 to 18 years in per cent of recommendation for the adult man 35 to 55 years; recommendation for girls 12 to 15 years in per cent of recommendation for the adult woman 35 to 55 years. (Natl. Acad. Sci.—Natl. Res. Council, Publ. 1146, 1964.)

for that individual and the child has firm muscles sufficiently well padded with fat, it can be concluded that caloric needs are being met. Tremendously wide differences must be expected among children in their growth patterns, with each still being a healthy individual. For most children, *what the appetite demands* is a fairly reliable guide to satisfying requirements.

The recommendations of the National Research Council for daily energy intake are intended to serve for individual children as approximate guides only, and are most useful when applied to groups of children (Table 24.5). The wide variation in body size and rate of growth during the years of adolescence have made it particularly difficult to establish caloric allowances that will not penalize some children by being too limited and at the same time prove too generous for others.

The recommendation for boys 12 to 15 years of age is 3000 Cal. daily; and to take care of the continuing rapid rate of growth in the 15 to 18 year period, 3400 Cal. For girls, 12 to 15 years, 2500 Cal. are recommended; with growth tapering off in the 15 to 18 year period the allowance is decreased to 2300 Cal.

It is not so easy to assess the adequacy of the protein, mineral, and vitamin intake as it is energy. Three extensive series of studies have contributed to the knowledge of nutritional needs and status of children. Macy and her coworkers in Detroit observed children 4 to 12 years of age, measuring the intake and excretion of eighteen chemical substances (25, 26). In a Southern regional experiment station project, the needs of the preadolescent girl were investigated for energy, protein, calcium, iron, phosphorus, magnesium, cobalt, copper, manganese, molybdenum, zinc, sulfur, vitamin A, carotene, riboflavin, folic acid, vitamin B_{12}, and pantothenic acid (15, 29, 31, 32, 35, 45, 47, 54). At the Washington Agricultural Experiment Station the nutritional status of adolescent children and the dietary intake of vitamin A, ascorbic acid, riboflavin, and niacin were determined (10, 11, 19, 20, 21, 22). These series of studies and other research are reflected in the Recommended Daily Allowances for children (Table 24.5).

Values for the minimum requirement for eight essential amino acids have been suggested by Nakagawa and his coworkers of Tokyo (33) for preadolescent boys. The investigators patterned the amino acid mixture used and the procedure followed after that of Rose (40). In brief, a negative nitrogen balance is induced by withdrawal of an essential amino acid from the mixture. On replacement of the amino acid, the least amount required to maintain a positive nitrogen balance is considered the minimal need. Removal of neither arginine nor histidine induced a negative balance. The findings are summarized in Table 24.8 with reported work for adults. With seven of the amino acids, all except tryptophan, the estimated minimal amino acid requirement for the boys, on the basis of total for the day, exceeded that for the adults. Amino acid needs have been investigated quantitatively only relatively recently. Further study of more persons may of course bring some changes in values.

Food Habits

Adequacy of Food Intake. To improve the food habits of children it must first be known what they eat, the good points and shortcomings of their usual food intake. As a rule when children start to school they enter an era of making more food choices on their own. By teenage time they wish, for the most part, to exercise full authority in matters of what they will and will not eat.

Table 24.8. Estimates of Minimal Amino Acid Requirements of Preadolescent
Boys[1] and Adults[2]

| Amino Acid | No. of Subjects | Preadolescent | | Adults | |
		Age Range in Years and Months	Value Defined Tentatively as Minimum, gm/Day	Male gm/Day	Female gm/Day
Isoleucine	3	11–0 to 11–6	1.00	0.70	0.45
Leucine	3	10–11 to 11–2	1.50	1.10	0.62
Lysine	5	10–7 to 11–0	1.60	0.80	0.50
Methionine	4	10–9 to 11–3	0.80	0.20[3]	0.35
Phenylalanine	4	10–9 to 12–3	0.80	0.30[4]	0.22
Threonine	4	10–4 to 12–6	1.00	0.50	0.30
Tryptophan	4	10–11 to 12–1	0.12	0.25	0.16
Valine	4	11–6 to 12–3	0.90	0.80	0.65

[1] From Nakagawa, Takahashi, Suzuki, and Kobayashi, *J. Nutrition* **80:** 310, 1963.
[2] From Food and Nutrition Board, Committee on Amino Acids, *Evaluation of Protein Nutrition.* Natl. Acad. Sci.—Natl. Res. Council Publ. 711, p. 10, 1959.
[3] With adequate cystine.
[4] With adequate tyrosine.

Dietary studies of school age and adolescent children in most sections of this country have been made (6, 13, 23, 30, 37, 38, 45, 46, 48, 50, 51, 52, 55). States have cooperated with each other and with federal agencies (the U.S. Department of Agriculture and the U.S. Public Health Service) in making observations that are sufficiently extensive to give a picture of the food consumption patterns of children in the United States during 1948 to 1963.

Certain nutrients in the diets of these children failed to meet the NRC recommendations more commonly than others. Calcium, ascorbic acid, and vitamin A meet the NRC recommendations least well. Iron in the diet of teenage girls commonly failed to meet the suggested allowance. Inadequate consumption of milk, citrus fruits, and other ascorbic-acid-rich foods, and green and yellow vegetables was chiefly responsible for the nutrient shortages. Protein was adequate in the diets more frequently than any other nutrient.

A unique record of food habits of children was obtained by Burke and her coworkers as part of a longitudinal study of the health of children from their first through their eighteenth year of life. One hundred twenty-five children (64 boys and 61 girls) from middle-class, economically independent families were observed. The average protein intake expressed as per cent of total Calories by age for boys and for girls (Table 24.9)

Table 24.9. Percentage Total Calories Derived from Total Protein by Age and Sex

Age, Years	Boys, Range in %	Girls, Range in %
1–4	13.0–13.5	13.2–13.9
4–11	12.9–13.1	12.9–13.3
11–18	12.2–12.6	12.4–12.8

Adapted from Burke, Reed, van den Berg, and Stuart, *Am. J. Clin. Nutr.* **9**: 732, 1961.

was found to be highest for the 1 to 4 year age group and least for the children 11 to 18 years of age. The protein intake of the majority of the children provided 12 to 14 per cent of the total Calorie value of the diet. Recommendations of the National Research Council are about 10 per cent of the total Calories.

Protein intake according to age and sex are shown in Table 24.10. As early as 5 years of age a difference in intake between the sexes begins

Table 24.10. Protein Intakes According to Age and Sex

Age, Years	Protein Intake (gm/day)							
	Boys				Girls			
	Mean	S. D.[1]	Lowest	Highest	Mean	S. D.[1]	Lowest	Highest
1–2	43.6	7.7	25.0	60.0	44.3	7.0	32.5	57.5
2–3	46.1	8.1	27.5	62.5	46.9	8.3	30.5	72.5
3–4	50.0	8.4	32.5	70.0	49.1	8.4	29.0	70.0
4–5	53.2	8.6	32.5	72.5	53.6	9.3	34.0	80.0
5–6	57.7	9.8	40.0	77.5	56.7	10.2	33.0	85.0
6–7	63.6	11.7	42.5	97.5	60.3	11.8	35.0	90.0
7–8	65.4	11.5	45.0	97.5	63.4	12.9	37.5	100.0
8–9	69.5	12.9	45.0	107.5	65.4	10.9	40.0	85.0
9–10	72.5	13.9	45.0	105.0	69.4	14.3	37.5	110.0
10–11	77.9	15.7	50.0	127.5	73.6	14.4	45.0	105.0
11–12	82.8	15.7	55.0	120.0	76.5	14.3	50.0	120.0
12–13	87.4	13.3	60.0	113.5	78.2	13.7	57.5	132.5
13–14	96.4	16.8	55.0	142.5	81.4	14.5	45.0	122.5
14–15	101.7	20.7	57.5	165.0	80.9	15.0	60.0	140.0
15–16	106.6	22.9	70.0	175.0	81.6	18.5	52.5	145.0
16–17	107.8	20.7	62.5	145.0	77.7	15.9	50.0	130.0
17–18	110.6	24.4	65.0	185.0	76.8	16.5	52.5	135.0

[1] S. D. = standard deviation.

From Burke, Reed, van den Berg and Stuart, *Pediatrics*, Part II, p. 926, 1959.

to appear and continues throughout the years of observation, with the boys consuming more than the girls (3, 4).

Calcium intakes of the same children (Table 24.11) were found to average approximately one gram or more daily (5). The Recommended Allowance for children up to 9 years of age is 0.8 gm daily; 9 to 12 years, 1.1 gm; 12 to 18 years for boys 1.4 gm, and for girls 1.3 gm daily.

Adolescent Girls. Much has been said and written about the nutritionally poor diets of adolescent girls, but little is known about the underlying influences affecting their eating behavior. A contributive study to this question was done at Iowa State University, by Hinton, Eppright, and coworkers (23). They found from observations of 140 girls, 12 to 14 years of age, that those who scored highest in a test measuring emotional stability, conformity, adjustment to reality, and family relationships had better diets and missed fewer meals than other girls. This finding is of particular significance for nutrition education.

Supplements to the Diet. Through the years it has interested nutritionists to find out how the addition of certain foods to the diet of children influences their physical status. Improvement in rate of growth was

Table 24.11. Calcium Intake (Grams per Day) According to Age and Sex

Age, Years	Boys				Girls			
	Mean	S. D.[1]	Lowest	Highest	Mean	S. D.[1]	Lowest	Highest
1–2	0.89	0.19	0.40	1.30	0.91	0.19	0.60	1.45
2–3	0.88	0.21	0.40	1.30	0.90	0.19	0.50	1.40
3–4	0.93	0.20	0.40	1.35	0.92	0.17	0.60	1.25
4–5	0.94	0.17	0.60	1.45	1.00	0.18	0.60	1.30
5–6	1.03	0.20	0.55	1.80	1.03	0.23	0.50	1.55
6–7	1.08	0.23	0.65	1.85	1.05	0.23	0.65	1.40
7–8	1.08	0.22	0.60	1.90	1.08	0.24	0.60	1.50
8–9	1.11	0.22	0.70	2.00	1.09	0.22	0.70	1.45
9–10	1.17	0.24	0.70	2.20	1.16	0.25	0.70	1.80
10–11	1.27	0.29	0.85	2.55	1.18	0.27	0.67	1.95
11–12	1.28	0.33	0.65	2.30	1.22	0.28	0.60	2.45
12–13	1.36	0.30	0.65	2.10	1.19	0.28	0.75	2.30
13–14	1.47	0.36	0.65	2.60	1.23	0.28	0.30	1.95
14–15	1.55	0.45	0.90	2.55	1.22	0.30	0.75	2.50
15–16	1.62	0.55	0.40	3.30	1.28	0.41	0.65	3.00
16–17	1.62	0.55	0.50	2.90	1.16	0.40	0.50	2.85
17–18	1.65	0.58	0.50	3.30	1.08	0.39	0.40	2.15

[1] S. D. = standard deviation.

From Burke, Reed, van den Berg and Stuart, *Am. J. Clin. Nutr.* **10**: 81, 1962.

the criterion most commonly used for assessing the beneficial effect of the added nutrients. No change in growth was interpreted as evidence that the current food intake supplied sufficient amounts of the dietary essentials, and providing more in the added food made no difference.

School feeding programs in childrens' institutions provided avenues for supplemental feeding. There are certain problems involved in getting precise information from such studies. It is difficult to find out about the "usual" diet and practically impossible to control it when children are living at home. It can be done with more ease when children live in institutions. The role of health, psychological influences, and whims of the appetite cannot be ruled out as factors. Nevertheless, these early observations did yield results which, without a doubt, led to better feeding of children—the ultimate goal of such nutrition studies.

Among the early recorded experiences was the one of Mann in England. He observed 350 boys over a period of 2 years; one group was kept on the usual diet and used as a control. An addition of approximately 336 Cal. was made to the usual diet of each of four groups, as a pint of milk to one, and sugar, margarine, and butter to the other three, respectively. To a fifth group, casein equivalent to the amount supplied by a pint of milk was used, and to the sixth group watercress was given. The supplement of a pint of milk produced the greatest growth, both in height and in weight (27).

Among the more recent investigations is one carried out with 185 Iowa school girls, 8 to 14 years of age (12). The food supplement consisted of milk, and fruits and vegetables high in vitamin A or vitamin C content. The control group was given fruits and vegetables providing a minimal amount of the vitamins. With supplementation of the diet so that the intakes of vitamin A and ascorbic acid ranged from 66 to 100 per cent of the Recommended Allowance, the blood levels of the carotenoids and ascorbic acid rose significantly above the levels in the unsupplemented period and above the levels of the control group.

A finding that has a bearing on the importance of providing an adequate diet for children is that as diets become more adequate, the consumption of sugar decreases. Macy and her collaborators (25) made this observation during their extensive investigations of nutrition during childhood. As the study progressed, the diets were adjusted as to quantity and quality to suit the needs of each particular child. Sugar could be used voluntarily as much or as little as desired, and as the diets became more adequate each child ate less sugar. This scientific finding confirms casual, everyday observations at home, at school, and at the county fair, that good diets are the best preventive to an abnormal craving for sweets.

Most important in the welfare of children today in many countries is protein supplementation to diets (28). Children of lower income groups in developing areas of the world almost always suffer protein malnutrition. Because of the magnitude of the problem, a Protein Advisory Group (PAG) was appointed by the Director General of the World Health Organization (WHO) in 1955, which was later established as a joint advisory group to WHO, the Food and Agriculture Organization (FAO), and the United Nations Children's Fund (UNICEF).

PAG has been instrumental in securing funds for research in the development of protein sources for use in areas of need. A publication of this Committee reports the gratifying progress that is being made in work with: soya protein in Brazil; fish flour in Mexico, Peru, and Chile; a cereal-cottonseed mixture (Incaparina) in Central America; leaf-protein concentration in Jamaica; peanut-cereal mixtures in Uganda and Nigeria; a protein-supplemental maize in South Africa; peanut flour in Senegal; various oil seed meals in the Congo; a chick pea-peanut flour mixture for India (India Multipurpose Food); and others (28, 42).

The Importance of Breakfast

Breakfast warrants special emphasis in view of the fact that it is the meal of the day most frequently skipped—not only by children but by adults as well. Furthermore, if not omitted entirely, it is apt to be scanty and hurried.

The breakfast problem is not new. In 1918 Roberts surveyed the dietary habits of 6000 preschool children in Gary, Indiana, finding one-third of them to have eaten no breakfast, or one that was wholly inadequate such as *one cup of coffee* or *one cup of coffee and a few cookies* (27). It is evident that poor breakfast habits begin at an early age.

Incidence of Poor Breakfasts. Studies of breakfast habits of children give ample evidence that many children are eating no breakfast at all or one that is inadequate (30, 37, 43, 44). The habits of 10,144 California students in 81 junior and senior high schools were obtained by questionnaire. Six per cent of the young people indicated that they never eat breakfast, 26 per cent that they do sometimes. The reason given by over half of those not eating breakfast or doing so irregularly was lack of time. In a Connecticut study, rural eighth graders omitted more meals than any of the other children in grades 5 through 8, from both town and country. Breakfast was the meal that over one-half of them skipped. Twelve per cent of 1300 Indiana children, 9 to 14 years of age, were found to be eating no breakfast or having coffee only. One-half to two-thirds of the 1188 Iowa school children whose food habits were studied had predominantly poor breakfasts.

Effects of Poor Breakfasts. Research studies show that without a good morning meal it is difficult to supply the recommended nutrient intake for the day. Only one child in five was found to make up in the other meals of the day the nutrient deficit caused by a poor breakfast (Fig. 24.11). Those who omit breakfast entirely invariably have a less adequate food intake for the day than those who eat a morning meal. In a study of the food habits of Montana students, the total day's food intake provided the needed nutrients in better supply when the breakfasts eaten were adequate, than when they were not (Fig. 24.12).

Poor breakfasts may interfere with achievement in school (16, 36). In a study in Toronto, Canada, teachers observed that children who reported eating inadequate breakfasts appeared to be more fatigued and less attentive to their school work than those who had eaten better breakfasts. Twelve- to fourteen-year-old boys in an Iowa study reacted in a similar manner; they were restless and inattentive in the late morning hours when they had eaten no breakfast. The same boys when they ate breakfast, improved in scholastic achievement and had sufficient energy for outside activity.

Findings from a contributive series of experiments at the University of Iowa give further evidence that whether or not breakfast is eaten, and the quality of the breakfast *does make a difference* with most people (9, 36). The observations were with young adults, for the most part; some with adolescent boys. Evenso, the studies are included in the discussion of children's food habits where evidence of the benefits of a good breakfast is needed for effective educational programs.

The general plan of the studies included feeding breakfasts of different nutritive quality, and in some series, omitting the meal entirely, accompanied by measurements of the effect on certain physical and

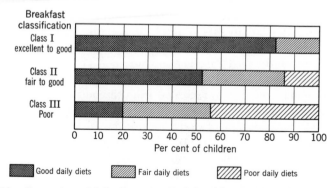

Fig. 24.11.   Comparison of daily diet ratings with breakfast classification. (Courtesy of Sidwell and Eppright, *J. Home Econ.*, **45**: 404, 1953.)

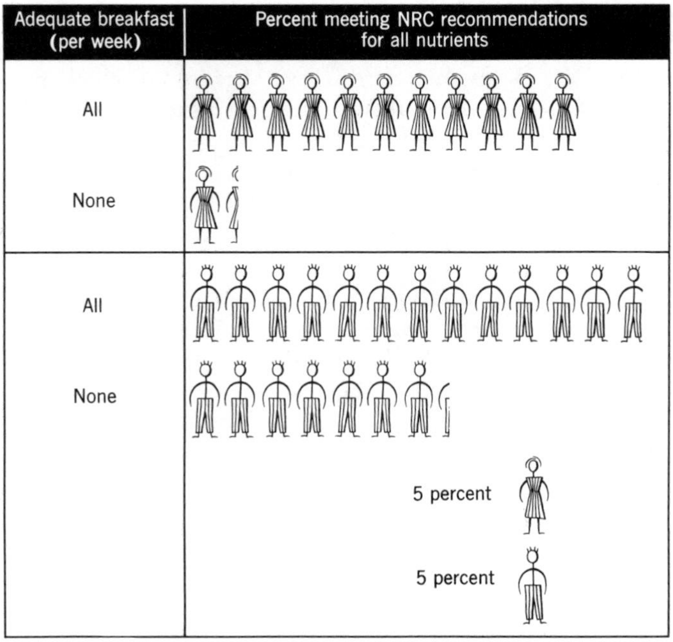

Fig. 24.12.   Effect of adequacy of breakfasts on success in meeting NRC Recommended Allowances for the day. (Adapted from Odland et al., *J. Am. Dietet. Assoc.*, 31: 1134, 1955.)

mental responses. The *basic breakfast*, an adequate morning meal, providing one-fourth of the daily caloric requirement (600 Cal. for the women; 750 for the men) contained the following foods: fruit, (100 gm), cereal (30 gm, 1 c), whole milk (360 gm, 12 oz, 1½ gl), sugar (5 gm, 1 tbsp), enriched white bread (60 gm, 2½ sl), butter (8 gm, 1 pat). The *heavy breakfast* supplied 1000 Cal. for the women, 1200 for the men, and provided in addition to the foods in the basic breakfast the following: bacon (20 gm, 2 sl), cream (60 gm, 2 oz), egg (50 gm, 1), and jelly (20 gm, 1 tbsp). With no *breakfast* no food was eaten between 8 o'clock in the evening and noon the next day. The measurements of behavior included *neuromuscular tremor, maximum work output,* and *reaction time.*

Neuromuscular tremor was recorded from the outstretched right arm, unsupported (except by voluntary resistance against the force of gravity) before and after one minute of strenuous exercise on a bicycle ergometer (an ordinary bicycle with instrument for measuring work output) (Fig. 24.13). Lower readings indicate less movement of the arm, and a more favorable response. Maximum work output was calculated from measurements taken as the subjects rode the bicycle ergometer at their maximum effort for one minute (Fig. 24.14). Reaction time to a stimulus of light was measured as the interval of time elapsing between the appearance of the light and the person's recognition of it, which he indicated by pressing a switch with the finger (Fig. 24.15). With reaction time, the shorter the time interval, the more favorable the response.

Effect of No Breakfast. By all three measures of individual efficiency *no breakfast* had an unfavorable effect on most persons. The tremor magnitude was greater and the reaction time slower in all subjects tested except adolescent boys. It is a tribute to the steady nerves and alertness of the 12 to 14 year olds that these responses were uninfluenced by omission of breakfast. However, all persons observed, including the boys, showed a decrease in maximum work output in the late morning hours when breakfast was omitted.

Effect of a Cup of Coffee. A cup of black coffee alone proved to be more detrimental to physical and mental efficiency than no breakfast at all. In the Iowa studies 10 women, 18 to 25 years of age, were given black

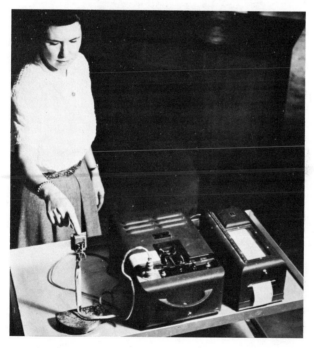

Fig. 24.13.   Determination of neuromuscular tremor magnitude. Index finger of unsupported arm lightly touches a pin. Tremor is thus transferred into an electric current which is amplified sufficiently to activate a recording pen. (Courtesy of␣W. W. Tuttle, Department of Physiology, College of Medicine, University of Iowa.)

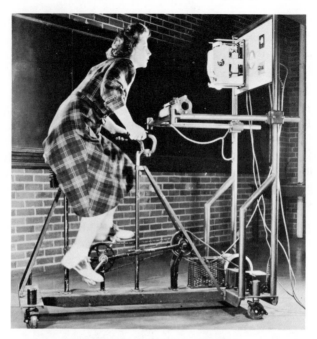

Fig. 24.14. Determination of maximum work output. Subject is shown riding a bicycle ergometer, which is a conventional bicycle with attachment for measuring work output. (Courtesy of W. W. Tuttle, Department of Physiology, College of Medicine, University of Iowa.)

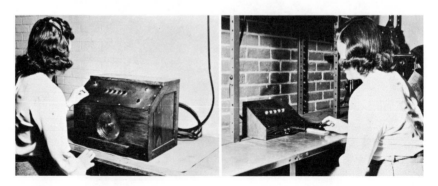

Fig. 24.15. Determination of reaction time. Operator (shown at left) presses switch to flash light before subject in the next room. Subject (shown at right) has hand on response key which is pressed when light flashes. (Courtesy of W. W. Tuttle, Department of Physiology, College of Medicine, University of Iowa.)

coffee without sugar. The tremor magnitude increased and the maximum work output decreased in all persons, and in 45 per cent of the cases the reaction time increased over those responses with no food or drink.

Effect of a Heavy Breakfast. A heavy breakfast decreased the maximum work output of the men studied but not of the adolescent boys. The men, 20 to 35 years of age, were fed a heavy breakfast of 1200 Cal. containing 38 to 40 gm of protein. In 75 per cent of the cases the men did significantly less work after eating the heavy breakfast than after the consumption of the regular basic breakfast of 750 Cal. with 25 gm of protein. The other two indices of physiological effect, tremor magnitude, and reaction time, registered no difference with the two types of breakfasts. The adolescent boys with their high nutrient needs could handle the heavy breakfast without evidence of detraction from their efficiency.

Effect of Amount of Protein in the Breakfast. Sufficient protein in the breakfast has been found to help prevent that hungry feeling before lunch. How much protein is enough to prevent the late forenoon lag? For young women 17 to 29 years of age a breakfast containing approximately 23 gm protein, with 20 gm fat, 46 gm carbohydrate, and providing 450 Cal., prevented hunger symptoms in all who ate it in a study at the University of Maine (7). The breakfast contained the following foods:

		protein, gm
Orange juice	½ c	1.0
Eggs	2	12.2
Bread	2 sl	4.0
Butter	1 tsp	0.0
Light cream	1 tbsp	0.4
Skim milk	⅔ c	5.7
Coffee	⅔ c	. . .
		23.3

What is the physiological explanation for protein in the breakfast allaying sensations of hunger and weakness before noontime? Breakfasts of equal caloric value, but low in protein content and high in carbohydrate or fat, do not appear to have this beneficial effect. The explanation lies in the difference in the effect the three foodstuffs have on the blood glucose level following the meal. Breakfasts sufficiently high in protein content elevate the blood glucose level above the fasting level for a period of approximately 4 hours after the meal; meals low in protein but high in fat and in carbohydrate elevate the level for only 2 and 3 hours respectively. Sensations of hunger and a feeling of weakness are associated with low blood sugar levels.

Is there a reason for the length of time that the blood glucose remains elevated after eating isocaloric breakfasts, some high in protein, some in fat, and some in carbohydrate? The explanation lies in the difference in the amount of glucose arising from the meal and the rate at which it enters the blood stream. Over half the protein in an average diet can be used as carbohydrate. It enters the blood stream slowly over an extended period because certain intermediary changes must be made before the protein can be used as glucose in the blood. With fat only the glycerol portion, which is considered to be about 10 per cent of the total, can be used as carbohydrate. Fat elevates the blood glucose least of the three foodstuffs. In the case of carbohydrate, it is more nearly ready to enter the blood stream as blood sugar than the protein and fat. Consequently, within the first hour after breakfast the blood glucose rises to a peak, but by the end of the second hour it has fallen almost to the prebreakfast (fasting) level. By then with a high carbohydrate breakfast, there is justification on a physiological basis for wanting to eat again.

The amount of protein in the meal is found to make a difference in the length of time the blood glucose can be held above fasting level (2, 7, 34, 36). The 23 gm of protein in the breakfasts of the young women in Maine, cited earlier in relation to allaying hunger, was sufficient to hold the blood glucose level above the fasting value for 4 hours. Numerous studies in the literature concur that approximately that amount of protein is needed; 15 gm was found to be insufficient in one study with young women to elevate the blood glucose for 3½ to 4 hours; 22 gm was sufficient in another. In observations with young men, 10 gm of protein was not enough whereas 25 gm was an adequate amount.

Good Breakfasts. Certain foods are commonly served for breakfast. That does not mean that other foods are not equally acceptable for the morning meal if they are wholesome and nutritious. It is reasonable to expect the foods of the morning meal to provide from one-quarter to one-fifth of the day's total nutritional requirements (with lunch and dinner each providing one-third and snacks the remainder). One pattern of an adequate breakfast for a school child includes the following foods:

Fruit
Whole-grain or enriched cereal
Egg or other protein food such as ham, sausage, or bacon
Bread, whole wheat or enriched
Butter or fortified margarine
Milk

The Role of Snacks

Contribution to Food Intake. Eating between meals is not in itself an offense to good nutrition; the kind of food eaten may be. We must accept the fact that the majority of children do eat snacks. The foods eaten for between-meal snacks are found consistently to provide energy to a greater extent than essential nutrients (Table 24.12) (14, 44). Unfortunately, snacks seem not to improve the diets that need improvement. Where the food intake was poor in quality, snacks contributed little to bolstering the nutrient content of the food for the day.

Snacking—A Social Custom. We recognize that between-meal snacks serve a dual function, first in providing a portion of the nutritional requirements of the day, and second in filling a social need. The gregarious aspect of snacking is no less important than the nutritional function. Members of groups, especially teenagers, influence the choices of one another through the tendency to follow the gang. It is an opportune situation to promote nutritious snacks as a popular selection.

Effect of Snacks on Meal-Time Eating. It is of interest to know whether eating snacks influences the quantity of food eaten at the following meal or the total intake for the day. Milk given between meals to children ranging from 3 to 14 years was found not to hamper their appetites for the next meal (53).

With teenage girls it has been noted that as the Calories from snacks increase, the Calories from breakfasts decrease. The girls who consumed the most candy and soft drinks tended to eat the smallest breakfasts (18).

Snack Foods. Good foods for snacks are those that provide at least as great a percentage of the day's total requirement for several of the essential nutrients as for energy and are not high in satiety value. All milk products, fruits, and sandwiches are good for in-between-meal eating (Fig. 24.16). Poor snack foods are those that provide "empty calories," that is, Calories and little else. Foods such as carbonated beverage, candy,

Table 24.12. Percentage of Total Day's Intake from Snacks

	Boys				Girls			
Age in Years	6–8	9–11	12–14	15+	6–8	9–11	12–14	15+
Calories	15	14	13	17	13	15	16	16
Protein	9	9	8	11	8	9	11	10
Calcium	11	9	11	14	9	10	12	13
Iron	10	9	8	11	9	10	11	10
Vitamin A value	8	7	6	8	7	8	9	8
Ascorbic acid	14	14	11	12	14	15	13	11
Thiamine	12	12	11	15	12	13	13	13
Riboflavin	11	11	12	15	10	12	14	14
Niacin	9	8	8	11	8	9	9	8

Adapted from Eppright and Swanson, *J. Am. Dietet. Assoc.* **31:** 257, 1955.

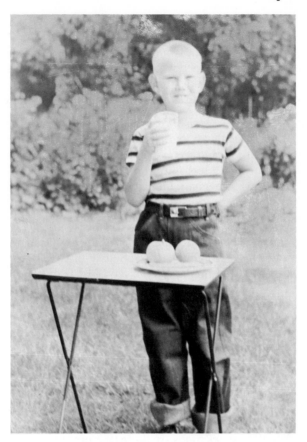

Fig. 24.16.   Enjoying a snack.

and crackerjack fall in that category. Concentrated sweets satisfy the appetite quickly; in other words, they are high in satiety value but jade the appetite.

Nibbling versus Eating Meals. Studies with experimental animals indicate that small frequent feedings bring about certain physiological responses that are beneficial; many animals of course are nibblers by nature. Rats fed an amount of food in two meals a day that would normally be consumed by nibbling become obese, with elevated blood glucose and blood cholesterol levels. In man changing his feeding regime from meal-eating (3 meals a day) to nibbling (as many as 10 meals a day) in which the nutrient intake was constant was found to lower blood cholesterol and phospholipids; returning to three meals a day was accompanied by a return of the lipids to higher levels. The reaction in man occurred in normal individuals and also those with hyperlipidemia (8, 17).

The Noon Meal

The midday meal, whether eaten at school or at home, should provide approximately one-third of the day's total Calories and nutrient needs. When the lunch is inadequate the total food intake for the day is apt to be inadequate also. The deficiencies caused by a poor lunch are not supplied by the other meals or by snacks.

Lunch at School. School feeding has been on the increase as judged by the extent of participation in the National School Lunch Program (Fig. 24.17). In 1944 a total of approximately 475 million lunches were served with 38 per cent the complete-meal type (Type A); in 1958, 1883 million lunches were served and 98 per cent were Type A. Currently (1965) 2.7 billion lunches are served each year in the schools (39).

Serving food at school is not a new venture. The practice was recorded

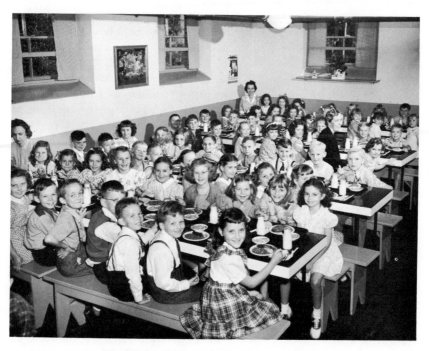

Fig. 24.17.   Children enjoying their school lunch.

long before the present-day feeding program was instigated. In the United States school feeding in the early days was initiated by voluntary societies and women's clubs, and was confined to cities, New York, Philadelphia, and others. Today, of course, it reaches rural and urban areas as well as cities.

School feeding is worldwide in scope. A survey made in 1949–1950 showed that in some countries a program had been organized on a nationwide scale, in others it was limited (41). In most countries some effort has been made at one time or another to provide some nourishment at school for the children.

Contributions of the School Lunch. A child's lunch at school should be a meal that will improve the nutritive value of his total food intake for the day. The complete-meal type of lunch, providing approximately one-third of the nutritional needs for the day, contributes the share of nutrients generally expected of the noonday meal. If only a partial meal is served, to be effective, those foods should supplement the nutrients provided by the remainder of the day's diet. It is an ill-advised practice to feed children at school the same foods provided in abundance in the family meals, and omit certain essential foods both at school and at home. Persons who assume responsibility for school feeding in local areas need to familiarize themselves with the prevailing food habits of families as a general guide for planning. Furthermore, the school lunch should provide for the child as good a meal as the one he would otherwise have had.

The school lunch is not only a means of providing nutritious food for children, but affords unique educational opportunities as well. Experiences in connection with the meal are natural situations for the teaching of certain health habits, the importance of good grooming, table manners, and nutrition. To fully realize the educational advantages, lunchroom practices may be related to classroom discussion and guidance in an integrated program. In this connection if the learning experiences are to be effective, they must be geared to the suitable educational level of the children.

It may be that for some few children it is not in their best interest to have lunch at school even though the program be of the finest caliber. We recognize that there are children who are readily over-stimulated and who benefit from being away from their classmates for a period of quiet at noontime.

Children's Enjoyment of the School Lunch. Although nutritive quality is an essential yardstick for planning the school lunch menus, within that framework cognizance of the food likes and dislikes of the children contribute much to the success of the program. Active participation in phases of menu planning, followed by serving foods that the children themselves have recommended, improves eating habits and general enjoyment of meal time.

It should be recognized too that children are sensitive to the quality of preparation of foods and the manner of serving. They like food well prepared but in simple ways, attractively but simply served, and in amounts suitable to their capacities. It has proved effective to take children behind scenes into the kitchen to see food in the process of preparation. First-hand experience with simple processes of food preparation has been found to whet disinterested appetites into accepting certain disliked foods. Sometimes it is forgotten that the school lunch is for the child and not the child for the school lunch. Success is certain to attend the program built around the child's needs and interests.

Nutritive Value of School Lunches. Reference was made in a preceding paragraph to the Type A complete lunch. The pattern for this meal as described in the National School Lunch Act of 1946 and later modifications specifies that one-third to one-half of the day's nutritive needs be provided and that at least the following foods be included:

(1) Fluid whole milk, one-half pint.

(2) A protein food such as two ounces (edible portion as served) of fresh or processed meat, poultry, fish, or cheese; or one-half cup cooked dry peas, beans, or soybeans; or four tablespoons of peanut butter; or one egg. To be counted in meeting this requirement, these foods must be served in a main dish or in a main dish and one other menu item.

(3) Vegetables and/or fruit—a three-fourth cup serving consisting of two or more vegetables or fruits, or both. Full-strength vegetable or fruit juice may be counted to meet not more than one-fourth cup of this requirement.

(4) Bread and cereal products as desired; one serving of whole-grain or enriched flour.

(5) Butter or fortified margarine—2 teaspoons.

Do meals planned following the five-point scheme listed provide at least one-third of the day's nutrient needs? Government research workers investigated that question (49). They found thiamine to be least well supplied, followed by ascorbic acid. These findings indicate that we should pay special attention to including foods that provide these vitamins when planning the school lunch menu.

A lunch without milk falls short of meeting the requirements of an adequate noonday meal. Calcium and riboflavin, in particular, and protein, thiamine, and energy value also were reduced in amount by the omission of milk.

Effect of School Lunch on Nutritional Status. Some children improve in nutritional status when provided a lunch at school, others show no change in physical condition. It is apparent that we cannot anticipate improvement in nutritional status unless the lunch provides essential nutrients that would otherwise be deficient in the total day's diet. Furthermore, children who are already well nourished cannot be expected to show striking improvement with school feeding.

An extensive study over a period of five years in Florida showed the school lunch to be of distinct benefit to the physical well-being of the children (1). The children showed symptoms of poor nutrition at the outset. During the school year these symptoms lessened. Notable among the changes during the period when the children were having lunch at school was the increase in hemoglobin values; during vacation the levels lowered again. Height and weight measurements charted on the Wetzel grid showed an advance in developmental level during the feeding period. On the other hand, children who were in fairly good physical condition prior to the program, as observed in two Maryland elementary schools, showed little difference in physical status with school feeding (49).

In a Pennsylvania study, the only children who showed improvement following their participation in the school lunch program were those whose lunches had been carefully planned by someone trained in nutrition and dietetics, who took care that the noon meal supplemented those served at home to provide a more adequate total daily food intake (24). The nutritive value of the lunches was computed and the nutritional status of the children assessed at intervals; medical and dental examinations were included.

The Evening Meal

The evening meal may also fail to supply its fair share of the day's dietary nutrients. Some families have their big meal for the day at noon and leftovers and snacks in the evening. Children who eat lunch away from home, and one that is not always adequate, have little opportunity to make up the deficiencies in the evening. A good evening meal, like breakfast and lunch, is essential in ensuring an adequate food intake for the day.

▶ SUGGESTIONS FOR GOOD DIETS FOR SCHOOL CHILDREN

Helpful suggestions are available in government publications for providing adequate meals for children.

A SAMPLE DAY'S MEALS FOR A 10-YEAR-OLD

BREAKFAST

Tomato juice (¾ c)
Hot whole wheat cereal (⅔ c) with milk (½ c)
Toast (2 sl) with butter or fortified margarine (2 tsp)
Milk (½ pt)

LUNCH

(If served at school or at home)
Creamed eggs (¾ c)
Green beans (½ c) with butter or fortified margarine (1 tsp)
Oatmeal muffins (2) with butter or fortified margarine (2 tsp)
Milk (½ pt)
(If brought from home)
Sandwich—peanut butter and raw carrot on buttered whole-grain or enriched
   bread
Supplemented at school by—
Orange
Milk soup (1 c) or cocoa (1 c)
Sandwich—chopped dried fruit on buttered whole-grain or enriched bread
Supplemented at school by—
Orange
Milk soup (1 c) or cocoa (1 c)

DINNER

Meat loaf (1 serving)
Scalloped potatoes (⅔ c)
Coleslaw with red and green peppers (½ c)
Whole wheat bread or enriched bread (2 sl) with butter or fortified margarine
   (2 tbsp)
Applesauce (½ c)
Molasses cookies (2 thin)
Milk (½ pt)

Snacks of fruit, milk, Graham crackers.

A SAMPLE DAY'S MEALS FOR AN ADOLESCENT BOY

BREAKFAST

Orange (1 med)
Shredded wheat with milk (½ c)
Eggs (2)
Muffins (3) with butter or fortified margarine (2 tbsp) and marmalade (2 tbsp)
Cocoa (2 c)

LUNCH

Macaroni and cheese (2 lg servings)
Sliced tomatoes (2) with mayonnaise (1 tbsp)
Rye bread (2 med sl) with butter or fortified margarine (1 tbsp)
Baked apple (1 lg) with sugar (1 tbsp) and cream (¼ c)
Cookies (2 large)
Milk (½ pt)

DINNER

Pot roast of beef (lg serving)
Baked potato with gravy
Cabbage (1 c) with butter or fortified margarine (2 tbsp)
Whole wheat bread (2 med sl) with butter or fortified margarine (1 tbsp)
Rice milk pudding (2 servings)
Milk (½ pt)

Snacks of fruit, milk, cookies, sandwiches.

REFERENCES

THE FIRST YEAR

1. Aitkin, F. C., and F. E. Hytten (1960). Infant feeding: Comparison of breast and artificial feeding. *Nutr. Abstr. Rev.* **30:** 341.
2. Aldrich, C. A. (1947). The advisability of breast feeding. A survey of the subcommittee on maternal and child feeding, National Research Council. *J. Am. Med. Assoc.* **135:** 915.
3. Bain, K. (1948). The incidence of breast feeding in hospitals in the United States. *Pediatrics* **2:** 313.
4. Bakwin, H. (1964). Feeding programs for infants. *Federation Proc.* **23:** 66.
5. Beal, V. A. (1956). Nutritional intake of children. IV. Vitamins A and D and ascorbic acid. *J. Nutr.* **60:** 335.
6. Beal, V. A., A. J. Meyers, and R. W. McCammon. (1962). Iron intake, hemoglobin, and physical growth during the first two years of life. *Pediatrics* **30:** 518.
7. Bothwell, T. H., and C. A. Finch (1962). *Iron Metabolism.* Little, Brown, and Co., Boston, p. 302.
8. Breast feeding (1956). Editorial. *J. Am. Med. Assoc.* **161:** 1569.
9. Deisher, R. W., and S. S. Goerr (1954). A study of early and later introduction of solids into the infant diet. *J. Pediat:* **45:** 191.
10. Filer, L. J., and G. A. Martinez (1963). Caloric and iron intake by infants in the United States: an evaluation of 4000 representative six-month-olds. *Clin. Pediat.* **2:** 470.
11. Gopalan, C., and B. Belavady (1960). Nutrition and lactation. In *Panel IV—Nutrition in Material and Infant Feeding.* Fifth Intern. Congr. Nutr., Washington, D.C.
12. Guthrie, H. A. (1963). Nutritional intake of infants. *J. Am. Dietet. Assoc.* **43:** 120.
13. Hansen, A. E., H. F. Wiese, A. N. Boelsche, H. E. Haggard, D. J. D. Adam, and H. Davis. (1963). Role of linoleic acid in infant nutrition. *Pediatrics* **31:** 171. Supplement.
14. Heinstein, M. I. (1963). Influence of breast feeding on children's behavior. *Children* **10:** 93.
15. Holt, L. E., P. Gyorgy, E. L. Pratt, S. E. Snyderman, and W. M. Wallace (1960). *Protein and Amino Acid Requirements in Early Life.* New York University Press, New York.

16. *Iron Deficiency Anemia* (1959). World Health Organ., WHO Tech. Rept. Series No. 182, Geneva.
17. Iron fortification of milk (1960). *Nutr. Rev.* **18:** 105.
18. Jeans, P. C., and G. Stearns (1938). The effect of vitamin D on linear growth in infancy. *J. Pediat.* **13:** 730.
19. Moore, C. V., and R. Dubach (1962). Iron. In *Mineral Metabolism*, Vol. 2, Pt. B. (C. L. Comar and F. Bonner, eds.) Academic Press, New York, p. 325.
20. *Recommended Dietary Allowances Sixth Revised Edition* (1964). Natl. Acad. Sci.—Natl. Res. Council, Publ. 1146, Washington, D.C.
21. Robertson, W. O. (1961). Breast feeding practices; some implications of regional variations. *Am. J. Public Health* **51:** 1035.
22. Schulman, I. (1962). Iron needs in infancy. *Pediatrics* **30:** 516.
23. Slyker, F., B. M. Hamil, M. W. Poole, T. B. Cooley, and I. G. Macy (1937). Relationship between vitamin D intake and linear growth in infants. *Proc. Soc. Exptl. Biol. Med.* **37:** 499.
24. Smith, C. A. (1961). Nutritional problems of children. *Nutr. Rev.* **19:** 353.
25. Smith, C. A., *et al.* (1955). Persistence and utilization of maternal iron for blood formation during infancy. *J. Clin. Invest.* **35:** 1391.
26. Spock, B., and M. E. Lowenberg (1955). *Feeding Your Baby and Child*. Duell, Sloan, and Pearce, New York, p. 55.
27. Stevenson, S. S. (1949). Comparison of breast and artificial feeding. *J. Am. Dietet. Assoc.* **25:** 752.

SUPPLEMENTARY READING

THE FIRST YEAR

Infant Care (1963). U.S. Dept. Health, Education, and Welfare, Children's Bureau Publ. 8, Washington, D.C.

Mellander, O., B. Vahlquist, T. Mellbin (1959). Breast feeding and artificial feeding. *Acta Paediatrica* **48:** 11. Suppl. 116.

Sargent, D. W. (1962). *An Evaluation of Basal Metabolism Data for Infants in the United States*. U.S. Dept. Agr., Home Econ. Res. Rept. 18, Washington, D.C.

Stitt, P. G., and M. M. Heseltine (1962). Some practical considerations of economy and efficiency in infant feeding. *Am. J. Public Health* **52:** 125.

Watson, E. H., and G. H. Lowrey (1962). *Growth and Development of Children*. 4th ed. Yearbook Medical Publishers, Chicago.

THE PRESCHOOL YEARS

1. Beal, V. A. (1954). Nutritional intake of children. II. Calcium, phosphorus, and iron. *J. Nutr.* **53:** 499.
2. Beal, V. (1961). Dietary intake of individuals followed through infancy and childhood. *Am. J. Public Health* **51:** 1107.
3. Bryan, M. S., and M. E. Lowenberg (1958). The father's influence on young children's food preferences. *J. Am. Dietet. Assoc.* **34:** 30.
4. Burke, B. S., R. B. Reed, H. S. van den Berg, and H. C. Stuart (1961). Relationships between animal protein, total protein, and total calorie intakes in diets of children from one to eighteen years of age. *Am. J. Clin. Nutr.* **9:** 729.
5. Burke, B. S., R. B. Reed, H. S. van den Berg, and H. C. Stuart (1959). Calcium and protein intakes of children between 1 and 18 years of age. *Pediatrics* **24:** 922. Supplement.

6. Davis, C. M. (1928). Self selection of diet by newly weaned infants. *Am. J. Diseases Children* **36:** 651.
7. Dudley, D. T., M. E. Moore, and E. M. Sunderlin (1960). Children's attitudes toward food. *J. Home Econ.* **54:** 297.
8. Lowenberg, M. E. (1948). Food preferences of young children. *J. Am. Dietet. Assoc.* **24:** 430.
9. *Mealtimes with Young Children* (1947). Rochester Child Health Institute, Rochester, Minnesota. Reprinted by permission, College of Home Economics, The Pennsylvania State University, Publ. 146. University Park, 1954.
10. Metheny, N. Y., F. E. Hunt, M. B. Patton, and H. Heye (1962). I. Nutritional sufficiency findings and family marketing practices II. Factors in food acceptance. *J. Home Econ.* **54:** 297, 303.
11. Stearns, G. (1952). Nutritional health of infants, children, and adolescents. *Proc. Natl. Food and Nutr. Institute*, U.S. Dept. Agr., Agr. Handbook 56, Washington, D.C. p. 59.

SUPPLEMENTARY READING

THE PRESCHOOL YEARS

Evaluation of Protein Quality (1963). Natl. Acad. Sci.—Natl. Res. Council, Publ. 1100. Washington, D.C.

Human Protein Requirements and Their Fulfillment in Practice (1955). Proc. of a Conf. in Princeton, N.J., Food and Agr. Organ. U.N., World Health Organ., and Josiah Macy Jr. Found., New York.

Sargent, D. W. (1961). *An Evaluation of Basal Metabolic Data for Children and Youth in the United States*. U.S. Dept. Agr., Home Econ. Res. Rept. 14, Washington, D.C.

Your Child from 1 to 6 (1962). U.S. Dept. Health, Education, and Welfare, Children's Bureau. Washington, D.C.

THE SCHOOL CHILD AND THE ADOLESCENT

1. Abbott, O. D., R. O. Townsend, R. B. French, and C. F. Ahmann (1946). *Effectiveness of the School Lunch in Improving the Nutritional Status of School Children*. Univ. Florida Agr. Expt. Sta. Bull. 426, Gainesville.
2. Addison, V. E., W. W. Tuttle, K. Daum, and R. Larsen (1953). Effect of amount and type of protein in breakfasts on blood sugar levels. *J. Am. Dietet. Assoc.* **29:** 674.
3. Burke, B. S., R. B. Reed, A. S. van den Berg and H. C. Stuart (1959). Longitudinal studies of child health and development, Harvard School of Public Health, Series II, No. 4. Calorie and protein intakes of children between one and eighteen years of age. *Pediatrics* **24:** 922.
4. —————— (1961). Longitudinal studies of child health and development, Harvard School of Public Health, Series II, No. 9. Relationships between animal protein, total protein, and total caloric intakes in the diets of children from one to eighteen years of age. *Am. J. Clin. Nutrition* **9:** 729.
5. —————— (1962). A longitudinal study of the calcium intake of children from one to eighteen years of age. *Am. J. Clin. Nutrition* **10:** 79.
6. Clayton, M. M. (1952). Food habits of Maine school children. *Am. J. Public Health*, **42:** 967.
7. Clayton, M. M., and S. W. Randall (1955). Blood changes following breakfasts of different types. *J. Am. Dietet. Assoc.* **31:** 876.
8. Cohn, C. (1961). Meal-eating, nibbling, and body metabolism. *J. Am. Dietet. Assoc.* **38:** 433.
9. Daum, K., W. W. Tuttle, C. Martin, and L. Myers (1950). Effect of various types of breakfasts on physiologic response. *J. Am. Dietet. Assoc.* **26:** 504.

10. Donald, E. A., N. C. Esselbaugh, and M. M. Hard (1958). Nutritional status of selected adolescent children. II. Vitamin A nutrition assessed by dietary intake and serum levels. *Am. J. Clin. Nutr.* **6:** 126.

11. Donald, E. A., N. C. Esselbaugh, and M. M. Hard (1962). Nutritional status of selected adolescent children. V. Riboflavin and niacin nutrition assessed by serum level and subclinical symptoms in relation to dietary intake. *Am. J. Clin. Nutr.* **10:** 68.

12. Eppright, E. S., C. Roderuck, P. Garcia, and K. Wessels (1963). Effects on girls of greater intake of milk, fruits, and vegetables. *J. Am. Dietet. Assoc.* **42:** 299.

13. Eppright, E. S., V. D. Sidwell, and P. P. Swanson (1954). Nutritive value of the diets of Iowa school children. *J. Nutr.* **54:** 371.

14. Eppright, E. S., and P. P. Swanson (1955). Distribution of nutrients among meals and snacks of Iowa school children. *J. Am. Dietet. Assoc.* **31:** 256.

15. Feeley, R. M., and Elsie Z. Moyer (1961). Metabolic patterns in preadolescent children. VI. Vitamin B$_{12}$ intake and urinary excretions. *J. Nutr.* **75:** 447.

16. Galloway, M. E., and E. C. Robertson (1948). Types of breakfasts eaten and their effect on the level of the blood sugar in school children. *J. Can. Dietet. Assoc.* **10:** 53.

17. Gwinup, G., R. C. Byron, W. H. Roush, F. A. Kruger, and G. J. Hamwi (1963). Effect of nibbling versus gorging on serum lipids in man. *Am. J. Clin. Nutr.* **13:** 209.

18. Hamilton, L. W. (1955). *Relationship of General Food Patterns to Breakfasts Eaten by a Group of Seventh Grade Students.* Master's Thesis, The Pennsylvania State University, University Park.

19. Hard, M. M., and N. C. Esselbaugh (1960). *Food Patterns of Washington Adolescent Children.* Wash. State Univ. Agr. Expt. Sta., Bull. 613, Pullman.

20. Hard, M. M., and N. C. Esselbaugh (1956). Nutritional status of selected adolescent children. I. Description of subjects and dietary findings. *Am. J. Clin. Nutr.* **4:** 261.

21. Hard, M. M., and N. C. Esselbaugh (1960). Nutritional status of selected adolescent children. IV. Cholesterol relationships. *Am. J. Clin. Nutr.* **8:** 346.

22. Hard, M. M., N. C. Esselbaugh, and E. A. Donald (1958). Ascorbic acid nutriture assessed by serum level and subclinical symptoms in relation to daily intake. *Am. J. Clin. Nutr.* **6:** 401.

23. Hinton, M. A., E. S. Eppright, H. Chadderdon, and L. Wolins (1963). Eating behavior and dietary intake of girls 12 to 14 years old. *J. Am. Dietet. Assoc.* **43:** 223.

24. Lowther, M. E., P. B. Mack, C. H. Logan, A. T. O'Brien, J. M. Smith, and P. K. Sprague (1940). The school lunch as a supplement to the home diet of grade school children. *Child Dev.* **11:** 203.

25. Macy, I. G. (1942). *Nutrition and Chemical Growths in Childhood.* Vol. I, Evaluation. Charles C Thomas, Springfield, Ill., p. 85.

26. Macy, I. G., and H. J. Kelly (1957). *Chemical Anthropology.* University of Chicago Press, Chicago, p. 2.

27. Martin, E. A. (1954). *Roberts' Nutrition Work with Children.* University of Chicago Press, Chicago, p. 142 and 170.

28. *Meeting Protein Needs of Infants and Children* (1961). Natl. Acad. Sci.—Natl. Res. Council, Publ. 843, Washington, D.C.

29. *Metabolic Patterns in Preadolescent Children* (1959). Southern Cooperative Series Bull. 64. Agr. Expt. Sta. of Georgia, Kentucky, Louisiana, Mississippi, Oklahoma, Tennessee, and Virginia.

30. Morgan, A. F. (ed) (1959). *Nutritional Status U.S.A.* Univ. Calif. Agr. Expt. Sta., Bull. 769, Berkeley.

31. Moschette, D. S. (1962). *Metabolic Patterns in Preadolescent Children. Blood Serum, Vitamin A, and Carotene Studies of Preadolescent Children.* Louisiana Agr. Expt. Sta., Bull. 552, Baton Rouge.

32. Moyer, E. Z., G. A. Goldsmith, O. N. Miller, and J. Miller (1963). Metabolic patterns in

preadolescent children. VII. Intake of niacin and tryptophan and excretion of niacin or tryptophan metabolites. *J. Nutr.* **79:** 423.

33. Nakagawa, I., T. Takahashi, T. Suxuki, and K. Kobayashi (1963). Amino acid requirements of children: Minimal needs of tryptophan, arginine, and histidine based on nitrogen balance method. *J. Nutr.* **80:** 305.

34. Orent-Keiles, E., and L. F. Hellman (1949). *The Breakfast Meal in Relation to Blood-sugar Values.* U.S. Dept. Agr., Cir. 827, Washington, D.C.

35. Pace, J. K., L. B. Stier, D. D. Taylor, and P. S. Goodman (1961). Metabolic patterns in preadolescent children. V. Intake and urinary excretion of pantothenic acid and of folic acid. *J. Nutr.* **74:** 345.

36. Physiologic results of breakfast habits (1957). *Nutr. Rev.* **15:** 196.

37. Potgieter, M., and E. H. Morse (1955). Food habits of children. *J. Am. Dietet. Assoc.* **31:** 794.

38. Reynolds, M. S., M. Dickson, M. Evans, and E. Olson (1948). Dietary practices of some Wisconsin children. *J. Home Econ.* **40:** 131.

39. Rorex, H. D. (1963). School lunch serves the nation—through food for learning. *Agr. Marketing* **8:** 12.

40. Rose, W. C., R. H. Wixom, H. B. Lockhart, and G. F. Lambert (1955). The amino acid requirements of man. XV. The valine requirement; summary and final observations. *J. Biol. Chem.* **217:** 987.

41. Scott, M. L. (1953). *School Feeding.* Food Agr. Organ. U.N., FAO Nutr. Studies No. 10, Rome.

42. Scrimshaw, N. S. (1963). Malnutrition and the health of children. *J. Am. Dietet. Assoc.* **42:** 203.

43. Spurling, D., M. Krause, N. Callaghan, and R. L. Huenemann (1954). Poor food habits are everybody's concern. *J. Home Econ.* **46:** 713.

44. Steele, B. F., M. M. Clayton, and R. E. Tucker (1952). Role of breakfast and of between-meal foods in adolescents' nutrient intake. *J. Am. Dietet. Assoc.* **28:** 1054.

45. Stier, L. B., D. D. Taylor, J. K. Pace, and J. N. Eisen (1961). Metabolic patterns in preadolescent children. IV. Fat intake and excretion. *J. Nutr.* **73:** 347.

46. Storvick, C. A., B. Schaad, R. E. Coffey, and M. B. Deardorff (1951). Nutritional status of selected population groups in Oregon. *Milbank Mem. Fund. Quart.* **29:** 165.

47. Symposium on metabolic patterns in preadolescent children. (1960). *Federation Proc.* **19:** 1007.

48. Trulson, M., D. M. Hegsted, and F. J. Stare (1949). New York State nutrition survey. I. A nutrition survey of public school children. *J. Am. Dietet. Assoc.* **25:** 595.

49. Velat, C., O. Mickelsen, M. L. Hathaway, S. F. Adelson, F. L. Meyer, and B. B. Peterkin (1951). *Evaluating School Lunches and Nutritional Status of Children.* U.S. Dept. Agr. and Fed. Sec. Agency, Cir. 859, Washington, D.C.

50. Warnick, K. P., S. V. Bring, and E. Woods (1955). Nutritional status of adolescent Idaho children. *J. Am. Dietet. Assoc.* **31:** 486.

51. Wharton, M. A. (1963). Nutritive intake of adolescents. *J. Am. Dietet. Assoc.* **42:** 306.

52. Whitehead, F. E. (1952). Dietary studies of school-age children in Ascension Parish, Louisiana. *Am. J. Public Health* **42:** 1547.

53. Wolman, I. J. (1946). Does milk between meals hamper the appetite or food intake of the child? *J. Pediat.* **28:** 703.

54. Wright, J. B., P. C. Martin, M. L. Skellenger, and D. S. Moschette (1960). Metabolic patterns in preadolescent children. III. Sulfur balance on three levels of nitrogen intake. *J. Nutr.* **72:** 314.

55. Young, C. M., V. L. Smudski, and B. F. Steele (1951). Fall and spring diets of school children in New York State. *J. Am. Dietet. Assoc.* **27:** 289.

SUPPLEMENTARY READING

THE SCHOOL CHILD AND THE ADOLESCENT

Breckenridge, M. E., and E. L. Vincent (1960). *Child Development.* 4th ed. W. B. Saunders Co., Philadelphia.

Eppright, E., M. Pattison, and H. Barbour (1963). *Teaching Nutrition.* 2nd ed. Iowa State University Press, Ames.

King, C. G., and G. Lam (1960). *Personality "Plus" Through Diet.* Public Affairs Pamphlet No. 299. The Public Affairs Committee, New York.

Leverton, R. (1960). *Food Becomes You.* Iowa State University Press, Ames.

Martin, E. A. (1963). *Nutrition in Action.* Holt, Rinehart, and Winston, New York.

Martin, E. A. (1963). *Nutrition Education in Action.* Holt, Rinehart, and Winston, New York.

CHAPTER 25

Nutrition during pregnancy, lactation, aging

▶ NUTRITION DURING PREGNANCY

During pregnancy the diet deserves special consideration to make sure that it will not be a limiting factor to the good health of both mother and child (21). The influence of nutrition begins prior to conception and continues throughout the gestation period. Many believe that the influence of nutrition on reproduction begins as early as the childhood years, when the character of the skeletal structure is being determined and the functional capacities of the organs and tissues are being established (25).

Whether or not the adequacy of the diet consumed by the mother bears a relationship to the absence or presence of complications of pregnancy is a controversial issue (2, 19). Certain ill effects have been associated with maternal consumption of a diet poor in nutritional quality. Toxemia in the mother and prematurity in the infant are found to be prevalent among women consuming inadequate diets. Thirty-five per cent of the women with poor diets, in a study of 186 mothers in Australia, suffered toxemia whereas the incidence was only 4 per cent among those selecting a good diet. The incidence of prematurity among their infants was 19 per cent for mothers eating poor diets, none for those consuming good diets (Fig. 25.1). Additional evidence of the ill effects of a poor diet comes from studies done in Canada and the United States (5, 11). Miscarriages and premature and still births were more

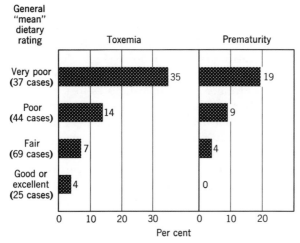

Fig. 25.1. Maternal diets in the latter half of pregnancy related to toxemia and prematurity. (From Woodhill et al., *Am. J. Obstet. Gynecol.*, **70**: 987, 1955.)

frequent if the maternal diet was inadequate. Illnesses and deaths resulting from the illnesses were more frequent among infants under 6 months of age, born to mothers eating poor diets.

One of the most extensive studies of prenatal nutrition was conducted at Vanderbilt University and included 2338 women of the lower income bracket (16). It was observed that when the mother's energy intake was 1500 Cal. or less or the protein less than 50 gm daily, the incidence of obstetric and fatal complications increased. However, the investigators indicated that the lessened dietary intake may have been the result of the complications rather than the cause of them.

The results of a study in India of 150 pregnant women of low socio-economic strata and 50 pregnant women of high economic strata show that the nutritional status of women during pregnancy and the condition of the offspring were not notably different for the two groups. The investigators pointed out that the women who were consuming a deficient diet during pregnancy had subsisted on this type of diet since birth, and that perhaps some physiological adaptation to conserve nutrients was in effect (1, 4).

Is there evidence that a good diet endows the mother with added assurance of a successful pregnancy and the infant with greater expectation of a good physical condition? The Harvard investigators found that mothers with diets of good quality not only suffered fewer complications during pregnancy but also had less difficulty during labor. Furthermore, the mother had better prospects of being able to nurse her infant if her diet had been of good quality during pregnancy (Fig. 25.2). As for the infant, the Harvard group found a definite all-over relationship between excellence of the mother's diet and superiority in the physical status of the newborn (Fig. 25.3). The Vanderbilt group (16), on the other hand, believe that "the obstetrician who assures his patient freedom from such complications as toxemia and prematurity by advocating an abundant nutrient intake must expect disappointment." However, the Vanderbilt investigators do not wish to be interpreted as concluding that nutrition is unimportant in pregnancy and add that "the necessity of insuring an adequate diet during pregnancy is unquestioned."

During the first eight weeks of the prenatal period the fetal organs are being formed. The second half is important because the major gain in weight of the fetus takes place during that period. As a consequence, the demands for building materials for the formation of new tissue are

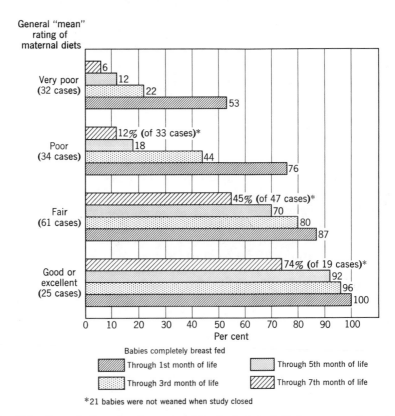

Fig. 25.2.   Breast feeding related to maternal diet in the latter half of pregnancy. Percentage of babies completely breast fed in each diet group. (From Woodhill et al., *Am. J. Obstet. Gynecol.*, **70:** 987, 1955.)

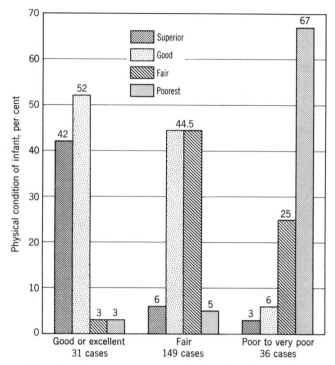

Fig. 25.3. Relationship of prenatal nutrition to the physical condition of the infant at birth and within first 2 weeks of life. (From Burke, Beal, Kirkwood, and Stuart, *Am. J. Obstet, Gynecol.,* **46:** 38, 1943.)

stepped up markedly. The maternal diet must provide for the additional requirements. It should be recognized also that not only is the fetal tissue increasing in amount but also the mother too is experiencing a growth of certain tissues; the mammary glands, and accessory tissues supporting the fetus, as well as certain other glands and tissues throughout the body increase in size during the prenatal period (15).

Energy

Calorie intake is of particular concern during pregnancy because of its relationship to maternal weight gain. The pattern of gain and amount are significant to the well-being of the mother. During the first trimester, although the absolute increase in weight is small, it is of prime importance for it is at this period that the fetus and placenta are being formed. Failure to gain weight in the first trimester, or to continue to do so in the second, increases the probability of premature birth (20, 25).

The size of the baby seems to be more influenced by the weight of the mother prior to pregnancy than on gain during the prenatal period. Obese mothers tend to give birth to heavy babies even though the gain in weight during pregnancy may not be high. Conversely, underweight mothers, despite a relatively high rate of gain, usually give birth to small babies.

Inadequate energy intakes are found to diminish the nitrogen retention of women during pregnancy. In a study of 38 women, Oldham (17) found that on the average more than twice as much nitrogen was retained by women whose protein intake was only 50 gm but whose Calorie intake was over 2100, than those whose protein intake was as much as 70 gm daily but their caloric intake was less than 2100. If Calories must be limited, particular attention must be paid to supplying adequate protein in the diet.

Although cognizant of the individual variability in energy need, the Food and Nutrition Board recommends a 200 Cal. increase daily over the usual intake in the second and third trimesters.

Protein

The amount of protein needed during pregnancy is greatly increased, particularly in the second half of pregnancy. The major portion of the protein acquisition by the fetus occurs in the three months prior to birth. The rate of protein deposition in the fetus, computed for the entire prenatal period, is around 1.4 gm per day. For the last three months of fetal life the rate is increased to 3.6 gm daily, and for the last month the increase reaches an average of 6.4 gm daily. Added to this are the needs of the mother, which are increased to take care of the enlargement of certain of her own body tissues during the prenatal period. For the mother who is in a state of good nutrition prior to pregnancy and whose protein intake during the early months of the prenatal period has been at least at the recommended level, the Food and Nutrition Board recommends an additional 20 gm protein daily during the second and third trimesters.

The quantitative need for protein has been studied by means of the nitrogen balance method. From observations of a person during the entire prenatal period, indications are that the body stores nitrogen to a greater extent than can be accounted for by the combined growth of the fetus and maternal tissues (10). Of course there are additional demands for nitrogen, for at birth nitrogen is lost from the body in fluids and tissue in addition to the fetus, and during lactation the nitrogen balance is customarily negative.

It has long been concluded, even though lacking precise experimental work with humans, that during pregnancy proteins of good quality should be eaten. Progress in identification of the amino acids essential for the human being, and the development of methods for the quantitative determination of them, has made it possible to investigate amino acid needs during pregnancy. Comparisons of the average excretions of amino acids by women in the pregnant and nonpregnant state show an increase during pregnancy. In a study of the eight indispensable amino acids, the magnitude of increase varied among them. The greatest average increases were for threonine and tryptophan, followed by lysine. An increase in excretion is interpreted as evidence of a greater need for that amino acid by the body (24).

Calcium

Factors influencing the calcium needs during pregnancy are considerably like those of protein. The amount required is influenced by the growth both of fetal and maternal tissues, with the greatest need coming in the last prenatal month. At birth the fetus contains approximately 22 gm of calcium, most of which is deposited in the last fetal month. The rate of accumulation of calcium in the fetus is about 50 mg per day at the third month; 120 mg daily by the seventh, and by the last month it reaches 450 mg per day.

Daily dietary needs for calcium have been determined by means of balance studies. For women in a state of good nutrition prior to the prenatal period, the Recommended Allowance for the second and third trimesters is an additional 0.5 gm per day more than the recommendation for a nonpregnant woman, amounting to a total of 1.3 gm. As with protein, calcium is retained during pregnancy beyond the needs estimated for the fetal and new maternal tissues. Such storage is not amiss, for during lactation the diet frequently supplies an insufficient amount of calcium to meet the augmented requirement.

In cases of undernutrition prior to the prenatal period, the intake of calcium, protein, and other nutrients should be increased at the outset and continued throughout (8). Women with histories of poor nutrition prior to pregnancy, when given an adequate diet, are found to store more calcium than women on the same diet who entered pregnancy in a good nutritional state.

Iron

The recommended intake for iron during the second and third trimesters of the prenatal period is 20 mg daily. As with the other nutrients, the quantitative need increases with the progress of pregnancy

(2, 7, 12). It is only by careful selection of foods that 20 mg of iron can be provided in the daily diet. Thus it becomes necessary to be on the watch to include iron-rich foods. Foods that are good sources of iron are liver, other meats, eggs, enriched or whole-grain cereals and breads, green and leafy vegetables, and some dried fruits.

Hypochromic anemia is common in pregnancy. The previous lifetime iron balance is of importance in determining the iron reserve and the capacity to meet the demands of pregnancy (3). Some believe it to be only a manifestation of hydremia (excess of water in the blood). It can be prevented fairly well by the ingestion of an adequate diet, although in some instances medicinal supplementation is prescribed by the physician. There are two physiological changes that help compensate for the added demands for iron. During the period of gestation the cessation of menstruation represents a saving of iron amounting to 200 to 300 mg. Also it has been demonstrated, using radioactive iron, that iron absorption is increased during pregnancy, particularly during the last trimester (2).

Iodine

During pregnancy the need for iodine is increased. In Switzerland, where a serious lack of iodine exists in the soil, it is observed that if mothers develop goiter due to an insufficient consumption of iodine, the possibilities of her child's also having goiter are ten times greater.

In regions where the incidence of goiter was highest among the mothers, cretinism was more apt to occur among the children. Where 55 per cent of the people in a village were afflicted with endemic goiter, the incidence of cretinism was around 1 per cent.

Under normal conditions the use of iodized salt can be depended upon to provide an adequate amount of iodine. However, with the increased need of pregnancy, and the possibility of the intake of salt being restricted, for medical reasons, it would seem wise to consult a physician concerning additional iodine intake. Such a practice is recommended particularly for persons living in areas where a lack of iodine is prevalent. (See Chapter 11.)

The Vitamins

The vitamin needs during pregnancy have been less thoroughly studied than the protein and mineral requirements. It is logical to assume that there is an increased demand for these nutrients during the prenatal period. Research that has been done supports this point of view. The recommendations of the Food and Nutrition Board for the daily allowances of the vitamins are greater than the recommendations for nonpregnant women.

Vitamins A and D. For vitamin A value the Recommended Allowance for the second and third trimesters of pregnancy is 6000 IU daily, based on the assumption that two-thirds of the total vitamin A activity of the diet is derived from carotene and related compounds, and one-third from the preformed vitamin. The 6000 IU allowance daily can be supplied easily by the combination of one quart of milk, butter or fortified margarine, a green vegetable, and occasionally liver.

Deprivation of vitamin A during pregnancy in experimental animals has been found to result in certain physical abnormalities. Newborn rats and pigs were found to have cleft palates, defects of the skeletal structure and of the eyes. To the other extreme, excessive intake has also caused physical abnormalities in rats. Such extremes have not been recorded for the human being.

The optimum intake of vitamin D during pregnancy is not definitely known. The level suggested is 400 IU daily for the second and third trimesters of the prenatal period. The diet cannot be depended upon to supply this amount unless milk with added vitamin D is used. Readily available sources of the vitamin on the market include fish liver oils and irradiated sterols of many kinds and potencies. Clinical symptoms of vitamin D deficiency are rare in the United States and Europe. In India, China, and other areas of the Far East symptoms of osteomalacia (late rickets) do occur during reproduction. Among the women in the Far East who can appear in public only if veiled, the source of vitamin D from the sun is completely eliminated.

Ascorbic Acid. One hundred mg daily is the Recommended Allowance for ascorbic acid during the second and third trimesters of pregnancy. Two servings of citrus fruit will supply the recommended intake. Tomatoes can be depended on to provide some of the vitamin; also cabbage, potatoes (under proper conditions of preparation), broccoli, strawberries, and cantaloup are among the good sources.

Evidence of an increased need for ascorbic acid is found in the study of maternal blood levels. As pregnancy progresses, the ascorbic acid concentration in the maternal blood tends to decrease. However, when the intake is maintained at a high level the customary progressive reduction does not occur (12).

Thiamine. The Recommended Allowance for thiamine for the second and third trimesters is 1 mg daily, which is slightly higher than the 0.4 mg per 1000 Cal. rate of the nonpregnant woman. Thiamine is supplied in good amounts by the following foods: whole-grain and enriched cereals containing approximately 0.8 mg per 1000 Cal.; whole milk, 0.5 mg per 1000 Cal.; and lean meats, an average of 0.3 mg per 1000 Cal.

The question of associating certain common symptoms manifested during pregnancy with an inadequate intake of thiamine arises periodically but remains controversial. Some investigators attribute the symptoms of general nervous fatigue, muscle cramps, neuritis, and toxemia to an insufficiency of thiamine; others disagree.

Riboflavin. The Recommended Allowance for riboflavin during the second and third trimesters is increased by 0.3 mg above the usual recommendation for women, making the daily allowance for pregnant women 18 to 35 years of age 1.6 mg. The daily intake of one quart of milk, together with enriched bread and cereals, and the other foods in an average mixed diet, will supply the riboflavin allowance without difficulty.

In experimental studies with the rat, a lack of riboflavin, particularly at the thirteenth or fourteenth embryo day, may interfere with normal cartilage formation and result in malformations of the skeletal structure. Cleft palates and shortening of the mandible, tibia, fibula, radius, and toes were observed (22).

Vitamin E. Although it is well established that vitamin E (alpha tocopherol) is essential for reproduction in animals, the need for the human being is controversial. Some investigators have reported that vitamin E is beneficial for women who have had histories of repeated abortions whereas others have found it to be ineffective even though given in high dosages over long periods of time. Most agree that the levels of total tocopherols in the blood rise as gestation progresses.

Vitamin K. At one time it was common practice to administer vitamin K routinely during pregnancy and also to the newborn for the prevention of hemorrhage in the newborn child. The practice is now being questioned on the grounds that it is uncertain whether the decreased prothrombin level characteristic of the newborn is a direct cause of hemorrhage. Furthermore, there is conflicting evidence as to whether or not vitamin K administration reduces the incidence of hemorrhage in the newborn. The more recent observations lend support to the belief that it is effective in reducing hemorrhage (18).

Foods Recommended in the Daily Diet

The following list of foods forms a basis for an adequate diet during pregnancy. It is wise to consult the family physician early to have individual guidance as to dietary needs.

Milk—3 or more cups of whole or skimmed milk.

Fruits and vegetables—5 to 7 servings of fruits and vegetables, including some green and leafy and some citrus fruits or tomatoes.

Lean meat, poultry, fish—at least one-quarter of a pound of meat or fish is desirable. It is well to include a serving of liver at intervals.

Eggs—at least one egg.

Cereals and bread—3 servings of enriched or whole-grained bread and cereals.

Butter and fortified margarine—should be used sparingly if weight is being watched.

Fluids and vitamin D are needed daily.

▶ NUTRITION DURING LACTATION

During lactation the increase in nutrient need is dependent primarily on the quantity of milk secreted. The production capacity is an individual physiologic characteristic, which is influenced by the environment. Among the influences which tend to diminish the secretion of milk, and may even suppress it completely, are such emotional factors as excitement, fear, and anxiety. Another factor we may call demand. The breast must be completely emptied at each nursing period if the secretion of milk is to be maintained. If the infant does not require the entire content, then removing the residual portion manually helps to assure continued secretion.

Another essential to maintenance of milk secretion is an adequate diet. Deficiencies in the food intake eventually cause a diminution in the quantity secreted and may even alter the composition.

The Recommended Allowances proposed by the Food and Nutrition Board were made on the basis of an average secretion of 850 ml of milk daily. The daily amounts recommended exceed those of any other period for women. Actually the quantity of milk secreted is markedly variable among individuals. On the average, the mother who is able to nurse her infant secretes around ½ liter of milk in the first week or two, increasing to as much as 1 liter by the fifth month of lactation.

Energy

The added energy allowance for lactation recommended by the National Research Council is 1000 Cal. above that for a nonlactating woman of similar size and activity. The average energy value of human milk is 70 Cal. per 100 ml (14). If the secretion is 850 ml daily, 600 Cal. is accounted for in the milk itself, leaving 400 of the 1000 Cal. allowance for other uses.

There is a question as to whether the actual process of milk formation requires sufficient energy to be measurable. An assessment of human requirements during lactation indicates that most likely the physiological processes of milk formation involve only a limited energy expenditure (6).

Insufficient energy in the diet will lead eventually to a diminished secretion of milk. Overfeeding, on the other hand, does not stimulate additional milk production and seems even in some cases to diminish the quantity.

The increase in the Recommended Allowances for lactation is not equally great for energy and the nutrients. As summarized in Fig. 25.4, the addition to the recommended caloric intake over that for women of 25 years is 48 per cent whereas for calcium, protein, and vitamin A the increase is much greater than that. It means that the foods added to supply the additional Calories must of necessity provide generously those nutrients needed in increased amounts; milk, and eggs are examples of good supplementary foods.

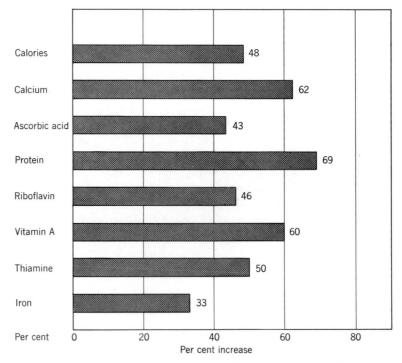

Fig. 25.4. Percentage increase in Recommended Allowances for women during lactation, over allowances for women 25 years of age. (Adapted from Recommended *Dietary Allowances Sixth Revised Edition,*Natl. Acad. Sci.—Natl. Res. Council, Publ. 1146, 1964.)

Protein

The Recommended Allowance for protein during lactation is a 20-gm daily increase over the recommendation for pregnancy and 40 gm greater daily than for the nonpregnant woman (Table A-1, Appendix). Inadequate protein in the diet will, as a general rule, cause a diminution in the quantity of milk secreted. There is evidence that supplying sufficient protein during both pregnancy and lactation favors milk production (10).

At an international conference on protein requirements in 1957, it was proposed that about 2.0 gm of food protein of high nutritive value may be needed to produce 1.0 gm of milk protein (23). These values apply to women who have been consuming an adequate diet and not to those who are undernourished. If the amount of milk secreted is 850 ml, with a protein content of approximately 10 gm, the need for the milk protein would be 20 gm of good quality food protein. The recommendation of 40 g is for total protein, without respect to quality.

A question frequently asked is whether pregnancy and lactation impose a drain on the protein stores of the mother. Continuous nitrogen balance studies with one woman through most of her pregnancy, and for several months after the birth of her infant, revealed no loss to the maternal tissues when the storage periods and periods of loss were totaled. During the prenatal period nitrogen was stored; at the time of birth some was lost; during lactation the maternal tissues continued to lose nitrogen. Nevertheless, in this case as in others observed, ample reserves deposited during pregnancy appear to be sufficient to take care of the nitrogen losses at parturition and during lactation, with no drain on maternal tissue (10).

Calcium and Phosphorus. The recommended amount of calcium daily is 1.3 gm. No recommendation is made for phosphorus, for if calcium and protein are adequate in the diet, phosphorus as a rule is adequate also.

During lactation there is a tendency for individuals to have a negative calcium and phosphorus balance (9). The losses can be offset to some extent by providing an adequate amount of the minerals in the diet together with a source of vitamin D (13).

Iron

Some iron is secreted in the milk, increasing the need to some extent for that element in the diet. The Food and Nutrition Board recommend that the allowance of 20 mg daily during pregnancy be continued through lactation.

The Vitamins

Less research has been done on the vitamin needs during lactation than for some of the other nutrients. The allowances proposed by the National Research Council, based on what research has been done and their own judgment, provides for sizable increases over the usual level for some of the vitamins. The actual amount needed by the mother is influenced by the quantity of milk produced.

The Recommended Allowances for the vitamins are: for vitamin A, 8000 IU daily, an increase of 60 per cent over the allowance recommended for women 25 to 45 years of age; for thiamine, 1.2 mg, an increase of 50 per cent; for riboflavin 1.9 mg, an increase of 46 per cent; and for ascorbic acid 100 mg, an increase of 43 per cent. For vitamin D the Food and Nutrition Board recommend 400 IU, the same as for pregnancy. In support of their recommendation for vitamin D they state: "The optimal amount of vitamin D for pregnancy and lactation is not known. On the basis of available evidence, 400 units is probably adequate."

▶ NUTRITION OF OLDER PERSONS

Grow old along with me!
The best is yet to be,
The last of life, for which the first was made.

It is of particular concern that older persons enjoy freedom from handicaps that may have resulted from poor nutrition in their earlier years, or ill effects that may be caused by poor eating habits during their later life. As King (11) explicitly states, "It is not enough to survive into the years from 60 to 80, they should be years of health and enjoyment, and mental vigor."

Concern for the nutrition of older people has continuously grown through the years, and justifiably so. The percentage of our population falling into the older age classification has progressively increased (17). In 1960 there were about 17 million persons 65 years of age and over in the United States, in 1900 there were 3 million. This group constituted 4 per cent of the total population in 1900; by 1960 it had increased to 9 per cent (4, 24). Several factors have contributed to this change in the composition of the population. Among them are the increase in the number of births, which in turn results in more persons to grow old. Another factor is international migration. Up to the time of the First World War, immigration to the United States increased steadily each decade, except during the Civil War and the depression years of the 1890's. Another influence, the decrease in death rate, has of course increased the number of older persons in the population.

Life expectancy at birth is predicted to be increased by 45 to 50 per cent in 1975 over that observed in 1900. In Fig. 25.5 the life expectancy of women and men in 1900, 1950, and 1975 at birth, at age 45, and at age 65 are presented. The life expectancy for women is increasing more rapidly than for men.

Certain physiological changes that inevitably accompany aging tend to decrease the functional capacity of the body. Changes that would be expected to have a direct effect on the utilization of food include a diminution in the size of the salivary glands, and a decrease in volume and acidity of gastric juice (5). Although there appears to be little information on changes in the small intestine with advancing age, there is some evidence of a decreased rate of absorption (3). Movements in

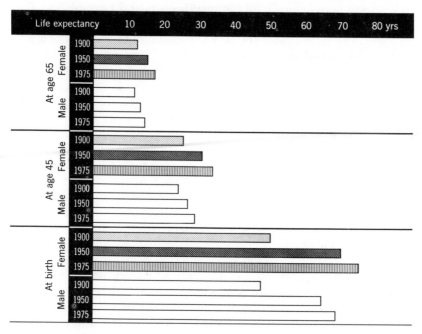

Fig. 25.5. Increase in life expectancy for women and men. (From *1961 White House Conference on Aging Chart Book*, U.S. Govt. Printing Office, p. 9.)

the colon seem to be unchanged. The gross weight of the liver is found to decrease between the fourth and seventh decades. A common difficulty that hinders normal eating in older persons is the loss of teeth and failure to replace them with dentures.

There is evidence of less adequate carbohydrate metabolism in the older years. After consumption of a sugar solution (glucose tolerance test) or following a meal that was chiefly carbohydrate, older persons (men and women over 50 years) were found to have blood glucose values that were higher than that expected for younger adults (9). Stieglitz (21), who has been particularly concerned with the processes of aging in individuals, explains that the "glucose tolerance test creates physiological stress" and with aging "tolerance for stresses of all sorts is diminished."

Nutrient Needs and Food Habits

Energy. In adults total energy needs decrease with aging. The Food and Nutrition Board (18) proposes a 5 per cent reduction in energy allowance per decade between ages 35 and 55 years; an 8 per cent reduction per decade from ages 55 to 75 years; and a further decrement of 10 per cent is recommended for age 75 years and beyond. The Daily Recommended Allowance for men 35 to 55 years of age is 2600 Cal.; for ages 55 to 75 years, 2200 Cal. For women 35 to 55 years of age the Daily Recommended Allowance is 1900 Cal.; for ages 55 to 75 years, 1600 Cal. The estimates are for persons normally active. The energy need is highly individual, varying widely from person to person.

Factors that contribute to the decreasing energy need with aging are a lowered basal rate and the lessened physical activity that customarily accompanies growing older. Causes for the progressive lowering of the basal rate, though not definitely known, are believed to be related to a combination of changes including (1) an alteration in body composition and (2) changes in the functioning of certain of the endocrine glands. With aging, the body tissues change in composition to relatively more fat and less muscular tissue. Estimates of the per cent of the body weight accounted for by fat in men ranging from 25 to 55 years of age are shown in Fig. 25.6.

In actual practice, as people grow older they tend to eat less and thus compensate to some extent for the reduced energy needs. A problem that was common to persons whose diets were very low in energy value was the lowering of the nutrient content of the diet (15). Observations of 2800 women and 250 men living in parts of the Middle and Far West show, however, that the problem of too many Calories in the daily diet does exist because many of the older persons weighed more than accepted levels considered best for their health (2).

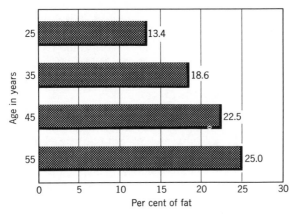

Fig. 25.6. Average estimated change in per cent of body weight accounted for by fat tissue. (Prepared from Brozek, *Federation Proc.*, 11: 787, 1952.)

Protein. The protein needs of older persons seem not to differ greatly from those of younger healthy adults (6, 10, 23). The Recommended Allowance is one gm per kg of body weight from young adulthood to old age, 18 to 75 years.

To supply the Recommended Allowance for protein, food relatively higher in protein content is needed as persons grow older. This is necessary because the energy need decreases. At ages 55 to 75 years, the Recommended Allowance for protein provides 13 to 14 per cent of the total Calories whereas at ages 18 to 35 years only 10 to 11 per cent of the Calories are provided by protein.

In a study of the food intake of "apparently healthy" persons ranging in age from 51 to 97 years who resided in the Boston area, the mean protein intake was 1.24 gm per kg (7). Information on diet history and current food intake was obtained by interview.

The essential amino acid content of the self-selected diets of 18 women ranging in age from 33 to 77 years was determined as a part of the study in the North Central Region of the nutritional status and dietary habits of older women (13). The diets were analyzed for isoleucine, leucine, lysine, threonine, valine, phenylalanine, and methionine, using microbiological methods. Methionine was least adequate in the diets, according to the present information on the quantitative needs for amino acids, followed by phenylalanine.

Minerals. The mineral needs of older persons have not been studied to any great extent. As with energy and protein, the investigations of mineral need have been chiefly with women thus far. The Recommended Allowance for calcium for the 55- to 75-year age group is 0.8 gm daily, which is the same amount as recommended for younger adults. Calcium and phosphorus intakes, sufficient in amount that equilibrium between intake and outgo could be expected, were computed by Ohlson, using results from studies that she and others had done. The values are summarized for ages 30 to 80, by decades, in Table 25.1. The need for calcium as predicted by Ohlson is less after 70 years than in the preceding decades, beginning at 30 years of age.

In the Boston study (7) cited earlier, approximately one-third of the group was consuming diets which provided between 0.7 and 1.0 gm of calcium daily (Fig. 25.7). Eighteen per cent consumed more than 1.3 gm daily, and 30 per cent less than 0.7 gm daily.

The importance of an adequate intake of calcium is expressed by the Food and Nutrition Board (18). The relatively high incidence of osteoporosis among older persons in the population of the United States is cited, and the possibility "that even minimal or moderate deficiency in calcium intake over a period of years may contribute to the occurrence or accentuation of this disease" (18).

The iron needs of women lessen after the menopause. As a consequence the Recommended Allowance in the 55- to 75-year age is reduced to 10 mg daily from the 15 mg recommended for younger adult women. For men of all age groups the recommendation is 10 mg daily.

In the Boston study (7) 63 per cent of the group were found to have total iron intakes from food and supplement of 8 to 14 mg daily, 6 per cent had less than 8 mg daily, and 14 per cent were ingesting over 20 mg daily (Fig. 25.7). Whether intakes above the estimated need are beneficial, detrimental, or indifferent has not been ascertained (14).

Vitamins. The vitamin needs of aging individuals are not well established as yet. The Food and Nutrition Board makes no age differentia-

Table 25.1. Intakes of Calcium and Phosphorus Predicted for Equilibrium for Successive Decades in Women, 30 to 80 Years

Age Range, Years	No.	Intake Predicted for Equilibrium	
		Calcium, gm/Day	Phosphorus, gm/Day
30–39	25	0.88	1.25
40–49	34	0.87	1.32
50–59	40	0.83	1.42
60–69	25	0.92	1.51
70–79	11	0.73	1.13

Adapted from Ohlson et al., *Federation Proc.* 11: 782, 1952.

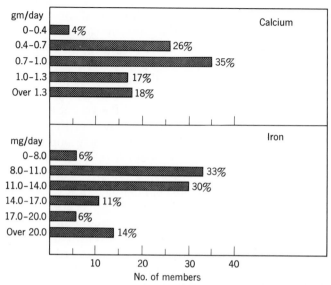

Fig. 25.7.   Calcium and iron intake, supplement included. (Courtesy of Davidson, Livermore, Anderson, and Kaufman, *Am. J. Clin. Nutr.*, **10**: 181, 1962.)

tion in the Recommended Allowances for adults for vitamin A and ascorbic acid but does recommend a decrease in thiamine, riboflavin, and niacin equivalent with increasing age and the concomitant lower energy need. The Recommended Allowances for vitamin A, ascorbic acid, thiamine, and riboflavin appear as a part of Table 25.2. For niacin equivalent the recommendation for men is 15 mg daily and for women 13 mg. There is evidence, however, that older women need more thiamine than younger women, from a study of 10 women 52 to 72 years of

Table 25.2. Vitamin Intake of 104 Aging Persons

	Recommended Allowance		Per Cent of Persons Consuming Vitamins at Various Levels					
	Men	Women	Amount	%	Amount	%	Amount	%
Vitamin A value IU	5000	5000	4000–6999	21	>4000	7	<7000	70
Thiamine mg	0.9	0.8	1–2	32	>1	21	<2	49
Riboflavin mg	1.3	1.2	1–2	33	>1	3	<2	64
Ascorbic acid mg	70	70	50–100	33	>50	16	<100	17

Compiled from Davidson, Livermore, Anderson, and Kaufman. *Am. J. Clin. Nutr.* **10**: 181, 1962.

age, and 8 women, 18 to 21 years. At all levels of intake the excretion of thiamine was less for the older than the younger group (16). Age was found not to be a factor in the mean concentration of ascorbic acid in the blood of women in a study of 569 persons ages 20 to 99 years (19).

Among the 104 persons of the Boston Age Center consumption of vitamins in excess of the Recommended Allowance was found to occur more frequently than failing to meet the recommendation (Table 25.2). The intake of vitamin A value is shown in Fig. 25.8. When a vitamin supplement was taken, 27 per cent of the group was consuming over 16,000 IU daily of vitamin A value. A total of 6 mg of thiamine and of riboflavin were consumed daily by 21 per cent and 25 per cent of the group, respectively, amounts approximately seven and five times the Recommended Allowances, respectively.

If the few studies on record can be considered indicative, aging persons use nutrient supplements to a notable extent. One-half the group of 104 persons in the Boston study, and over one-third of the 283 older persons studied in Rochester, New York used supplements. An analysis of the contributions of the supplements for meeting dietary needs was made in the Rochester study (1). Of the 104 persons using supplements, 48 were consuming diets that met the Recommended Allowances without supplements. An additional 13 persons were not consuming diets that met the Recommended Allowances in all nutrients, but even so the supplement did not provide the nutrients needed. Only 12 of the 104 per-

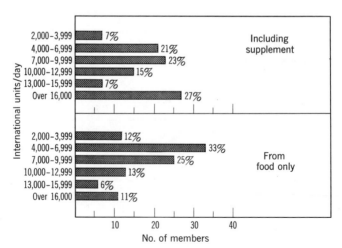

Fig. 25.8. Intake of vitamin A value. (Courtesy of Davidson, Livermore, Anderson, and Kaufman, *Am. J. Clin. Nutr.*, **10:** 181, 1962.)

sons using supplements had preparations that provided all the nutrients needed to bolster the nutrient content of the diet.

The Older Person and His Food

There are important considerations in the nutrition of the aging other than merely seeing that they have a nutritionally adequate food supply. The habits of eating, food likes and dislikes, and notions about food and diet are most likely long standing and will not be readily amenable to change. Stieglitz (22) sounds the watchword of success in planning dietaries for older persons, when he states that, "It is essential to individualize." Consequently, their fixed habits should demand some respect. Keeping this in mind, we can find many ways to provide an adequate diet. In a practical sense it means pleasing the appetite of the aging person, and making the diet adequate within that framework.

Diet and Longevity

Experimental work with animals has demonstrated that kind and amount of food and manner of feeding have an influence on length of life. Sherman (20), in his laboratory at Columbia University, found that when diets adequate for growth and reproduction in the white rat were improved, the animals responded with increased growth, a prolonged reproductive period, and a longer life. The nutrients added were calcium, riboflavin, and vitamin A.

Another approach to lengthening the life span through diet is that of retarding the rate of growth in young animals by limiting the caloric intake. McCay (12), at Cornell University, fed diets planned to provide an abundance of food essentials but limited in energy value. Animals on this dietary regime grew slowly, matured late, and outlived the animals who ate an adequate diet *ad libitum.*

Alteration in the fat content of the diet tends to influence the life span of experimental animals. Rats fed a ration containing 22.7 per cent fat had a shorter life span than those fed diets that were 3.4 per cent fat. The two groups of animals grew at essentially the same rate (8).

These experimental studies on the relationship of diet to length of life are fundamental to our understanding of the far-reaching influence of diet on life processes. At present we do not see a direct application to human beings but, on the other hand, we do not summarily dismiss them as having no significance for man. Studies with the human take longer, particularly those concerned with longevity!

REFERENCES

NUTRITION DURING PREGNANCY AND LACTATION

1. Bagchi, K., and A. K. Bose. (1962). Effect of low nutrient intake during pregnancy on obstetrical performance and offspring. *Am. J. Clin. Nutr.* **11**: 586.
2. Beaton, G. H. (1961). Nutritional and physiological adaptations in pregnancy. *Federation Proc.* **20**: 196.
3. Bothwell, T. H., and C. A. Finch (1962). *Iron Metabolism.* Little, Brown, and Co., Boston. p. 314.
4. Burgess, A., and R. F. A. Dean. (1962). *Malnutrition and Food Habits.* The Macmillan Co., New York, p. 30.
5. Ebbs, J. H., F. F. Tisdall, and W. A. Scott (1941). The influence of prenatal diet on the mother and child. *J. Nutr.* **22**: 515.
6. Garry, R. C., and D. Stiven (1936). A review of recent work on dietary requirements in pregnancy and lactation, with an attempt to assess human requirements. *Nutr. Abstr. Rev.* **5**: 855.
7. Hahn, P. F., et al. (1951). Iron metabolism in human pregnancy as studied with radioactive isotope Fe^{59}. *Am. J. Obstet. Gynecol.* **61**: 477.
8. Hummel, F. C., H. A. Hunscher, M. F. Bates, P. Bonner, I. G. Macy, and J. A. Johnston (1937). A consideration of the nutritive state in the metabolism of women during pregnancy. *J. Nutr.* **13**: 263.
9. Hunscher, H. A. (1930). Metabolism of women during the reproductive cycle. II. Calcium and phosphorus utilization in two successive lactation periods. *J. Biol. Chem.* **86**: 37.
10. Hunscher, H. A., F. C. Hummel, B. N. Erickson, and I. G. Macy (1935). Metabolism of women during the reproductive cycle. VI. A case of the continuous nitrogen utilization of a multipara during pregnancy, parturition, puerperuium and lactation. *J. Nutr.* **10**: 579.
11. Jeans, P. C., M. D. Smith, and G. Stearns (1955). Incidence of prematurity in relation to maternal nutrition. *J. Am. Dietet. Assoc.* **31**: 576.
12. Macy, I. G. 1958. Metabolic and biochemical changes in normal pregnancy. *J. Am. Med. Assoc.* **168**: 2265.
13. Macy, I. G., H. A. Hunscher, S. S. McCosh, and B. Nims (1930). Metabolism of women during the reproductive cycle. III. Calcium, phosphorus, and nitrogen utilization in lactation before and after supplementing the usual home diets with cod liver oil and yeast. *J. Biol. Chem.* **86**: 59.
14. Macy, I. G., H. J. Kelly, and R. E. Sloan (1953). *The Composition of Milks.* Natl. Acad. Sci.—Natl. Res. Council, Publ. 254, Washington, D.C.
15. Macy, I. G., E. Z. Moyer, H. J. Kelly, H. C. Mack, P. C. DiLoreto, and J. P. Pratt (1954). Physiological adaptation and nutritional status during and after pregnancy. *J. Nutr.* **52**: Supplement 1, 3.
16. McGanity, W. J., E. B. Bridgforth, and W. J. Darby (1958). Vanderbilt Cooperative Study of maternal and infant nutrition. XII. Effect of reproductive cycle on nutritional status and requirements. *Symposium IV. Council on Foods and Nutrition.* American Medical Association, Chicago.
17. Oldham, H., and B. B. Sheft (1951). Effect of calorie intake on nitrogen utilization during pregnancy. *J. Am. Dietet. Assoc.* **27**: 847.
18. *Recommended Dietary Allowances Sixth Revised Edition* (1964). Natl. Acad. Sci.—Natl. Res. Council, Publ. 1146, Washington, D.C.
19. Seifert, E. (1961). Changes in beliefs and food practices in pregnancy. *J. Am. Dietet. Assoc.* **39**: 455.

20. Tompkins, W. T. (1955). Nutrition in pregnancy. In *Modern Nutrition in Health and Disease*. (M. G. Wohl and R. S. Goodhart, eds.) Lea and Febiger, Philadelphia, p. 885.
21. Toverud, K. U., G. Stearns, and I. G. Macy (1950). *Maternal Nutrition and Child Health, an Interpretative Review*. Natl. Res. Council, Publ. 123, Washington, D.C.
22. Warkany, J. (1945). Manifestations of prenatal nutritional deficiency. In *Vitamins and Hormones*. Vol. III. Academic Press, New York, p. 73.
23. Waterlow, J. C., and J. M. L. Stephens (eds.) (1957). *Human Protein Requirements*. Conference sponsored by F.A.C., WHO, and the Josiah Macy Jr. Found., New York, p. 130.
24. Wertz, A. W., M. B. Derby, P. K. Ruttenberg, and G. P. French (1959). Urinary excretion of amino acids by the same women during and after pregnancy. *J. Nutr.* **68:** 583.
25. Wishik, S. M. (1959). Nutrition in pregnancy and lactation. *Federation Proc.* **18:** 4.

NUTRITION DURING AGING

1. Baker, D. A., and C. LeBovit (1963). The nutritional adequacy of diets of older people. *Family Econ. Rev.* June, p. 10.
2. Batchelder, E. L. (1957). Nutritional status and dietary habits of older people. *J. Am. Dietet. Assoc.* **33:** 471.
3. Becker, G. H., J. Meyer, and H. Necheler (1950). Fat absorption in young and old age. *Gastroenterology* **14:** 80.
4. Britton, V. (1963). Age groups in the population and consumer needs. *Family Econ. Rev.*, June p. 12.
5. Carlson, A. J. (1949). Physiologic changes of normal aging. *Geriatric Medicine*, 2nd ed., E. J. Stieglitz, ed. W. B. Saunders Co., Philadelphia, p. 47.
6. Daum, K., W. W. Tuttle, B. Warren, M. Sabin, C. J. Imig, and M. T. Schumacher (1952). Nitrogen utilization in older men. *J. Am. Dietet. Assoc.* **28:** 305.
7. Davidson, C. S., J. Livermore, P. Anderson, and S. Kaufman (1962). The nutrition of a group of apparently healthy aging persons. *Am. J. Clin. Nutr.* **10:** 181.
8. French, C., R. H. Ingram, J. A. Uram, G. P. Barron, and R. W. Swift (1953). The influence of dietary fat and carbohydrate on growth and longevity in rats. *J. Nutr.* **51:** 329.
9. Gillum, H. L., A. F. Morgan, and R. I. Williams (1955). Nutritional status of the aging. II. Blood glucose levels. *J. Nutr.* **55:** 289.
10. Horwitt, M. K. (1953). Dietary requirements of the aged. *J. Am. Dietet. Assoc.* **29:** 443.
11. King, C. G. (1952). Trends in the science of food and its relation to life and health. *Nutr. Rev.* **10:** 1.
12. McCay, C. M., M. F. Crowell, and L. A. Maynard (1935). The effect of retarded growth upon the length of life span and upon the ultimate body size. *J. Nutr.* **10:** 63.
13. Mertz, E. T., E. J. Baxter, L. E. Jackson, C. E. Roderuck, and A. Weis (1952). Essential amino acids in self-selected diets of older women. *J. Nutr.* **46:** 313.
14. Moore, C. V., and R. Dubach (1962). Iron. In *Mineral Metabolism*. Vol. 2, Pt. B. (C. L. Comar and F. Bronner, eds.) Academic Press, New York.
15. Ohlson, M. A., P. H. Roberts, S. A. Joseph, and P. M. Nelson (1948). Dietary practices of 100 women from 40 to 75 years of age. *J. Am. Dietet. Assoc.* **24:** 286.
16. Oldham, H. G. (1962). Thiamine requirements of women. *Ann. N.Y. Acad. Sci.* **98:** 542.
17. Population. (1955). *Rural Family Living*, U.S. Dept. Agr., Washington, D.C., March, p. 19.
18. *Recommended Dietary Allowances Sixth Revised Edition* (1964). Natl. Acad. Sci.—Natl. Res. Council, Publ. 1146, Washington, D.C.
19. Roderuck, C., L. Burrill, L. J. Campbell, B. E. Brakke, M. T. Childs, R. Leverton, M. Chaloupka, E. H. Jebe, and P. P. Swanson (1958). Estimated dietary intake, urinary excretion, and blood vitamin C in women of different ages. *Am. J. Nutr.* **66:** 15.

20. Sherman, H. C. (1952). *Chemistry of Food and Nutrition.* 8th ed. The Macmillan Co., New York, p. 275.
21. Stieglitz, E. J. (1951). Nutrition problems of geriatric medicine. In *Handbook of Nutrition.* 2nd ed. The Blakiston Co., Philadelphia, p. 327.
22. Stieglitz, E. J. (1952). Nutritional problems in later maturity. In *Proc. Natl. Food and Nutr. Inst.* U.S. Dept. Agr., Agr. Handbook 56, Washington, D.C., p. 64.
23. Watkin, D. M. (1958). The assessment of protein nutrition in aged man. *Ann. N.Y. Acad. Sci.* **60:** 982.
24. *White House Conference on Aging. Chart Book* (1961). Federal Council on Aging, U.S. Dept. Health, Education, and Welfare, Washington, D.C., p. 78.

SUPPLEMENTARY REFERENCES

Food Guide for Older Folks (1961). U.S. Dept. Agr., Home Garden Bull. 17, Washington, D.C.

Jahnke, K. (1960). Nutrition in old age. In *Recent Advances in Human Nutrition.* (J. F. Brock, ed.) Little, Brown, and Co., Boston, p. 316.

King, C. G., and G. Britt (1962). *Food Hints for Mature People.* Public Affairs Pamphlet No. 336. The Public Affairs Committee, New York.

Mitchell, H. H. (1962). *Comparative Nutrition.* Vol. I. Academic Press, New York, p. 411.

The Nutritional Ages of man (1958). *Proceedings of the Borden Symposium on Nutrition,* New York.

CHAPTER 26

New developments
in foods and nutrition

Many new areas of research have emerged in the field of foods and nutrition during the last twenty-five years. The feeding problems encountered by military personnel during the Second World War have initiated the search for newer methods of food preservation. The use of additives in foods has become a subject of national and international interest. The effect on the world's food supply of one of the by-products of atomic blasts, strontium-90, has precipitated an entirely new area of scientific investigation. Also, ways to harness atomic energy for the benefit of mankind have been explored for application to the fields of foods and nutrition. More recently, man's venture into space has created new research challenges for the food technologist, the physiologist, the biochemist, and the nutritionist.

The topics presented in this chapter include newer methods of food preservation, additives to foods, strontium-90 in the diet, and food and nutriture for man in space.

▶ NEWER METHODS OF FOOD PRESERVATION

Until the middle of the nineteenth century, food and food products were preserved by drying, pickling, or salting. The invention of preserving food by the process now known as canning is credited to the Frenchman François Appert, who in the early 1800's devised this process for the armies of Napoleon. He referred to the food sealed in a complex arrangement of glass and corks as the "sealing of the seasons." The process of freezing, which is used to preserve both raw and prepared foods, is a discovery of the twentieth century. The newer methods of food preservation include dehydration, freeze-drying and irradiation.

To highlight the progress that has been made in the preservation of food within recent years, the food inventories of two historic voyages are presented: Columbus' trip to the "New World" in 1492, and the 2405-mile submerged voyage of the nuclear-propelled submarine, U.S.S. Skate, across the North Pole in 1958 (Table 26.1).

Dehydrated Foods

The objective in dehydration is to remove most of the water from a food without changing its color, flavor, or texture. The dehydrated foods of today are quite superior to those of the past because of newer methods of technology and modern equipment (3). Different types of foods are processed by dehydration: eggs, potato products, fruits, citrus fruit juices, soups, and others. Skimmilk powder, however, is probably the most widely known and used of the dehydrated foods.

Dehydrated foods have several advantages over their fresh, canned, or frozen counterparts. They are usually economical and easy to prepare, require no specialized equipment for storage, and are easy and economical to transport.

Freeze-Dried Foods

The preservation method of freeze-drying involves the removal of water from a food by *sublimation* after it has been frozen (8). Sublimation is a physical process whereby a solid substance is vaporized or a vapor is condensed without first changing to a liquid. In freeze-drying, the frozen water or ice crystals in the food tissues vaporize and condense, leaving the tissues as water vapor without forming water.

Freeze-dried food products have several desirable qualities not found in food products dried from the liquid state (dehydration). They retain their natural shape, are least altered chemically, and are readily reconstituted with water.

Many types of foods have been subjected to the freeze-dried process on an experimental basis. However, until recently only limited numbers of these products have been sold for civilian use. As of May 1963, there were only 33 freeze-dried foods on the commercial market (2).

The U.S. Department of Agriculture has initiated a series of studies to evaluate the acceptability and economics of freeze-dried food

Table 26.1. Food Lists for Pioneer Voyages

	Niña, Pinta, Santa Maria	U.S.S. *Skate*
Milk group:	Cheese	Milk (fresh, dried, evaporated) Cheese (canned)ˈ Butter Cream (dried, stabilized) Ice cream paste
Meat group:	Salt meat (beef and pork) Salt fish (barreled sardines and anchovies) (*fishing tackle*)	Pork cuts (frozen) Prefried bacon, pullman hams, brown-and-serve sausage (canned) Beef, boneless (fresh, frozen, canned, corned, dehydrated) Veal, boneless (frozen) Liver, prefabricated (frozen) Luncheon meats (fresh, canned) Chile con carne (dehydrated) Poultry (chicken cuts, frozen; turkey legs, canned) Fish (frozen, canned dehydrated) Eggs (fresh, frozen, dried)
Vegetable-fruit group:	Chickenpeas Lentils Beans Rice Raisins Almonds Garlic	Potatoes (fresh, canned, dehydrated granules, dehydrated diced) Cabbage, string beans, peppers, onions (dehydrated) Peas (dehydrofrozen) Beans (dried) Other vegetables and fruit (fresh, frozen, canned, dried) Tomato juice, concentrated (canned) Orange, grapefruit juice (dehydrated crystals) Lemon, concentrated (frozen) Apples, pie style (dehydrated) Applesauce (instant) Soups: Potato, onion, vegetable (dehydrated) Soup bases Jellies, jams (canned) Sauces (canned) Peanut butter
Bread-cereal-wheat group:	Flour (salted at milling) Biscuit (well-seasoned, good, not old)	Flour Flour mixes; bread, rolls, doughnut, cake, pancake Oatmeal Cornmeal Breakfast cereal, assorted Bread (fresh) Brown bread (canned) Cookies Macaroni, spaghetti, noodles Crackers
Other foods:	Olive oil Honey Wine Vinegar	Shortening, hydrogenated Salad oil Dessert powders Catsup, chili sauce Pickles, olives Vinegar Sugar, sirups Candies Spices, condiments Coffee (ground, instant) Tea Cocoa

From *Power to Produce. The Yearbook of Agriculture 1960*. U.S. Dept. Agr., p. 453, 1960.

483

products. The first publication of this series reports on the results of a
palatability test on twenty-eight freeze-dried foods now available commercially (2). The foods studied were beef, pork, chicken, seafoods,
soups, and several mixtures of foods. In these tests similar food items
processed by either canning or freezing were used as a basis of
comparison. The taste panel scored three of the freeze-dried foods
superior, fifteen equal to, and ten poorer than their food counterparts
in either the canned or frozen form. The foods that scored superior
were beef noodle soup, chicken noodle soup, and shrimp creole.
In general, the scores for the freeze-dried foods were higher when
served as mixtures than when served plain.

Like dehydrated foods, freeze-dried foods require no special equipment for storage, are easy to prepare, and are economical to transport.
However, at this time freeze-dried foods are expensive and not readily
available in the average grocery store or supermarket.

Irradiated Foods

The research and development directed to the preservation of foods
by irradiation are outgrowths of a program directed to finding peace-
ful uses for atomic energy following the Second World War. Since 1953
the U.S. Army has undertaken the testing of the wholesomeness of
irradiated foods as part of a program to study the possible uses of
ionizing radiation in food processing. Radiation preservation is still in
the experimental stage, and before irradiated food products are sold on
the commercial market, their wholesomeness, as judged by toxicity and
nutritional adequacy tests with animals and man, must be established
under the requirements of the Food Additives Amendment of 1958.

The irradiation process is sometimes referred to as "cold sterilization"
because the microorganisms in the food are destroyed or inactivated by
nuclear ionization rather than by heat. In heat sterilization a food must
be processed at about 240°F for an hour or more to produce a sterile
product, whereas in irradiation the heat produced amounts to only a
small rise in temperature (not more than 10°C) for a very short period
of time (11, 14).

Two types of radiation sources are being tested for food preservation:
those from radioactive isotopes or gamma rays and those produced by
machines or electron sources. The U.S. Army Radiation Laboratory at
Natick, Massachusetts, uses cobalt-60 gamma radiation in their experimental irradiation studies (Fig. 26.1). Doses of radiation used on foods
are expressed by a unit called the *rad*, which represents 100 ergs
of energy per gm of irradiated material.

In theory, radiation sterilization should provide a fresh or cooked

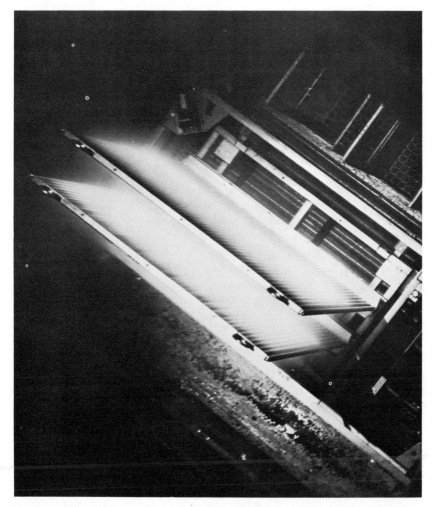

Fig. 26.1. World's largest Cobalt-60 gamma radiation source concentration at the U.S. Army Radiation Laboratory used in the experimental preservation processing of meat, fish, and other foods. The concentration source looks like a neon sign as it rests on the bottom of the 25-foot deep storage pool. (U.S. Army photograph, courtesy of U.S. Army Natick Laboratory, Natick, Massachusetts.)

sterile product with a better taste and texture than foods processed by heat sterilization. In practice, however, this does not always occur because large doses of radiation may produce marked off-flavors and changes in color and texture in some foods. For example, foods may develop an off-flavor resembling a scorched taste, cooked meats may turn pink in color, and lettuce wilts (13).

Kraybill (6) has summarized some of the undesirable effects of radiation on foods and has presented information on procedures that have been instituted to alleviate these effects. For example, the off-flavors and odors produced in meats and foods high in fat can be controlled by irradiation under vacuum or in an atmosphere of nitrogen, and during the irradiation of milk the off-flavors and metallic flavor can be eliminated by simultaneous irradiation and vacuum distillation.

Research studies are still under way to prove the wholesomeness of irradiated foods. In this presentation, only generalities concerning the effects of irradiation on food nutrients and human studies will be discussed.

The nutritional value of irradiated foods has been evaluated by chemical, microbiological, and animal feeding studies. As a general statement, the vitamins in foods are more sensitive to destruction by ionizing radiation than are the other nutrients (1, 7, 12). The fat-soluble vitamins (A, E, and K) are easily destroyed by irradiation whereas ascorbic acid, thiamine, and pyridoxine are reduced to somewhat the same level as in processing by heat sterilization.

Short-time human feeding studies have been conducted with irradiated foods (9). In these seven fifteen-day feeding trials, healthy young men served as experimental subjects. The experimental diets varied in per cent of Calories from irradiated foods, in the number of irradiated foods in the diet, and in the storage condition of the foods, either frozen or at room temperature. As examples, in Test 1, 35 per cent of the Calories of the diet came from 11 irradiated foods stored in the frozen state whereas in Test 4, the 30 irradiated foods stored frozen represented 100 per cent of the caloric value of the diet. During each feeding trial and for a one-year period thereafter, clinical examinations and laboratory tests were made on each subject to check for the presence of any toxic effects. None of the subjects, however, showed any evidence of toxicity from eating irradiated foods.

It appears that small or medium doses of ionizing radiation may have a more immediate application to food preservation than the large dose of the "cold sterilization" technique (4, 5). Small doses of radiation (less than 100 thousand rads) have been used successfully to deinfest flour and spices, to prevent sprouting in stored potatoes, and to delay the ripening of fruit (Table 26.2). The same treatment may have a significant use to destroy the organism in pork that causes trichinosis (6). Medium doses of radiation (about 100 thousand to 1 million rads) now referred to as "pasteurization" or "radiopasteurization" have been shown to extend the shelf life of some foods stored under refrigeration. Meats have had their shelf life increased fivefold when treated with 100 to 500 thousand rads. Fruits treated with 100 to 150 thousand rads,

Table 26.2. The Use and Effect of Varying Levels of Ionizing Radiation on Food and Related Products

Level of Ionizing Radiation	Use	Effect on Finished Product
Small Exposure (less than 100 thousand rads)	Prevents sprouting of potatoes, destroys insects in flour and spices, and delays ripening of fruit.	Products not sterile but little or no effect on flavor or color of foods.
Medium Exposure or *"Pasteurization"* (about 100 thousand to 1 million rads)	Extends the shelf life of meats, fish, fruits, and vegetables under refrigeration.	Products not completely sterile but little or no effect on flavor or color of foods.
Large Exposure or *"Sterilization"* (a few million rads)	Sterilizes foods so they can be stored as canned foods when properly packaged.	Products completely sterile but often causes marked off-flavors and changes in color and texture.

Adapted from text of "Modern food processing," in *Food. The Yearbook of Agriculture 1959.* U.S. Dept. Agr., p. 421, 1959.

packed under vacuum, and stored at refrigerator temperature were quite acceptable for a period of four or five months.

In 1963 two irradiated foods were approved by the Food and Drug Administration for public consumption: irradiated bacon and wheat processed by irradiation to destroy infestation (15). Neither of these products is on sale in the commercial market at this time, and it is unlikely that they will be available to the civilian consumer until about 1970. In Canada and the U.S.S.R., however, irradiated potatoes are available in limited quantities, as approved by these governments.

Ionizing energy preservation studies for the wholesomeness of twenty-one other foods are now being conducted by the U.S. Army Radiation Laboratory (15). Petitions for the use of ionizing radiation to prevent the sprouting of potatoes and to control microorganisms on oranges and lemons are now under consideration by the Food and Drug Administration (10).

▶ ADDITIVES TO FOODS

Additives to foods demand the attention of the student of nutrition today. Many of the food products on the market have had chemicals added; these are known as additives (3, 7, 8, 13, 14). As defined by The Food Protection Committee of the National Academy of Science—National Research Council, an additive to food is "a substance or mixture of substances, other than a basic foodstuff, which is present in food as a result of any aspect of production, processing, storage, or packaging" (11). Although some of the substances are introduced intentionally for the purpose of improving the nutritive value or quality of the product, others are present as a residue after some stage of production or manufacture. The latter type of substance is essential in modern agricultural production and food technology.

Additives to Improve Nutritive Value

A limited number of foods have had nutrients added to them to improve the nutritive value. The addition of iodine to salt in 1924 was the first important addition of an essential nutrient to a staple article of food for nutritional purposes. Increasing the vitamin D content of milk by adding irradiated ergosterol was a second milestone. Next was the enrichment of white flour and bread, which began in the United States on a voluntary basis in 1941 with the addition of specified amounts of thiamine, riboflavin, niacin, and iron, and the addition of specified amounts of vitamin D and calcium optional (2, 14). In 1947 standards for the enrichment of corn meal and corn grits with the same nutrients as are added to the wheat products were established by the Food and Drug Administration. More recently, rice also is being enriched. Margarine may be fortified with vitamin A; if represented as containing the vitamin, the concentration must be 15,000 IU of the vitamin per pound, which equals the estimated average vitamin A potency of butter.

The introduction of the specified additives to the respective foods has the approval of nutritionists and persons concerned with the health and well-being of the populace. These nutrients had been found at one time to occur in less than the recommended amounts in the diets of the general population or in segments of it. The beneficial effects realized by the consumption of foods enhanced in nutritive value through additives are discussed in the chapters devoted to the respective nutrients.

It should be kept in mind that bolstering the nutritive value of staple foods, beneficial as it may be, is not a substitute for education in the proper choice and preparation of foods. It is wise to continuously exert effort toward improving methods of production, processing, and storage, attempting to preserve more fully the nutrients present in the native products.

The common viewpoint of the Food and Nutrition Board of the National Research Council and the Council on Foods and Nutrition of the American Medical Association on additives to improve the nutritive value of foods is set forth here in an abbreviated form (9). The requirements for the endorsement of the addition of a specific nutrient to a particular food are as follows:

1. The principle of the addition of specific nutrients to certain foods is endorsed, with defined limitations, for the purpose of maintaining good nutrition in all segments of the population at all economic levels. The requirements which should be met for the addition of a particular nutrient to a given food include (a) acceptable evidence that the supplemented food would be physiologically or economically advantageous for a significant segment of the consumer population, (b) assurance that the food item concerned would be an effective vehicle of distribution for the nutrient to be added, and (c) evidence that such addition would not be prejudicial to the achievement of a diet good in other respects.

2. The desirability of meeting nutritional needs by the use of an adequate variety of foods as far as practicable is emphasized strongly. To that end, research and education are encouraged to insure the proper choice and preparation of foods and to improve food production, processing, storage, and distribution so as to retain their essential nutrients.

3. Foods suitable as vehicles for the distribution of additional nutrients are those which have a diminished nutritive content as a result of loss in refining or other processing or those which are widely and regularly consumed. The nutrients added to such foods should be the kinds and quantities associated with the class of foods involved. The addition of other than normally occurring levels of nutrients to these foods may be favored when properly qualified judgment indicates that the addition will be advantageous to public health and other methods for effecting the desired purpose appear to be less feasible.

4. Scientific evaluation of the desirability of restoring an essential nutrient or nutrients to the diet is necessary whenever technologic or economic changes lead to a nutritionally significant reduction in the intake of a nutrient or nutrients. Such reduction might result either from a marked decrease in the consumption of an important food or from a considerable increase in the consumption of foods of diminished nutritive quality.

Similar evaluation is desirable, with the limitations defined in the preceding Section 1, whenever advances in nutritional science and in food technology make possible the preparation of nutrient-enriched products which are likely to make important contributions to good nutrition.

5. The endorsement of the following is affirmed: the enrichment of flour, bread,

degerminated corn meal, corn grits, whole grain corn meal, and white rice; the retention or restoration of thiamine, riboflavin, niacin, and iron in processed food cereals; the addition of vitamin D to milk, fluid skim milk, and nonfat dry milk; the addition of vitamin A to margarine, fluid skim milk, and nonfat dry milk; and the addition of iodine to table salt. The protective action of fluoride against dental caries is recognized and the standardized addition of fluoride to water is endorsed in areas in which the water supply has a low fluoride content.

6. The above statements of policy and of endorsement apply to conditions existing in the United States. Recommendations for additions of nutrients to foods for export should be based on similar physiological or economic advantages expected to accrue to the respective consumers.

Increasing in use, particularly in beverages, are non-nutritive sweeteners as sugar substitutes (1). Saccharin and the calcium and sodium cyclamates (cyclohexyl sulfamates) are commonly used. Such sweeteners were permitted in foods in the first place for persons who needed to restrict their intake of carbohydrate. Now widespread use has been made of the products by persons who wish to reduce caloric intake.

Additives to Improve the Quality of Products

The more complicated the processing of foods, the greater is the need for additives. More and more foods appear on the market with built-in preparation. For highly processed foods to be acceptable in keeping quality, flavor, and standard characteristics, the addition of certain chemicals has been necessary.

Ascorbic acid is added to some fruit to prevent browning in freezing; sulfur dioxide is added to dried apricots and apples to prevent discoloration.

Emulsifiers are added to bakery products to improve volume, uniformity, and fineness of grain; to dairy products for smoothness; and to confectionery for homogeneity and keeping quality. Among the common emulsifiers are lecithin, the mono- and diglycerides, and propylene glycol. Chemists sometimes call the emulsifiers "surfactants"—short for "surface active agents" (16)

Preservatives are added to extend the keeping quality of the product. The kind added is influenced by the properties of the product. Antioxidants are added to fats to delay the onset of rancidity. Examples of antioxidants are butylated hydroxyanisole (BHA), butylated hydroxytoluene (BHT), nordihydroguariaretic acid (NDGA), and propyl gallate.

The preservatives used in bread are called mold and rope inhibitors, or antimycotic agents. Those permitted in bread include sodium and calcium propionate, sodium diacetate, acetic acid, lactic acid, and monocalcium phosphate. Sorbic acid and sodium and potassium sorbates are antimycotic agents for cheeses (16).

Preservatives that prevent physical or chemical changes which affect color, flavor, texture, or appearance are called sequestrants. Those used in dairy products include sodium, calcium, and potassium salts of citric, tartaric, metaphosphoric, and pyrophosphoric acids. Other common preservatives are benzoic acid, sodium benzoate, sulfur dioxide, sugar, salt, and vinegar.

Stabilizers and thickeners are used to improve smoothness of texture of confectionery, ice cream, and other frozen desserts; uniformity of color, flavor, and viscosity of chocolate milk; "body" of artificially sweetened beverages. Stabilizing and thickening agents include pectins, vegetable gums (carob bean, carragheen, guar), gelatin, and agar agar.

Acids, alkalies, buffers, and neutralizing agents are added to influence the degree of acidity or alkalinity, which is important in many classes of processed foods. For example,

The acid ingredient acts on the leavening agent in baked goods, and releases the gas which causes rising. The taste of many soft drinks is due largely to an organic acid. Acidity of churning cream must be controlled for flavor and keeping quality of the butter. Acids contribute flavor to confectionery and help to prevent a "grainy" texture. Buffers and neutralizing agents are chemicals added to control acidity or alkalinity, just as acids and alkalies may be added directly. Some common chemicals in this class are ammonium bicarbonate, calcium carbonate, potassium acid tartarate, sodium aluminum phosphate, and tartaric acid (16).

Flavoring agents are added to improve the taste in such products as soft drinks, bakery goods, confectionery, and ice cream. Synthetic flavors are provided by such chemicals as amyl acetate, benzaldehyde, carvone, ethyl butyrate, and methyl salicylate.

Coloring matter is added to improve the appearance.

Even though extensive, this is not an exhaustive list of chemicals added to foods to improve the quality of products. These additives are introduced with no concern for nutritive value but with concern for the quality of the product, which of course influences the consumers' choice (8).

Incidental Additives

Incidental additives are chemical substances remaining in foods from some stage of production or manufacture of the product. The most important additives in this classification are the "pesticides." Included in this general grouping are insecticides, fungicides, and rodenticides, each of which helps in the control of pests harmful to crops and food. Through the use of these chemicals, the production of food is facilitated; there is less loss of crops and food during storage; also the product produced is of higher quality.

Federal legislation has been enacted for consumer protection from pesticide residues in foods. All commercial pesticides must be registered with the U.S. Department of Agriculture before they can be shipped in interstate commerce. Review of labels is a significant part of the registration process. "This review makes it possible for scientists in the department to see that label directions and warnings are adequate, if followed, to assure safe and effective use of the product. To be sure that users of pesticides have dependable guidance, the Department of Agriculture will accept for registration only those products, which, when used according to directions, will leave no residues at all or residues that come safely within official tolerances" (3, p. 98).

Control of Additives to Foods in the United States

The agency of the government with the primary responsibility for regulating the use of chemical additives in food and monitoring compliance with these regulations in interstate commerce is the Food and Drug Administration (FDA) (5, 10, 11). In 1954 Congress enacted the Pesticide Chemicals Amendment to the Food, Drug, and Cosmetic Law, which places responsibility on the manufacturer to demonstrate that the residues are harmless under conditions of use. Thus in the case of commercially canned or frozen foods, the processor is responsible for using products that comply with the established tolerances.

"As an administrative principle, tolerances are set by FDA at 1/100 of the lowest level which causes effects in the most sensitive test animals whenever data on human toxicity are not available" (15, p. 17). In the case of some pesticides no amount of residue is permitted because of their high toxicity; for others no tolerances are established because the residues are harmless.

The Federal Food and Drug Administration, in cooperation with the state administrations, is concerned that wholesome food of good nutritive quality, accurately labeled be provided for the public. The federal agency operates under the provisions of the Food, Drug, and Cosmetic Act of 1938, which provided for the promulgation of standards for certain foods and for the labeling of products for special dietary uses. The standard of identity for a particular food includes a definition of the food, stipulations as to kinds and amounts of ingredients permissible, and the quality of the product. The standard is established and made effective only after public hearings and after the proposed recommendations have been published to allow any who are interested to challenge its accuracy, accomplishment of desired purpose, and legality.

Since the enactment of the Food, Drug, and Cosmetic Act in 1938, three important amendments have been made to it. One of the amendments is the Pesticide Chemical Amendment enacted in 1954; another is the Food Additives Amendment of 1958, which "requires that food additives be tested for safety prior to use and that government approval must be obtained for their use." Prior to the passage of the Additives Amendment only those additives that were proved in court to be deleterious to health could be forbidden (4).

The third amendment to the Act, the Color Additive Amendment of 1960, "regulates the listing and certification of colors which are to be used in foods, drugs, and cosmetics, and in addition provides for testing both existing colors and new colors for safety" (12).

The law requires that chemicals for use in processing food must be proved by the industry to be safe for that purpose *before* they can be sold. The manufacturer or promoter of a new food additive must test it for safety on animals and submit the results to the Food and Drug Administration. If the Food and Drug Administration is satisfied as to the safety of the additive, it will issue a regulation specifying the amount which may be used, the foods in which it may be used, and any other necessary conditions of use. If the safety of the additive is not established, its use will be prohibited.

Additives—An International Problem

The use of additives is an international problem, so much so that a joint Food and Agriculture Organization—World Health Organization Expert Committee on Food additives was established in 1955 and has functioned actively ever since. The Expert Committee has concerned itself chiefly with the evaluation of "the evidence on the toxicological aspects of a number of antimicrobials and antioxidants used as food additives" (7). Such substances "are widely used in many countries, because they can play an important part in reducing food wastage by improving storage efficiency and distribution. . . ." In some countries there are departments responsible for the control of the use of these drugs. "In many others, however, there is no adequate machinery by which those responsible for public health can usefully handle these problems" (7).

At the 1961 meeting of the Expert Committee, particular attention was paid to food for babies. The Committee strongly recommended that "baby foods should be prepared without food additives, if possible." If not possible, it was urged that "great caution should be exercised both in the choice of additive and in the level of use." Special consideration for infants is explained on the basis that "the detoxicating mechanisms that are effective in the more mature individual may be ineffective in the baby" (7).

► STRONTIUM-90 IN THE DIET

One of the hazardous by-products of fission piles and atomic blasts is the radioactive form of strontium, strontium-90. This contamination product may be a potential cause of sarcomas in the animal organism. Because of the long half-life of this "bone-seeking" radionuclide (about 28 years) there is a worldwide interest in the present rates of strontium-90 accumulation in plants, animals, and man due to the contamination of the earth's atmosphere from bomb tests within recent years.

Generalities on Strontium

Strontium belongs to the same group of elements as does the mineral calcium. Thus the behavior of either its stable or radioactive forms is controlled by and closely allied to calcium. Both minerals move in the "food chain" from soil to plant to animal to man. Strontium, like calcium, is deposited for the most part in the bones and teeth. However, in the animal organism, there is a preferential absorption of calcium rather than strontium from the digestive tract, and there is a preferential excretion of strontium from the body (8). This biological preference actually helps to protect the body against the accumulation of excess strontium.

Man ingests small amounts of strontium in the food he eats because it is one of the trace elements normally found in biological material. Harrison and his group (3) have reported that from a normal diet their subjects ingested about 1.99 mg of strontium per day and excreted nearly the same amount (about 1.97 mg per day). The body load of strontium in man has been demonstrated to be about four to six times higher after an intravenous dose than after an oral dose (8).

Radiostrontium in the Diet

Strontium-90 is measured in units known as *micromicrocuries* ($\mu\mu$c) or *picocuries* (pc). The Food Protection Committee of the National Research Council (6) has suggested that the values for dietary strontium-90 be expressed in two ways: the amount of strontium-90 per unit of calcium and the amount of strontium-90 per unit of product. For example, the 1959 wheat crop grown in the United States averaged about 113 $\mu\mu$c (or pc) of strontium-90 per gm of calcium and 46 $\mu\mu$c (or pc) of strontium-90 per kg of wheat (5).

For almost a decade, the Health and Safety Laboratory of the Atomic

Energy Commission, the United States Public Health Service, and other research units in this country have conducted regular analyses for strontium-90 and other radionuclides in the American food and water supply. Data from similar analyses are available from other parts of the world.

Indices of the strontium-90 content of the American food supply at any one time are determined in several ways. One procedure is to use the radioactivity in milk as a guide to strontium-90 in the diet, another procedure is to present data in terms of amounts of food typical for various age groups, and a newer approach is to present data in terms of the food need for the group with the largest nutritive requirement in the United States population (the male teenager).

Milk has been singled out as a food indicator of the strontium-90 in the diet because year-around samples can be procured. The average strontium-90 concentration in milk for selected cities in the United States for the period of September 1962 to August 1963 is shown in Table 26.3 (1). Higher strontium-90 values for milk were found in the eastern than in the western section of the country. Phoenix, Austin, and Honolulu had the lowest values whereas New Orleans and Chattanooga had the highest in this listing. The average value for all the cities tested in the network during this period was 20.4 pc of strontium-90 per liter of milk.

Values for the strontium-90 content of samples of a variety of foods

Table 26.3. Average Strontium-90 Concentration in Milk, September 1962 to August 1963, in Selected Cities in the United States

City	Strontium-90, pc/liter	City	Strontium-90, pc/liter
Atlanta, Ga.	25	Laramie, Wyo.	18
Austin, Texas	8	Minneapolis, Minn.	25
Boston, Mass.	27	New Orleans, La.	36
Chattanooga, Tenn.	31	New York, N.Y.	23
Chicago, Ill.	18	Oklahoma City, Okla.	22
Cleveland, Ohio	18	Palmer, Alaska	15
Dallas, Texas	20	Phoenix, Ariz.	4
Denver, Colo.	14	Pittsburgh, Pa.	24
Detroit, Mich.	18	St. Louis, Mo.	19
Hartford, Conn.	18	San Francisco, Calif.	12
Honolulu, Hawaii	8	Seattle, Wash.	21
Kansas City, Mo.	22	Washington, D.C.	19

From "Annual average radionuclide concentration in pasteurized milk, September 1962—August 1963." *Radiol. Health Data* **5:** 603, 1963.

collected in four regions of the United States during May to June 1961 have been reported (4). The test cities were New York and Boston (Northeast); Chicago and Sioux Falls (North Central); El Paso, Knoxville, and New Orleans (South); and Denver, Los Angeles, and Spokane (West). The compilation of values reported did not represent diets or amounts of food consumed, but rather approximate amounts of food typical for various age groups (infants, low- and middle-income teenagers, and middle-income adults). Among the types of food composites analyzed, the average values for strontium-90 ranged from 13 to 4.3 $\mu\mu c$ per gm of calcium. The higher strontium-90-calcium ratios were found in the Northeast and the low ones in the West. In general, it was concluded that these values were in agreement with findings from other studies.

The Food and Drug Administration study of radionuclides in diets for teenagers began in 1961 with Washington, D.C. as the test area. In 1962, Atlanta, Minneapolis, St. Louis, and San Francisco were added to expand the testing to a national basis. At present, food samples are collected and analyzed quarterly. To assure representative food samples from each of the five test areas, a well-designed purchasing procedure is followed. From a list of 82 items of food and drink, a two-week food supply is purchased in each city that duplicates the diet of a 19-year-old male. These foods are then cooked and prepared as they would be in the home before the samples are taken for strontium-90 analyses.

The strontium-90 concentration in the total diet, including drinking water, for the period May 1962 through February 1963 in the five test cities is shown in Table 26.4 (2). The resumption of nuclear testing in 1961 is reflected in an increase of strontium-90 in the food and water during this ten-month period. In May 1962 the strontium-90 values of the total diet ranged from 11.3 to 37.6 pc per day whereas in February 1963 the values ranged from 26.7 to 47.1 pc per day. According to the Federal Radiation Council Range II maximum value for strontium-90 of 200 pc per day, the value of 47.1 pc per day found in the Atlanta food samples in February 1963 was well within the range of safety proposed at this time.

Food analyses have shown that milk and milk products carry an appreciable portion of the total strontium-90 in the diet. This fact, however, does not warrant a decrease in milk consumption in this country. The Food Protection Committee of the National Research Council has emphasized

... that the important parameter is the level of contamination of the total diet. The use of milk as an indicator food does not imply that a decrease in the consumption of milk would result in a decrease in the total strontium-90 intake. Foods substituted for milk would probably result in higher intakes of strontium-90 because of the higher Sr-90/Ca ratio in such foods (6).

Table 26.4. Strontium-90 Concentration in the Total Diet (Including Drinking Water)

Sampling Locations	May 1962 pc/kg	May 1962 pc/Day[1]	August 1962 pc/kg	August 1962 pc/Day[1]	November 1962 pc/kg	November 1962 pc/Day[1]	February 1963 pc/kg	February 1963 pc/Day[1]
San Francisco, Calif.	3.0	11.3	3.4	12.8	4.8	18.1	8.0	30.1
Washington, D.C.	6.4	24.0	6.9	26.0	8.4	31.6	12.0	45.1
Atlanta, Ga.	9.7	36.4	7.2	27.1	9.2	34.6	12.5	47.1
Minneapolis, Minn.	5.2	19.5	9.0	33.8	7.9	29.7	8.8	33.1
St. Louis, Mo.	10.0	37.6	8.8	33.1	9.5	35.7	7.1	26.7

[1] Estimated intake for the 19-year age group.

From "Radionuclides in diets for teen-agers, May 1962–February 1963." Division of Pharmacology, Food and Drug Administration, *Radiol. Health Data* **5**: 286, 1963.

Although methods have been suggested and developed for the remedial modification of foods to remove radiostrontium (7), in the 1962 report of the Food Protection Committee of the National Research Council (6) it is stated that "the present extent of environmental contamination does not warrant extraordinary measures for the decontamination of foods."

▶ FOOD AND NUTRITURE FOR MAN IN SPACE

History undoubtedly will record the research and development directed to the accomplishment of manned space flight as one of the greatest scientific and engineering feats of all times.

The manned balloon flights conducted prior to the suborbital and orbital flights of Project Mercury gave significant information on man's performance at high altitudes (11). It was found that man could exist for more than a day in a sealed cabin at high altitudes, approximately 100,000 feet (19 miles) in the atmosphere. These pioneer test pilots breathed an artificial atmosphere and ate a ration composed of specially prepared foods.

Some Studies Directed to Nutriture for Space Travel

Only a resume of some of the studies directed to nutriture for man's exploration of space is presented here. Tubed foods, freeze-dried foods, unconventional-type foods, equipment for feeding the space traveler, and feeding concepts for Projects Mercury and Gemini are the topics discussed.

Tubed Foods. These types of food products were developed for personnel performing in high-flying aircraft and space vehicles where pressure suits and other conditions might interfere with normal feeding procedures. Tubed foods can be eaten without the removal of a pressure helmet, do not require refrigeration, are ready to eat, are not affected by high altitudes, and require little storage and disposal space.

The food, either in the liquid or semisolid form, is packed in a pliable aluminum tube to which is fitted a screw-on, five-inch plastic tube called a pontube. When the tube is squeezed by hand, food passes into the mouth via the pontube (Fig. 26.2). Welbourn and Lachance (15)

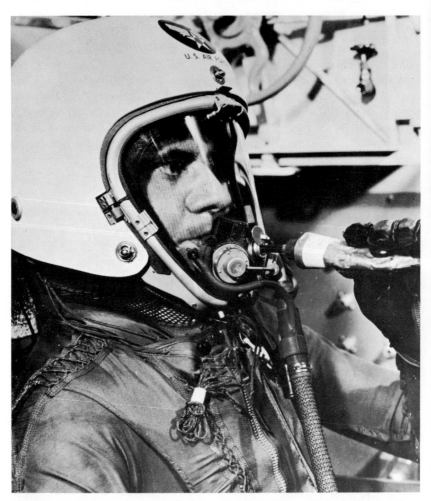

Fig. 26.2. Subject eating tubed food while wearing MA-2 oxygen helmet. (U.S. Air Force photograph.)

have measured the palatability of nineteen different tubed foods with human subjects. The twelve tubed foods found to warrant consideration for operational use were applesauce, peaches, vegetable juice, fruit dessert, semisolid beef, chocolate, semisolid chicken, pork dinner, semisolid ham, veal dinner, beef dinner, and beef noodle soup.

Freeze-dried Foods. The proposed use of freeze-dried foods in the fourteen-day flights of Project Gemini and Apollo has given impetus to an intensive research and development program of this type of food preservation (2, 9, 11). Details on freeze-dried food products are presented in a preceding section of this chapter.

Unconventional Types of Foods. The need to supply adequate nutrition in future long-range space flights, where it no longer will be possible to carry sufficient supplies for life support, has led to the initiation of studies to find unconventional food products that may be used as sources of Calories, amino acids, minerals, and vitamins for the space traveler. Although bacteria and vegetable tissues grown in tissue cultures have been proposed as "potential space food" (4), the two examples of unconventional food sources presented here are the high-energy metabolites and algae.

High-energy metabolites are long-chained compounds which have a caloric value greater than that of the conventional energy nutrients: carbohydrate, 4 Cal. per gm; fat, 9 Cal. per gm; and protein, 4 Cal. per gm. Two high-energy metabolites now under study are 1, 3-butanediol and 2, 4-dimethyl heptanoic acid (1, 8). It has been reported that in diets of rats, 1,3-butanediol was utilized for energy at about 6 Cal. per gm to replace dietary carbohydrate and to increase the caloric density of high-fat rations. The applicability of high-energy metabolites for human diets remains to be demonstrated.

The use of algae as a food supplement is not new. People in various parts of the world, particularly in the Far East, have used small portions of algae in their diets for centuries. There are various kinds of algae: green, blue-green, red, and brown. In general, a 100-gm portion of powdered green algae contains about 59 gm of protein, 19 gm of fat, 13 gm of carbohydrate, and 550 Cal. (10). Analytical data in terms of protein, amino acids, certain vitamins, lipids, ash, and energy in various algae and mixtures of algae have been reported (5, 6, 7).

There is interest in this unicellular plant for space travel because of its photosynthetic properties where-by algae may be useful both as a food and a respiratory gas exchanger. In the process of photosynthesis, carbon dioxide is used by the plant to synthesize nutrients, and oxygen is produced as a by-product in these reactions (see Chapter 9). Thus the carbon dioxide of the expired air may be exchanged for oxygen in this cycle. Also there is considerable interest in the possible production and use of algae in the overpopulated countries of the world to bolster the nutritive value of their inadequate food supplies.

Although many studies have been conducted on the culture and growth of algae, the use of the plant in algal gas exchange systems, the composition of algae, and other related topics, data on the acceptability and tolerance of algae feeding in man are scarce. Powell, Nevels, and McDowell (10) have conducted a short-time feeding study on man's acceptability and tolerance to algae feeding. The algae, a mixture of *Chlorella* and *Scenedesmus,* was added to the basal diet in increasing amounts during the six-week period of the study (10, 20, 50, 100, 200, and 500 gm per man per day). In an attempt to mask the strong, bitter taste of the algae, the plant product was incorporated into such foods as gingerbread, chocolate cookies, and chocolate cake. It was found that algae intakes up to a level of 100 gm per day, incorporated into the basal diet, were tolerated by all subjects. Early in the study, however, some of the subjects manifested gastrointestinal symptoms which increased at algae intakes above 100 gm per day. Some subjects experienced headaches, vomiting, and malaise at these higher levels of intake. Despite the reduced tolerance for algae at levels above 100 gm per day, no abnormalities were detected by either the physical or the clinical measurements in this study.

The recent work of Vanderveen and his group (14) suggests that some of the poor acceptability and lack of tolerance associated with algae as a food may be related to bacterial contamination. They have found that in a "self-nourishing" (autotrophic) algae culture as much as one-third of the culture population may be bacteria.

Work is now under way to investigate the potential of decolorized algae as a food source. The strong taste and odor of green algae can be removed to yield a product quite bland in taste and odor. However, the nutrient value of decolorized algae has not been reported as yet.

In addition to the work with algae, there is an interest in the possible use of higher plants as food sources for the permanent space stations of the future (12, 13, 16). Some of the plants being studied are cabbage, cauliflower, Chinese cabbage, dandelion, endive, kale, lettuce, sweet potato, and tampala.°

Equipment for Feeding the Space Traveler. Many types of equipment have been designed, fabricated, and tested for the purpose of feeding man during high-altitude flight and space travel. A plastic water-container, a feeding system using aluminum cans, a solar-powered oven, and feeding ports for tubed foods are just a few examples of types of

° The tampala leaf is used like spinach.

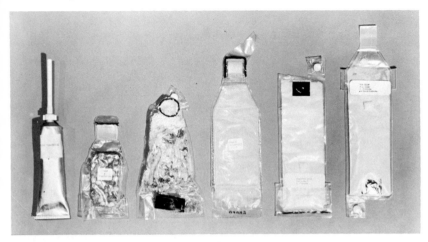

Fig. 26.3. Evolution of the design of rehydratable food containers used for feeding man in space. (National Aeronautics and Space Administration photograph, courtesy of the Manned Spacecraft Center, Houston, Texas.)

feeding equipment that have been developed (11). Of particular interest is the development and evolution of the design of the feeder and dispenser used for space feeding (9). Figure 26.3 shows the evolution of the design of feeders from the aluminum tube with a pontube (on the left) to the film food package of dehydrated pea soup (on the right). The dispenser shown in Fig. 26.4 has two openings called ports; one for the entrance of water for rehydration of the food and the other, which opens and closes as needed, is the feeding port.

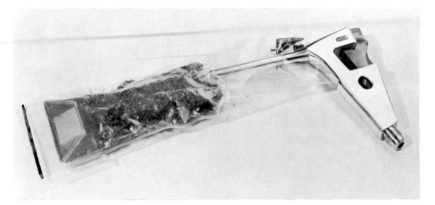

Fig. 26.4. Current Gemini rehydratable food container and water probe. (National Aeronautics and Space Administration photograph, courtesy of the Manned Spacecraft Center, Houston, Texas.)

The Life Support System and Feeding Concept of Project Mercury

One of the important research areas in the Manned Space Program has been and still is the undertakings directed to provide the astronaut with an adequate life support balance from the time he leaves until he returns to earth. This balance includes the life support needs for pressure, oxygen, water, as well as food, and the removal of the products of metabolism (carbon dioxide, water, heat, urine, and feces).

A sketch of the general features of the life support system used in the space flights of Project Mercury is shown in Fig. 26.5 (2). Because of the need to conserve weight and space in these initial space flights, a supply of oxygen and water was carried in these missions for the closed environmental system designed for Project Mercury. In this type of system the astronaut wore a pressure suit continually, ventilated with 5 pounds per square inch of oxygen in the pressurized cabin of the vehicle. The end products of metabolism were collected and treated in the following manner: carbon dioxide was removed by absorption with lithium hydroxide; water was removed by a water separator, and that condensed in the heat exchanger removed mechanically; heat was removed by a water-evaporative heat exchanger; odors were absorbed by activated charcoal; urine was collected in a device worn in the pressure suit; and fecal production was controlled by the ingestion of a low-residue preflight diet.

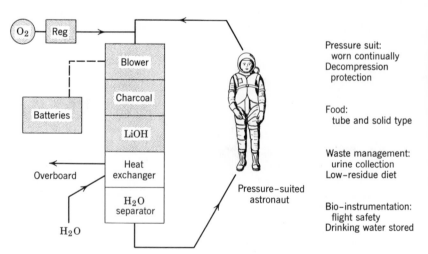

Fig. 26.5. Mercury life support system. (Courtesy of National Aeronautics and Space Administration—Manned Space Center, material cited from *Bioastronautics*, NASA-SP-18, December 1962.)

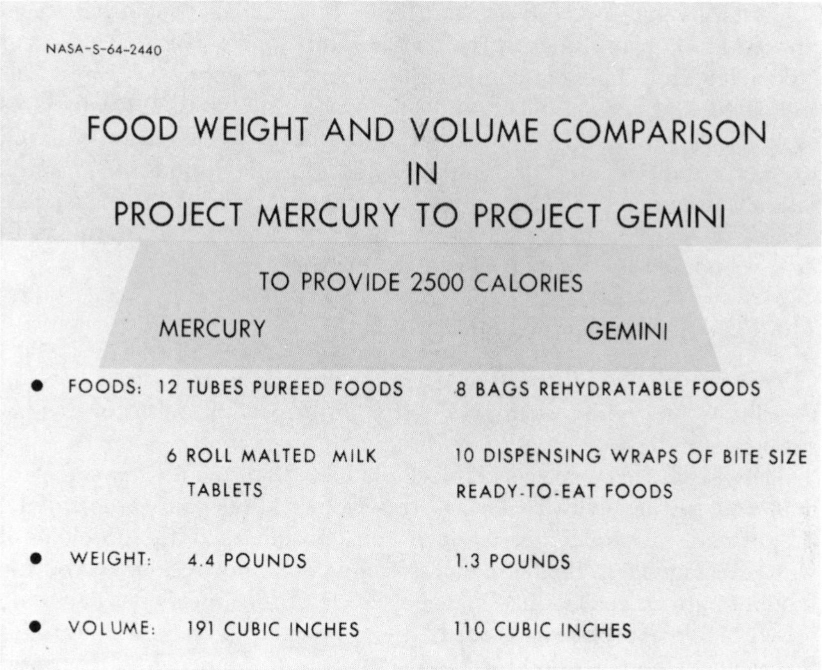

NASA-S-64-2440

FOOD WEIGHT AND VOLUME COMPARISON
IN
PROJECT MERCURY TO PROJECT GEMINI

TO PROVIDE 2500 CALORIES

	MERCURY	GEMINI
• FOODS:	12 TUBES PUREED FOODS	8 BAGS REHYDRATABLE FOODS
	6 ROLL MALTED MILK TABLETS	10 DISPENSING WRAPS OF BITE SIZE READY-TO-EAT FOODS
• WEIGHT:	4.4 POUNDS	1.3 POUNDS
• VOLUME:	191 CUBIC INCHES	110 CUBIC INCHES

Fig. 26.6. A comparison of the food weight and volume in the space flights of Project Mercury and Project Gemini. (National Aeronautics and Space Administration protograph, courtesy of the Manned Spacecraft Center, Houston, Texas.)

Because of the short duration of the Project Mercury flights, food was not mandatory except in the multi-orbital flight (MA-9) of Astronaut Cooper (9). No food was carried on board the spaceships in the first two short-time suborbital flights. In the later orbital flights, however, the handling of food and food containers was an experimental phase of the flight plan and information was also collected on gastrointestinal function during periods of weightlessness. The food items used in the early orbital flights were pureed foods (meats, vegetables, and fruits), malted milk tablets, and bite-size food cubes (Fig. 26.6). Dehydrated foods were included in the food pattern of flight MA-9.

The Feeding Concept of Russian Spaceflights

Little information is available on the feeding concept used in the Russian spaceflights. Nevertheless, some interesting facts concerning Russian space feeding have been found in documents from the Library of Congress (3).

Gargarin and Titov, the first of the Russian cosmonauts, ingested pureed foods from tubes in their flights into space. The space diets of Nikolayev and Popovich contained ordinary-type foods (i.e., meat cutlets, fried veal, chicken fillet, and sandwiches) prepared in small pieces as well as tubed foods. Water, coffee, and fruit juices have been reported to have complemented the semisolid and bite-sized foods of the space ration. Large doses of vitamins also were important in the Russian space diet. The space feeding pattern of the Russian cosmonauts appears to be a scheduled food intake every four or five hours.

The Feeding Concept of Project Gemini

Two astronauts will travel in space for periods up to fourteen days in the flights of Project Gemini. Food is an important cargo in this life support system.

The feeding concept for Project Gemini (9) provides for a diet of 2500 Cal. per day, with a caloric distribution of 51 per cent carbohydrate, 32 per cent fat, and 17 per cent protein. To minimize the problems of waste management, the flight diet is composed of low-residue foods. The feeding pattern consists of a four-day cycle of four meals per day using rehydratable and bite-sized, ready-to-eat foods (Fig. 26.6). The drinking water and water needed for food rehydration are provided by water produced by a fuel cell (water⁻production from oxygen and hydrogen gases) and stored at cabin temperature.

REFERENCES

NEWER METHODS OF FOOD PRESERVATION

1. Ballamy, W. D. (1959). Progress in food and drug sterilization by ionizing radiations. *Military Med.* **124:** 270.
2. Bird, K. (1963). *Freeze-Dried Foods: Palatability Tests.* U.S. Dept. Agr., Marketing Res. Rept. 617, Washington, D.C.
3. Boggs, M. M., and C. L. Rasmussen (1959). Modern food processing. In *Food. The Yearbook of Agriculture, 1959* (A. Stefferud, ed.) U.S. Dept. Agr., Washington, D.C., p. 418.
4. Clifcorn, L. E. (1959). Preservation of foods by irradiation. *Am. J. Public Health* **49:** 493.
5. Enkel, W. W., and W. Haber (1960). Tooling-up for low-dose irradiation processing of fresh foods. *Food Technol.* **14:** 198.
6. Kraybill, H. F. (1958). Nutritional and biochemical aspects of foods preserved by ionizing radiation. *J. Home Econ.* **50:** 695.
7. McDowell, M. E., and N. Raica, Jr. (1962). *Review of the United States Army's Irradiated Food Wholesomeness Program.* U.S. Army Med. Res. and Nutr. Lab Rept. 268.
8. Meryman, H. T. (1960). Principles of freeze-drying. *Ann. N.Y. Acad. Sci.* **85:** 630.
9. Plough, I. C., E. L. Bierman, L. M. Lenz, and N. F. Witt (1960). Human feeding studies with irradiated foods. *Federation Proc.* **19:** 1052.
10. Radiation and food (1964). *FDA Memo for Consumers from the Food and Drug Administration,* U.S. Dept. of Health, Education, and Welfare, CM-24, Washington, D.C.

11. *Radiation Sterilization of Foods* (1955). Hearing Before the Subcommittee on Research and Development of the Joint Committee on Atomic Energy, Congress of the United States, Washington, D.C.
12. Read, M. S. (1960). A summary of the wholesomeness of gamma-irradiated foods. *Federation Proc.* **19:** 1055.
13. Robinson, H. E., and W. M. Urbain (1960). Radiation preservation of foods. *J. Am. Med. Assoc.* **174:** 1310.
14. Ryer, R., III (1956). Influence of radiation preservation of foods on military feeding. *Food Technol.* **10:** 516.
15. U.S. Army Natick Laboratories (1964). Personal communication.

ADDITIVES TO FOODS

1. Ballinger, R. A., and L. C. Larkin (1964). *Sweeteners Used by Food Processing Industries.* U.S. Dept. Agr., Agr. Econ. Rept. 48, Washington, D.C.
2. *Bread Facts for Consumer Education* (1955). U.S. Dept. Agr., Agr. Inf. Bull. 142, Washington, D.C.
3. *Chemicals in Modern Food and Fiber Production* (1962). Natl. Acad. Sci.—Natl. Res. Council, Publ. 1033, Washington, D.C.
4. Darby, W. J., and G. Lam (1961). *Food and Science . . . Today and Tomorrow.* Public Affairs Pamphlet 320. The Public Affairs Committee, New York.
5. Day, P. L. (1960). The Food and Drug Administration faces new responsibilities. *Nutr. Rev.* **18:** 1.
6. Effects of Processing and Additives on Foods (1961). Panel V. Fifth Inter. Congr. on Nutr. *Federation Proc.* **20:** 207.
7. *Evaluation of the Toxicity of a Number of Antimicrobials and Antioxidants* (1962). Sixth Report of the Joint FAO-WHO Expert Committee on Food Additives. World Health Organ., WHO Tech. Rept. Series 228, Geneva.
8. *Food Additives. What They Are/How They Are Used* (1960). Manufacturing Chemists' Assoc., Washington, D.C.
9. General policy on addition of specific nutrients to foods. A Council on Foods and Nutrition statement (1961). *J. Am. Med. Assoc.* **178:** 1024.
10. Larrick, G. P. (1961). The nutritive adequacy of our food supply. *J. Am. Dietet. Assoc.* **39:** 117.
11. *Principles and Procedures for Evaluating the Safety of Intentional Chemical Additives in Foods* (1954). Natl. Acad. Sci.—Natl. Res. Council, Washington, D.C.
12. Safe use of chemicals in foods. A Council on Foods and Nutrition statement (1961). *J. Am. Med. Assoc.* **178:** 749.
13. *Science and Food: Today and Tomorrow* (1961). Natl. Acad. Sci.—Natl. Res. Council, Publ. 877, Washington, D.C.
14. Taylor, L. C., and M. C. Burk (1954). Review of cereal food enrichment in the United States 1950–1953. *Natl. Food Situation* **69:** 17, U.S. Dept. Agr., Washington, D.C.
15. *Use of Pesticides.* (1963). A Report of the Presidents Advisory Committee. U.S. Government Printing Office. Washington, D.C.
16. *What Consumers Should Know about Food Additives.* U.S. Dept. Health, Education, and Welfare. Food and Drug Administration, Washington, D.C.

STRONTIUM-90 IN THE DIET

1. Annual average radionuclide concentration in pasteurized milk, September 1962–August 1963. *Radiol. Health Data* **5:** 603.
2. Food and Drug Administration (1963). Radionuclides in diets for teenagers—May 1962–February 1963. *Radiol. Health Data* **5:** 285.

3. Harrison, G. E., W. H. A. Raymond, and H. C. Tretheway (1955). The metabolism of strontium in man. *Clin. Sci.* **14:** 681.
4. Michelson, I., J. C. Thompson, Jr., B. W. Hess, and C. L. Comar (1962). Radioactivity in total diet. *J. Nutr.* **78:** 371.
5. Olson, T. A., Jr. (1962). Strontium-90 in the 1959 United States wheat crop. *Science* **135:** 1064.
6. *Radionuclides in Foods* (1962). Food and Protection Committee, Natl. Acad. Sci.—Natl. Res. Council, Publ. 988, Washington, D.C.
7. Read, M. S. (1963). Countermeasures against radionuclides in foods. *Federation Proc.* **22:** 1418.
8. Spencer, H., D. Laszlo, and M. Brothers (1957). Strontium-85 and calcium-45 metabolism in man. *J. Clin. Invest.* **36:** 680.

FOOD AND NUTRITURE FOR MAN IN SPACE

1. Goldblith, S. A., S. A. Miller, E. Wick, P. M. Richardson, and H. Dymsza (1960). *High-Energy Metabolites.* WADD Tech. Rept. 60-575, Wright-Patterson AFB, Ohio.
2. Johnson, R. S. (1962). Bioengineering. In *Bioastronautics,* NASA SP-18, Washington, D.C.
3. Lachance, P. A. (1963). Palatable food can aid moon bound man. *Good Taste Magazine* **2:** 5.
4. Lachance, P. A., and J. E. Vanderveen (1963). Problems in space foods and nutrition— food for extended space travel and habitation. *Food Technol.* **17:** 59.
5. Leveille, G. A., H. E. Sauberlich, and M. E. McDowell (1962). Nutrient content of various algae and amino acid adequacy for growth of rats and chicks. In *Biologistics for Space System Symposium—May 1962.* AMRL-TDR-62-116, Wright-Patterson AFB, Ohio, p. 405.
6. Lubitz, J. A. (1962). Animal nutrition studies with *Chlorella* 71105. Part I. Protein quality, digestibility, and composition. In *Biologistics for Space System Symposium— May 1962.* AMRL-TDR-62-116, Wright-Patterson AFB, Ohio, p. 331.
7. McDowell, M. E., and G. A. Leveille (1963). Feeding experiments with algae. *Federation Proc.* **22:** 1431.
8. Miller, S. A., H. A. Dymsza, E. L. Wick, and S. A. Goldblith (1962). *Investigations of Compounds of High Caloric Density.* MRL-TDR-62-35, Wright-Patterson AFB, Ohio.
9. Nanz, R. A., E. L. Michel, and P. A. Lachance (1964). *The Evolution of a Space Feeding Concept for Project Gemini.* Institute of Food Technologists, 24th Annual Meeting, May 26, 1964, Washington, D.C.
10. Powell, R. C., E. M. Nevels, and M. E. McDowell (1961). Algae feeding in humans. *J. Nutr.* **75:** 7.
11. Taylor, A. A., B. Finkelstein, and R. E. Hayes (1960). *Food for Space Travel.* ARDC Tech. Rept. 60-8, Andrews AFB, Va.
12. The Boeing Company, Bioastronautics Section (1962). Investigations of selected higher plants as gas exchange mechanisms for closed ecological systems. In *Biologistics for Space Systems Symposium—May 1962.* AMRL-TDR-62-116, Wright-Patterson AFB, Ohio, p. 213.
13. The Boeing Company, Bioastronautics Section (1962). *Investigations of Selected Higher Plants as Gas Exchange Mechanisms for Closed Ecological Systems.* AMRL-TDR-62-127, Wright-Patterson, AFB, Ohio.
14. Vanderveen, J. E., E. G. Sander, C. M. Cox, and K. M. Offner (1962). Nutritional value of algae grown under sterile conditions. In *Biologistics for Space Systems Symposium— May 1962.* AMRL-TDR-62-116, Wright Patterson AFB, Ohio, p. 357.

15. Welbourn, J. L., and P. A. Lachance (1961). *Suitability of Tube Foods for In-Flight Feeding.* ASD Tech. Rept. 61-456, Wright-Patterson, AFB, Ohio.
16. Wilks, S. S. (1962). Preliminary report on the photosynthetic gas exchange potentialities of the family *Lemnaceae* (duckweed). In *Biologistics for Space Systems Symposium— May 1962.* AMRL-TDR-62-116, Wright Patterson AFB, Ohio, p. 265.

SUPPLEMENTARY REFERENCES

Bing, F. C. (1964). Chemical and other additives to foods. In *Modern Nutrition in Health and Disease,* 4th ed. (M. G. Wohl and R. S. Goodhart, Eds.), Lea and Febiger, Philadelphia.

Federal Food, Drug, and Cosmetic Act as amended and General Regulations for its Enforcement. (1963). U.S. Dept. Health, Education, and Welfare. Food and Drug Administration. Washington, D.C.

Report of the Second Joint FAO/WHO Conference on Food Additives. (1963). Food Agr. Organ. U.N., Rome.

Freeze-Drying of Foods (1962). Advisory Board on Quartermaster Research and Development, Natl. Acad. Sci.—Natl. Res. Council, Washington, D.C.

Nutrition Symposium—Fallout, Food, and Man (1963). *Federation Proc.* **22:** 1389.

Nutrition Symposium—Food and Nutritional Problems in Prolonged Space Travel (1963). *Federation Proc.* **22:** 1424.

Symposium on New Aspects of Nutrition Uncovered in Studies with Irradiated Foods (1960). *Federation Proc.* **19:** 1023.

Glossary

Acerola fruit is the tropical West Indian cherry, which is a rich food source of the vitamin, ascorbic acid.

Acid is a chemical compound that contains hydrogen and an electronegative element or radical, whose water solution turns litmus red and usually has a sour taste. It neutralizes a base or alkali to form a salt and water.

Acid-base balance is a hypothetical relationship of acid to alkali (base) in the body. Proteins and certain minerals aid in the maintenance of the acid-base balance. The reaction in the body is just on the alkaline side of neutrality.

Adrenal glands are a pair of endocrine glands, located near the kidneys, that secrete a variety of substances, one of which is epinephrine or adrenalin.

Alopecia is a condition of baldness.

Amino group is a characteristic group in amino acids and other compounds comprised of nitrogen and hydrogen (NH_2).

Androgens are male sex hormones.

Anorexia is the term used to describe the lack of appetite for food.

Antagonist is a chemical substance that counteracts the effects of another chemical substance.

Antibody is any substance in the blood serum or other fluids of the body that exerts a destructive action on bacteria.

Antivitamin is a chemical substance structurally similar to a vitamin which produces symptoms of vitamin deprivation on administration.

Aphagia is loss of the power of swallowing.

Ariboflavinosis is the term used to describe the condition resulting from a deficiency of the vitamin, riboflavin.

Arteriole is a minute vessel of the circulatory system carrying arterial blood.

Ascites is an accumulation of fluid in the abdominal cavity.

Atherosclerosis is a disease in which the walls of the arteries become narrowed as a result of the deposition of lipid-containing material.

Atrophy is the wasting away of a cell, tissue, organ, or part.

Avidin is the protein found in uncooked egg white that has an affinity to combine with the vitamin, biotin, resulting in a compound that no longer has vitamin activity.

Base is a chemical compound that contains a hydroxyl group (OH), an electropositive group, whose water solution turns litmus blue. Sometimes called an alkali or hydroxide, it neutralizes an acid to form a salt and water.

Bicarbonate group is a chemical group (HCO_3), which contains 1 carbon, 1 hydrogen, and 3 oxygen atoms. As a unit, the group carries a negative charge of electricity.

Blood is the fluid which circulates through the body bringing nourishment to and removing waste products from the cells.

Blood platelets or thrombocytes are components of the blood that aid in the coagulation of the blood.

Blood volume is the total amount of blood in the body.

Buffer is any substance which tends to prevent or lessen the change in acidic or basic concentration.

Calorie is the standard unit used to measure energy; it is defined as the quantity of heat required to raise the temperature of 1 kg of water 1 degree centigrade.

Calorimetry is the measurement of the amount of heat given off or absorbed.

Capillaries are very small blood vessels that extend into the tissue and cells; they begin at the end of the smallest arteries and end at the beginning of the smallest veins.

Carbonic anhydrase is an enzyme that contains the element zinc in its molecule; catalyzes the decomposition of carbonic acid into carbon dioxide and water and thus facilitates the exchange of carbon dioxide for oxygen in the lungs.

Carboxyl group is the acid group in organic acids (—COOH).

Catalyst, in the physiological sense, is a substance essential to a reaction but does not enter into the final products formed.

Cell is the smallest individual unit that makes up all living tissue.

Cellulose is the complex carbohydrate which makes up the skeletal parts of all plants.

Centimeter (cm) is a metric unit of length that is equivalent to ⅖ of an inch or 10 millimeters.

Cheilosis is the condition characterized by lesions of the lips and at the angles of the mouth, which is caused by a deficiency of the vitamin, riboflavin.

Coenzyme is a substance that combines with an inactive form of an enzyme to form a new compound that has enzyme activity.

Collagen is a comparatively insoluble protein present in connective tissue, bone and cartilage.

Compound is a substance which can be made from or changed into two or more elements.

Conjunctiva is the tissue that covers the eyeball and lines the eyelids.

Convulsion is a condition marked by involuntary contraction of the muscles.

Cornea is the transparent external covering of the front portion of the eyeball.

Costochondral relates to the cartilages at the end of the ribs.

Cretin is a person suffering with a chronic condition characterized by arrested physical and mental development caused by a lack of thyroid secretion prior to and after birth.

Cytoplasm is the semiliquid substance found inside the cell.

Delirium is a temporary mental state characterized by illusions and violent excitement.

Dermatitis is an inflammation of the skin.

Diathesis exudative, is a change in body tissues including thickening of the mucous membrane of the tongue, increased secretion of sebum on the scalp, severe itching, and edema.

Dicoumarol is the trade name for the compound dicoumarin, which delays coagulation of blood.

Disaccharide is a carbohydrate composed of two simple sugars.

Dystrophy is progressive weakening of a muscle.

Edema is the presence of an abnormally large amount of fluid in the tissue spaces of the body.

Electrocardiogram is a tracing made with an electrocardiograph, which records the electric current produced by the contraction of the heart muscle.

Element is a substance which cannot be subdivided by ordinary physical or chemical means.

Endemic is a term meaning prevalent in a particular region or locality.

Endocrine gland is the general name of a gland that produces a hormone or internal secretion.

Enzyme is a protein secreted by living cells inducing chemical changes in other substances without entering into a reaction itself.

Epithelial tissue is the protective covering on the outside of the body and forms the mucous membranes lining the cavities of the body.

Ergometer is an instrument for measuring the force of muscular contraction.

Erythrocyte is the mature red cell of the blood that contains hemoglobin, the carrier of oxygen to the tissues and cells.

Erythropoiesis is the process of production of red blood cells by the bone marrow.

Essential fatty acids are those fatty acids needed for good health that the body cannot synthesize and must be obtained in food.

Essential mineral is an inorganic substance which is needed by at least two species of animals for good health.

Estrogens are hormones secreted by the ovaries.

Etiology is the study or theory of the causation of any disease.

Exudation is the outpouring of an abnormal substance which becomes deposited in or on the tissues.

Fasting level is a quantitative physiological measurement taken after a number of hours without food, usually before breakfast.

Fat-soluble vitamins are those vitamins grouped together because of their solubility in fat solvents and include vitamins A, D, E, and K.

Fatty acid is a chained carbon compound containing a carboxyl (COOH) group that is found in every fat molecule.

Fetus is the developing young in the mammalian uterus.

Fibula is the outer and the smaller of the two bones of the legs.

Flavin is a yellow pigmented compound found in plant and animal materials.

Fluoridation is the term used to describe the addition of fluorides to drinking water (one part of fluoride per million parts of water) as a protective agent in tooth hygiene.

Fluorosis is the chronic poisoning caused by ingesting too much fluoride and is characterized by mottling of the enamel of the teeth.

Folinic acid is one of the active forms of the vitamin, folacin.

Food and Agriculture Organization of the United Nations (FAO) with head-quarter offices in Rome, Italy, is concerned with the problems of nutrition of the people, of the world. Through FAO the pooled efforts of nations are directed to the problems of increasing production and providing food for people who do not have enough. The world situation of food and agriculture is reviewed at regular intervals and reported to the member nations for their use.

Food and Nutrition Board, founded in 1940, is the advisory group in the area of food and nutrition in the National Research Council of the National Academy of Sciences.

Fortified food has had added to it nutrients such as vitamins or other dietary essentials in an amount sufficient to make the total content greater than the natural (unprocessed) food of its class, as in the addition of vitamin D to milk.

Gingivitis is an inflammation of the gums.

Globin is the protein in hemoglobin.

Globulin is a class of proteins.

Glossitis is an inflammation of the tongue.

Glucose tolerance test is used to indicate the efficiency of the body to use glucose by observing the changes in the concentration of glucose in the blood after a large amount of the sugar has been ingested.

Glycerol, also called glycerin, is the alcohol found in all fats.

Goitrogenic is a term meaning goiter-producing.

Gram (gm) is a metric unit of weight that is equivalent to about ⅛₈ of an ounce (1 oz = 28.4 gm), 1/1000 of a kilogram, or 1000 milligrams.

Ground-substance is the semifluid or gelatinous substance between cells.

Heme is the nonprotein, iron-containing portion of hemoglobin.

Hemeralopia is a condition of defective vision in a bright light.

Hemoglobin is the red coloring matter found in the red blood cells that transports the oxygen from the lungs to the tissues.

Hemolysis is the process whereby the red cell bursts, releasing the hemoglobin from it.

Hemopoiesis is the process whereby the constituents of the blood are formed.

Hemorrhage is a condition in which blood escapes from the vessels. The term is also used synonymously with bleeding.

Hemosiderin is an iron-containing pigment that is a storage form of iron.

Homeostasis is a term coined by physiologist Cannon to express the tendency of the body to maintain the normal state.

Hormone or endocrine is a chemical substance, produced by one of the ductless glands of the body, that passes directly into the blood stream or lymph and thence to the various cells and tissues where it acts.

Hydrolysis is a process whereby a complex substance takes up water and in the process is broken down into simpler units.

Hyperlipidemia is a condition of excess lipids in the blood.

Hyperphagia is the ingestion of a greater than optimal quantity of food.

Hypervitaminosis describes the condition or disorder caused by an intake of too much of a vitamin.

Hypochromic is a term meaning low pigment, a deficiency of hemoglobin in the red blood cells.

Hypoplastic means marked by defective or incomplete development.

Hypopotassemia is a disorder in which the level of the blood potassium is below normal.

Hypoproteinemia is an abnormally small amount of protein in the blood.

Inanition is the condition which results from a complete lack of food.

Inorganic acid is one that has no carbon atoms in its chemical structure; examples are hydrochloric, sulfuric, and phosphoric acids.

Inorganic compound is one that contains no carbon in its chemical structure; examples are water, table salt, and iron rust.

Insulin is the hormone secreted by certain cells of the pancreas and is involved in the metabolism of carbohydrate in the body.

Intravenous means within a vein.

Ion is an atom or group of atoms that carries a charge of positive or negative electricity.

Irradiation is exposure to rays, such as ultraviolet or x-ray.

Islets of Langerhans are a group of cells found in the pancreas that are responsible for the production of insulin.

Isocaloric means of equal energy value.

Keratin is an insoluble protein found in skin, hair, and finger nails.

Keratomalacia is a dryness with ulceration and perforation of the cornea.

Kilogram (kg) is a metric unit of weight that is equivalent to 2.2 pounds or 1000 grams.

Kwashiorkor is a dietary deficiency disease of infants and children due primarily to an inadequate intake of protein. *Kwashiorkor* is one of the original African tribal names, meaning *red boy,* which refers to the characteristic (but not always present) feature of skin and hair discoloration with the disease.

Labile implies something that easily decomposes or is not stable.

Laboratory determination involves a laboratory process which may be chemical, physical, microbiological, or observations of the behavior of experimental animals.

Lacrimation is the term used to describe the discharge of tears.

Lactalbumin is one of the proteins in milk.

Lesion is an injury or loss of function of a part of the body.

Leucocyte is the white cell of the blood which aids in the body's defense against invading bacteria.

Leukemia is a disease characterized by an overproduction of white cells and a decrease in the number of red cells of the blood. The cause of this disease is not known.

Lipid is an inclusive term for fat and fat-like substances.

Liter (1) is a metric unit of liquid measure that is equivalent to 1.056 quarts or 1000 milliliters.

Lymph is the liquid material of the lymphatic system which drains the tissue spaces of the body.

Macrocytic anemia is a type of anemia in which the red blood cells are unusually large.

Maize is corn.

Mandible is the bone forming the lower jaw.

Marine plankton is a collective name for the minute organisms which live in sea waters.

Median is the midpoint of a series of values with half above and half below.

Meter (m) is a metric unit of length that is equivalent to 39.371 inches or 100 centimeters.

Microcytic anemia is a type of anemia in which the red cells are abnormally small.

Microgram (µg) is a metric unit of weight that is equivalent to a millionth of a gram or 1/1000 milligram.

Milligram (mg) is a metric unit of weight that is equivalent to 1/1000 gram or 1000 micrograms.

Milliliter (ml) is a metric unit of liquid measure that is equivalent to 1/1000 liter.

Millimeter (mm) is a metric unit of length that is equivalent to 1/10 centimeter.

Mineral is an inorganic substance.

Miscarriage is expulsion of the fetus before it is capable of independent existence.

Monoiodotyrosine is an iodine-containing compound in the thyroid gland.

Monosaccharide is a carbohydrate composed of one simple sugar.

Mucous membrane is modified epithelial tissue lining the canals and cavities of the body, such as the gastrointestinal and respiratory tracts.

Muscles, striated are for the most part voluntary muscles, that is, under the control of the will. Striated refers to the striped appearance of the muscle.

National Academy of Sciences is a national scientific group, founded over a century ago, to serve science and the government in the United States.

National Research Council, founded in 1916 by the National Academy of Sciences, is an organization of leading scientists, in cooperation with major scientific and technical societies of this country, whose purpose is to coordinate their efforts to serve science and the government.

Necrosis is death of a circumscribed area of tissue.

Neuromuscular pertains to nerves and muscles.

Nitrogen is a chemical element with the symbol "N," found free in air and combined in protein and other compounds.

Norm is a standard which has been established.

Nucleoprotein is a conjugated protein which contains both nitrogen and phosphorus.

Nutrient is a substance that furnishes nourishment.

Nutriment is nutritious material.

Nutrition and Consumer-Use Research, U.S. Department of Agriculture, develops through research new knowledge about nutrition, consumer use of foods, fibers, and other products, and efficient household management. The research is carried on in three Divisions: Human Nutrition; Clothing and Housing; both headquartered at Beltsville, Md., and the Consumer and Food Economics Research Division headquartered at Hyattsville, Md.

Nyctalopia is night blindness; failure or imperfection of vision at night or in a dim light.

Occlusion refers to the contact of teeth of both jaws when closed.

Odontoblasts are the tooth cells that form the outer surface of the dental pulp adjacent to the dentin.

Oral pertains to the mouth; an oral feeding is given by mouth as opposed to some other method, as intravenous or intramuscular.

Organ is a part of the body composed of a group of tissues that perform several functions.

Organic acid is one that has carbon atoms in its chemical structure; examples are acetic, butyric, and linoleic acids.

Organic compound is one that contains carbon atoms in its chemical structure; examples are carbohydrates, fats, and proteins.

Osmotic pressure within the cell and of the tissue fluid surrounding it is a regulating factor of the normal water content of all living cells.

Osteoid tissue is bone tissue previous to calcification.

Osteomalacia is a softening of the bones, chiefly in adults, due to faulty calcium and phosphorus utilization.

Oxalic acid is an organic acid occurring in some foods which combines with calcium to form an insoluble salt.

Parakeratosis is an abnormality of the skin in which there is failure to form keratin.

Parathyroid glands are pairs of small endocrine glands located on the lateral lobes of the thyroid that are involved in the metabolism of calcium.

Parturition is the act or process of giving birth to a child.

Pentosuria is the occurrence of pentose (5 carbon atom) sugar in the urine.

Pernicious anemia is a type of anemia characterized by large immature red cells and caused by an inadequate supply of vitamin B_{12} to the body.

Phytic acid is a phosphorus-containing compound found chiefly in whole grain.

Pituitary gland often termed the "master gland of the endocrine system," is a small gland located at the base of the brain; among its functions, it controls the activity of the thyroid, adrenals, and parathyroid glands.

Placenta is a round, flat organ in the uterus that is the means of joining the mother and the fetus through the umbilical cord.

Plasma is the fluid portion of the circulating blood.

Polycythemia is a disorder where an above-normal number of red cells is present in the blood stream.

Polyneuritis is a condition which involves the inflammation of many nerves.

Polysaccharide is a carbohydrate composed of more than two simple sugars.

Precursor in nutrition means a substance that is converted into another, such as ergosterol, which can be changed to vitamin D.

Preformed vitamin is ready for use by the body, in contrast to a provitamin which must first be converted to the vitamin.

Prenatal is existing before birth.

Prophylactic is a tendency to ward off disease.

Proteolysis is the process of breaking proteins to simpler compounds, proteoses, peptones, and other products.

Prothrombin is a substance in blood necessary for blood clot formation.

Provitamin is a substance that can be converted into a vitamin; the carotenes are provitamins A, ergosterol is a provitamin D.

Purine is a chemical compound that is an end product of nucleoprotein metabolism.

Pyrimidines are organic compounds containing carbon, hydrogen, and nitrogen, some of which are constituents of nucleic acid.

Pyruvic acid is one of the acids formed during the metabolism of the energy nutrients.

Radioactive elements or isotopes are substance that give off particles of matter that can penetrate a solid material and can be measured by suitable instruments. These substances are elements whose atoms are similar to the "parent element" but differ in atomic weight; the atomic weight of hydrogen is 1 whereas that of its isotope, deuterium, is 2. Certain radioactive elements such as carbon, hydrogen, iron, and calcium, have been used to study biological reactions because these elements can be used to "tag" the compound under study.

Rancidity is a condition in fats that have undergone oxidative changes, a process of decomposition.

Red blood cells or erythrocytes are components of the blood that contain hemoglobin, the substance that carries oxygen to the cells.

Rennet is an extract of a calf's stomach containing rennin, which is used for curdling milk as in cheese making.

Retina is the sensitive membrane of the eye that receives the image formed by the lens, and is connected with the brain by the optic nerve.

Rhodopsin is a pigment in the retina of the eye which contains vitamin A; also known as visual purple.

Sarcoma is a malignant connective tissue growth.

Scintillation counter is an instrument that indicates the amount of radiation emitted by radioactive material.

Serum is the colorless fluid portion of blood that separates when blood clots.

Skeletal means pertaining to the bony framework of the body.

Standard deviation is a measure of the dispersion of individual numerical values around the mean value.

Sterols are a group of compounds complex in structure, soluble in fat solvents; important among the sterols are the provitamins D.

Still birth is the birth of a dead child.

Subcutaneous means beneath the skin.

Synthesis is the process whereby a chemical or biological substance is built up from its individual parts.

Synthetic means artificial, in contrast to natural.

Systemic denotes pertaining to or affecting the body as a whole.

Tetany is a condition characterized by muscle twitching, cramps and convulsions as a result of abnormal calcium metabolism.

Therapeutic is an adjective meaning curative, describing the art of healing in reference to disease.

Thrombocyte is the platelet constituent of the blood that aids in blood coagulation.

Thrombosis is the formation or presence of a clot (thrombus) in a blood vessel or in one of the cavities of the heart.

Thyroid gland is a large endocrine gland located in front of the trachea that stores iodine and manufactures thyroxine and thyroglobulin.

Tissue is a group of similar cells working together to perform a particular function.

Transplacental means carried through the placenta.

United States Pharmacopoeia (USP) is a publication containing a list of chemicals used in medicine, their properties, and dosage.

Uterus is the hollow muscular organ in which the fetus develops.

Visual purple is a pigment in the retina of the eye that contains vitamin A; also known as rhodopsin.

Water-soluble vitamins are a family of vitamins grouped together because of their solubility in water and include ascorbic acid, thiamine, riboflavin, niacin, vitamin B_6, pantothenic acid, biotin, folacin (folic acid), vitamin B_{12}, and choline.

White blood cells or leucocytes are components of the blood that serve as the body's defense against invading bacteria.

World Health Organization of the United Nations (WHO) with headquarters offices in Geneva, Switzerland, is concerned with the health problems of the world's population. The main nutritional target of the WHO is protein malnutrition. In the WHO's Region for the Americas, a vegetable protein mixture— "Incaparina"—has been developed by the Institute of Nutrition of Central America and Panama (INCAP) and is being distributed to children with low-protein diets.

Xerophthalmia is an abnormally dry and lusterless condition of the conjunctiva of the eye caused by a deficiency of vitamin A.

Appendix

Table A-1. Food and Nutrition Board, National Academy of Sciences—National Research Council

Recommended Daily Dietary Allowances,[1] Revised 1963

Designed for the maintenance of good nutrition of practically all healthy persons in the U.S.A.

(Allowances are intended for persons normally active in a temperate climate)

	Age[2] Years from to	Weight, kg (lb)	Height, cm (in.)	Calories[3]	Protein, gm	Calcium, gm	Iron, mg	Vitamin A Value, IU	Thiamine, mg	Riboflavin, mg	Niacin Equiv.[4] mg	Ascorbic Acid, mg	Vitamin D, IU
Men	18–35	70 (154)	175 (69)	2,900	70	0.8	10	5,000*	1.2	1.7	19	70	
	35–55	70 (154)	175 (69)	2,600	70	0.8	10	5,000	1.0	1.6	17	70	
	55–75	70 (154)	175 (69)	2,200	70	0.8	10	5,000	0.9	1.3	15	70	
Women	18–35	58 (128)	163 (64)	2,100	58	0.8	15	5,000	0.8	1.3	14	70	
	35–55	58 (128)	163 (64)	1,900	58	0.8	15	5,000	0.8	1.2	13	70	
	55–75	58 (128)	163 (64)	1,600	58	0.8	10	5,000	0.8	1.2	13	70	
	Pregnant (2nd and 3rd trimester)			+ 200	+20	+0.5	+ 5	+1,000	+0.2	+0.3	+3	+30	400
	Lactating			+1,000	+40	+0.5	+5	+3,000	+0.4	+0.6	+7	+30	400
Infants[5]	0– 1	8 (18)		kg x 115 ±15	kg x 2.5 ±0.5	0.7	kg x 1.0	1,500	0.4	0.6	6	30	400
Children	1– 3	13 (29)	87 (34)	1,300	32	0.8	8	2,000	0.5	0.8	9	40	400
	3– 6	18 (40)	107 (42)	1,600	40	0.8	10	2,500	0.6	1.0	11	50	400
	6– 9	24 (53)	124 (49)	2,100	52	0.8	12	3,500	0.8	1.3	14	60	400
Boys	9–12	33 (72)	140 (55)	2,400	60	1.1	15	4,500	1.0	1.4	16	70	400
	12–15	45 (98)	156 (61)	3,000	75	1.4	15	5,000	1.2	1.8	20	80	400
	15–18	61 (134)	172 (68)	3,400	85	1.4	15	5,000	1.4	2.0	22	80	400
Girls	9–12	33 (72)	140 (55)	2,200	55	1.1	15	4,500	0.9	1.3	15	80	400
	12–15	47 (103)	158 (62)	2,500	62	1.3	15	5,000	1.0	1.5	17	80	400
	15–18	53 (117)	163 (64)	2,300	58	1.3	15	5,000	0.9	1.3	15	70	400

[1] The allowance levels are intended to cover individual variations among most normal persons as they live in the United States under usual environmental stresses. The recommended allowances can be attained with a variety of common foods, providing other nutrients for which human requirements have been less well defined. See Publ. 1146 for more detailed discussion of allowances and of nutrients not tabulated.

[2] Entries on lines for age range 18–35 years represent the 25-year age. All other entries represent allowances for the midpoint of the specified age periods, i.e., line for children 1–3 is for age 2 years (24 months); 3–6 is for age 4½ years (54 months); etc.

[3] Tables 1 and 2 and figures 1 and 2 in Publ. 1146 show calorie adjustments for weight and age.

[4] Niacin equivalents include dietary sources of the preformed vitamin and the precursor, tryptophan. 60 mg tryptophan represents 1 mg niacin.

[5] The calorie and protein allowances per kg for infants are considered to decrease progressively from birth. Allowances for calcium, thiamine, riboflavin, and niacin increase proportionately with calories to the maximum values shown.

* 1000 IU from preformed Vitamin A and 4000 IU from beta-carotene.

520

Table A-2. Nutrient Intake Recommended for Adults of Different Body Size and Degree of Activity, Canada
(Weights illustrated are the 25th, 50th, and 75th percentiles of the 25–29 year age group in the Canadian population)

Weight, lb[1]	Activity[2]	Calories	Protein, gm[3]	Calcium, gm	Iron, mg	Vitamin A, IU[4]	Vitamin D, IU	Ascorbic Acid, mg	Thiamine, mg	Riboflavin, mg	Niacin, mg
Males:											
144	Maintenance	2150	46	0.5	6	3700	—	30	0.6	1.1	6
	A	2650	46	0.5	6	3700	—	30	0.8	1.3	8
	B	3400	46	0.5	6	3700	—	30	1.0	1.7	10
	C	4000	46	0.5	6	3700	—	30	1.2	2.0	12
	D	4600	46	0.5	6	3700	—	30	1.4	2.3	14
158	Maintenance	2300	50	0.5	6	3700	—	30	0.7	1.2	7
	A	2850	50	0.5	6	3700	—	30	0.9	1.4	9
	B	3650	50	0.5	6	3700	—	30	1.1	1.8	11
	C	4250	50	0.5	6	3700	—	30	1.3	2.1	13
	D	4900	50	0.5	6	3700	—	30	1.5	2.5	15
176	Maintenance	2500	55	0.5	6	3700	—	30	0.8	1.3	8
	A	3100	55	0.5	6	3700	—	30	0.9	1.5	9
	B	3950	55	0.5	6	3700	—	30	1.2	2.0	12
	C	4600	55	0.5	6	3700	—	30	1.4	2.3	14
	D	5350	55	0.5	6	3700	—	30	1.6	2.7	16

Table A-2. Nutrient Intake Recommended for Adults of Different Body Size and Degree of Activity, Canada

Weight, lb[1]	Activity[2]	Calories	Protein, gm[3]	Calcium, gm	Iron, mg	Vitamin A, IU[4]	Vitamin D, IU	Ascorbic Acid, mg	Thiamine, mg	Riboflavin, mg	Niacin, mg
Females:											
111	Maintenance	1750	35	0.5	10	3700	—	30	0.5	0.9	5
	A	2200	35	0.5	10	3700	—	30	0.7	1.1	7
	B	2800	35	0.5	10	3700	—	30	0.8	1.4	8
	C	3300	35	0.5	10	3700	—	30	1.0	1.7	10
	D	3800	35	0.5	10	3700	—	30	1.2	1.9	12
124	Maintenance	1900	39	0.5	10	3700	—	30	0.6	1.0	6
	A	2400	39	0.5	10	3700	—	30	0.7	1.2	7
	B	3000	39	0.5	10	3700	—	30	0.9	1.5	9
	C	3550	39	0.5	10	3700	—	30	1.1	1.8	11
	D	4100	39	0.5	10	3700	—	30	1.2	2.0	12
136	Maintenance	2050	43	0.5	10	3700	—	30	0.6	1.0	6
	A	2550	43	0.5	10	3700	—	30	0.8	1.3	8
	B	3250	43	0.5	10	3700	—	30	1.0	1.6	10
	C	3800	43	0.5	10	3700	—	30	1.1	1.9	11
	D	4400	43	0.5	10	3700	—	30	1.3	2.2	13
Pregnancy—during											
3rd trimester add		up to 500	10	0.7	3	500	400	10	0.15	0.25	1.5
Lactation—add		500 to 1000	10 to 20	0.7	3	1500	400	20	0.3	0.5	3

[1] Weights include indoor clothing without shoes.
[2] See "Description of Categories of Energy Expenditure," Table A-2'.
[3] Protein recommendation is based on normal mixed Canadian diet. Vegetarian diets may require a higher protein content.

From Dietary Standard for Canada. *Can. Bull. Nutr.* vol. 6, No. 1, 1964.

[4] Vitamin A is based on mixed Canadian diet supplying both vitamin A and carotene. As preformed vitamin A the suggested intake would be about two-thirds of that indicated.

Table A-2′. Description of Categories of Energy Expenditure, Canada

Category	Home or Household	Office	Industry	Recreation
Maintenance	Ablutions, dressing, brushing hair, etc; washing dishes, knitting, mending	Work at desk requiring little movement	Supervising, monitoring	Spectator at games, theatre, etc; playing cards, chess, billiards, etc; reading, driving car
A	Most household chores, repairing appliances, mowing the lawn, wiping windows, laundering, cooking, normal housecleaning	Office work involving typing, filing, computing, drafting, working on ledgers, walking from desk to desk, etc; salesclerk, barbering, hairdressing, nursing, laboratory work	Shop and mill work, operating lathe, assembly line work, driving truck, tractor or bull-dozer, operating dragline, most mechanical trades and crafts, cooking for restaurant, hotel, or short order; sewing	Golf, walking, bowling, fishing, hunting, most hobbies and crafts, (e.g., woodworking, metal work, leather work, photography, painting), ballroom dancing, Ping-Pong
B	Digging or spading in garden, rolling lawn, moving furniture within house, scrubbing floors and walls, polishing floors by hand	Moving files, furniture, heavy packages, etc; stooping and lifting	Masonry, carpentry, loading and unloading trucks, power-equipped mining, commercial cooking and baking, military marching and drilling, commercial laundering, maid service such as making beds and cleaning rooms	Sports such as hockey, football, basketball, field hockey, field and track, fast Ping-Pong or tennis, dancing with much action or movement, gymnastics, swimming or skiing for pleasure
C	Farm chores, spading heavy clay, moving clay or stones in wheelbarrow		Felling trees in lumbering, mining without power equipment, harvesting and haying by manual methods, manual handling of wheelbarrow in construction work, military marching with full pack	Training for professional athletics or Olympic sports, vigorous activity in football, basketball, etc; difficult mountain climbing
D			Hand felling trees, shoveling gravel, coal, etc.	Training for weight lifting, marathon sports such as cross-country running or skiing, long bicycle races, rowing races, marathon swimming races

From Dietary Standard for Canada. *Can. Bull. on Nutr.*, vol. 6, No. 1, 1964.

523

Table A-3. Recommended Daily Nutrient Intakes for Boys and Girls, Canada

Sex	Age, Years	Weight, lb	Activity Category	Calories	Protein, gm[1]	Calcium, gm	Iron, mg	Vitamin A, IU[2]	Vitamin D, IU	Ascorbic Acid, mg	Thiamine, mg	Riboflavin, mg	Niacin, mg
Both	0-1	7-20	Usual	360-900	12-24	0.5	5	1000	400	20	0.3	0.5	3
Both	1-2	20-26	Usual	900-1200	25-30	0.7	5	1000	400	20	0.4	0.6	4
Both	2-3	31	Usual	1400	30	0.7	5	1000	400	20	0.4	0.7	4
Both	4-6	40	Usual	1700	30	0.7	5	1000	400	20	0.5	0.9	5
Both	7-9	57	Usual	2100	40	1.0	5	1500	400	30	0.7	1.1	7
Both	10-12	77	Usual	2500	50	1.2	12	2000	400	30	0.8	1.3	8
Boy	13-15	108	Usual	3100	75	1.2	12	2700	400	30	0.9	1.6	9
Girl	13-15	108	Usual	2600	75	1.2	12	2700	400	30	0.8	1.3	8
Boy	16-17	136	B[3]	3700	55	1.2	12	3200	400	30	1.1	1.9	11
Girl	16-17	120	A[4]	2400	50	1.2	12	3200	400	30	0.7	1.2	7
Boy	18-19	144	B[3]	3800	60	0.9	6	3200	400	30	1.1	1.9	11
Girl	18-19	124	A[4]	2450	50	0.9	10	3200	400	30	0.7	1.2	7

[1] Protein recommendation is based on normal mixed Canadian diet. Vegetarian diets may require a higher protein content.
[2] Vitamin A is based on the mixed Canadian diet supplying both vitamin A and carotene. As preformed vitamin A the suggested intake would be about two-thirds of that indicated.

[3] Expenditure assessed as being 113% of that of a man of same weight and engaged in same degree of activity.
[4] Expenditure assessed as being 104% of that of a woman of the same weight and engaged in the same degree of activity.

From Dietary Standard for Canada. *Can. Bull. on Nutr.* vol. 6, No. 1, 1964.

Table A-4. Daily Nutrient Allowances for Selected Groups, United Kingdom

	Adolescent Male, 15–19 yr	Men on Light Work	Men on Heavy Work	Adolescent Female, 15–19 yr	Women on Light Work
Energy (Cal.)	3500	2750	3500	2500	2250
Protein (gm)	130	80	102	93	66
Iron (mg)	15.0	12.0	12.0	15.0	12.0
Calcium (gm)	1.4	0.8	0.8	1.1	0.8
Vitamin A (IU)	5000	5000	5000	5000	5000
Vitamin D (IU)	400	—	—	400	—
Thiamine (mg)	1.4	1.1	1.4	1.0	0.9
Niacin (mg)	14	11	14	10	9
Riboflavin (mg)	2.1	1.6	2.1	1.5	1.4
Ascorbic acid (mg)	30	20	20	30	20
Iodine (μg)	150	100	100	150	100

From *Report of the Committee on Nutrition* (1950). British Medical Association, London.

Table A-5. Desirable Weights for Men of Ages 25 and Over

Height (with shoes, 1-in. heels)		Weight in Pounds According to Frame (as ordinarily dressed)		
Feet	Inches	Small Frame	Medium Frame	Large Frame
5	2	112–120	118–129	126–141
5	3	115–123	121–133	129–144
5	4	118–126	124–136	132–148
5	5	121–129	127–139	135–152
5	6	124–133	130–143	138–156
5	7	128–137	134–147	142–161
5	8	132–141	138–152	147–166
5	9	136–145	142–156	151–170
5	10	140–150	146–160	155–174
5	11	144–154	150–165	159–179
6	0	148–158	154–170	164–184
6	1	152–162	158–175	168–189
6	2	156–167	162–180	173–194
6	3	160–171	167–185	178–199
6	4	164–175	172–190	182–204

From Metropolitan Life Insurance Company. Derived previously from data of the Build and Blood Pressure Study, 1959, Society of Actuaries.

Table A-6. Desirable Weights for Women of Ages 25 and Over

Height (with shoes, 2-in. heels)		Weights in Pounds According to Frame (as ordinarily dressed)		
Feet	Inches	Small Frame	Medium Frame	Large Frame
4	10	92–98	96–107	104–119
4	11	94–101	98–110	106–122
5	0	96–104	101–113	109–125
5	1	99–107	104–116	112–128
5	2	102–110	107–119	115–131
5	3	105–113	110–122	118–134
5	4	108–116	113–126	121–138
5	5	111–119	116–130	125–142
5	6	114–123	120–135	129–146
5	7	118–127	124–139	133–150
5	8	122–131	128–143	137–154
5	9	126–135	132–147	141–158
5	10	130–140	136–151	145–163
5	11	134–144	140–155	149–168
6	0	138–148	144–159	153–173

From Metropolitan Life Insurance Company. Derived previously from data of the Build and Blood Pressure Study, 1959, Society of Actuaries.

Table A-7. Food Composition Table for Short Method of Dietary Analysis (3rd revisi

Food and Approximate Measure	Weight, gm	Food Energy, Cal.	Protein, gm
Milk, cheese, cream; related products			
Cheese: blue, cheddar (1 cu in., 17 gm),			
cheddar process (1 oz), Swiss (1 oz)	30	105	6
cottage (from skim) creamed (½ c)	115	120	16
Cream: half-and-half (cream and milk) (2 tbsp)			
For light whipping add 1 pat butter	30	40	1
Milk: whole (3.5% fat) (1 c)	245	160	9
fluid, nonfat (skim) and buttermilk (from skim)	245	90	9
milk beverages, (1 c) cocoa, chocolate drink made with skim milk. For malted milk add 4 tbsp half-and-half (270 gm)	245	210	8
milk desserts, custard (1 c) 248 gm, ice cream (8 fl oz) 142 gm		290	8
cornstarch pudding (248 gm), ice milk (1 c) 187 gm		280	9
White sauce, med (½ c)	130	215	5
Egg: 1 large	50	80	6
Meat, poultry, fish, shellfish, related products			
Beef, lamb, veal: lean and fat, cooked, inc. corned beef (3 oz) (all cuts)	85	245	22
lean only, cooked; dried beef (2 + oz) (all cuts)	65	140	20
Beef, relatively fat, such as steak and rib, cooked (3 oz)	85	350	18
Liver: beef, fried (2 oz)	55	130	15
Pork, lean & fat, cooked (3 oz) (all cuts)	85	325	20
lean only, cooked (2 + oz) (all cuts)	60	150	18
ham, light cure, lean & fat, roasted (3 oz)	85	245	18
Luncheon meats: bologna (2 sl), pork sausage, cooked (2 oz), frankfurter (1), bacon, broiled or fried crisp (3 sl)		185	9
Poultry			
chicken: flesh only, broiled (3 oz)	85	115	20
fried (2 + oz)	75	170	24
turkey, light & dark, roasted (3 oz)	85	160	27
Fish and shellfish			
salmon (3 oz) (canned)	85	130	17
fish sticks, breaded, cooked (3–4)	75	130	13
mackerel, halibut, cooked	85	175	19
blue fish, haddock, herring, perch, shad, cooked (tuna canned in oil, 20 gm)	85	160	19
clams, canned; crab meat, canned; lobster; oyster, raw; scallop; shrimp, canned	85	75	14
Mature dry beans and peas, nuts, peanuts, related products			
Beans: white with pork & tomato, canned (1 c)	260	320	16
red (128 gm), Lima (96 gm), cowpeas (125 gm), cooked (½ c)		125	8

Fat, gm	Carbo-hy-drate, gm	Cal-cium, mg	Iron, mg	Vita-min A Value, IU	Thia-mine, mg	Ribo-flavin, mg	Niacin, mg	Ascor-bic Acid, mg
9	1	165	0.2	345	0.01	0.12	trace	0
5	3	105	0.4	190	0.04	0.28	0.1	0
4	2	30	trace	145	0.01	0.04	trace	trace
9	12	285	0.1	350	0.08	0.42	0.1	2
trace	13	300	trace	—	0.10	0.44	0.2	2
8	26	280	0.6	300	0.09	0.43	0.3	trace
17	29	210	0.4	785	0.07	0.34	0.1	1
10	40	290	0.1	390	0.08	0.41	0.3	2
16	12	150	0.2	610	0.06	0.22	0.3	trace
6	trace	25	1.2	590	0.06	0.15	trace	0
16	0	10	2.9	25	0.06	0.19	4.2	0
5	0	10	2.4	10	0.05	0.16	3.4	0
30	0	10	2.4	60	0.05	0.14	3.5	0
6	3	5	5.0	30,280	0.15	2.37	9.4	15
24	0	10	2.6	0	0.62	0.20	4.2	0
8	0	5	2.2	0	0.57	0.19	3.2	0
19	0	10	2.2	0	0.40	0.16	3.1	0
16	—	5	1.3	—	0.21	0.12	1.7	0
3	0	10	1.4	80	0.05	0.16	7.4	0
6	1	10	1.6	85	0.05	0.23	8.3	0
5	0	—	1.5	—	0.03	0.15	6.5	0
5	0	165	0.7	60	0.03	0.16	6.8	0
7	5	10	0.3	—	0.03	0.05	1.2	0
10	0	10	0.8	515	0.08	0.15	6.8	0
8	2	20	1.0	60	0.06	0.11	4.4	0
1	2	65	2.5	65	0.10	0.08	1.5	0
7	50	140	4.7	340	0.20	0.08	1.5	5
—	25	35	2.5	5	0.13	0.06	0.7	—

Food and Approximate Measure	Weight, gm	Food Energy, Cal.	Pro- tein, gm
Nuts: almonds (12), cashews (8), peanuts (1 tbsp), pea- nut butter (1 tbsp), pecans (12), English walnuts (2 tbsp), coconut (¼ c)	15	95	3
Vegetables and vegetable products			
Asparagus, cooked, cut spears (⅔ c)	115	25	3
Beans: green (½ c) cooked 60 gm; canned 120 gm		15	1
Lima, immature, cooked (½ c)	80	90	6
Broccoli spears, cooked (⅔ c)	100	25	3
Brussels sprouts, cooked (⅔ c)	85	30	3
Cabbage (110 gm); cauliflower, cooked (80 gm); and sauerkraut, canned (150 gm) (reduce ascorbic acid value by one-third for kraut) (⅔ c)		20	1
Carrots, cooked (⅔ c)	95	30	1
Corn, 1 ear, cooked (140 gm); canned (130 gm) (½ c)		75	2
Leafy greens: collards (125 gm), dandelions (120 gm), kale (75 gm), mustard (95 gm), spinach (120 gm), turnip (100 gm cooked, 150 gm canned) (⅔ c cooked and canned) (reduce ascorbic acid one-half for canned)		30	3
Peas, green (½ c)	80	60	4
Potatoes-baked, boiled (100 gm), 10 pc French fried (55 gm) (for fried, add 1 tbsp cooking oil)		85	3
Pumpkin, canned (½ c)	115	40	1
Squash, winter, canned (½ c)	100	65	2
Sweetpotato, canned (½ c)	110	120	2
Tomato, 1 raw, ⅔ c canned, ⅔ c juice	150	35	2
Tomato catsup (2 tbsp)	35	30	1
Other, cooked (beets, mushrooms, onions, turnips) (½ c)	95	25	1
Others commonly served raw, cabbage (½ c, 50 gm), celery (3 sm stalks, 40 gm), cucumber (¼ med, 50 gm), green pepper (½, 30 gm), radishes (5, 40 gm)		10	trace
carrots, raw (½ carrot)	25	10	trace
lettuce leaves (2 lg)	50	10	1
Fruits and fruit products			
Cantaloup (½ med)	385	60	1
Citrus and strawberries: orange (1), grapefruit (½), juice (½ c), strawberries (½ c), lemon (1), tangerine (1)		50	1
Yellow, fresh: apricots (3), peach (2 med); canned fruit and juice (½ c) or dried, cooked, unsweetened: apri- cot, peaches (½ c)		85	—
Other, dried: dates, pitted (4), figs (2), raisins (¼ c)	40	120	1
Other, fresh: apple (1), banana (1), figs (3), pear (1)		80	—
Fruit pie: to 1 serving fruit add 1 tbsp flour, 2 tbsp sugar, 1 tbsp fat			

Fat, gm	Carbo-hy-drate, gm	Cal-cium, mg	Iron, mg	Vita-min A Value, IU	Thia-mine, mg	Ribo-flavin, mg	Niacin, mg	Ascor-bic Acid, mg
8	4	15	0.5	5	0.05	0.04	0.9	—
trace	4	25	0.7	1,055	0.19	0.20	1.6	30
trace	3	30	0.4	340	0.04	0.06	0.3	8
1	16	40	2.0	225	0.14	0.08	1.0	14
trace	4	90	0.8	2,500	0.09	0.20	0.8	90
trace	5	30	1.0	450	0.07	0.12	0.7	75
trace	4	35	0.5	80	0.05	0.05	0.3	37
trace	7	30	0.6	10,145	0.05	0.05	0.5	6
trace	18	5	0.4	315	0.06	0.06	1.1	6
trace	5	175	1.8	8,570	0.11	0.18	0.8	45
1	10	20	1.4	430	0.22	0.09	1.8	16
trace	30	10	0.7	trace	0.08	0.04	1.5	16
1	9	30	0.5	7,295	0.03	0.06	0.6	6
1	16	30	0.8	4,305	0.05	0.14	0.7	14
—	27	25	0.8	8,500	0.05	0.05	0.7	15
trace	7	14	0.8	1,350	0.10	0.06	1.0	29
trace	8	10	0.2	480	0.04	0.02	0.6	6
—	5	20	0.5	15	0.02	0.10	0.7	7
trace	2	15	0.3	100	0.03	0.03	0.2	20
trace	2	10	0.2	2,750	0.02	0.02	0.2	2
trace	2	34	0.7	950	0.03	0.04	0.2	9
trace	14	25	0.8	6,540	0.08	0.06	1.2	63
—	13	25	0.4	165	0.08	0.03	0.3	55
—	22	10	1.1	1,005	0.01	0.05	1.0	5
—	31	35	1.4	20	0.04	0.04	0.5	—
—	21	15	0.5	140	0.04	0.03	0.2	6

531

Food and Approximate Measure	Weight, gm	Food Energy, Cal.	Pro- tein, gm
Grain products			
Enriched and whole grain: bread (1 sl, 23 gm), biscuit (½), cooked cereals (½ c), prepared cereals (1 oz), Graham crackers (2 lg), macaroni, noodles, spaghetti (½ c, cooked), pancake (1, 27 gm), roll (½), waffle (½, 38 gm)		65	2
Unenriched: bread (1 sl, 23 gm), cooked cereal (½ c), macaroni, noodles, spaghetti (½ c), popcorn (½ c), pretzel sticks, small (15), roll (½)		65	2
Desserts			
Cake, plain (1 pc), doughnut (1). For iced cake or doughnut add value for sugar (1 tbsp). For choco- late cake add chocolate (30 gm)	45	145	2
Cookies, plain (1)	25	120	1
Pie crust, single crust (½ shell)	20	95	1
Flour, white, enriched (1 tbsp)	7	25	1
Fats and Oils			
Butter, margarine (1 pat, ½ tbsp)	7	50	trace
Fats and oils, cooking (1 tbsp), French dressing (2 tbsp)	14	125	0
Salad dressing, mayonnaise type (1 tbsp)	15	80	trace
Sugars, sweets			
Candy, plain (½ oz), jam and jelly (1 tbsp), sirup (1 tbsp), gelatin dessert, plain (½ c), beverages, carbonated (1 c)		60	0
Chocolate fudge (1 oz), chocolate sirup (3 tbsp)		125	1
Molasses (1 tbsp), caramel (⅓ oz)		40	trace
Sugar (1 tbsp)	12	45	0
Miscellaneous			
Chocolate, bitter (1 oz)	30	145	3
Sherbet (½ c)	96	130	1
Soups: bean, pea (green) (1 c)		150	7
noodle, beef, chicken (1 c)		65	4
clam chowder, minestrone, tomato, vegetable (1 c)		90	3

The use of the short method of dietary analysis reduces the time required to com- pute the nutritive value of a diet. In the evaluation of a mixed dietary using this method the accuracy approximates that of computations using the conventional food table.

Fat, gm	Carbo-hy-drate, gm	Cal-cium, mg	Iron, mg	Vita-min A Value, IU	Thia-mine, mg	Ribo-flavin, mg	Niacin, mg	Ascor-bic Acid, mg
1	16	20	0.6	10	0.09	0.05	0.7	—
1	16	10	0.3	5	0.02	0.02	0.3	—
5	24	30	0.4	65	0.02	0.05	0.2	—
5	18	10	0.2	20	0.01	0.01	0.1	—
6	8	3	0.3	0	0.04	0.03	0.3	—
trace	5	1	0.2	0	0.03	0.02	0.2	0
6	trace	1	0	230	—	—	—	—
14	0	0	0	0	0	0	0	0
9	1	2	0.1	45	trace	trace	trace	0
0	14	3	0.1	trace	trace	trace	trace	trace
2	30	15	0.6	10	trace	0.02	0.1	trace
trace	8	20	0.3	trace	trace	trace	trace	trace
0	12	0	trace	0	0	0	0	0
15	8	20	1.9	20	0.01	0.07	0.4	0
1	30	15	trace	55	0.01	0.03	trace	2
4	22	50	1.6	495	0.09	0.06	1.0	4
2	7	10	0.7	50	0.03	0.04	0.9	trace
2	14	25	0.9	1,880	0.05	0.04	1.1	3

The values in Table A-7 were computed chiefly from the figures compiled by Watt and Merrill in Agriculture Handbook 8, *Composition of Foods—Raw, Processed, Prepared*, revised 1963.
Courtesy of Leichsenring and Wilson, *J. Am. Dietet. Assoc.* Nov., 1965.

The source of the data in Table A-8 is *Nutritive Value of Foods,* Home and Garden Bulletin 72, revised, U.S. Department of Agriculture, Washington, D.C. Data for some cooked and prepared foods are taken from Church and Church, *Food Values of Portions Commonly Used—Bowes and Church,* 9th ed., J. B. Lippincott Co., Philadelphia.

The abbreviation for trace (tr) is used to indicate fatty acid and vitamin values that would round to zero with the number of decimal places carried in these tables. For other components that would round to zero, a zero is used.

Dashes show that no basis could be found for imputing a value although there was some reason to believe that a measurable amount of the constituent might be present.

Other abbreviations used in Table A-8 are:

av —average	oz —ounce
c —cup	% —per cent
diam —diameter	pc —piece
hp —heaping	qt —quart
jc —juice	sc —section
lb —pound	serv —serving
lg —large	sl —slice
lv —leaves	sm —small
med —medium	sq —square
	tbsp —tablespoon

Table A-8. Nutritive Value of Foods in Common Household Units

Food	Weight, gm	Approximate Measure	Food Energy, Cal.	Pro- tein, gm	Fat (total lipid), gm
Almonds, shelled	142	1 c	850	26	77
Apple, raw	150	1 med	70	tr	tr
Apple brown betty	230	1 c	345	4	8
Apple butter	20	1 tbsp	37	tr	tr
Apple juice, bottled or canned	249	1 c	120	tr	tr
Applesauce, sweetened	254	1 c	230	1	tr
Apricots:					
raw	114	3 apricots	55	1	tr
sirup pack	259	1 c	220	2	tr
dried, uncooked	150	1 c	390	8	1
dried, cooked	285	1 c	240	5	1
Asparagus:					
fresh, cooked	175	1 c	35	4	tr
canned, green	96	6 spears	20	2	tr
Bacon:					
broiled or fried	16	2 sl	100	5	8
Canadian, cooked	21	1 sl	65	6	4
Banana, raw	150	1 med	85	1	tr
Beans:					
baked, with tomato sauce, with pork	261	1 c	320	16	7
baked, with tomato sauce, without pork	261	1 c	310	16	1
green snap, fresh cooked	125	1 c	30	2	tr
green snap, canned	239	1 c	45	2	tr
Lima, fresh, cooked	160	1 c	180	12	1
red kidney, canned	256	1 c	230	15	1
wax, canned	125	1 c	27	2	tr
Beef, cooked:					
cuts, braised, simmered, pot-roasted	72	2.5 oz, lean	140	22	5
cuts, braised, simmered, pot-roasted	85	3 oz, lean and fat	245	23	16
hamburger, ground lean	85	3 oz	185	23	10
hamburger, regular	85	3 oz	245	21	17
rib roast	51	1.8 oz, lean	125	14	7
rib roast	85	3 oz, lean and fat	375	17	34
round	78	2.7 oz, lean	125	24	3
round	85	3 oz, lean and fat	165	25	7
steak, sirloin	56	2 oz, lean	115	18	4
steak, sirloin	85	3 oz, lean and fat	330	20	27
Beef, canned:					
corned beef	85	3 oz	185	22	10
corned beef hash	85	3 oz	155	7	10

Fatty Acids										
Satur-ated (total), gm	Unsaturated		Carbo-hydrate, gm	Cal-cium, mg	Iron, mg	Vitamin A Value, IU	Thia-mine, mg	Ribo-flavin, mg	Niacin, mg	Ascorbic Acid, mg
	Oleic, gm	Lino-leic, gm								
6	52	15	28	332	6.7	0	0.34	1.31	5.0	tr
—	—	—	18	8	0.4	50	0.04	0.02	0.1	3
4	3	tr	68	41	1.4	230	0.13	0.10	0.9	3
—	—	—	9	3	0.1	0	tr	tr	tr	tr
—	—	—	30	15	1.5	—	0.01	0.04	0.2	2
—	—	—	60	10	1.3	100	0.05	0.03	0.1	3
—	—	—	14	18	0.5	2890	0.03	0.04	0.7	10
—	—	—	57	28	0.8	4510	0.05	0.06	0.9	10
—	—	—	100	100	8.2	16350	0.02	0.23	4.9	19
—	—	—	62	63	5.1	8550	0.01	0.13	2.8	8
—	—	—	6	37	1.0	1580	0.27	0.32	2.4	46
—	—	—	3	18	1.8	770	0.06	0.10	0.8	14
3	4	1	1	2	0.5	0	0.08	0.05	0.8	—
—	—	—	3	4	—	0	0.18	0.03	1.1	0
—	—	—	23	8	0.7	190	0.05	0.06	0.7	10
3	3	1	50	141	4.7	340	0.20	0.08	1.5	5
—	—	—	60	177	5.2	160	0.18	0.09	1.5	5
—	—	—	7	62	0.8	680	0.08	0.11	0.6	16
—	—	—	10	81	2.9	690	0.08	0.10	0.7	9
—	—	—	32	75	4.0	450	0.29	0.16	2.0	28
—	—	—	42	74	4.6	tr	0.13	0.10	1.5	—
—	—	—	6	45	2.1	150	0.05	0.06	0.5	6
2	2	tr	0	10	2.7	10	0.04	0.16	3.3	—
8	7	tr	0	10	2.9	30	0.04	0.18	3.5	—
5	4	tr	0	10	3.0	20	0.08	0.20	5.1	—
8	8	tr	0	9	2.7	30	0.07	0.18	4.6	—
3	3	tr	0	6	1.8	10	0.04	0.11	2.6	—
16	15	1	0	8	2.2	70	0.05	0.13	3.1	—
1	1	tr	0	10	3.0	tr	0.06	0.18	4.3	—
3	3	tr	0	11	3.2	10	0.06	0.19	4.5	—
2	2	tr	0	7	2.2	10	0.05	0.14	3.6	—
13	12	1	0	9	2.5	50	0.05	0.16	4.0	—
5	4	tr	0	17	3.7	20	0.01	0.20	2.9	—
5	4	tr	9	11	1.7	—	0.01	0.08	1.8	—

Food	Weight, gm	Approximate Measure	Food Energy, Cal.	Pro- tein, gm	Fat (total lipid), gm
Beef, dried or chipped	57	2 oz	115	19	4
Beef and vegetable stew	235	1 c	210	15	10
Beef potpie	227	1 pie, 4¼" diam	560	23	33
Beer, av 3.6% alcohol	240	1 c	100	1	0
Beets, cooked, diced	165	1 c	50	2	tr
Beet greens, cooked	100	½ c	27	2	tr
Beverages, carbonated:					
cola type	240	1 c	95	0	0
gingerale	230	1 c	70	0	0
Biscuit, enriched flour	38	1, 2½" diam	140	3	6
Blackberries, raw	144	1 c	85	2	1
Blueberries, raw	140	1 c	85	1	1
Bluefish, baked or broiled	85	3 oz	135	22	4
Bouillon cubes	4	1 cube	5	1	tr
Brains, all kinds, raw	85	3 oz	106	9	7
Bran, raisin	28	⅔ c	99	2	tr
Bran flakes, 40%	28	1 oz	85	3	1
Brazilnuts, shelled	140	1 c	915	20	94
Bread:					
Boston, enriched	48	1 sl	100	3	1
cracked-wheat	23	1 sl	60	2	1
French or Vienna, enriched	454	1 lb	1315	41	14
Italian, enriched	454	1 lb	1250	41	4
raisin, enriched	23	1 sl	60	2	1
rye, American	23	1 sl	55	2	tr
rye, pumpernickle	454	1 lb	1115	41	5
white, enriched	23	1 sl	60	2	1
white, unenriched	23	1 sl	60	2	1
whole wheat	23	1 sl	55	2	1
Breadcrumbs, dry	88	1 c	345	11	4
Broccoli, cooked	150	1 c	40	5	tr
Brussels sprouts, cooked	130	1 c	45	5	1
Buckwheat flour, light	98	1 c	342	6	1
Butter:					
stick, ⅛	14	1 tbsp	100	tr	11
pat or square	7	1 pat	50	tr	6
Buttermilk, cultured, skim	246	1 c	90	9	tr
Cabbage:					
raw	100	1 c	25	1	tr
cooked	170	1 c	35	2	tr
Chinese, raw	100	1 c	15	1	tr

[1] Calcium may not be usable because of presence of oxalic acid.
[2] Year-round average.

Saturated (total), gm	Unsaturated		Carbohydrate, gm	Calcium, mg	Iron, mg	Vitamin A Value, IU	Thiamine, mg	Riboflavin, mg	Niacin, mg	Ascorbic Acid, mg
	Oleic, gm	Linoleic, gm								
2	2	tr	0	11	2.9	—	0.04	0.18	2.2	—
5	4	tr	15	28	2.8	2310	0.13	0.17	4.4	15
9	20	2	43	32	4.1	1860	0.25	0.27	4.5	7
—	—	—	9	12	tr	—	0.01	0.07	1.6	—
—	—	—	12	23	0.8	40	0.04	0.07	0.5	11
—	—	—	6	118[1]	3.2	6700	0.08	0.18	0.4	34
—	—	—	24	—	—	0	0	0	0	0
—	—	—	18	—	—	0	0	0	0	0
2	3	1	17	46	0.6	tr	0.08	0.08	0.7	tr
—	—	—	19	46	1.3	290	0.05	0.06	0.5	30
—	—	—	21	21	1.4	140	0.04	0.08	0.6	20
—	—	—	0	25	0.6	40	0.09	0.08	1.6	—
—	—	—	tr	—	—	—	—	—	—	—
—	—	—	1	14	3.1	0	0.20	0.22	3.7	15
—	—	—	22	0	1.0	0	0.10	—	1.1	0
—	—	—	23	20	1.2	0	0.11	0.05	1.7	0
19	45	24	15	260	4.8	tr	1.34	0.17	2.2	—
—	—	—	22	43	0.9	0	0.05	0.03	0.6	0
—	—	—	12	20	0.3	tr	0.03	0.02	0.3	tr
3	8	2	251	195	10.0	tr	1.26	0.98	11.3	tr
tr	1	2	256	77	10.0	0	1.31	0.93	11.7	0
—	—	—	12	16	0.3	tr	0.01	0.02	0.2	tr
—	—	—	12	17	0.4	0	0.04	0.02	0.3	0
—	—	—	241	381	10.9	0	1.05	0.63	5.4	0
tr	tr	tr	12	16	0.6	tr	0.06	0.04	0.5	tr
tr	tr	tr	12	16	0.2	tr	0.02	0.02	0.3	tr
tr	tr	tr	11	23	0.5	tr	0.06	0.03	0.7	tr
1	2	1	65	107	3.2	tr	0.19	0.26	3.1	tr
—	—	—	7	132	1.2	3750	0.14	0.29	1.2	135
—	—	—	8	42	1.4	680	0.10	0.18	1.1	113
—	—	—	78	11	1.0	0	0.08	0.04	0.4	0
6	4	tr	tr	3	0	460[2]	—	—	—	0
3	2	tr	tr	1	0	230[2]	—	—	—	0
—	—	—	13	298	0.1	10	0.09	0.44	0.2	2
—	—	—	5	49	0.4	130	0.05	0.05	0.3	47
—	—	—	7	75	0.5	220	0.07	0.07	0.5	56
—	—	—	3	43	0.6	150	0.05	0.04	0.6	25

Food	Weight, gm	Approximate Measure	Food Energy, Cal.	Pro- tein, gm	Fat (total lipid), gm
Cakes:					
angelfood	40	2″ sc, ¹⁄₁₂ of 8″ diam	110	3	tr
chocolate, chocolate icing	120	2″ sc, ¹⁄₁₆ of 10″ diam	445	5	20
cupcake, with chocolate					
icing	50	1, 2¾″ diam	185	2	7
cupcake, without icing	40	1, 2¾″ diam	145	2	6
fruitcake, dark	30	1 pc, 2″ x 2″ x ½″	115	1	5
plain, with chocolate icing	100	2″ sc, ¹⁄₁₆ of 10″ diam	370	4	14
plain, without icing	55	1 pc, 3″ x 2″ x 1½″	200	2	8
pound	30	1 sl, 2¾″ x 3″ x ⅝″	140	2	9
sponge	40	2″ sc, ¹⁄₁₂ of 8″ diam	120	3	2
Candy:					
butterscotch	5	1 pc	21	0	tr
caramels	28	1 oz	115	1	3
chocolate almond bar	32	1 bar	176	3	12
chocolate, milk	28	1 oz	150	2	9
chocolate cream	13	1 pc	51	1	2
fondant	11	1 av	4	—	—
fudge, plain	28	1 oz	115	1	3
hard	28	1 oz	110	0	tr
marshmallow	28	1 oz	90	1	tr
peanut brittle	25	1 pc	110	2	4
Cantaloupe, raw	385	½ of 5″ melon	60	1	tr
Carrots:					
raw	110	1 c, grated	45	1	tr
cooked	145	1 c, diced	45	1	tr
Cashew nuts	135	1 c	760	23	62
Cauliflower:					
raw	100	1 c	25	2	tr
cooked	120	1 c	25	3	tr
Celery:					
raw	100	1 c, diced	15	1	tr
cooked	65	½ c, diced	12	1	tr
Cheese:					
blue or Roquefort type	28	1 oz	105	6	9
Camembert	28	1 oz	84	5	7
Cheddar or American	17	1″ cube	70	4	5
Cheddar or American	112	1 c, grated	445	28	36
Cheddar, process	28	1 oz	105	7	9

[3] If the fat used in the recipe is butter or fortified margarine, the vitamin A value for choco-late cake with fudge icing will be 490 IU; 100 IU for fruit cake; 300 IU for plain cake with-out icing; 220 IU per cupcake; 400 IU for plain cake with icing; 220 IU per cupcake with icing; and 300 IU for pound cake.

Fatty Acids										
Satur-	Unsaturated					Vitamin				
ated (total), gm	Oleic, gm	Lino-leic, gm	Carbo-hydrate, gm	Cal-cium, mg	Iron, mg	A Value, IU	Thia-mine, mg	Ribo-flavin, mg	Niacin, mg	Ascorbic Acid, mg
—	—	—	24	4	0.1	0	tr	0.06	0.1	0
8	10	1	67	84	1.2	190[3]	0.03	0.12	0.3	tr
2	4	tr	30	32	0.3	90[3]	0.01	0.04	0.1	tr
1	3	tr	22	26	0.2	70[3]	0.01	0.03	0.1	tr
1	3	1	18	22	0.8	40[3]	0.04	0.04	0.2	tr
5	7	1	59	63	0.6	180[3]	0.02	0.09	0.2	tr
2	5	1	31	35	0.2	90[3]	0.01	0.05	0.1	tr
2	5	1	14	6	0.2	80[3]	0.01	0.03	0.1	0
1	1	tr	22	12	0.5	180[3]	0.02	0.06	0.1	tr
—	—	—	4	1	0.1	0	0	tr	tr	0
2	1	tr	22	42	0.4	tr	0.01	0.05	tr	tr
—	—	—	16	68	0.9	40	0.03	0.16	0.3	tr
5	3	tr	16	65	0.3	80	0.02	0.09	0.1	tr
—	—	—	9	—	—	—	—	—	—	—
—	—	—	10	—	—	—	—	—	—	—
2	1	tr	21	22	0.3	tr	0.01	0.03	0.1	tr
—	—	—	28	6	0.5	0	0	0	0	0
—	—	—	23	5	0.5	0	0	tr	tr	0
—	—	—	18	10	0.5	7	0.02	0.12	1.2	0
—	—	—	14	27	0.8	6540[4]	0.08	0.06	1.2	63
—	—	—	11	41	0.8	12100	0.06	0.06	0.7	9
—	—	—	10	48	0.9	15220	0.08	0.07	0.7	9
10	43	4	40	51	5.1	140	0.58	0.33	2.4	—
—	—	—	5	22	1.1	90	0.11	0.10	0.6	69
—	—	—	5	25	0.8	70	0.11	0.10	0.7	66
—	—	—	4	39	0.3	240	0.03	0.03	0.3	9
—	—	—	2	33	0.3	0	0.03	0.02	0.2	3
5	3	tr	1	89	0.1	350	0.01	0.17	0.1	0
—	—	—	1	29	0.1	286	0.01	0.21	0.3	0
3	2	tr	tr	128	0.2	220	tr	0.08	tr	0
20	12	1	2	840	1.1	1470	0.03	0.51	0.1	0
5	3	tr	1	219	0.3	350	tr	0.12	tr	0

[4] Value based on varieties with orange-colored flesh, for green-fleshed varieties value is about 540 IU per ½ melon.

Food	Weight, gm	Approximate Measure	Food Energy, Cal.	Pro-tein, gm	Fat (total lipid), gm
foods, Cheddar	28	1 oz	90	6	7
cottage, creamed	225	1 c	240	31	9
cream	15	1 tbsp	55	1	6
Limburger	28	1 oz	97	6	8
Parmesan	28	1 oz	110	10	7
Swiss	28	1 oz	105	8	8
Cherries:					
raw, sweet, with stems[5]	130	1 c	80	2	tr
canned, red, sour, pitted,					
heavy sirup	260	1 c	230	2	1
Chicken:					
broiled	85	3 oz, flesh only	115	20	3
canned, boneless	85	3 oz	170	18	10
creamed	118	½ c, sm serv	208	18	12
fryer, breast, fried	94	½ breast, with bone	155	25	5
fryer, leg, fried	59	with bone	90	12	4
potpie	227	1 pie, 4¼″ diam	535	23	31
roasted	80	2 sl, 3″ x 3″ x ¼″	158	23	7
Chili con carne (no beans)	255	1 c	510	26	38
Chili sauce	17	1 tbsp	20	tr	tr
Chocolate:					
bitter or baking	28	1 oz	145	3	15
sweet	28	1 oz	150	1	10
Chocolate-flavored milk drink	250	1 c	190	8	6
Chocolate sirup	20	1 tbsp	50	tr	tr
Clams:					
raw	85	3 oz	65	11	1
canned, solids and liquid	85	3 oz	45	7	1
Cocoa beverage with milk	242	1 c	235	9	11
Coconut:					
dried, sweetened	62	1 c, shredded	340	2	24
fresh	97	1 c, shredded	335	3	34
Coleslaw	120	1 c	120	1	9
Cookies:					
plain and assorted	25	1 cooky, 3″ diam	120	1	5
wafers	10	2 wafers, 2⅛″ diam	49	1	2
Corn:					
fresh, cooked	140	1 ear, 5″ long	70	3	1
canned	256	1 c	170	5	2
Corn flakes	28	1 oz	110	2	tr

[5] Measure and weight apply to entire vegetable or fruit including parts not usually eaten.

Fatty Acids										
Satur-ated (total), gm	Unsaturated		Carbo-hydrate, gm	Cal-cium, mg	Iron, mg	Vitamin A Value, IU	Thia-mine, mg	Ribo-flavin, mg	Niacin, mg	Ascorbic Acid, mg
	Oleic, gm	Lino-leic, gm								
4	2	tr	2	162	0.2	280	0.01	0.16	tr	0
5	3	tr	7	212	0.7	380	0.07	0.56	0.2	0
3	2	tr	tr	9	tr	230	tr	0.04	tr	0
—	—	—	1	165	0.2	358	0.02	0.14	0.1	0
—	—	—	1	325	0.1	297	tr	0.20	0.1	0
4	3	tr	1	262	0.3	320	tr	0.11	tr	0
—	—	—	20	26	0.5	130	0.06	0.07	0.5	12
—	—	—	59	36	0.8	1680	0.07	0.06	0.4	13
1	1	1	0	8	1.4	80	0.05	0.16	7.4	—
3	4	2	0	18	1.3	200	0.03	0.11	3.7	3
—	—	—	7	83	1.1	328	0.04	0.18	3.8	tr
1	2	1	1	9	1.3	70	0.04	0.17	11.2	—
1	2	1	tr	6	0.9	50	0.03	0.15	2.7	—
10	15	3	42	68	3.0	3020	0.25	0.26	4.1	5
—	—	—	0	16	1.7	0	0.06	0.14	7.2	0
18	17	1	15	97	3.6	380	0.05	0.31	5.6	—
—	—	—	4	3	0.1	240	0.02	0.01	0.3	3
8	6	tr	8	22	1.9	20	0.01	0.07	0.4	0
6	4	tr	16	27	0.4	tr	0.01	0.04	0.1	tr
3	2	tr	27	270	0.4	210	0.09	0.41	0.2	2
tr	tr	tr	13	3	0.3	—	tr	0.01	0.1	0
—	—	—	2	59	5.2	90	0.08	0.15	1.1	8
—	—	—	2	47	3.5	—	0.01	0.09	0.9	—
6	4	tr	26	286	0.9	390	0.09	0.45	0.4	2
21	2	tr	33	10	1.2	0	0.02	0.02	0.2	0
29	2	tr	9	13	1.6	0	0.05	0.02	0.5	3
2	2	5	9	52	0.5	180	0.06	0.06	0.3	35
—	—	—	18	9	0.2	20	0.01	0.01	0.1	tr
—	—	—	7	—	—	—	—	—	—	—
—	—	—	16	2	0.5	310[6]	0.09	0.08	1.0	7
—	—	—	40	10	1.0	690[6]	0.07	0.12	2.3	13
—	—	—	24	5	0.4	0	0.12	0.02	0.6	0

[6] Based on yellow varieties; white varieties contain only a trace of cryptoxanthin and carotenes, the pigments in corn that have biological activity.

Food	Weight, gm	Approximate Measure	Food Energy, Cal.	Protein, gm	Fat (total lipid), gm
Corn grits:					
enriched, cooked	242	1 c	120	3	tr
unenriched, cooked	242	1 c	120	3	tr
Corn muffin, enriched	48	1 med, 2¾″ diam	150	3	5
Cornmeal, white or yellow, dry:					
enriched	145	1 c	525	11	2
unenriched	118	1 c	420	11	5
Crabmeat, canned	85	3 oz	85	15	2
Crackers:					
Graham	14	2 med	55	1	1
saltines	8	2 crackers	35	1	1
soda, plain	11	2 crackers	50	1	1
Cranberry sauce, sweetened	277	1 c	405	tr	1
Cream:					
half-and-half	15	1 tbsp	20	tr	2
heavy or whipping	15	1 tbsp	55	tr	6
light or coffee	15	1 tbsp	30	tr	3
Cucumber, raw	50	6 sl	5	tr	tr
Custard, baked	248	1 c	285	13	14
Dandelion greens, cooked	180	1 c	60	4	1
Dates, fresh and dried	178	1 c	490	4	1
Doughnut, cake type	32	1 doughnut	125	1	6
Eggs:					
raw, whole	50	1 med	80	6	6
boiled	100	2 med	160	13	12
scrambled	64	1 med	110	7	8
Farina, enriched, cooked	238	1 c	100	3	tr
Fats, cooking, vegetable	12.5	1 tbsp	110	0	12
Figs, dried	21	1 fig	60	1	tr
Fig bars	16	1 sm	55	1	1
Fishsticks, breaded, cooked	227	10 sticks	400	38	20
Fruit cocktail, canned	256	1 c	195	1	1
Gelatin, dry, plain	10	1 tbsp	35	9	tr
Gelatin dessert:					
plain	239	1 c	140	4	0
with fruit	241	1 c	160	3	tr
Gingerbread	55	1 pc, 2″ x 2″ x 2″	175	2	6

[7] Vitamin A value based on yellow product; white product contains only a trace.

[8] Iron, thiamine, riboflavin, and niacin are based on the minimal level of enrichment specified in standards of identity promulgated under the Federal Food, Drug, and Cosmetic Act.

[9] Based on recipe using white cornmeal; if yellow cornmeal is used, the vitamin A value is 140 IU per muffin.

Fatty Acids						Vitamin				
Satur-ated (total), gm	Unsaturated		Carbo-hydrate, gm	Cal-cium, mg	Iron, mg	A Value, IU	Thia-mine, mg	Ribo-flavin, mg	Niacin, mg	Ascorbic Acid, mg
	Oleic, gm	Lino-leic, gm								
—	—	—	27	2	0.7[8]	150[7]	0.10[8]	0.07[8]	1.0[8]	0
—	—	—	27	2	0.2	150[7]	0.05	0.02	0.5	0
2	2	tr	23	50	0.8	80[9]	0.09	0.11	0.8	tr
tr	1	1	114	9	4.2[8]	640[7]	0.64[8]	0.38[8]	5.1[8]	0
1	2	2	87	24	2.8	600[7]	0.45	0.13	2.4	0
—	—	—	1	38	0.7	—	0.07	0.07	1.6	—
—	—	—	10	6	0.2	0	0.01	0.03	0.2	0
—	—	—	6	2	0.1	0	tr	tr	0.1	0
tr	1	tr	8	2	0.2	0	tr	tr	0.1	0
—	—	—	104	17	0.6	40	0.03	0.03	0.1	5
1	1	tr	1	16	tr	70	tr	0.02	tr	tr
3	2	tr	tr	11	tr	230	tr	0.02	tr	tr
2	1	tr	1	15	tr	130	tr	0.02	tr	tr
—	—	—	2	8	0.2	tr	0.02	0.02	0.1	6
6	5	1	28	278	1.0	870	0.10	0.47	0.2	1
—	—	—	12	252	3.2	21060	0.24	0.29	—	32
—	—	—	130	105	5.3	90	0.16	0.17	3.9	0
1	4	tr	16	13	0.4[10]	30	0.05[10]	0.05[10]	0.4[10]	tr
2	3	tr	tr	27	1.1	590	0.05	0.15	tr	0
4	5	1	1	54	2.3	1180	0.09	0.28	0.1	0
3	3	tr	1	51	1.1	690	0.05	0.18	tr	0
—	—	—	21	10	0.7[11]	0	0.11[11]	0.07[11]	1.0[11]	0
3	8	1	0	0	0	—	0	0	0	0
—	—	—	15	26	0.6	20	0.02	0.02	0.1	0
—	—	—	12	12	0.2	20	0.01	0.01	0.1	tr
5	4	10	15	25	0.9	—	0.09	0.16	3.6	—
—	—	—	50	23	1.0	360	0.04	0.03	1.1	5
—	—	—	—	—	—	—	—	—	—	—
—	—	—	34	—	—	—	—	—	—	—
—	—	—	40	—	—	—	—	—	—	—
1	4	tr	29	37	1.3	50	0.06	0.06	0.5	0

[10] Based on product made with enriched flour. With unenriched flour, approximate values per doughnut are: iron, 0.2 mg; thiamine, 0.01 mg; riboflavin, 0.03 mg; niacin, 0.2 mg.

[11] Iron, thiamine, riboflavin, and niacin are based on the minimum levels of enrichment specified in standards of identity promulgated under the Federal Food, Drug, and Cosmetic Act.

Table A-8 (continued)

Food	Weight, gm	Approximate Measure	Food Energy, Cal.	Pro-tein, gm	Fat (total lipid), gm
Grapefruit:					
raw, white	285	½ med, 4¼" diam	55	1	tr
raw, white	194	1 c, sc	75	1	tr
juice, canned	247	1 c, unsweetened	100	1	tr
juice, dehydrated,					
water added	247	1 c	100	1	tr
Grapes:					
Concord, Niagara	153	1 c	65	1	1
Muscat, Thompson, Tokay	160	1 c	95	1	tr
Grape juice, bottled	254	1 c	165	1	tr
Grapenut flakes	28	1 oz	110	3	tr
Gravy, meat, brown	18	1 tbsp	41	tr	4
Haddock, fried	85	3 oz	140	17	5
Heart, beef, lean, braised	85	3 oz	160	27	5
Herring:					
Atlantic, broiled	85	1 med	217	21	14
smoked, kippered	100	½ fish	211	22	13
Honey, strained or extracted	21	1 tbsp	65	tr	0
Honeydew melon	150	1 wedge, 2" x 6½"	48	1	0
Ice cream, plain	71	1 sl, or ⅛ qt brick	145	3	9
Ice milk	187	1 c	285	9	10
Jams and preserves	20	1 tbsp	55	tr	tr
Jellies	20	1 tbsp	55	tr	tr
Kale, cooked	110	1 c	30	4	1
Kohlrabi, cooked	75	½ c	23	2	tr
Lamb:					
chop, cooked	137	1 chop, 4.8 oz	400	25	33
leg, roasted	71	2.5 oz, lean	130	20	5
shoulder, roasted	64	2.3 oz, lean	130	17	6
Lard	14	1 tbsp	125	0	14
Lemon	106	1 med	20	1	tr
Lemon juice, fresh	15	1 tbsp	5	tr	tr
Lettuce:					
head, Iceberg	454	1 head, 4¼" diam	60	4	tr
leaves	50	2 lg	10	1	tr
Lime juice, fresh	246	1 c	65	1	tr
Liver:					
beef, fried	57	2 oz	130	15	6
calf, cooked	72	2 sl, 3" x 2¼" x ⅜"	147	16	7
pork, fried	74	2 sl, 3" x 2¼" x ⅜"	170	18	7
Lobster:					
boiled or broiled	334	1 (¾ lb) + 2 tbsp			
		butter	308	20	25
canned	85	½ c	75	15	1

546

	Fatty Acids									
		Unsaturated								
Saturated (total), gm	Oleic, gm	Lino-leic, gm	Carbo-hydrate, gm	Cal-cium, mg	Iron, mg	Vitamin A Value, IU	Thia-mine, mg	Ribo-flavin, mg	Niacin, mg	Ascorbic Acid, mg
—	—	—	14	22	0.6	10	0.05	0.02	0.2	52
—	—	—	20	31	0.8	20	0.07	0.03	0.3	72
—	—	—	24	20	1.0	20	0.07	0.04	0.4	84
—	—	—	24	22	0.2	20	0.10	0.05	0.5	92
—	—	—	15	15	0.4	100	0.05	0.03	0.2	3
—	—	—	25	17	0.6	140	0.07	0.04	0.4	6
—	—	—	42	28	0.8	—	0.10	0.05	0.6	tr
—	—	—	23	—	1.2	0	0.13	—	1.6	0
—	—	—	2	—	0.2	0	0.15	0.01	tr	—
1	3	tr	5	34	1.0	—	0.03	0.06	2.7	2
—	—	—	1	5	5.0	20	0.21	1.04	6.5	1
—	—	—	0	—	1.2	130	0.01	0.15	3.3	0
—	—	—	0	66	1.4	0	tr	0.28	2.9	0
—	—	—	17	1	0.1	0	tr	0.01	0.1	tr
—	—	—	13	26	0.6	60	0.08	0.05	0.3	34
5	3	tr	15	87	0.1	370	0.03	0.13	0.1	1
6	3	tr	42	292	0.2	390	0.09	0.41	0.2	2
—	—	—	14	4	0.2	tr	tr	0.01	tr	tr
—	—	—	14	4	0.3	tr	tr	0.01	tr	1
—	—	—	4	147	1.3	8140	—	—	—	68
—	—	—	5	35	0.5	tr	0.03	0.03	0.2	28
18	12	1	0	10	1.5	—	0.14	0.25	5.6	—
3	2	tr	0	9	1.4	—	0.12	0.21	4.4	—
3	2	tr	0	8	1.0	—	0.10	0.18	3.7	—
5	6	1	0	0	0	0	0	0	0	0
—	—	—	6	18	0.4	10	0.03	0.01	0.1	38
—	—	—	1	1	tr	tr	tr	tr	tr	7
—	—	—	13	91	2.3	1500	0.29	0.27	1.3	29
—	—	—	2	34	0.7	950	0.03	0.04	0.2	9
—	—	—	22	22	0.5	30	0.05	0.03	0.3	80
—	—	—	3	6	5.0	30280	0.15	2.37	9.4	15
—	—	—	3	5	9.0	19130	0.13	2.39	11.7	15
—	—	—	8	10	15.6	12070	0.25	2.30	12.4	10
—	—	—	1	80	0.7	920	0.11	0.06	2.3	0
—	—	—	0	55	0.7	—	0.03	0.06	1.9	—

Food	Weight, gm	Approximate Measure	Food Energy, Cal.	Pro-tein, gm	Fat (total lipid), gm
Macaroni:					
enriched, cooked	130	1 c	190	6	1
unenriched, cooked	130	1 c	190	6	1
Macaroni & cheese, baked	220	1 c	470	18	24
Mackerel, canned	85	3 oz	155	18	9
Malted milk beverage	270	1 c	280	13	12
Mangos	100	1 sm	66	1	tr
Margarine:					
stick, ⅛	14	1 tbsp	100	tr	11
pat or sq	7	1 pat	50	tr	6
Metrecal	237	8 oz	225	18	5
Milk:					
whole	244	1 c	160	9	9
nonfat, skim	246	1 c	90	9	tr
dry, nonfat, instant	70	1 c	250	25	tr
condensed	306	1 c	980	25	27
evaporated	252	1 c	345	18	20
Molasses:					
light	20	1 tbsp	50	—	—
blackstrap	20	1 tbsp	45	—	—
Muffins, white, enriched	48	1 med, 2¾″ diam	140	4	5
Mushrooms, canned	244	1 c	40	5	tr
Mustard greens, cooked	140	1 c	35	3	1
Noodles:					
enriched, cooked	160	1 c	200	7	2
unenriched, cooked	160	1 c	200	7	2
Oats, puffed	28	1 oz	115	3	2
Oatmeal, cooked	236	1 c	130	5	2
Oils, salad, corn	14	1 tbsp	125	0	14
Okra, cooked	85	8 pods	25	2	tr
Olives:					
green, pickled	16	4 med	15	tr	2
ripe, pickled	10	3 sm	15	tr	2
Onions:					
raw	110	1 onion, 2½″ diam	40	2	tr
cooked	210	1 c	60	3	tr
young green	50	6 onions	20	1	tr
Orange:					
navel	180	1 med	60	2	tr

[12] Iron, thiamine, riboflavin, and niacin are based on the minimum levels of enrichment specified in standards of identity promulgated under the Federal Food, Drug, and Cosmetic Act.

[13] Based on the average vitamin A content of fortified margarine. Federal specifications for

Satur-ated (total), gm	Unsaturated Oleic, gm	Unsaturated Lino-leic, gm	Carbo-hydrate, gm	Cal-cium, mg	Iron, mg	Vitamin A Value, IU	Thia-mine, mg	Ribo-flavin, mg	Niacin, mg	Ascorbic Acid, mg
—	—	—	39	14	1.4[12]	0	0.23[12]	0.14[12]	1.9[12]	0
—	—	—	39	14	0.6	0	0.02	0.02	0.5	0
11	10	1	44	398	2.0	950	0.22	0.44	2.0	tr
—	—	—	0	221	1.9	20	0.02	0.28	7.4	—
—	—	—	32	364	0.8	670	0.17	0.56	0.2	2
—	—	—	17	9	0.2	6350	0.06	0.06	0.9	41
2	6	2	tr	3	0	460[13]	—	—	—	0
1	3	1	tr	1	0	230[13]	—	—	—	0
—	—	—	28	500	3.8	1250	0.50	0.75	3.8	25
5	3	tr	12	288	0.1	350	0.08	0.42	0.1	2
—	—	—	13	298	0.1	10	0.10	0.44	0.2	2
—	—	—	36	905	0.4	20	0.24	1.25	0.6	5
15	9	1	166	802	0.3	1090	0.23	1.17	0.5	3
11	7	1	24	635	0.3	820	0.10	0.84	0.5	3
—	—	—	13	33	0.9	—	0.01	0.01	tr	—
—	—	—	11	137	3.2	—	0.02	0.04	0.4	—
1	3	tr	20	50	0.8	50	0.08	0.11	0.7	tr
—	—	—	6	15	1.2	tr	0.04	0.60	4.8	4
—	—	—	6	193	2.5	8120	0.11	0.19	0.9	68
1	1	tr	37	16	1.4[14]	110	0.23[14]	0.14[14]	1.8[14]	0
1	1	tr	37	16	1.0	110	0.04	0.03	0.7	0
tr	1	1	21	50	1.3	0	0.28	0.05	0.5	0
tr	1	1	23	21	1.4	0	0.19	0.05	0.3	0
1	4	7	0	0	0	—	0	0	0	0
—	—	—	5	78	0.4	420	0.11	0.15	0.8	17
tr	2	tr	tr	8	0.2	40	—	—	—	—
tr	2	tr	tr	9	0.1	10	tr	tr	—	—
—	—	—	10	30	0.6	40	0.04	0.04	0.2	11
—	—	—	14	50	0.8	80	0.06	0.06	0.4	14
—	—	—	5	20	0.3	tr	0.02	0.02	0.2	12
—	—	—	16	49	0.5	240	0.12	0.05	0.5	75

fortified margarine require a minimum of 15000 IU of vitamin A per pound.

[14] Iron, thiamine, riboflavin, and niacin are based on the minimum levels of enrichment specified in standards of identity promulgated under the Federal Food, Drug, and Cosmetic Act.

Food	Weight, gm	Approximate Measure	Food Energy, Cal.	Pro-tein, gm	Fat (total lipid), gm
other varieties	210	1 med	75	1	tr
sections	97	½ c	44	1	tr
juice, fresh	247	1 c	100	1	tr
juice, frozen	248	1 c	110	2	tr
juice, dehydrated,					
water added	248	1 c	115	1	tr
Orange and grapefruit					
juice, frozen	248	1 c	110	1	tr
Ocean perch, breaded, fried	85	3 oz	195	16	11
Oyster meat, raw	240	1 c	160	20	4
Oyster stew	230	1 c with 3–4 oysters	200	11	12
Pancakes:					
white, enriched	27	1 cake, 4″ diam	60	2	2
buckwheat	27	1 cake, 4″ diam	55	2	2
Papayas, raw	182	1 c	70	1	tr
Parsley, raw, chopped	3.5	1 tbsp	1	tr	tr
Parsnips, cooked	155	1 c	100	2	1
Peaches:					
raw	114	1 med	35	1	tr
raw	168	1 c, sliced	65	1	tr
canned, sirup pack	257	1 c	200	1	tr
dried, cooked	270	1 c	220	3	1
frozen	340	12-oz carton	300	1	tr
Peanuts, roasted	9	1 tbsp	55	2	4
Peanut butter	16	1 tbsp	95	4	8
Pears:					
raw	182	1 med	100	1	1
canned, sirup pack	255	1 c	195	1	1
Peas, green:					
fresh, cooked	160	1 c	115	9	1
canned	249	1 c	165	9	1
Pecans, chopped	7.5	1 tbsp	50	1	5
Peppers, green, raw	62	1 med	15	1	tr
Pickles:					
dill	135	1 pickle, 4″ long	15	1	tr
relish	13	1 tbsp	14	tr	tr
sour	30	1 sl, 1½″ diam x 1″	3	tr	tr
sweet	20	1 pickle, 2¾″ long	30	tr	tr
Pies:					
apple	135	⅐ of 9″ pie	345	3	15

[15] Based on yellow-fleshed varieties; for white-fleshed varieties value is about 50 IU per 114-gm peach and 80 IU per cup of sliced peaches.

[16] Average weight in accordance with commercial freezing practices. For products without

| Fatty Acids | | | | | | | | | | |
| Satur-ated (total), gm | Unsaturated | | Carbo-hydrate, gm | Cal-cium, mg | Iron, mg | Vitamin A Value, IU | Thia-mine, mg | Ribo-flavin, mg | Niacin, mg | Ascorbic Acid, mg |
	Oleic, gm	Lino-leic, gm								
—	—	—	19	67	0.3	310	0.16	0.06	0.6	70
—	—	—	11	32	0.4	180	0.08	0.03	0.3	48
—	—	—	23	25	0.5	490	0.22	0.06	0.9	127
—	—	—	27	22	0.2	500	0.21	0.03	0.8	112
—	—	—	27	25	0.5	500	0.20	0.06	0.9	108
—	—	—	26	20	0.2	270	0.16	0.02	0.8	102
—	—	—	6	28	1.1	—	0.08	0.09	1.5	—
—	—	—	8	226	13.2	740	0.33	0.43	6.0	—
—	—	—	11	269	3.3	640	0.13	0.41	1.6	—
tr	1	tr	9	27	0.4	30	0.05	0.06	0.3	tr
1	1	tr	6	59	0.4	60	0.03	0.04	0.2	tr
—	—	—	18	36	0.5	3190	0.07	0.08	0.5	102
—	—	—	tr	7	0.2	300	tr	0.01	tr	6
—	—	—	23	70	0.9	50	0.11	0.13	0.2	16
—	—	—	10	9	0.5	1320[15]	0.02	0.05	1.0	7
—	—	—	16	15	0.8	2230[15]	0.03	0.08	1.6	12
—	—	—	52	10	0.8	1100	0.02	0.06	1.4	7
—	—	—	58	41	5.1	3290	0.01	0.15	4.2	6
—	—	—	77	14	1.7	2210	0.03	0.14	2.4	135[16]
1	2	1	2	7	0.2	—	0.03	0.01	1.5	0
2	4	2	3	9	0.3	—	0.02	0.02	2.4	0
—	—	—	25	13	0.5	30	0.04	0.07	0.2	7
—	—	—	50	13	0.5	tr	0.03	0.05	0.3	4
—	—	—	19	37	2.9	860	0.44	0.17	3.7	33
—	—	—	31	50	4.2	1120	0.23	0.13	2.2	22
tr	3	1	1	5	0.2	10	0.06	0.01	0.1	tr
—	—	—	3	6	0.4	260	0.05	0.05	0.3	79
—	—	—	3	35	1.4	140	tr	0.03	tr	8
—	—	—	3	2	0.2	14	0	tr	tr	1
—	—	—	1	8	0.4	93	tr	0.02	tr	2
—	—	—	7	2	0.2	20	tr	tr	tr	1
4	9	1	51	11	0.4	40	0.03	0.02	0.5	1

added ascorbic acid, value is about 37 mg per 12-oz carton and 50 mg per 16-oz carton; for those with added ascorbic acid, 139 mg per 12-oz carton and 186 mg per 16-oz carton.

Food	Weight, gm	Approximate Measure	Food Energy, Cal.	Pro- tein, gm	Fat (total lipid), gm
cherry	135	½ of 9″ pie	355	4	15
custard	130	½ of 9″ pie	280	8	14
lemon meringue	120	½ of 9″ pie	305	4	12
mince	135	½ of 9″ pie	365	3	16
pumpkin	130	½ of 9″ pie	275	5	15
Piecrust, plain, baked	135	1, 9″ crust	675	8	45
Pimentos, canned	38	1 med	10	tr	tr
Pineapple:					
raw	140	1 c, diced	75	1	tr
canned, sirup pack	260	1 c, crushed	195	1	tr
canned, sirup pack	122	2 sm sl + 2 tbsp jc	90	tr	tr
juice, canned	249	1 c	135	1	tr
Pizza, cheese	75	5½″ sector	185	7	6
Plums:					
raw	60	1 plum, 2″ diam	25	tr	tr
canned, sirup pack	122	3 plums + 2 tbsp jc	100	tr	tr
Popcorn, popped	14	1 c	65	1	3
Pork:					
chop, cooked	98	1 chop, 3.5 oz	260	16	21
ham, cured	85	3 oz	245	18	19
ham, fresh, lean	107	2 sl, 2″ x 1½″ x 1″	254	40	9
boiled ham	57	2 oz	135	11	10
Potatoes:					
baked	99	1 med	90	3	tr
French fried	57	10 pc	155	2	7
hash-browned	100	½ c	241	3	12
mashed	195	1 c with milk	125	4	1
mashed	195	1 c with milk & butter	185	4	8
Potato chips	20	10 chips	115	1	8
Pretzels	5	5 sm sticks	20	tr	tr
Prunes:					
dried, uncooked	32	4 prunes	70	1	tr
dried, cooked, sirup	270	1 c (17–18 prunes)	295	2	1
juice, canned	256	1 c	200	1	tr
Puddings:					
chocolate	144	½ c	219	5	7
lemon snow	130	1 serv	114	3	tr
tapioca	132	½ c	181	5	5
vanilla	248	1 c	275	9	10
Pumpkin, canned	228	1 c	75	2	1
Radishes, raw	40	4 sm	5	tr	tr
Raisins, dried	160	1 c	460	4	tr
Raspberries, red, raw	123	1 c	70	1	1
Rhubarb, cooked, sugar added	272	1 c	385	1	tr

Fatty Acids										
Saturated (total), gm	Unsaturated		Carbohydrate, gm	Calcium, mg	Iron, mg	Vitamin A Value, IU	Thiamine, mg	Riboflavin, mg	Niacin, mg	Ascorbic Acid, mg
	Oleic, gm	Linoleic, gm								
4	10	1	52	19	0.4	590	0.03	0.23	0.6	1
5	8	1	30	125	0.8	300	0.07	0.21	0.4	0
4	7	1	45	17	0.6	200	0.04	0.10	0.2	4
4	10	1	56	38	1.4	tr	0.09	0.05	0.5	1
5	7	1	32	66	0.6	3210	0.04	0.15	0.6	tr
10	29	3	59	19	2.3	0	0.27	0.19	2.4	0
—	—	—	2	3	0.6	870	0.01	0.02	0.1	36
—	—	—	19	24	0.7	100	0.12	0.04	0.3	24
—	—	—	50	29	0.8	120	0.20	0.06	0.5	17
—	—	—	24	13	0.4	50	0.09	0.03	0.2	8
—	—	—	34	37	0.7	120	0.12	0.04	0.5	22
2	3	tr	27	107	0.7	290	0.04	0.12	0.7	4
—	—	—	7	7	0.3	140	0.02	0.02	0.3	3
—	—	—	26	11	1.1	1470	0.03	0.02	0.5	2
2	tr	tr	8	1	0.3	—	—	0.01	0.2	0
8	9	2	0	8	2.2	0	0.63	0.18	3.8	—
7	8	2	0	8	2.2	0	0.40	0.16	3.1	—
—	—	—	0	7	2.5	0	0.69	0.33	5.4	0
4	4	1	0	6	1.6	0	0.25	0.09	1.5	—
—	—	—	21	9	0.7	tr	0.10	0.04	1.7	20
2	2	4	20	9	0.7	tr	0.07	0.04	1.8	12
—	—	—	32	18	1.2	30	0.08	0.06	1.7	7
—	—	—	25	47	0.8	50	0.16	0.10	2.0	19
4	3	tr	24	47	0.8	330	0.16	0.10	1.9	18
2	2	4	10	8	0.4	tr	0.04	0.01	1.0	3
—	—	—	4	1	0	0	tr	tr	tr	0
—	—	—	18	14	1.1	440	0.02	0.04	0.4	1
—	—	—	78	60	4.5	1860	0.08	0.18	1.7	2
—	—	—	49	36	10.5	—	0.02	0.03	1.1	4
—	—	—	37	147	0.2	196	0.05	0.22	0.2	0
—	—	—	27	4	0.1	0	tr	0.02	tr	10
—	—	—	28	151	0.6	195	0.05	0.21	0.6	0
5	3	tr	39	290	0.1	390	0.07	0.40	0.1	2
—	—	—	18	57	0.9	14590	0.07	0.12	1.3	12
—	—	—	1	12	0.4	tr	0.01	0.01	0.1	10
—	—	—	124	99	5.6	30	0.18	0.13	0.9	2
—	—	—	17	27	1.1	160	0.04	0.11	1.1	31
—	—	—	98	212	1.6	220	0.06	0.15	0.7	17

Food	Weight, gm	Approximate Measure	Food Energy, Cal.	Pro- tein, gm	Fat (total lipid), gm
Rice:					
parboiled, cooked	176	1 c	185	4	tr
puffed	14	1 c	55	1	tr
white, cooked	168	1 c	185	3	tr
Rice flakes	30	1 c	115	2	tr
Rolls:					
plain, enriched	38	12 per lb	115	3	2
plain, unenriched	38	12 per lb	115	3	2
sweet	43	1 roll	135	4	4
Rutabagas, cooked	100	½ c	38	1	tr
Rye flour, light	80	1 c	285	8	1
Salads:					
apple, celery, walnut	154	3 hp tbsp, 2 lv lettuce	137	2	8
carrot & raisin	134	3 hp tbsp, 2 lv lettuce	153	2	6
fruit, fresh	195	3 hp tbsp, 2 lv lettuce	174	2	11
gelatin with fruit	188	1 sq, 2 lv lettuce	139	2	6
gelatin with vegetable	164	1 sq, 2 lv lettuce	115	2	6
lettuce, tomato,		4 lv lettuce,			
mayonnaise	115	3 sl tomato	80	2	6
potato	123	½ c, French dressing	184	2	11
Salad dressings:					
blue cheese	16	1 tbsp	80	1	8
commercial, plain	15	1 tbsp	65	tr	6
French	15	1 tbsp	60	tr	6
home cooked, boiled	17	1 tbsp	30	1	2
mayonnaise	15	1 tbsp	110	tr	12
Thousand Island	15	1 tbsp	75	tr	8
Salmon, pink, canned	85	3 oz	120	17	5
Sardines, Atlantic	85	3 oz	175	20	9
Sauerkraut, canned	235	1 c	45	2	tr
Sausage:					
bologna	227	8 sl	690	27	62
frankfurter, cooked	51	1 frankfurter	155	6	14
liverwurst	30	1 sl, 3″ diam x ¼″	79	5	6
pork, links or patty, cooked	113	4 oz	540	21	50
Vienna	18	1 av, 2″ x ¾″ diam	39	3	3
Scallops, fried	145	5–6 med pc	427	24	28
Shad, baked	85	3 oz	170	20	10
Sherbet, orange	193	1 c	260	2	2
Shortbread	16	2 pc, 58 per lb	78	1	3

[17] Iron, thiamine, and niacin are based on the minimum levels of enrichment specified in standards of identity promulgated under the Federal Food, Drug, and Cosmetic Act. Ribo- flavin based on unenriched rice. When the minimum level of enrichment for riboflavin speci-

| Fatty Acids | | | | | | | | | | |
| Satur-ated (total), gm | Unsaturated | | Carbo-hydrate, gm | Cal-cium, mg | Iron, mg | Vitamin A Value, IU | Thia-mine, mg | Ribo-flavin, mg | Niacin, mg | Ascorbic Acid, mg |
	Oleic, gm	Lino-leic, gm								
—	—	—	41	33	1.4[17]	0	0.19[17]	0.02[17]	2.0[17]	0
—	—	—	13	3	0.3	0	0.06	0.01	0.6	0
—	—	—	41	17	1.5[17]	0	0.19[17]	0.01[17]	1.6[17]	0
—	—	—	26	9	0.5	0	0.10	0.02	1.6	0
tr	1	tr	20	28	0.7	tr	0.11	0.07	0.8	tr
tr	1	tr	20	28	0.3	tr	0.02	0.03	0.3	tr
1	2	tr	21	37	0.3	30	0.03	0.06	0.4	0
—	—	—	9	55	0.4	330	0.07	0.08	0.9	36
—	—	—	62	18	0.9	0	0.12	0.06	0.5	0
—	—	—	16	32	0.8	355	0.08	0.08	0.4	5
—	—	—	28	48	1.5	4708	0.08	0.08	0.5	6
—	—	—	21	45	0.8	685	0.08	0.09	0.4	32
—	—	—	22	23	0.5	391	0.04	0.05	0.3	16
—	—	—	15	24	0.5	1977	0.04	0.06	0.3	8
—	—	—	7	20	0.8	1115	0.06	0.07	0.5	19
—	—	—	21	21	0.8	243	0.07	0.04	0.8	16
2	2	4	1	13	tr	30	tr	0.02	tr	tr
1	1	3	2	2	tr	30	tr	tr	tr	—
1	1	3	3	2	0.1	—	—	—	—	—
1	1	tr	3	15	0.1	80	0.01	0.03	tr	tr
2	3	6	tr	3	0.1	40	tr	0.01	tr	—
1	2	4	2	2	0.1	50	tr	tr	tr	tr
1	1	tr	0	167[18]	0.7	60	0.03	0.16	6.8	—
—	—	—	0	372	2.5	190	0.02	0.17	4.6	—
—	—	—	9	85	1.2	120	0.07	0.09	0.4	33
—	—	—	2	16	4.1	—	0.36	0.49	6.0	—
—	—	—	1	3	0.8	—	0.08	0.10	1.3	—
—	—	—	1	3	1.6	1725	0.05	0.34	1.4	0
18	21	5	tr	8	2.7	0	0.89	0.39	4.2	—
—	—	—	0	2	0.4	0	0.02	0.02	0.6	0
—	—	—	19	41	3.1	0	0.09	0.17	2.3	0
—	—	—	0	20	0.5	20	0.11	0.22	7.3	—
—	—	—	59	31	tr	110	0.02	0.06	tr	4
—	—	—	11	2	tr	0	0.01	tr	tr	0

fied in the standards of identity becomes effective the value will be 0.12 mg per cup of par-boiled rice and of white rice.

[18] Based on total contents of can. If bones are discarded, value will be greatly reduced.

Food	Weight, gm	Approximate Measure	Food Energy, Cal.	Pro- tein, gm	Fat (total lipid), gm
Shrimp, canned	85	3 oz	100	21	1
Sirups, table blends	20	1 tbsp	60	0	0
Soups:					
bean	250	1 c	170	8	6
beef	250	1 c	100	6	4
beef noodle	250	1 c	70	4	3
beef bouillon, broth,					
consomme	240	1 c	30	5	0
chicken	250	1 c	75	4	2
chicken noodle	250	1 c	65	4	2
clam chowder	255	1 c	85	2	3
cream, mushroom	240	1 c	135	2	10
pea, green	245	1 c	130	6	2
tomato	245	1 c	90	2	2
vegetable with beef broth	250	1 c	80	3	2
vegetable-beef	203	1 serv, 3 from can	64	6	2
Soy flour, medium fat	88	1 c	232	37	6
Spaghetti:					
enriched, cooked	140	1 c	155	5	1
unenriched, cooked	140	1 c	155	5	1
in tomato sauce	250	1 c with cheese	260	9	9
Italian style	292	1 serv, with meat sauce	396	13	21
Italian style	302	1 serv, as above with grated cheese	436	15	24
Spinach	180	1 c	40	5	1
Squash:					
summer, cooked	210	1 c	30	2	tr
winter, cooked	205	1 c	130	4	1
Strawberries:					
raw	149	1 c	55	1	1
frozen	284	10-oz carton	310	1	1
Sugar:					
brown	14	1 tbsp	50	0	0
maple	15	1 pc, 1¼″ x 1″ x ½″	52	—	—
white, granulated	12	1 tbsp	45	0	0
white, powdered	8	1 tbsp	30	0	0
Sweet potatoes:					
baked	110	1 med, 5″ x 2″	155	2	1
candied	175	1 sm, 3½″ x 2¼″	295	2	6
Tangerine	114	1 med	40	1	tr

[19] Iron, thiamine, riboflavin, and niacin are based on the minimum levels of enrichment specified in standards of identity promulgated under the Federal Food, Drug, and Cosmetic Act.

Fatty Acids										
Saturated (total), gm	Unsaturated Oleic, gm	Linoleic, gm	Carbohydrate, gm	Calcium, mg	Iron, mg	Vitamin A Value, IU	Thiamine, mg	Riboflavin, mg	Niacin, mg	Ascorbic Acid, mg
—	—	—	1	98	2.6	50	0.01	0.03	1.5	—
—	—	—	15	9	0.8	0	0	0	0	0
1	2	2	22	62	2.2	650	0.14	0.07	1.0	2
2	2	tr	11	15	0.5	—	—	—	—	—
1	1	1	7	8	1.0	50	0.05	0.06	1.1	tr
0	0	0	3	tr	0.5	tr	tr	0.02	1.2	—
1	1	tr	10	20	0.5	—	0.02	0.12	1.5	—
tr	1	1	8	10	0.5	50	0.02	0.02	0.8	tr
—	—	—	13	36	1.0	920	0.03	0.03	1.0	—
1	3	5	10	41	0.5	70	0.02	0.12	0.7	tr
1	1	tr	23	44	1.0	340	0.05	0.05	1.0	7
tr	1	1	16	15	0.7	1000	0.06	0.05	1.1	12
—	—	—	14	20	0.8	3250	0.05	0.02	1.2	—
—	—	—	6	5	0.5	2340	0.03	0.04	0.8	—
—	—	—	33	215	11.4	100	0.72	0.30	2.3	0
—	—	—	32	11	1.3[19]	0	0.19[19]	0.11[19]	1.5[19]	0
—	—	—	32	11	0.6	0	0.02	0.02	0.4	0
2	5	1	37	80	2.2	1080	0.24	0.18	2.4	14
—	—	—	39	27	2.1	901	0.12	0.12	3.0	24
—	—	—	40	99	2.2	1041	0.12	0.16	3.0	24
—	—	—	6	167	4.0	14580	0.13	0.25	1.0	50
—	—	—	7	52	0.8	820	0.10	0.16	1.6	21
—	—	—	32	57	1.6	8610	0.10	0.27	1.4	27
—	—	—	13	31	1.5	90	0.04	0.10	0.9	88
—	—	—	79	40	2.0	90	0.06	0.17	1.5	150
—	—	—	13	12	0.5	0	tr	tr	tr	0
—	—	—	14	27	0.5	—	—	—	—	—
—	—	—	12	0	tr	0	0	0	0	0
—	—	—	8	0	tr	0	0	0	0	0
—	—	—	36	44	1.0	8910	0.10	0.07	0.7	24
2	3	1	60	65	1.6	11030	0.10	0.08	0.8	17
—	—	—	10	34	0.3	350	0.05	0.02	0.1	26

Food	Weight, gm	Approximate Measure	Food Energy, Cal.	Pro-tein, gm	Fat (total lipid), gm
Tomatoes:					
raw	150	1 med	35	2	tr
canned	242	1 c	50	2	tr
Tomato juice, canned	242	1 c	45	2	tr
Tomato catsup	17	1 tbsp	15	tr	tr
Tongue, beef, simmered	85	3 oz	210	18	14
Tuna, canned, drained	85	3 oz	170	24	7
Turkey, roasted	100	3 sl, 3″ x 2½″ x ¼″	200	31	8
Turnips, cooked, diced	155	1 c	35	1	tr
Turnip greens, cooked	145	1 c	30	3	tr
Veal:					
chop, loin, cooked	122	1 med	514	28	44
cutlet, broiled	85	3 oz	185	23	9
roast	85	3 oz	230	23	14
Vinegar	15	1 tbsp	2	0	—
Waffles, baked	75	1 waffle, ½″ x 4½″ x 5½″	210	7	7
Walnuts, English	8	1 tbsp, chopped	50	1	5
Watermelon:					
raw	100	½ c cubes	28	1	tr
raw	925	1 wedge, 4″ x 8″	115	2	1
Wheat:					
puffed	28	1 oz	105	4	tr
shredded	28	1 oz	100	3	1
Wheat flakes	28	1 oz	100	3	tr
Wheat flours:					
all-purpose or family, enriched	110	1 c, sifted	400	12	1
all-purpose or family, unenriched	110	1 c, sifted	400	12	1
cake or pastry flour	110	1 c, sifted	365	8	1
self-rising, enriched	110	1 c	385	10	1
whole wheat	120	1 c	400	16	2
Wheat germ	68	1 c	245	18	7
White sauce, medium	265	1 c	430	10	33
Yeast, brewer's, dry	8	1 tbsp	25	3	tr
Yoghurt	246	1 c	120	8	4

[20] Year-round average. Samples marketed from November through May average around 15 mg per 150-gm tomato; from June through October, around 39 mg.

[21] Iron, thiamine, riboflavin, and niacin are based on the minimum level of enrichment specified in the standards of identity promulgated under the Federal Food, Drug, and Cosmetic Act.

Fatty Acids

Satur-ated (total), gm	Unsaturated		Carbo-hydrate, gm	Cal-cium, mg	Iron, mg	Vitamin A Value, IU	Thia-mine, mg	Ribo-flavin, mg	Niacin, mg	Ascorbic Acid, mg
	Oleic, gm	Lino-leic, gm								
—	—	—	7	20	0.8	1350	0.10	0.06	1.0	34[20]
—	—	—	10	15	1.2	2180	0.13	0.07	1.7	40
—	—	—	10	17	2.2	1940	0.13	0.07	1.8	39
—	—	—	4	4	0.1	240	0.02	0.01	0.3	3
—	—	—	tr	6	1.9	—	0.04	0.25	3.0	—
—	—	—	0	7	1.6	70	0.04	0.10	10.1	—
—	—	—	0	30	5.1	tr	0.08	0.17	9.8	0
—	—	—	8	54	0.6	tr	0.06	0.08	0.5	33
—	—	—	5	267	1.6	9140	0.21	0.36	0.8	100
—	—	—	0	7	3.5	0	0.17	26	5.8	0
5	4	tr	—	9	2.7	—	0.06	0.21	4.6	—
7	6	tr	0	10	2.9	—	0.11	0.26	6.6	—
—	—	—	1	1	0.1	—	—	—	—	—
2	4	1	28	85	1.3	250	0.13	0.19	1.0	tr
tr	1	3	1	8	0.2	tr	0.03	0.01	0.1	tr
—	—	—	7	7	0.2	590	0.05	0.05	0.2	6
—	—	—	27	30	2.1	2510	0.13	0.13	0.7	30
—	—	—	22	8	1.2	0	0.15	0.07	2.2	0
—	—	—	23	12	1.0	0	0.06	0.03	1.3	0
—	—	—	23	12	1.2	0	0.18	0.04	1.4	0
tr	tr	tr	84	18	3.2[21]	0	0.48[21]	0.29[21]	3.8[21]	0
tr	tr	tr	84	18	0.9	0	0.07	0.05	1.0	0
tr	tr	tr	79	17	0.5	0	0.03	0.03	0.7	0
tr	tr	tr	82	292	3.2[21]	0	0.49[21]	0.29[21]	3.9[21]	0
tr	1	1	85	49	4.0	0	0.66	0.14	5.2	0
1	2	4	32	49	6.4	0	1.36	0.46	2.9	0
18	11	1	23	305	0.5	1220	0.12	0.44	0.6	tr
—	—	—	3	17	1.4	tr	1.25	0.34	3.0	tr
2	1	tr	13	295	0.1	170	0.09	0.43	0.2	2

▶ AMINO ACID CONTENT OF FOODS

The source of the data in Table A-9 is *Amino Acid Content of Foods*, Home Economics Research Report 4. The values given are for 100-gm edible portions of food. In addition to the eight essential amino acids, values are listed for cystine and tyrosine because of their sparing action to methionine and phenylalanine, respectively. Values for arginine, histidine, alanine, aspartic acid, glutamic acid, glycine, proline, and serine have not been included in Table A-9 but can be found in the source material.

A simple problem is presented to show the reader how these data may be used:

The Problem:

What is the tryptophan value of 1 pint of whole milk?

Solution of the Problem:

1 pint whole milk = 2 cups whole milk
2 cups whole milk = 488 gm (from Table A-5)
100 gm whole milk contains 0.049 gm tryptophan (from Table A-9)

$$1 \text{ pint whole milk} = \frac{488 \text{ gm} \times 0.049 \text{ gm}}{100 \text{ gm}} = 0.239 \text{ gm tryptophan}$$

| Food | Trypto-phan, gm | Threo-nine, gm | Isoleu-cine, gm | Leu-cine, gm | Lysine, gm | Sulfur Containing | | | Phenyl-alanine, gm | Tyro-sine, gm | Valine, gm |
						Meth-ionine, gm	Cystine, gm	Total, gm			
Almonds	0.176	0.610	0.873	1.454	0.582	0.259	0.377	0.636	1.146	0.618	1.124
Asparagus, canned	0.023	0.057	0.069	0.083	0.089	0.027	—	—	0.060	—	0.092
Bacon	0.095	0.306	0.399	0.728	0.587	0.141	0.106	0.247	0.434	0.234	0.434
Banana	0.018	—	—	—	0.055	0.011	—	—	—	0.031	—
Beans, baked	0.057	0.274	0.291	0.486	0.354	0.059	0.018	0.077	0.333	0.165	0.312
Beans, Lima, canned	0.049	0.171	0.233	0.306	0.240	0.041	0.042	0.083	0.197	0.131	0.246
Beans, snap, canned	0.014	0.038	0.045	0.058	0.052	0.014	0.010	0.024	0.024	0.021	0.048
Beef, ground	0.187	0.707	0.837	1.311	1.398	0.397	0.202	0.599	0.658	0.543	0.888
Beef, Porterhouse	0.192	0.724	0.858	1.343	1.433	0.407	0.207	0.614	0.674	0.556	0.911
Beef, rib roast	0.203	0.768	0.910	1.425	1.520	0.432	0.220	0.652	0.715	0.590	0.966
Bread	0.091	0.282	0.429	0.668	0.225	0.142	0.200	0.342	0.465	0.243	0.435
Broccoli	0.037	0.122	0.126	0.163	0.147	0.050	—	—	0.119	—	0.170
Brussel sprouts	0.044	0.153	0.186	0.194	0.197	0.046	—	—	0.148	—	0.193
Cabbage	0.011	0.039	0.040	0.057	0.066	0.013	0.028	0.041	0.030	0.030	0.043
Carrot, raw	0.010	0.043	0.046	0.065	0.052	0.010	0.029	0.039	0.042	0.020	0.056
Cauliflower	0.033	0.102	0.104	0.162	0.134	0.047	—	—	0.075	0.034	0.144
Celery	0.012	—	—	—	0.021	0.015	0.006	0.021	—	0.016	—
Cheese, Cheddar	0.341	0.929	1.685	2.437	1.834	0.650	0.141	0.791	1.340	1.195	1.794
Cheese, cottage	0.179	0.794	0.989	1.826	1.428	0.469	0.147	0.616	0.917	0.917	0.978
Chicken	0.250	0.877	1.088	1.490	1.810	0.537	0.277	0.814	0.811	0.725	1.012
Corn, canned	0.012	0.082	0.074	0.220	0.074	0.039	0.033	0.072	0.112	0.067	0.125
Cornflakes	0.052	0.275	0.306	1.047	0.154	0.135	0.152	0.157	0.354	0.283	0.386
Cornmeal, whole, ground	0.056	0.367	0.425	1.192	0.265	0.171	0.119	0.290	0.418	0.562	0.470
Egg	0.211	0.637	0.850	1.126	0.819	0.401	0.299	0.700	0.739	0.551	0.950
Frankfurter	0.120	0.582	0.688	1.018	1.143	0.300	0.177	0.477	0.518	0.461	0.713
Grapefruit	0.001	—	—	—	0.006	0.000	—	—	—	—	—
Haddock	0.181	0.789	0.923	1.374	1.596	0.530	0.245	0.775	0.676	0.492	0.970
Ham, boiled	0.219	0.934	1.135	1.762	1.915	0.554	0.368	0.923	0.872	0.879	1.186
Hominy	0.084	0.316	0.349	0.810	0.358	0.099	—	—	0.333	0.331	0.398
Kale	0.042	0.139	0.133	0.252	0.121	0.035	0.036	0.071	0.158	—	0.184
Lamb, leg	0.233	0.824	0.933	1.394	1.457	0.432	0.236	0.668	0.732	0.625	0.887
Lettuce	0.012	—	—	—	0.070	0.004	—	—	—	—	—

Table A-9 (continued)

Food	Tryptophan, gm	Threonine, gm	Isoleucine, gm	Leucine, gm	Lysine, gm	Sulfur Containing			Phenylalanine, gm	Tyrosine, gm	Valine, gm
						Methionine, gm	Cystine, gm	Total, gm			
Liver, beef or pork	0.296	0.936	1.031	1.819	1.475	0.463	0.243	0.706	0.993	0.738	1.239
Milk, whole and nonfat	0.049	0.161	0.233	0.344	0.272	0.086	0.031	0.117	0.170	0.178	0.240
Milk, dried, nonfat	0.502	1.641	2.271	3.493	2.768	0.870	0.318	1.188	1.724	1.814	2.444
Milk, human	0.023	0.062	0.075	0.124	0.090	0.028	0.027	0.055	0.060	0.071	0.086
Mustard greens	0.037	0.060	0.075	0.062	0.111	0.024	0.035	0.059	0.074	0.121	0.108
Oatmeal	0.183	0.470	0.733	1.065	0.521	0.209	0.309	0.518	0.758	0.524	0.845
Onions	0.021	0.022	0.021	0.037	0.064	0.013	–	–	0.039	0.046	0.031
Orange juice	0.003	–	–	–	0.021	0.002	–	–	–	–	–
Peanut butter	0.330	0.803	1.228	1.816	1.066	0.263	0.449	0.712	1.510	1.071	1.487
Peas, canned	0.028	0.125	0.156	0.212	0.160	0.027	0.037	0.064	0.131	0.083	0.139
Peppers	0.009	0.050	0.046	0.046	0.051	0.016	–	–	0.055	–	0.033
Pineapple	0.005	–	–	–	0.009	0.001	–	–	–	–	–
Pork, loin	0.213	0.716	0.842	1.207	1.346	0.409	0.192	0.601	0.646	0.585	0.853
Pork, sausage	0.092	0.442	0.524	0.774	0.869	0.228	0.135	0.363	0.394	0.351	0.543
Potatoes, raw	0.021	0.079	0.088	0.100	0.107	0.025	0.019	0.044	0.088	0.036	0.107
Rice, white and converted	0.082	0.298	0.356	0.655	0.300	0.137	0.103	0.240	0.382	0.347	0.531
Salmon, canned	0.200	0.876	1.025	1.526	1.771	0.588	0.271	0.859	0.750	0.546	1.076
Shrimp, canned	0.186	0.811	0.948	1.412	1.640	0.545	0.251	0.796	0.694	0.506	0.996
Soybeans	0.526	1.504	2.054	2.946	2.414	0.513	0.678	1.191	1.889	1.216	2.005
Spinach	0.037	0.102	0.107	0.176	0.142	0.039	0.046	0.085	0.099	0.073	0.126
Squash, summer	0.005	0.014	0.019	0.027	0.023	0.008	–	–	0.016	–	0.022
Sweet potatoes, raw	0.031	0.085	0.087	0.103	0.085	0.033	0.029	0.062	0.100	0.081	0.135
Tomatoes	0.009	0.033	0.029	0.041	0.042	0.007	–	–	0.028	0.014	0.028
Turkey	–	1.014	1.260	1.836	2.173	0.664	0.330	0.994	0.960	–	1.187
Turnip greens	0.045	0.125	0.107	0.207	0.129	0.052	0.045	0.097	0.146	0.105	0.149
Veal, round	0.256	0.846	1.030	1.429	1.629	0.446	0.231	0.677	0.792	0.702	1.008
Walnuts	0.175	0.589	0.767	1.228	0.441	0.306	0.320	0.626	0.767	0.583	0.974
Wheat flour, white	0.129	0.302	0.483	0.809	0.239	0.138	0.210	0.348	0.577	0.359	0.453
Wheat germ	0.265	1.343	1.177	1.708	1.534	0.404	0.287	0.691	0.908	0.882	1.364
Wheat, shredded	0.085	0.405	0.449	0.684	0.331	0.139	0.204	0.343	0.481	0.236	0.577
Yeast, dried, brewer's	0.710	2.353	2.398	3.226	3.300	0.836	0.548	1.384	1.902	1.902	2.723

Table A-10. The Phosphorus, Sodium, Potassium, and Magnesium Content of Some Typical Foods

Food	Phosphorus, mg/100 gm	Sodium, mg/100 gm	Potassium, mg/100 gm	Magnesium, mg/100 gm
Apples, raw	10	1	110	8
Asparagus, frozen, cooked	64	1	220	14
Bacon, broiled or fried	224	1021	236	25
Beans, green, canned	25	236[1]	95	14
Beef, T-bone steak, cooked	166	60	370	28
Beef, ground, cooked	194	47	450	21
Bread, white, enriched	97	507	105	22
Broccoli, frozen, cooked	62	10	267	21
Butter	16	987	23	2
Carrots, raw	36	47	341	23
Cheese, Cheddar	478	700	82	45
Chicken, broiler, cooked	201	66	274	19
Coffee, instant, dry powder	383	72	3256	456
Corn, canned	49	236[1]	97	19
Cream, light	80	43	122	11
Egg	205	122	129	11
Grapefruit sections, canned	14	1	135	11
Ham, canned	156	1100	340	17
Ice cream	115	63[2]	181	14
Lettuce	25	9	264	11
Liver, beef, cooked	476	184	380	18
Milk, whole	92	50	140	13
Oatmeal, cooked	57	218	61	21
Orange juice, frozen	16	1	186	12
Peanut butter	395	606	652	173
Peas, canned	76	236[1]	96	20
Pork loin, cooked	256	65	390	27
Potato, white, mashed	49	301	261	12
Shrimp, French-fried[3]	191	186	229	51
Spinach, frozen	44	52	333	65
Tomatoes, canned	19	130	217	12
Tomato juice, canned	18	200	227	10
Veal cutlet, cooked	203	80	500	18
Walnuts, shelled	380	2	450	131

[1] Estimated average based on addition of salt in the amount of 0.6 per cent.
[2] Values for product without added salt.
[3] Dipped in egg, bread crumbs, and flour or in batter. From *Composition of Foods—Raw, Processed, Prepared.* U.S. Dept. Agr., Agr. Handbook 8, revised 1963.

Table A-11. Low-Cost Family Food Plan, Revised 1964

	Weekly Quantities of Food² for Each Member of Family										
Sex-Age Group¹	Milk, Cheese, Ice Cream,³	Meat, Poultry, Fish,⁴	Eggs,	Dry Beans, Peas, Nuts,	Flour, Cereals, Baked Goods,⁵	Citrus Fruit, Tomatoes,	Dark-Green and Deep-Yellow Vegetables,	Potatoes,	Other Vegetables and Fruits,	Fats, Oils,	Sugars, Sweets,
	qt	lb oz	no.	lb oz	lb oz	lb oz	lb oz	lb oz	lb oz	lb oz	lb oz
Children											
7 months to 1 year	4	1 4	5	0 0	1 0	1 8	0 4	0 8	1 0	0 1	0 2
1 to 3 years	4	1 12	5	0 1	1 8	1 8	0 4	0 12	2 4	0 4	0 4
3 to 6 years	4	2 0	5	0 2	2 0	1 12	0 4	1 4	3 4	0 6	0 6
6 to 9 years	4	2 4	6	0 4	2 12	2 0	0 8	2 4	4 4	0 8	0 10
Girls											
9 to 12 years	5½	2 8	7	0 6	2 8	2 4	0 12	2 4	5 0	0 8	0 10
12 to 15 years	7	2 8	7	0 6	2 12	2 4	1 0	2 8	5 0	0 8	0 12
15 to 20 years	7	2 12	7	0 6	2 8	2 4	1 4	2 4	4 12	0 6	0 10
Boys											
9 to 12 years	5½	2 8	6	0 6	3 0	2 0	0 12	2 8	5 0	0 8	0 12
12 to 15 years	7	2 8	6	0 6	4 4	2 0	0 12	3 4	5 4	0 12	0 12
15 to 20 years	7	3 8	6	0 6	4 12	2 0	0 12	4 4	5 8	0 14	0 14

Women

20 to 35 years	3½	3	4	7	0	6	2	8	1	12	1	8	2	0	5	0	0	6	0	10
35 to 55 years	3½	3	4	7	0	6	2	4	1	12	1	8	1	8	4	8	0	4	0	10
55 to 75 years	3½	2	8	5	0	4	2	0	2	0	1	0	1	4	3	12	0	4	0	6
75 years and over	3½	2	4	5	0	4	1	8	2	0	1	0	1	4	3	0	0	4	0	4
Pregnant[6]	5½	3	12	7	0	6	2	12	3	4	2	0	1	8	5	8	0	6	0	6
Lactating[6]	8	3	12	7	0	6	3	12	3	4	1	8	3	4	5	8	0	10	0	10

Men

20 to 35 years	3½	3	8	6	0	6	4	4	1	12	0	12	3	4	5	8	1	12	1	0
35 to 55 years	3½	3	4	6	0	6	3	12	1	12	0	12	3	0	5	0	0	10	0	12
55 to 75 years	3½	3	0	6	0	4	2	12	1	12	0	12	2	4	4	8	0	10	0	10
75 years and over	3½	2	12	6	0	4	2	8	1	8	0	12	2	0	4	4	0	8	0	8

[1] Age groups include the persons of the first age listed up to but not including those of the second age listed.

[2] Food as purchased or brought into the kitchen from garden or farm.

[3] Fluid whole milk, or its calcium equivalent in cheese, evaporated milk, dry milk, or ice cream.

[4] Bacon and salt pork should not exceed ⅓ pound for each 5 pounds of meat group.

[5] Weight in terms of flour and cereal. Count 1½ pounds bread as 1 pound flour.

[6] Three additional quarts of milk are suggested for pregnant and lactating teenagers.

From *Family Economics Review*. U.S. Dept. Agr. Washington D.C., Oct. 1964.

Table A-12. Economy Family Food Plan, Revised 1964
(Designed for temporary use when funds are limited)

Sex-Age Group[1]	Milk, Cheese, Ice Cream,[3] qt	Meat, Poultry, Fish,[4] lb	oz	Eggs, no.	Dry Beans, Peas, Nuts, lb	oz	Flour, Cereals, Baked Goods,[5] lb	oz	Citrus Fruit, Tomatoes, lb	oz	Dark-Green and Deep-Yellow Vegetables, lb	oz	Potatoes, lb	oz	Other Vegetables and Fruits, lb	oz	Fats, Oils, lb	oz	Sugars, Sweets, lb	oz
Children																				
7 months to 1 year	4	1	0	4	0	0	1	0	1	0	0	4	0	12	1	0	0	2	0	2
1 to 3 years	4	1	4	4	0	0	1	12	1	0	0	4	1	0	2	0	0	4	0	4
3 to 6 years	3½	1	8	4	0	0	2	4	1	4	0	4	1	8	2	8	0	6	0	6
6 to 9 years	3½	1	12	5	0	0	3	0	1	8	0	8	2	8	3	0	0	10	0	10
Girls																				
9 to 12 years	5	1	12	5	0	10	2	12	1	12	0	12	2	8	3	4	0	8	0	10
12 to 15 years	6	2	0	6	0	10	3	0	1	12	1	0	3	0	3	8	0	10	0	10
15 to 20 years	6	2	0	6	0	8	2	12	1	12	1	4	2	8	3	4	0	8	0	10
Boys																				
9 to 12 years	5	2	0	5	0	8	3	4	1	8	0	12	2	12	3	4	0	10	0	10
12 to 15 years	6	2	0	5	0	10	4	4	1	12	0	12	3	8	3	8	0	14	0	12
15 to 20 years	6	2	8	5	0	10	5	0	1	12	0	12	4	12	3	8	1	0	0	14

Weekly Quantities of Food[2] for Each Member of Family

Women

20 to 35 years	3	1 12	6	0 10	2 12	1 8	1 8	2 12	3 0	0 8 0 12
35 to 55 years	3	1 12	6	0 10	2 8	1 8	1 8	2 8	2 12	0 6 0 8
55 to 75 years	3	1 8	4	0 6	2 0	1 12	1 0	2 8	2 12	0 6 0 6
75 years and over	3	1 4	4	0 6	1 12	1 12	1 0	2 0	2 4	0 4 0 6
Pregnant[6]	5½	2 0	7	0 10	3 0	3 0	2 0	2 8	4 8	0 6 0 6
Lactating[6]	8	2 0	6	0 10	4 0	3 0	1 8	3 12	4 8	0 12 0 12

Men

20 to 35 years	3	2 0	5	0 8	4 8	1 8	1 0	4 4	3 8	0 14 1 2
35 to 55 years	3	1 12	5	0 8	4 4	1 8	1 0	3 8	3 4	0 12 0 14
55 to 75 years	3	1 8	5	0 6	3 4	1 8	1 0	2 12	3 0	0 12 0 10
75 years and over	3	1 8	5	0 6	3 0	1 8	1 0	2 8	2 12	0 10 0 6

[1] Age groups include the persons of the first age listed up to but not including those of the second age listed.

[2] Food as purchased or brought into the kitchen from garden or farm.

[3] Fluid whole milk, or its calcium equivalent in cheese, evaporated milk, dry milk, or ice cream.

[4] Bacon and salt pork should not exceed ⅓ pound for each 5 pounds of meat group.

[5] Weight in terms of flour and cereal. Count 1½ pounds bread as 1 pound flour.

[6] Three additional quarts of milk are suggested for pregnant and lactating teenagers.

From *Family Economics Review.* U.S. Dept. Agr. Washington D.C., Oct. 1964.

Table A-13. Moderate-Cost Family Food Plan, Revised 1964

	Weekly Quantities of Food[2] for Each Member of Family										
Sex-Age Group[1]	Milk, Cheese, Ice Cream,[3]	Meat, Poultry, Fish,[4]	Eggs,	Dry Beans, Peas, Nuts,	Flour, Cereals, Baked Goods,[5]	Citrus Fruit, Tomatoes,	Dark-Green and Deep-Yellow Vegetables,	Potatoes,	Other Vegetables and Fruits,	Fats, Oils,	Sugars, Sweets,
	qt	lb oz	no.	lb oz	lb oz	lb oz	lb oz	lb oz	lb oz	lb oz	lb oz
Children											
7 months to 1 year	5	1 8	6	0 0	0 14	1 8	0 4	0 8	1 8	0 1	0 2
1 to 3 years	5	2 4	6	0 1	1 4	1 8	0 4	0 12	2 12	0 4	0 4
3 to 6 years	5	2 12	6	0 1	1 12	2 0	0 4	1 0	4 0	0 6	0 8
6 to 9 years	5	3 4	7	0 2	2 8	2 4	0 8	1 12	4 12	0 10	0 14
Girls											
9 to 12 years	5½	4 4	7	0 4	2 8	2 8	0 12	2 0	5 8	0 8	0 12
12 to 15 years	7	4 8	7	0 4	2 8	2 8	1 0	2 4	5 12	0 12	0 14
15 to 20 years	7	4 8	7	0 4	2 4	2 8	1 4	2 0	5 8	0 8	0 12
Boys											
9 to 12 years	5½	4 4	7	0 4	2 12	2 4	0 12	2 4	5 8	0 10	0 14
12 to 15 years	7	4 12	7	0 4	4 0	2 4	0 12	3 0	6 0	0 14	1 0
15 to 20 years	7	5 4	7	0 6	4 8	2 8	0 12	4 0	6 8	1 2	1 2

	Milk³ (qt.)	Meat⁴ (lb.)	Eggs (no.)								
Women											
20 to 35 years	3½	4 12	8	0 4	2 4	2 4	1 8	1 8	5 12	0 8	0 14
35 to 55 years	3½	4 12	8	0 4	2 4	2 4	1 8	1 4	5 0	0 6	0 8
55 to 75 years	3½	4 4	6	0 2	1 8	2 4	0 12	1 4	4 4	0 6	0 8
75 years and over	3½	3 8	6	0 2	1 4	2 4	0 12	1 0	3 12	0 4	0 8
Pregnant[6]	5½	5 8	8	0 4	2 12	3 4	2 0	1 8	5 12	0 6	0 8
Lactating[6]	8	5 8	8	0 4	3 12	3 8	1 8	2 12	6 4	0 12	0 12
Men											
20 to 35 years	3½	5 0	7	0 4	4 0	2 4	0 12	3 0	6 8	1 0	1 4
35 to 55 years	3½	4 12	7	0 4	3 8	2 4	0 12	2 8	5 12	0 14	1 0
55 to 75 years	3½	4 8	7	0 2	2 8	2 4	0 12	2 4	5 8	0 12	0 14
75 years and over	3½	4 8	7	0 2	2 4	2 4	0 12	2 0	5 4	0 8	0 12

[1] Age groups include the persons of the first age listed up to but not including those of the second age listed.

[2] Food as purchased or brought into the kitchen from garden or farm.

[3] Fluid whole milk, or its calcium equivalent in cheese, evaporated milk, dry milk, or ice cream.

[4] Bacon and salt pork should not exceed ⅓ pound for each 5 pounds of meat group.

[5] Weight in terms of flour and cereal. Count 1½ pounds bread as 1 pound flour.

[6] Three additional quarts of milk are suggested for pregnant and lactating teenagers.

From *Family Economics Review.* U.S. Dept. Agr. Washington D.C., Oct. 1964.

Table A-14. Liberal Family Food Plan, Revised 1964

Weekly Quantities of Food[2] for Each Member of Family

Sex-Age Group[1]	Milk, Cheese, Ice Cream,[3]	Meat, Poultry, Fish,[4]		Eggs,	Dry Beans, Peas, Nuts,		Flour, Cereals, Baked Goods,[5]		Citrus Fruit, Toma-toes,		Dark-Green and Deep-Yellow Vege-tables,		Pota-toes,		Other Vege-tables and Fruits,		Fats, Oils,		Sugars, Sweets,	
	qt	lb	oz	no.	lb	oz	lb	oz	lb	oz	lb	oz	lb	oz	lb	oz	lb	oz	lb	oz
Children																				
7 months to 1 year	5	1	8	7	0	0	0	14	1	12	0	4	0	8	1	8	0	1	0	2
1 to 3 years	5	2	12	7	0	1	1	4	1	12	0	4	0	12	2	12	0	4	0	4
3 to 6 years	5	3	4	7	0	1	1	8	2	4	0	8	0	12	4	8	0	8	0	10
6 to 9 years	5½	4	4	7	0	2	2	4	2	12	0	8	1	8	5	4	0	10	1	0
Girls																				
9 to 12 years	5½	4	12	7	0	4	2	4	3	0	0	12	1	12	6	0	0	10	0	14
12 to 15 years	7	5	12	7	0	2	2	4	3	0	1	0	2	0	6	0	0	12	1	2
15 to 20 years	7	5	8	7	0	2	2	0	3	0	1	4	1	12	5	12	0	10	0	14
Boys																				
9 to 12 years	5½	5	0	7	0	4	2	12	2	12	0	12	2	4	6	0	0	10	1	0
12 to 15 years	7	5	8	7	0	4	3	12	3	0	0	12	3	0	6	8	0	14	1	4
15 to 20 years	7	6	4	7	0	6	4	4	3	4	0	12	4	4	7	4	1	4	1	2

Women

20 to 35 years	4	5	8	0	4	2	0	3	0	1	8	1	4	6	4	0	8	1	2
35 to 55 years	4	5	8	0	4	1	12	3	0	1	8	1	0	6	0	0	6	0	12
55 to 75 years	4	4	12	0	1	1	4	3	0	0	12	1	0	4	8	0	6	0	12
75 years and over	4	4	4	0	1	1	0	3	0	0	12	0	12	4	0	0	4	0	10
Pregnant[6]	5½	6	4	0	4	2	8	4	0	2	0	1	4	6	4	0	6	0	12
Lactating[6]	8	6	0	0	4	3	12	4	0	1	8	2	8	6	4	0	14	1	4

Men

20 to 35 years	4	6	0	0	4	3	12	3	0	0	12	2	12	7	12	1	0	1	8
35 to 55 years	4	5	8	0	4	3	4	3	0	0	12	2	4	6	8	0	14	1	4
55 to 75 years	4	5	0	0	2	2	8	3	0	0	12	2	0	6	0	0	10	1	2
75 years and over	4	5	0	0	2	2	4	2	12	1	12	1	12	5	12	0	8	0	14

[1] Age groups include the persons of the first age listed up to but not including those of the second age listed.

[2] Food as purchased or brought into the kitchen from garden or farm.

[3] Fluid whole milk, or its calcium equivalent in cheese, evaporated milk, dry milk, or ice cream.

[4] Bacon and salt pork should not exceed ⅓ pound for each 5 pounds of meat group.

[5] Weight in terms of flour and cereal. Count 1½ pounds bread as 1 pound flour.

[6] Three additional quarts of milk are suggested for pregnant and lactating teenagers.

From *Family Economics Review.* U.S. Dept. Agr. Washington D.C., Oct. 1964.

INDEX